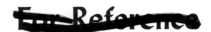

Mental Retardation

Lewis B. Holmes, M.D.

Assistant Professor of Pediatrics, Harvard Medical School; Genetics Unit, Children's Service, Massachusetts General Hospital; Clinical Geneticist, Eunice Kennedy Shriver Center, Walter E. Fernald State School, Waverley, Massachusetts

Hugo W. Moser, M.D.

Associate Professor of Neurology, Harvard Medical School; Neurologist, Massachusetts General Hospital; Assistant Superintendent, Walter E. Fernald State School; Co-Director, Eunice Kennedy Shriver Center, Walter E. Fernald State School, Waverley, Massachusetts

Saevar Halldórsson, M.D.

Consultant in Pediatrics, Department of Pediatrics, University Hospital, Reykjavík, Iceland; Consultant Kópavogshaeli, Central Institution for the Mentally Retarded in Iceland; Pediatrician, Department of Pediatrics, St. Joseph's Hospital, Reykjavík, Iceland. Formerly, Clinical and Research Fellow in Pediatrics, Children's Service, Massachusetts General Hospital, and Department of Pediatrics, Harvard Medical School

Cornelia Mack, M.S.

Program Specialist, Division of Family Health Services, Department of Public Health, Commonwealth of Massachusetts. Formerly, Research Assistant, Genetics Unit, Children's Service, Massachusetts General Hospital

Shyam S. Pant, M.D.

Neurologist, Holy Family Hospital and Tirathram Shah Hospital, New Delhi, India. Formerly, Clinical and Research Fellow in Neurology and Neuropathology, Neurology Service, Massachusetts General Hospital and Department of Neurology, Harvard Medical School

Benjamin Matzilevich, M.D.

Instructor in Neurology, Harvard Medical School; Clinical Director, Walter E. Fernald State School, Waverley, Massachusetts

Mental Retardation

An Atlas of Diseases with Associated Physical Abnormalities

The Macmillan Company, New York · Collier-Macmillan Limited, London

THE MACMILLAN COMPANY
866 THIRD AVENUE, NEW YORK, NEW YORK 10022
COLLIER-MACMILLAN CANADA, LTD., TORONTO, ONTARIO

Library of Congress catalog card number: 71-172671

Printing: 1 2 3 4 5 6 7 8   Year: 2 3 4 5 6 7 8

Preface

Anyone who has tried to establish a medical diagnosis for mentally retarded individuals knows what frustration is. The clinician continually encounters individuals who presumably fit a diagnosis of which he (or she) is not aware—perhaps a disease already delineated, perhaps not. So many syndromes and diseases have been described that no one can remember them all, nor would there be any point in trying. Authoritative information on the diseases associated with mental retardation is scattered throughout many medical books* and journals, some of which are hard to find. Thus, we have attempted to bring together the pertinent data in this comprehensive clinical atlas. We have described 173 disorders characterized by mental retardation and physical abnormalities.

The emphasis herein is visual. More than 1000 photographs depict major physical features of the mentally retarded and are used to convey the fact that not every individual with a particular disease has the same physical features. The changes with age in progressive diseases are also illustrated. Such information should be of inestimable value to the examining physician, especially pediatricians, internists, and neurologists, in addition to other professionals—pathologists, cytogeneticists, psychologists, social workers, and educators—who want to know more about a specific disease or syndrome.

Mental Retardation is divided into seven chapters based on an etiologic classification: metabolic and endocrine diseases, progressive diseases of the nervous system, acquired conditions, chromosomal abnormalities, central nervous system malformations, multiple deformity syndromes, and neurocutaneous syndromes. The introduction to each chapter provides a perspective on the diseases discussed, in relation to similar diseases that either are not associated with mental retardation or do not have attendant physical abnormalities. A concise but complete summary of each disorder is presented on a left-hand page and illustrated by four to six photographs on the opposite right-hand page. Physical features are discussed in a sequence similar to the standard physical examination: head, eyes, ears, etc. Special emphasis is given to neurologic findings and data on the incidence and severity of the mental retardation. Following the description of physical features, pathology, recent diagnostic studies, and other relevant laboratory data, there are discussions—under separate headings—of treatment and prognosis, genetics, and differential diagnosis. Each description is followed by a list of selected references, which include the original description of the disorder and some of the important recent papers in the world biomedical literature.

The scope of the medical problems discussed herein includes many complex and rapidly changing areas of research. To make certain that our text was factually accurate, balanced in areas of controversy, and complete, we enlisted the assistance of many of our colleagues. Their advice has greatly improved the quality of the book, and we wish to thank each one: Drs. Leonard Atkins, John Crawford, Allen Crocker, William DeMyer, Lowell Goldsmith, Frederick Hecht, Dick Hoefnagel, Gwendolyn Hogan, Thomas Kemper, Edwin

*Excellent books in which some of the disorders are discussed include the following:
1. Gorlin, R. J., and Pindborg, J. J. *Syndromes of the Head and Neck.* Blakiston Division, McGraw-Hill Book Co., New York, 1964.
2. Stanbury, J. B., Wyngaarden, J. B., and Fredrickson, D. S. *The Metabolic Basis of Inherited Disease,* 3rd ed. McGraw-Hill Book Co., New York, 1972.
3. Gellis, S. S., and Feingold, M. *Atlas of Mental Retardation Syndromes.* U.S. Department of Health, Education, and Welfare, U.S. Government Printing Office, No. 0-310-072, 1968.
4. Aita, J. A. *Congenital Facial Anomalies with Neurologic Defects.* Charles C Thomas, Publisher, Springfield, Ill., 1969.
5. Goodman, R. M., and Gorlin, R. J. *The Face in Genetic Disorders.* C. V. Mosby Co., St. Louis, 1970.
6. Smith, D. W. *Recognizable Patterns of Human Malformation. Genetic, Embryologic, and Clinical Aspects.* W. B. Saunders Co., Philadelphia, 1970.

Kolodny, Harvey Levy, Gerald Medoff, Vincent Riccardi, E. P. Richardson, Jr., Paul Rosman, Vivian Shih, Priscilla Taft, David Walton, Alfred Weber, and Paul Yakovlev. Any inaccuracies, imbalances, or deficiencies are, of course, the responsibility of the authors.

Like most clinical atlases, the work expanded far beyond our original expectations. Essential to the completion of the project was the assistance over four years of several different secretaries and assistants. Those most important in our work were Mr. William C. Allen, Mrs. Judie Beard, Mrs. Catherine Cook, Mrs. Jeanne Ells, Mrs. Virginia Fanara, Mrs. Dorothy Gillis, Mrs. Janet Parker, and Miss Carol Schmidt.

The work on this book was supported in part by Maternal and Child Health Service, Project 906.

The illustrations in *Mental Retardation* are a source of pride to all of us. Most of the photography, copying, reprinting, and composite work was undertaken by Miss Virginia Taylor. Much of the superb quality is due to her efforts to improve tone, contrast, and clarity of hundreds of illustrations. The photography in the early stages of manuscript development was done by Mr. Robert McEnany.

We could not have compiled illustrations of 173 syndromes without the generous cooperation of physicians throughout the world who sent us several thousand prints, slides, and negatives. From the pictures received we selected several hundred illustrations and added many of our own. Listed below are the 317 individuals who sent us photographs which appear in this book.

Argentina

Sebastian A. Rosasco   *Buenos Aires*

Australia

Janos Brody   *Gordonvale, N. Queensland*
Athel Hockey   *W. Perth, Western Australia*
Brian Turner   *North Ryde*

Belgium

Anne Marie De Barsy   *Antwerp*
C. Hooft   *Ghent*
Jules G. Leroy   *Antwerp*
H. Loeb   *Brussels*

Canada

Murray L. Barr   *London, Ontario*
Peter Bowen   *Edmonton, Alberta*
P. E. Conen   *Toronto, Ontario*
André La France   *Montreal, Quebec*
J. C. Boileau Grant   *Toronto, Ontario*
R. B. Lowry   *Vancouver, British Columbia*
D. C. McFarlane   *London, Ontario*
James R. Miller   *Vancouver, British Columbia*
F. R. Sergovich   *London, Ontario*
Irene A. Uchida   *Winnipeg, Manitoba*
Witold Zaleski   *Saskatoon, Saskatchewan*

Colombia

Federico Lopez   *Medellin*

Denmark

G. Asboe-Hansen   *Copenhagen*
E. Graven Nielsen   *Odense*
Mette Warburg   *Copenhagen*

England

Harry Angelman	*Warrington*
John A. Black	*Sheffield*
L. J. Butler	*London*
David N. Challacombe	*Bristol*
L. Crome	*Carshalton, Surrey*
Margaret E. B. Davies	*Birmingham*
C. E. Dent	*London*
R. R. Gordon	*Sheffield*
J. Insley	*Birmingham*
Irene M. Irving	*Liverpool*
J. Jancar	*Bristol*
P. M. Jeavons	*Birmingham*
Brian H. Kirman	*Epsom, Surrey*
J. Lorber	*Sheffield*
T. P. Mann	*Brighton*
Alan McDermott	*Birmingham*
H. H. Nixon	*London*
B. W. Richards	*Caterham, Surrey*
Dorothy S. Russell	*Dorking, Surrey*
Michael A. Salmon	*Maidstone, Kent*
J. M. Tanner	*London*
Angela I. Taylor	*London*
J. M. Walshe	*Cambridge*
John N. Walton	*Newcastle-Upon-Tyne*

Finland

Matti Sulamaa	*Helsinki*

France

Jean DeGrouchy	*Paris*
Simone Gilgenkrantz	*Nancy*
Pierre Maroteaux	*Paris*
A. Rossier	*Paris*

Germany

K. D. Ebel	*Cologne*
Walter Fuhrmann	*Giessen*
W. Lenz	*Munster*
Carl Mietens	*Wurzburg*
Eberhard Passarge	*Hamburg*
R. A. Pfeiffer	*Munster*
J. W. Spranger	*Kiel*
Walter M. Teller	*Ulm*
H.-R. Wiedemann	*Kiel*
Ulrich Wolf	*Freiburg*

Greece

Christos S. Bartsocas	*Athens*
Spyros Doxiadis	*Athens*

Hungary

A. Kallo	*Budapest*
Stephen Kornyey	*Pecs*

Iran

Mohsen Mahloudji	*Shiraz*

Israel

Moshe Berant	*Hadera*
David Kahana	*Hadera*
U. Sandbank	*Petah Tigva*

Italy

Paolo Durand	*Genova*

Netherlands

W. H. D. DeHaas	*Amsterdam*
E. H. Hermans	*Rotterdam*
A. Th. M. van Balen	*Rotterdam*
L. H. B. M. van Benthem	*Heemskerk*

Northern Ireland

Nina A. J. Carson	*Belfast*

Norway

Martin Seip	*Oslo*

Scotland

J. Stanley Cant	*Glasgow*
Wallace M. Dennison	*Glasgow*

South Africa

Robert McDonald	*Cape Town*

Sweden

Hans Forssman	*St. Jorgen*
Ingrid Gamstorp	*Jonkoping*
Bengt Hagberg	*Uppsala*
Bertil Hall	*Lund*
Lennart Juhlin	*Uppsala*
Rolf Zetterstrom	*Stockholm*

Switzerland

Erica M. Buhler	*Basel*
W. Schmid	*Zürich*
Alexander Todorov	*Geneva*
F. Vassella	*Berne*
D. Vischer	*Zürich*

United Arab Republic

H. El-Hefnawi	*Cairo*
Samia A. Temtamy	*Cairo*

United States

Jon M. Aase	*Seattle, Washington*
William A. Akers	*San Francisco, California*
Penelope W. Allderdice	*New York, New York*
Milton Alter	*Minneapolis, Minnesota*
Frank M. Anderson	*Los Angeles, California*
Carol R. Angle	*Omaha, Nebraska*
Leonard Atkins	*Boston, Massachusetts*
James H. Austin	*Denver, Colorado*
Sidney M. Baker	*New Haven, Connecticut*
Betty Q. Banker	*Cleveland, Ohio*
Fred A. Baughman, Jr.	*Grand Rapids, Michigan*
Edwin Beckman	*Boston, Massachusetts*
Patricia H. Benedict	*Boston, Massachusetts*
Peter H. Berman	*Philadelphia, Pennsylvania*
Josette Bianchine	*Baltimore, Maryland*
Joseph Bittenbender	*Harrisburg, Pennsylvania*
David Bixler	*Indianapolis, Indiana*
Elena Boder	*Beverly Hills, California*
Patricia Borns	*Philadelphia, Pennsylvania*
W. Roy Breg	*Southbury, Connecticut*
William J. Brown	*Atlanta, Georgia*
Randolph K. Byers	*Boston, Massachusetts*
David L. Chadwick	*San Diego, California*
Joe C. Christian	*Indianapolis, Indiana*
Eugene C. Ciccarelli	*Hyannis, Massachusetts*
William D. Cochran	*Boston, Massachusetts*
Grange S. Coffin	*Berkeley, California*

David G. Cogan	Boston, Massachusetts	Frederic M. Kenny	Pittsburgh, Pennsylvania
Jonathan Cohen	Boston, Massachusetts	Irwin J. Kerber	Memphis, Tennessee
William H. Coles	New Orleans, Louisiana	Sidney Kibrick	Boston, Massachusetts
David E. Comings	Duarte, California	Bernard Kliman	Boston, Massachusetts
John P. Connelly	Charlestown, Massachusetts	Richard Koch	Los Angeles, California
Peggy J. Copple	Portland, Oregon	Edwin H. Kolodny	Boston, Massachusetts
Henry R. Cowell	Wilmington, Delaware	Bruce W. Konigsmark	Baltimore, Maryland
John D. Crawford	Boston, Massachusetts	Stephen M. Krane	Boston, Massachusetts
Allen C. Crocker	Boston, Massachusetts	Gerald J. Kurlander	Indianapolis, Indiana
Harold E. Cross	Baltimore, Maryland	Theodore Kushnick	Jersey City, New Jersey
Felix De la Cruz	Bethesda, Maryland	David J. Lang	Durham, North Carolina
Arthur C. Curtis	Ann Arbor, Michigan	Leonard O. Langer, Jr.	Minneapolis, Minnesota
Jasper R. Daube	Rochester, Minnesota	James B. Lee	St. Louis, Missouri
Noble J. David	Miami, Florida	Frederick H. Lovejoy, Jr.	Boston, Massachusetts
Anatole S. Dekaban	Bethesda, Maryland	Charles U. Lowe	Bethesda, Maryland
William DeMyer	Indianapolis, Indiana	Henry T. Lynch	Omaha, Nebraska
Bennett M. Derby	New York, New York	John I. Lynch	Portsmouth, Virginia
Murdina M. Desmond	Houston, Texas	Joseph D. Mann	Grand Rapids, Michigan
Louis K. Diamond	San Francisco, California	Philip Marden	Madison, Wisconsin
Angelo M. DiGeorge	Philadelphia, Pennsylvania	Andrew M. Margileth	Washington, D.C.
Philip R. Dodge	St. Louis, Missouri	Charles H. Markham	Los Angeles, California
Theodore C. Doege	Seattle, Washington	Richard E. Marshall	Seattle, Washington
David D. Donaldson	Boston, Massachusetts	Donald D. Matson	Boston, Massachusetts
George N. Donnell	Los Angeles, California	Gilbert W. Mellin	New York, New York
Elizabeth Dooling	Boston, Massachusetts	Barbara R. Migeon	Baltimore, Maryland
Daniel B. Drachman	Baltimore, Maryland	James Q. Miller	Charlottesville, Virginia
Philip P. Ellis	Denver, Colorado	Aubrey Milunsky	Boston, Massachusetts
Stanley M. Elmore	Richmond, Virginia	Henry L. Nadler	Chicago, Illinois
Eric Engel	Nashville, Tennessee	Andre J. Nahmias	Atlanta, Georgia
Arthur Falek	Atlanta, Georgia	Walter E. Nance	Indianapolis, Indiana
Daniel D. Federman	Boston, Massachusetts	P. F. J. New	Boston, Massachusetts
Pierre E. Ferrier	Seattle, Washington	David S. Newcombe	Burlington, Vermont
Thomas B. Fitzpatrick	Boston, Massachusetts	Jacqueline A. Noonan	Lexington, Kentucky
Patrick B. Flynn	San Francisco, California	James J. Nora	Houston, Texas
Vincent J. Fontana	New York, New York	William L. Nyhan	San Diego, California
Allan H. Fradkin	Galveston, Texas	Sidney Olansky	Atlanta, Georgia
George R. Fraser	Seattle, Washington	John M. Opitz	Madison, Wisconsin
Donald S. Fredrickson	Bethesda, Maryland	Richard M. Paddison	New Orleans, Louisiana
Jose Galindo	Glens Falls, New York	Charles E. Parker	Los Angeles, California
Lytt I. Gardner	Syracuse, New York	Carlos E. Pena	Washington, D.C.
Park S. Gerald	Boston, Massachusetts	Ernest H. Picard	Boston, Massachusetts
James L. German	New York, New York	Daniel W. Pieroni	Indianapolis, Indiana
Walter R. Gilbert, Jr.	Jacksonville, Florida	Arthur L. Prensky	St. Louis, Missouri
Frederick D. Gillespie	Parkersburg, West Virginia	Hope H. Punnett	Philadelphia, Pennsylvania
James P. Gills	Durham, North Carolina	Galen W. Quinn	Durham, North Carolina
Sid Gilman	New York, New York	Elizabeth W. Rauschkolb	Houston, Texas
Rolando V. Goco	Laurel, Maryland	William B. Reed	Burbank, California
Morton F. Goldberg	Arlington, Virginia	Leonard E. Reisman	Philadelphia, Pennsylvania
Robert J. Gorlin	Minneapolis, Minnesota	Jack S. Remington	Palo Alto, California
William C. Grabb	Ann Arbor, Michigan	Retina Associates	Boston, Massachusetts
Robert M. Greenstein	Hartford, Connecticut	Vincent M. Riccardi	Boston, Massachusetts
Herman Grossman	New York, New York	E. P. Richardson, Jr.	Boston, Massachusetts
Dupont Guerry III	Richmond, Virginia	Harris D. Riley, Jr.	Oklahoma City, Oklahoma
Catherine Haberland	Chicago, Illinois	Meinhard Robinow	Dayton, Ohio
Hannibal Hamlin	Boston, Massachusetts	Blair O. Rogers	New York, New York
James B. Hanshaw	Rochester, New York	N. Paul Rosman	Boston, Massachusetts
Janet B. Hardy	Baltimore, Maryland	Robert E. Rossman	Tyler, Texas
Rita G. Harper	Brooklyn, New York	Albert B. Sabin	Cincinnati, Ohio
Gerald W. Hazard	Hyannis, Massachusetts	Mannie M. Schechter	Bronx, New York
Albert F. Heck	Baltimore, Maryland	I. Herbert Scheinberg	Bronx, New York
Dick Hoefnagel	Hanover, New Hampshire	Alan L. Schiller	Boston, Massachusetts
Gwendolyn R. Hogan	Boston, Massachusetts	Larry Schneck	Brooklyn, New York
J. B. Howell	Dallas, Texas	C. Ronald Scott	Seattle, Washington
R. Rodney Howell	Baltimore, Maryland	Heddie Sedano	Minneapolis, Minnesota
William F. Hoyt	San Francisco, California	Morton Seelenfreund	Boston, Massachusetts
Y. E. Hsia	New Haven, Connecticut	N. T. Shahidi	Madison, Wisconsin
Peter R. Huttenlocher	New Haven, Connecticut	Edward M. Shapiro	Pasadena, Texas
Carl H. Ide	Columbia, Missouri	Edward B. Shaw	San Francisco, California
J. T. Jabbour	Memphis, Tennessee	Carol S. Shear	Miami, Florida
Laird G. Jackson	Philadelphia, Pennsylvania	Jack G. Shiller	Westport, Connecticut
Sture A. M. Johnson	Madison, Wisconsin	John Shillito, Jr.	Boston, Massachusetts
Richard C. Juberg	Shreveport, Louisiana	Stanton E. Shuler	New Orleans, Louisiana
R. H. Kampmeir	Nashville, Tennessee	Henry K. Silver	Denver, Colorado
Ellen S. Kang	Boston, Massachusetts	Joe Leigh Simpson	New York, New York
Thomas Kemper	Waverley, Massachusetts	E. B. Singleton	Houston, Texas

Evelyn Siris
Alfred A. Smith
David W. Smith
J. Lawton Smith
Richard L. Sogg
Arthur R. Sohval
G. B. Solitaire
Juan F. Sotos
Maryann South
J. W. Spranger
John B. Stanbury
Janet M. Stewart
William B. Strong
H. Saul Sugar
Gerald I. Sugarman
Robert L. Summitt
Leonard Sussman
Sidney J. Sussman
Kunihiko Suzuki
August G. Swanson
Philip D. Swanson
Mihran O. Tachdjian
Priscilla Taft
Hooshang Taybi
Mary A. Telfer
Robert Touloukian
H. Richard Tyler

Eldridge, California
New York, New York
Seattle, Washington
Miami, Florida
Campbell, California
New York, New York
New Haven, Connecticut
Columbus, Ohio
Houston, Texas
Madison, Wisconsin
Cambridge, Massachusetts
Denver, Colorado
Cleveland, Ohio
Detroit, Michigan
Los Angeles, California
Memphis, Tennessee
New York, New York
Philadelphia, Pennsylvania
Philadelphia, Pennsylvania
Seattle, Washington
Seattle, Washington
Chicago, Illinois
Boston, Massachusetts
Oakland, California
Elwyn, Pennsylvania
New Haven, Connecticut
Boston, Massachusetts

Lieven J. Van Riet
Bruno W. Volk
David S. Walton
Josef Warkany
Gordon V. Watters
Felice M. Weber
Eugene S. Welter
Derek W. Williams
Hibbard E. Williams
Miriam G. Wilson
J. Windmiller
Paul V. Woolley, Jr.
Herman Yannet
Jorge J. Yunis
Hans Zellweger
Wolfgang Zeman
Gabriele M. ZuRhein

Houston, Texas
Brooklyn, New York
Boston, Massachusetts
Cincinnati, Ohio
Boston, Massachusetts
Los Angeles, California
Joliet, Illinois
Denver, Colorado
San Francisco, California
Los Angeles, California
Dallas, Texas
Detroit, Michigan
Southbury, Connecticut
Minneapolis, Minnesota
Iowa City, Iowa
Indianapolis, Indiana
Madison, Wisconsin

Wales

T. S. Davies
K. M. Laurence

Cwmbran, Monmouthshire
Penarth, Glamorgan

West Indies

Marigold J. Thorburn

Kingston, Jamaica

Contents

Mental Retardation

Introduction

Mental retardation is defined as "subaverage general intellectual functioning which originates during the developmental periods and is associated with impairment in adaptive behavior" [1].* This definition does not attempt to specify a cutoff point in terms of intellectual function below which individuals are classified as retarded. Furthermore, it emphasizes that a person should not be so classified unless he is unable to adapt his behavior to the setting in which he lives. Finally, the definition specifies that the deficit in intellectual and adaptive behavior must have been present before adulthood. Intellectual deficits that develop after that period are referred to as dementia.

A number of more or less standardized tests have been designed to measure intellectual function. These tests indicate that in the general population intelligence is distributed along a continuous Gaussian curve. The mean intelligence quotient is set, by definition, at 100. The standard deviation, depending upon what test is used, varies between 12 and 17 points and is commonly set at 15 [2].

In the past, individuals were classified as mentally retarded if their intelligence fell short of normal by more than two standard deviations. With the standard deviation set at 15, individuals whose intelligence quotient was below 70 would then be considered retarded. Such dependence upon a number score has obvious limitations and dangers. Individual tests are subject to error. Tests are standardized in reference to particular population groups, and their validity in diverse cultural settings has not been established. Most important, the uncritical assignment of the label "mental retardation" on the basis of a test score may cause serious harm to the individual so labeled. Realizing these limitations, but needing to establish the magnitude of the problem, the prevalence of mental retardation in the United States and England has been estimated to be about 3 percent [2].

The causes of the mental retardation are many. The largest portion, about 75 to 90 percent, represents the mildly, familial, or "physiologically" retarded whose intelligence test scores usually vary between 50 and 70. Important etiologic factors for many of these individuals are poverty and disadvantaged community settings [3]. The majority of these individuals do not have demonstrable brain pathology [4]. This book is concerned with the smaller portion of the mentally retarded, those with associated physical abnormalities. Some of these individuals are only mildly retarded, but many have intelligence quotients below 50.

This book began as part of an effort to properly diagnose and classify mentally retarded patients at the Walter E. Fernald State School in Waverley, Massachusetts. In evaluating these patients, it soon became evident that no specific diagnosis could be given for many of them. As is shown in the accompanying summary of clinical evaluations of 1378 individuals at this institution, many (39.3 percent) could not be classified in any diagnostic category [5]. Spurred on by the difficulty in diagnosing many of these patients, a compilation was begun of all the clinically recognizable causes of mental retardation. When this effort began in 1966, there were no available reference books that showed the complete list of diagnostic possibilities. So what began as a local effort to properly diagnose mentally retarded patients expanded into an attempt to write a comprehensive clinical reference book. It was apparent then, and even more so in subsequent years, that the nosology of mental retardation is rapidly expanding.

Clinical Evaluations of 1378 Individuals at Walter E. Fernald State School, Waverley, Massachusetts

Disease Category	Number of Patients		% of Surveyed Population
	IQ <50	IQ >50	
1. Metabolic and endocrine diseases	38	5	3.1
2. Progressive diseases of the nervous system	5	7	0.9
3. Acquired conditions	278	79	25.9
4. Chromosomal abnormalities	247	10	18.7
5. Central nervous system abnormalities	49	16	4.7
6. Multiple congenital deformities	64	16	5.8
7. Neurocutaneous diseases	4	0	0.3
8. Psychosis	7	6	0.9
9. Mentally retarded, cause unknown	385	156	39.3
10. Not mentally retarded	0	6	0.4
Total	1077	301	100.0

In order to include as many as possible of the reported diseases, the world's literature was scanned and pictures were borrowed from investigators throughout the world.

The rapid increase in the number of newly recognized causes of mental retardation is the result of both recent advances in laboratory methodology and increased interest by physicians. We have subdivided our book to reflect the current understanding of the many types of diseases that cause mental retardation and have associated physical abnormalities. Chapters I, III, and IV contain the diseases for which the etiology is best understood. Many of the endocrine and metabolic diseases in Chapter I are caused by specific biochemical abnormalities. The progressive diseases in Chapter II follow Chapter I because it is anticipated that the biochemical abnormalities in many will soon be established. Two conditions, globoid cell leukodystrophy and Wolman's disease, were initially included in Chapter II and subsequently moved to Chapter I because of the delineation of the primary biochemical abnormality during the writing of this book. We expect that with time the number of diseases in Chapter I will increase and those in Chapter II will diminish. The acquired diseases included in Chapter III reflect both recent progress in the methodology for infectious diseases and increased awareness of teratogens. The chromosomal abnormalities in Chapter IV have all been delineated since 1959. In contrast to the conditions dealt with in the early chapters, those in Chapters V, VI, and VII—the central nervous system abnormalities, multiple deformity syndromes, and neurocutaneous diseases—are still diagnosed by clinical and histopathologic criteria; there are few, if any, diagnostic laboratory tests.

In compiling the diseases discussed in all of these chapters, we have been eager "splitters" [6] in recognizing new diseases. As much attention is given to rare diseases as to well-known, carefully studied conditions. We run certain calculated risks in including as specific genetic syndromes the many "new diseases" that have been reported only in one family or a few unrelated patients. Future experience may prove that what appears to be a separate disease is only part of the spectrum of another disease. Furthermore, the association with mental retardation in the first patients may be misleading. Many syndromes are first identified among patients in institutions for the mentally retarded, which is an obviously biased method of ascertainment. Another problem is in knowing the role of an individual's deformities and social isolation in determining his performance on intelligence tests.

We believe that this compilation of most of the reported diseases will pay dividends in several ways. The practicing physician familiar with this list may be able to solve several of his immediate diagnostic problems. We have already found this to be true during the course of writing this book. Several of our own patients have been recognized as having diseases of which we were previously unaware. The recognition of additional cases acts as a spur to the more detailed clinical and laboratory studies and leads to improved understanding of the disease. This is especially true of the diseases caused by genetic biochemical defects for which laboratory methods are rapidly being improved and expanded. An important dividend is the value of a precise diagnosis for the family. Some of the hereditary diseases can be successfully treated. In other instances, more specific family planning can be followed through the use of prenatal diagnosis from cultured amniotic cells [7]. For the many unfortunate situations where neither treatment nor prenatal diagnosis is possible, there is some comfort for the family in at least knowing the diagnosis, whether the disease is hereditary, and, if hereditary, the risk of its recurrence.

This book will soon be out of date. This is inevitable in such a rapidly changing field of biologic research. We anticipate the delineation of many new biochemical abnormalities. Possibly, the current concept of the chromosomal abnormality syndromes will be revised with the use of several new staining techniques [8]. No doubt many new syndromes with multiple deformities will be delineated. Even at this time we are aware of several, such as Biemond's syndrome [9], X-linked microphthalmia with mental deficiency [10], and the multiple deformity syndrome in the second family described by Bowen and coworkers [11], which we are unable to include in this book. Furthermore, several new disorders were described in 1971 while this book was being printed [12–20]. No doubt there are many others of which we are not aware. Also, we are currently evaluating several patients or families with "new" mental retardation syndromes. This group of unpublished studies could be multiplied several times by combining it with work being done by investigators throughout the world.

References

1. Heber, R. (ed.). A Manual on terminology and classification in mental retardation. *Am. J. Ment. Defic.,* **64** (monogr. suppl.), 1959.
2. Penrose, L. S. *The Biology of Mental Defect,* 3rd ed. Grune & Stratton, New York, 1963.
3. Zigler, E. Familial mental retardation: a continuing dilemma. *Science,* **155:**292–98, 1967.
4. Crome, L. The brain and mental retardation. *Br. Med. J.,* 1:897–904, 1960.
5. Moser, H. W., and Wolf, P. A. The nosology of mental retardation. Including the report of a survey of 1378 mentally retarded individuals at the Walter E. Fernald State School. *Birth Defects: Original Article Series,* Vol. VII, No. 1, February, 1971, pp. 117–34. Williams & Wilkins Co., Baltimore.
6. McKusick, V. A. On lumpers and splitters, or the nosology of genetic disease. *Birth Defects: Original Article Series,* Vol. V, No. 1, January, 1969, pp. 23–32. Williams & Wilkins Co., Baltimore.
7. Milunsky, A., Littlefield, J. W., Kanfer, J. N., Kolodny, E. H., Shih, V. E., and Atkins, L. Prenatal genetic diagnosis. *N. Engl. J. Med.,* **382:**1370–81, 1441–47 and 1498–1504, 1970.
8. Hecht, F., Wyandt, H. E., and Erbe, R. W. Revolutionary cytogenetics. *New Engl. J. Med.,* **285:**1482–84, 1971.
9. Biemond, A. Het syndroom van Laurence-Biedl en een aanverwant, nieuw syndroom. *Ned. Tijdschr. Geneeskd.,* **78:**1801–1809, 1934.
10. Cuendet, J. F. La microphtalmie compliquée. *Ophthalmologica,* **141:**380–85, 1961.
11. Bowen, P., Lee, C. S. N., Zellweger, H., and Lindenberg, R. A familial syndrome of multiple congenital defects. *Bull. Johns Hopkins Hosp.,* **114:**402–14, 1964.
12. Kaufman, R. L., Rimoin, D. L., Prensky, A. L., and Sly, W. S. An oculo-cerebrofacial syndrome. *Birth Defects: Original Article Series,* Vol. VII, No. 1, February, 1971, pp. 135–38. Williams & Wilkins Co., Baltimore.
13. Scott, C. R., Bryant, J. I., and Graham, C. B. A new craniodigital syndrome with mental retardation. *J. Pediatr.,* **78:**658–63, 1971.
14. Palant, D. I., Feingold, M., and Berkman, M. D. Unusual facies, cleft palate, mental retardation, and limb abnormalities in siblings—a new syndrome. *J. Pediatr.,* **78:**686–89, 1971.
15. Telfer, M. A., Sugar, M., Jaeger, E. A., and Mulcahy, J. Dominant piebald trait (white forelock and leukoderma) with neurological impairment. *Am. J. Hum. Genet.* **23:**383–89, 1971.
16. Lowry, R. B., MacLean, R., McLean, D. M., and Tischler, B. Cataracts, microcephaly, kyphosis, and limited joint movement in two siblings: a new syndrome. *J. Pediatr.,* **79:**282–84, 1971.
17. Dawson, G., Matalon, R., and Stein, A. O. Lactosylceramidosis: lactosylceramide galactosyl hydrolase deficiency and accumulation of lactosylceramide in cultured skin fibroblasts. *J. Pediatr.,* **79:**423–29, 1971.
18. Ruvalcaba, R. H. A., Reichert, A., and Smith, D. W. A new familial syndrome with osseous dysplasia and mental deficiency. *J. Pediatr.,* **79:**450–55, 1971.
19. Johanson, A., and Blizzard, R. A syndrome of congenital aplasia of the alae nasi, deafness, hypothyroidism, dwarfism, absent permanent teeth, and malabsorption. *J. Pediatr.,* **79:**982–87, 1971.
20. Tay, C. H. Ichthyosiform erythroderma, hair shaft abnormalities, and mental and growth retardation. A new recessive disorder. *Arch. Dermatol.,* **104:**4–13, 1971.

Chapter I
Metabolic and Endocrine Diseases

Introduction

Even though they account for only a relatively small proportion of cases of mental retardation, the metabolic disorders are of intense current interest. This is because recent advances in biochemistry and genetics have made it possible to clarify their pathogenesis, and conversely study of these disorders has contributed a great deal to the understanding of normal metabolism.

Since this book deals with conditions in which there is abnormal physical appearance, not all of the metabolic disorders associated with mental retardation will be covered here. In some metabolic disorders there is a pathognomonic physical abnormality such as the Kayser-Fleischer ring in Wilson's disease. In others, such as the mucopolysaccharidoses, an abnormal physical appearance, while not pathognomonic, almost always represents the first diagnostic clue. Phenylketonuria illustrates another situation: there is reduced pigmentation, but this physical abnormality is of limited diagnostic importance, and laboratory studies are of paramount importance. Finally, there is a large number of disorders, such as maple syrup urine disease and methyl malonic aciduria, in which there are no specific physical abnormalities. [1].

The frequency with which metabolic disorders are the cause of mental retardation has not been determined exactly, since systematic studies have not been done of a representative group of mentally retarded individuals. Present estimates depend upon three indirect approaches, each of which has serious limitations in terms of sampling. These approaches are (1) surveys of residents of institutions for the mentally retarded, (2) large-scale metabolic surveys, and (3) utilization of hospital and clinic records to assess the prevalence of disorders known to be associated with mental retardation.

Metabolic disorders are the cause of mental retardation in approximately 3 percent of residents of institutions for the retarded. The most common disorder is untreated phenylketonuria, which accounts for approximately 1 percent of the institutionalized population. Hypothyroidism is the second most common (approximately 0.5 percent). A large variety of rare disorders together make up the remainder (approximately 1 to 1.5 percent) [2]. These figures are subject to variation with time and place. Thus, because of the success of early therapeutic intervention, the frequency with which disorders such as phenylketonuria cause mental retardation is expected to diminish. A high frequency of homocystinuria—second only to that of phenylketonuria—has been found among the mentally retarded in Northern Ireland, but this condition appears to be less frequent in other parts of the world.

The metabolic surveys of newborn infants conducted in Massachusetts since 1962 are a useful tool for assessing the frequency of various metabolic disorders in the general population. In Massachusetts the incidence of phenylketonuria is approximately 1:14,000. Other relatively common metabolic abnormalities are iminoglycinuria (1:15,000), Hartnup disease (1:16,000), and histidinemia (1:16,000). Iminoglycinuria appears not to be of clinical significance. Although Hartnup disease was discovered in mentally retarded children, experience with newborn screening programs suggests that many, if not most, patients with Hartnup disease are clinically normal. Histidinemia was initially considered to be associated with mild mental retardation or specific speech defects; however, the experience with mass screening suggests that this condition is usually benign [3].

There are many disorders associated with mental retardation which cannot as yet be detected by mass screening methods, and in which other clinical abnormalities overshadow the mental retardation. In some of these disorders, such as Pompe's disease, globoid cell leukodystrophy, or Tay-Sachs disease, death occurs at an early age, and the patients are usually not admitted to institutions for the retarded. Estimates of the frequency of these disorders depend upon surveys of the records of a large number of facilities which provide health services, and this has only rarely been done.

In the understanding of a genetic disorder there are five levels of sophistication [4]:

1. Description of the phenotype
2. Delineation of the mendelian nature of the condition
3. Discovery of the general biochemical nature of the disorder
4. Identification of a defect in a specific enzyme or other protein gene product
5. Determination of the precise nature of the genic change

On this scale the understanding of most of the metabolic disorders included in this chapter is at level 4; i.e., the enzymatic defect has been defined. Knowledge of the mucopolysaccharidoses is at this time at the third level; we have included them in this chapter because so much is now known about the substances that are accumulated and because it appears likely that the enzymatic defect will be clarified in the near future. Knowledge about most of the endocrine disorders is at level 3. Even though the biochemical cause of the endocrine defects may be unknown, they have been included here because of the extensive knowledge about their metabolic consequences.

An understanding of the basic biochemical disturbance is required for meaningful classification and precise diagnosis of metabolic and endocrine disorders. More important, it offers promise for therapy and prevention. In most instances, specific therapeutic approaches can be developed only after the biochemical nature of the disease is clarified, and then require detailed evaluation of efficacy and safety. Prevention of metabolic disorders is facilitated if the heterozygous state can be detected and if the disorder can be diagnosed prenatally [5]. In our discussions of the metabolic disorders we have included summaries of recent knowledge about therapy and prevention.

References

1. Stanbury, J. B., Wyngaarden, J. B., and Fredrickson, D. S. (eds.). *The Metabolic Basis of Inherited Disease*, 3rd ed. McGraw-Hill Book Co., New York, 1972.
2. Moser, H. W., and Wolf, P. A. The nosology of mental retardation. *Birth Defects: Original Article Series*, Vol. VII, No. 1, February, 1971, pp. 117–34. Williams & Wilkins Co., Baltimore.
3. Levy, H. L., Madigan, P. M., and Shih, V. E. Massachusetts metabolic disorder screening program. I. Techniques and results of urine screening. *Pediatrics* (1972, in press).
4. O'Brien, J. S. Cited in McKusick, V. A. The nosology of the mucopolysaccharidoses. *Am. J. Med.*, **47**:730–47, 1969.
5. Milunsky, A., Littlefield, J. W., Kanfer, J. N., Kolodny, E. H., Shih, V. E., and Atkins, L. Prenatal genetic diagnosis. *N. Engl. J. Med.*, **283**:1370–81, 1441–47, 1498–1504, 1970.

Argininosuccinic Aciduria

In 1958 Allen, Cusworth, Dent, and Wilson [1] reported a mentally retarded 3½-year-old girl with convulsions, transient ataxia, and friable hair. Her brother was similarly affected. Both had large quantities of argininosuccinic acid in their urine. More than 15 additional patients have since been described [2–7]. The disorder is due to deficient activity of argininosuccinase [8]. This is one of the enzymes of the Krebs-Henseleit urea cycle, the main pathway for ammonia detoxication.

Physical Features

ABDOMEN: Enlargement of the liver has been noted in a few patients, primarily severely ill infants [5].

HAIR: Most patients have sparse dull, stubby, friable scalp hair (trichorrhexis nodosa) (*Figures A and D*). The eyebrows, eyelashes, and hair on the arms and legs may also be involved. Microscopic examination of the hair shows transverse fractures with fraying of the broken ends, torsion, and variations in the diameter of different hairs [9] (*Figure E*).

Nervous System

Almost all of the reported patients have been mentally retarded to either a moderate or severe degree. Most have had grand mal seizures, particularly in early childhood. Intermittent cerebellar ataxia and nystagmus have occurred in several patients. The ataxia may be disabling for brief periods, but most of the time there is little or no disturbance in coordination. Episodes of short-lived coma associated with a very dysrhythmic electroencephalogram and an elevated blood ammonia have occurred in two patients [4,7].

Pathology

Autopsies have been performed on two infants—one 8 days old [5] and the other 8 months old [6]—and on one 16-year-old boy [7]. The principal finding in the infants was delay in myelination (*Figure F*). The 16-year-old boy showed no abnormality in the white matter. However, as is true in other diseases associated with hyperammonemia, the astrocytic nuclei were abnormal and resembled Alzheimer type II cells [7]. He also had a gross neuronal loss in the thalamus.

Laboratory Studies

A deficiency of argininosuccinase has been demonstrated in red blood cells [8], liver [6], and cultured skin fibroblasts [10]. Large quantities of argininosuccinic acid are present in the urine (0.9 to 9 g per 24 hours), brain, liver, and spinal fluid. The blood ammonia level may be normal or only slightly elevated in the fasting state, but marked elevations occur after meals or after an ammonia load is given [4]. Abnormal liver function is usually evident in patients with hepatomegaly.

Treatment and Prognosis

Two patients died at 6 days of age. Those who survive infancy have only moderate disability; the main risks to their survival are seizures or episodes of hyperammonemia. The latter may be controlled by restricting protein intake. Theoretically, prevention of hyperammonemia beginning soon after birth might reduce the severity of mental retardation. Supplementation of the diet with arginine can restore the hair to normal (*Figures B and C*). This is probably because the enzymatic defect may lead to arginine deficiency, and arginine is an important constituent of hair [4].

Genetics

Autosomal recessive. The heterozygote state can be diagnosed by measuring the level of argininosuccinase in red blood cells [9]. Prenatal diagnosis is possible [11].

Differential Diagnosis

1. Trichorrhexis nodosa, seizures, and severe mental retardation are also features of patients with kinky hair disease, but these patients have neither elevated blood ammonia nor argininosuccinic aciduria. As it is an X-linked recessive disorder, only males are affected (see page 100).
2. The combination of trichorrhexis nodosa and mental retardation has occurred in two patients who did not have argininosuccinic aciduria (see page 350).
3. Trichorrhexis nodosa and mental retardation were features of the siblings reported by Tay [12], but they also had skin lesions and short stature.

References

1. Allen, J. D., Cusworth, D. C., Dent, C. E., and Wilson, V. K. A disease, probably hereditary, characterized by severe mental deficiency and a constant gross abnormality of amino acid metabolism. *Lancet,* 1:182–87, 1958.
2. Westall, R. G. Argininosuccinic aciduria. Identification and reactions of abnormal metabolite in a newly described form of mental disease, with some preliminary metabolic studies. *Biochem. J.,* 77:135–44, 1960.
3. Coryell, M. E., Hall, W. K., Thevaos, T. G., Welter, D. A., Gatz, A. J., Horton, B. F., Sisson, B. D., Looper, J. W., Jr., and Farrow, R. T. A familial study of a human enzyme defect, argininosuccinic aciduria. *Biochem. Biophys. Res. Commun.,* 14:307–12, 1964.
4. Moser, H. W., Efron, M. L., Brown, H., Diamond, R., and Neumann, C. G. Argininosuccinic aciduria. Report of two new cases and demonstration of intermittent elevation of blood ammonia. *Am. J. Med.,* 42:9–26, 1967.
5. Baumgartner, R., Scheidegger, S., Stalder, G., and Hottinger, A. Arginin-bernsteinsäure—Krankheit des Neugeborenen mit letalem Verlauf (Neonatal death due to argininosuccinic aciduria). *Helv. Paediatr. Acta.,* 23:77–106, 1968.
6. Solitaire, G. B., Shih, V. E., Nelligan, D. J., and Dolan, T. F., Jr. Argininosuccinic aciduria: clinical, biochemical, anatomical and neuropathological observations. *J. Ment. Defic. Res.,* 13:153–70, 1969.
7. Lewis, P. D., and Miller, A. L. Argininosuccinic aciduria. Case report with neuropathological findings. *Brain,* 93:413–22, 1970.
8. Tomlinson, S., and Westall, R. G. Argininosuccinic aciduria, argininosuccinase and arginase in human blood cells. *Clin. Sci.,* 26:261–69, 1964.
9. Rauschkolb, E. W., Freeman, R. G., and Farrell, G. Hair fragility—an important clue to aminoacidopathy in mental retardation. *Cutis,* 4:1315–18, 1968.
10. Shih, V. E., Littlefield, J. W., and Moser, H. W. Argininosuccinase deficiency in fibroblasts cultured from patients with argininosuccinic aciduria. *Biochem. Genet.,* 3:81–83, 1969.
11. Jacoby, L. B., Littlefield, J. W., Milunsky, A., Shih, V. E., and Wilroy, R. S., Jr. A microassay for argininosuccinase in cultured cells. *Am. J. Hum. Genet.* (1972, in press).
12. Tay, C. H. Ichthyosiform erythroderma, hair shaft abnormalities, and mental and growth retardation. A new recessive disorder. *Arch. Dermatol.,* 104:4–13, 1971.

Plate I-1. *A:* A 7-year-old girl with short, thin, light-colored hair. *B* and *C:* Show growth of her hair after 3 months' dietary supplementation with arginine. *D:* A 20-year-old girl with sparse, dull, short hair. *E:* Shows the irregularities in the diameter of this girl's hair and one area of twisting and bending (*arrow*). *F:* A coronal section of the cerebrum of an 8-month-old infant at the level of the third ventricle, showing the lack of sharp distinction between gray and white matter due to an extensive defect in myelination. (*A–C:* Courtesy of Dr. A. Hockey, Perth, Australia. *D:* From G. Farrell *et al., Tex. Med.,* **65:**90–101, 1969. *E:* Courtesy of Dr. E. W. Rauschkolb, Houston, Tex. *F:* From G. B. Solitare *et al., J. Ment. Defic. Res.,* **13:**153–70, 1969.)

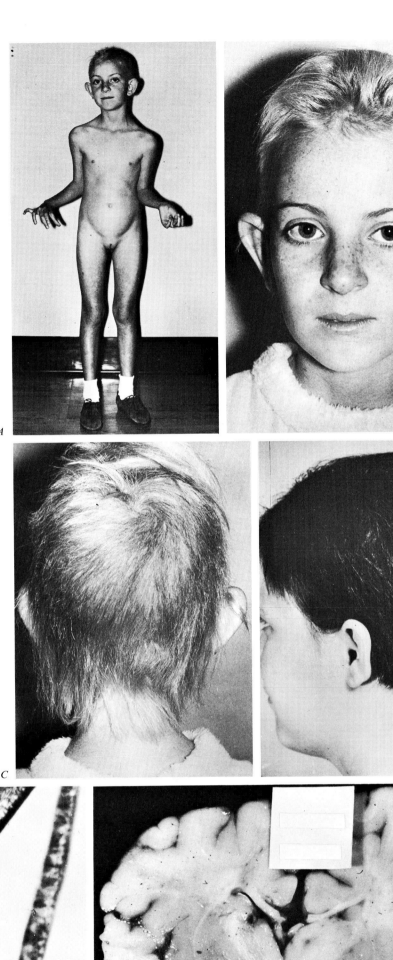

A

B

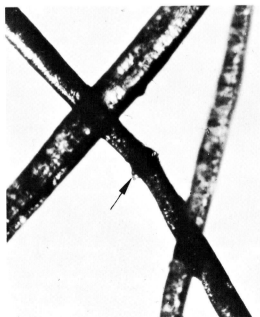

C

D

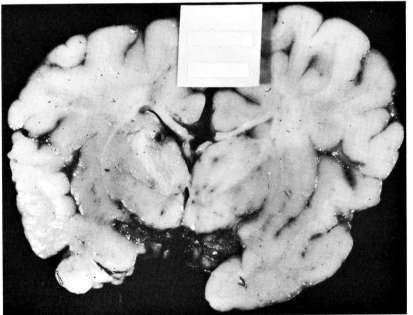

E

F

Cerebral Gigantism

In 1964 Sotos, Dodge, Muirhead, Crawford, and Talbot [1] described 5 children with rapid growth, acromegalic features, and nonprogressive cerebral dysfunction. More than 40 additional patients have since been described [2–6].

Physical Features

HEAD: The head is large (greater than the 90th percentile for age), and the anteroposterior diameter is increased. The characteristic posture is with the head and neck thrust forward (*Figures E and F*).

FACE: The face is long, the hairline is receding, the forehead is high and prominent, the eyes are widely spaced, the eyelids are droopy, and the palpebral fissures slant downward (*Figures A and D*). The brow protrudes anteriorly and the chin is often prognathic. Some patients have a sad, blank facial expression; they appear to be looking up through drooping eyelids.

EARS: The ears often are large, rotated posteriorly, and protruding.

MOUTH: The palate has a high, narrow arch. Early teething is common.

BACK: In one review 8 of 24 patients had kyphosis or scoliosis [5]. Some patients have a slumped stance with increased lumbar lordosis.

LIMBS: The hands and feet are disproportionately large in patients of all ages (*Figure C*).

HEIGHT AND WEIGHT: At birth and throughout childhood the height and weight of most patients are above the 90th percentile of the normal range. Some patients have the greatest linear growth in the first years of life and others in the teen-age years. Adults may have normal height or they may be excessively tall [7] (*Figure B*).

GROWTH AND DEVELOPMENT: The age at puberty is usually appropriate for the patient's height, weight, and bone age, but is earlier than in normal children [1,7].

Nervous System

General clumsiness, an awkward gait, and ataxia are frequent. Most patients are slow in learning to walk and talk. About one third have seizures. Most patients are mildly retarded, but some have normal intelligence and others are severely retarded [2,5].

Laboratory Studies

Growth hormone and insulin levels before and after stimulation with arginine and hypoglycemia are usually normal. A few patients have had hypothyroidism [7]. Urinary gonadotropin and ketosteroid levels are compatible with the height age and pubertal development. The concentration of certain essential amino acids in the plasma was elevated in two patients [6]. Pneumoencephalograms show in many patients both dilated cerebral ventricles and increased width of the cerebral mass. Skull x-rays show no evidence of increased intracranial pressure. The sella turcica is large but within the normal range. The frontal sinuses are enlarged. The distal phalanges show tufting, similar to that seen in acromegaly [7].

Treatment and Prognosis

These patients usually have a mild degree of mental retardation and can do well once they are adults. The ventricular enlargement and macrencephaly are not an indication for a ventriculoatrial shunt.

Genetics

These patients usually do not have any similarly affected relatives. Exceptions that have been reported include concordance of identical twins [2] and affected first cousins [8].

Differential Diagnosis

1. Excessively tall stature, prognathism, large hands and feet, and tufting of the phalanges are also features of acromegaly, but acromegalic patients have elevated serum growth hormone levels and evidence of a pituitary tumor.
2. Large hands, hypertelorism, prognathism, kyphoscoliosis, and mental retardation are features of patients with the syndrome of acromegaloid features, hypertelorism, and pectus carinatum, but they also have coarse facial features and short stature (see page 316).

References

1. Sotos, J. F., Dodge, P. R., Muirhead, D., Crawford, J. D., and Talbot, N. B. Cerebral gigantism in childhood. *N. Engl. J. Med.,* **271:**109–16, 1964.
2. Hook, E. B., and Reynolds, J. W. Cerebral gigantism: endocrinological and clinical observations of six patients including a congenital giant, concordant monozygotic twins, and a child who achieved adult gigantic size. *J. Pediatr.,* **70:**900–14, 1967.
3. Milunsky, A., Cowie, V. A., and Donoghue, E. C. Cerebral gigantism in childhood. *Pediatics,* **40:**395–402, 1967.
4. Gaudier, B., Ponte, C., Dehaene, Ph., Nuyts, J. P., and Ryckewaert, Ph. Encéphalopathie infantile et dysmorphies complexes: III.—Le gigantisme cérébral. *Lille Med.,* **13:**760–65, 1968.
5. Abraham, J. M., and Snodgrass, G. J. A. I. Sotos' syndrome of cerebral gigantism. *Arch. Dis. Child.,* **44:**203–10, 1969.
6. Bejar, R. L., Smith, G. F., Park, S., Spellacy, W. N., Wolfson, S. L., and Nyhan, W. L. Cerebral gigantism: concentrations of amino acids in plasma and muscle. *J. Pediatr.* **76:**105–11, 1970.
7. Crawford, J. D. Personal communication, 1970.
8. Hooft, C., Schote, H., and Van Hoover, G. Familial cerebral gigantism. *Acta Paediatr. Belg.,* **22:**173–86, 1968.

Plate I-2. *A–C:* A girl at 16 months and 27 years, showing the high forehead in infancy and gigantism in adulthood. She is shown standing next to her mother and with her hand next to her mother's hand. Her adult height is 6 feet 3 inches and weight 250 pounds. *D:* An 8-month-old infant with a high forehead, drooping eyelids, and increased anteroposterior skull diameter. Head circumference was 19½ inches. *E:* A 4½-year-old boy with stooped posture and forward thrust of his head and neck. He was 50 inches tall and weighed 48 pounds. *F:* An 8½-year-old girl with similar posture. She had large hands and was 56¾ inches tall· and weighed 94 pounds. (*A, D–F:* Courtesy of Dr. J. D. Crawford, Boston, Mass. *B* and *C:* Courtesy of Dr. E. Picard, Boston, Mass.)

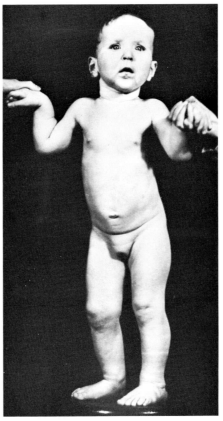

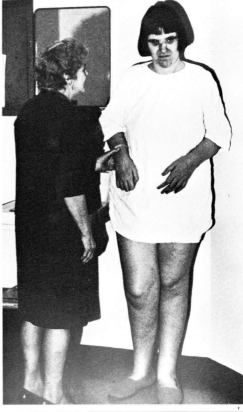

A

B

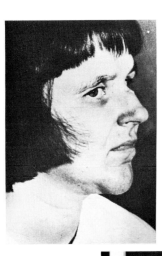

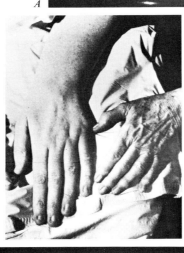

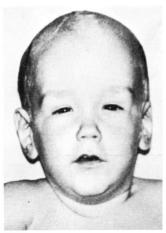

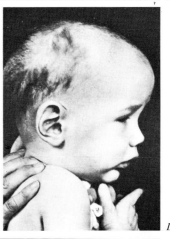

C

D

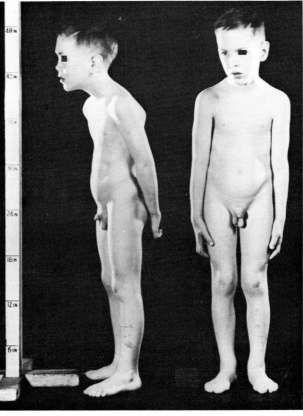

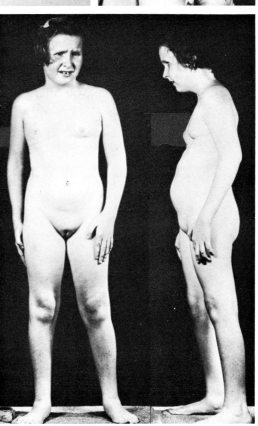

E

F

Congenital Hypothyroidism (Cretinism)

Congenital hypothyroidism is one of the best known and most studied causes of mental retardation. Many different causes, most of which are hereditary metabolic defects, have been identified:

1. Aplasia, hypoplasia, or maldescent of thyroid
   a. Embryonic defect of development
   b. Maternal radioiodine
2. Defective synthesis of thyroid hormone (nonendemic goitrous cretinism)
   a. Iodide transport defect
   b. Iodide organification defect
   c. Failure of coupling of iodotyrosines
   d. Failure of iodotyrosine deiodinase
   e. Releasing defect
   f. Abnormal iodinated polypeptides in serum [1]
3. Impaired thyroid response to thyrotropin [2]
4. Maternal ingestion of medications during pregnancy
   a. Goitrogens, such as propylthiouracil
   b. Iodides [3]
5. Iodide deficiency (endemic cretinism) (*Figure F*)
6. Hereditary syndromes with specific defect unknown
   a. Familial goiter and cretinism (Pendred's syndrome)
   b. Familial syndrome of deaf-mutism, stippled epiphyses, goiter, and abnormally high PBI [4]
   c. Hypothyroidism and vertebral anomalies [5]

Except for the presence or absence of a goiter (*Figure E*), patients with congenital hypothyroidism of different causes have the same physical features. Not all goiters are palpable at the same age. For example, the goiters of patients with thyroid ectopia and with defective synthesis of thyroid hormone are often not appreciated until the latter half of the first decade.

Physical Features

HEAD: The anterior fontanel remains open much longer than is normal.

FACE: The nasal bridge is flat, the eyelids puffy, and the palpebral fissures narrow; the mouth is kept open and the thick, broad tongue protrudes (*Figure A*). In older children and adults the features are coarse (*Figure C*) and the face is often expressionless.

VOICE: The voice is hoarse.

NECK: The neck is short and thick.

CHEST: The heart is often large and the rate slow. Murmurs are often audible.

ABDOMEN: The abdomen is large and an umbilical hernia usually develops in the first few weeks of life (*Figure B*).

LIMBS: The hands are broad and the fingers are short.

SKIN: The infant's skin is dry, scaly, and cold and often has a mottled appearance in the newborn (*Figure A*). Carotenemia causes yellow discoloration of the skin but not of the sclera. Older children and adults develop myxedema and have rough, dry skin and doughy, indurated subcutaneous tissue (*Figure D*).

HAIR: In adults, the scalp is thickened and the hair is coarse and brittle and may be sparse. In infants, the hair is fine and straight; the hairline extends far down on the forehead, and lanugo hair is prominent over the upper back, shoulder, and deltoid areas.

HEIGHT: Shortness of stature is often severe (*Figures B and F*).

WEIGHT: Relative to their height, these patients are at all ages average in weight.

GROWTH AND DEVELOPMENT: If the hypothyroidism is untreated, sexual maturation is delayed or does not occur at all. In some patients isosexual precocity has been observed.

Nervous System

Infants have muscular hypotonia, weakness, and diminished deep tendon reflexes. A few have firm, large muscles (the Kocher-Debré–Sémélaigne syndrome) [6]. Both mental and motor development are retarded. The more profound the deficiency of thyroid hormone, both during fetal development and in the early months of life, the poorer the prognosis for mental development [7].

Laboratory Studies

In addition to abnormal thyroid function tests, x-rays are most useful, showing a retarded bone age and epiphyseal dysgenesis throughout the skeleton.

Treatment and Prognosis

In general, adequate replacement of thyroid hormone results in a reversal of the signs and symptoms of congenital hypothyroidism. Thyroidectomy is often necessary for large goiters. There are two general principles for establishing the prognosis for ultimate intelligence of an infant or child at the time the diagnosis of hypothyroidism is first made. First, the extent of delay in bone maturation at the time of diagnosis is the most useful prognostic tool in the neonate. Development less than the normal for 30 weeks gestation forecasts an ominous outcome for the term infant [8]. Second, the prognosis for patients with no thyroid tissue identifiable clinically or by radioiodine or technitium scanning is much worse than that for patients with some tissue, either normally placed or ectopic [8]. The usefulness of thyroid replacement in improving mental capabilities has long been debated. In one study [9] it was shown that only one half of the infants treated at less than 6 months of age had IQ's above 90.

Differential Diagnosis

1. A flat nasal bridge, a protruding tongue, and muscular hypotonia are features of infants with Down's syndrome, but they do not have hypothermia, mottled skin, carotenemia, or abnormal thyroid function tests (see page 150).
2. A large tongue and umbilical hernia are features of patients with the syndrome of macroglossia, omphalocele, visceromegaly, and neonatal hypoglycemia (Beckwith-Wiedemann syndrome) (see page 56).
3. Patients with Hurler's syndrome have a flat nasal bridge and coarse facial features, but they are differentiated by corneal opacities, increased urinary glycosaminoglycan levels, and different x-ray changes (see page 38).
4. Severe hypotonia, stippled epiphyses, and a flat nasal bridge are features of patients with the cerebrohepatorenal syndrome, but they also have a high brow, eye anomalies, flexion contractures, and hepatomegaly (see page 270).

References

1. Stanbury, J. B. Familial goiter. In *The Metabolic Basis of Inherited Disease*, Stanbury, J. B., Wyngaarden, J. B., and Fredrickson, D. S. (eds.), 2nd ed. McGraw-Hill Book Co., New York, 1966, pp. 215–57.
2. Stanbury, J. B., Rocmans, P., Buhler, U. K., and Ochi, Y. Congenital hypothyroidism with impaired thyroid response to thyrotropin. *N. Engl. J. Med.*, **279**:1132–36, 1968.
3. Carswell, F., Kerr, M. M., and Hutchison, J. H. Congenital goiter and hypothyroidism produced by maternal ingestion of iodides. *Lancet*, **1**:1241–43, 1970.
4. Retetoff, S., DeWind, L. T., and DeGroot, L. J. Familial syndrome combining deaf-mutism, stippled epiphyses, goiter and abnormally high PBI: possible target organ refractoriness to thyroid hormone. *J. Clin. Endocrinol. Metab.*, **27**:279–94, 1967.
5. Lintermans, J. P., and Seyhnaeve, V. Hypothyroidism and vertebral anomalies: a new syndrome? *Am. J. Roentgenol. Radium Ther. Nucl. Med.*, **109**:294–98, 1970.
6. Najjar, S. S., and Nachman, H. S. The Kocher-Debré-Sémélaigne syndrome. Hypothyroidism with muscular "hypertrophy." *J. Pediatr.*, **66**:901–908, 1965.
7. Man, E. B., Mermann, A. C., and Cooke, R. E. The development of children with congenital hypothyroidism. *J. Pediatr.*, **63**:926–41, 1963.
8. Crawford, J. D. Personal communication, 1970.
9. Wilkins, L. *The Diagnosis and Treatment of Endocrine Disorders in Childhood and Adolescence*, 3rd ed. Charles C Thomas, Springfield, Ill., 1965, p. 114.

Plate I-3. *A:* An infant with puffy eyelids, a protruding tongue, and mottled skin. The bandage covers a large umbilical hernia. *B:* The 4-year-old child on the right has a protuberant abdomen and short stature. The child on the left is a normal age control. *C* and *D:* A 50-year-old woman with coarse facial features and dry, doughy skin with indurated subcutaneous tissue. *E:* A 16-year-old girl with a large goiter due to a peroxidase deficiency. The excised thyroid weighed 97 g. *F:* An Ecuadorian woman with endemic goitrous cretinism due to iodide deficiency. She had marked shortness of stature and dysplasia of both proximal femoral epiphyses. (*A* and *B:* Courtesy of Dr. J. D. Crawford, Boston, Mass. *E* and *F:* Courtesy of Dr. J. B. Stanbury, Cambridge, Mass.)

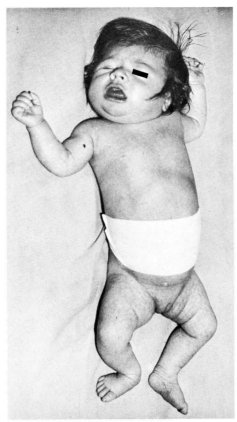

A

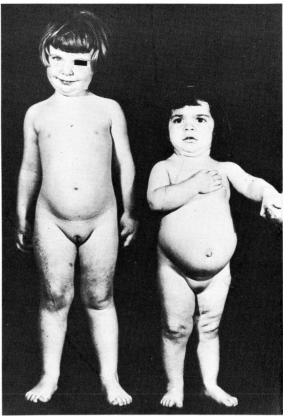

B

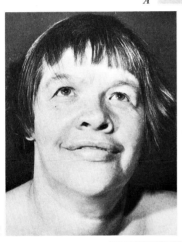

C

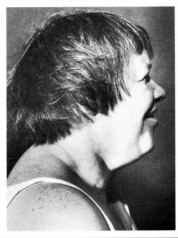

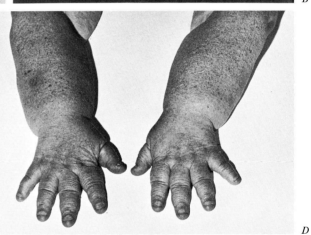

D

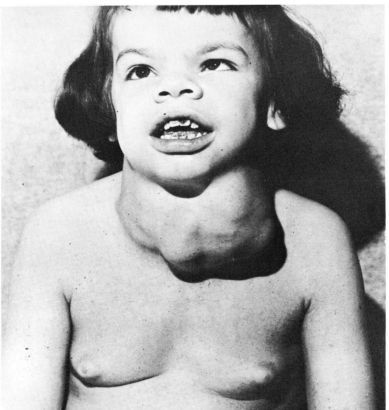

E

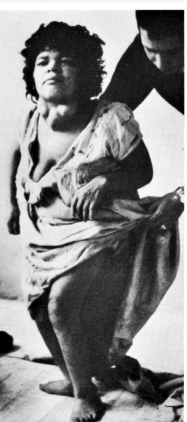

F

11

Fucosidosis (Mucopolysaccharidosis F)

In 1966, 1967, and 1969 Durand and associates [1–3] reported two siblings with progressive neurologic deterioration, enlarged heart and salivary glands, thick skin, and, on x-ray, beaking of the lumbar vertebrae. Van Hoof and Hers subsequently showed [4] that these two patients had deficient activity of the lysosomal enzyme alpha-fucosidase and accumulated certain fucose-containing compounds. Two additional patients had the same biochemical abnormalities [5,6].

Physical Features

FACE: Two patients had a broad nose, thick lips, and enlarged tongue [5,6] (*Figure E*).
MOUTH: The two siblings had enlarged salivary glands [3].
ABDOMEN: One patient had slight hepatosplenomegaly [3] and another a small umbilical hernia.
BACK: All had dorsolumbar kyphosis.
SKIN: Thick skin and abundant sweating were noted in two patients [3].

Nervous System

The siblings developed normally for the first several months and began to show a regression in mental development at about one year of age. They first became hypotonic and later hypertonic and spastic; finally they showed decerebrate rigidity and dementia [3] (*Figures A and B*). The other two patients had somewhat delayed early development and then showed signs of mental regression. Spasticity, hyperreflexia, and loss of contact with surroundings were noted during the third or fourth year [5,6].

Pathology

Cells in the cerebrum, liver, heart, and skin were enlarged; the cytoplasm was distended with a homogeneous, eosinophilic material [3,5] (*Figure C*). Electron microscopy showed cytoplasmic vacuoles which were surrounded by a membrane. Within these vacuoles, and also in the mitochondria, there were lamellar bodies [5] (*Figure F*). The siblings' brains showed loss of neurons in the cerebral cortex, thalamus, hypothalamus, and cerebellum. Myelin was deficient. The adrenal glands were atrophic with thin cortical and medullary areas.

Laboratory Studies

The tissues of all four patients showed a deficiency of alpha-fucosidase. There was an accumulation of fucose-containing glycolipids and mucopolysaccharides. The levels of polysaccharides and sulfatides in the urine were normal.

Peripheral lymphocytes showed many vacuoles. The concentration of sodium and of chloride in the sweat and saliva in the two siblings was two to five times normal. On x-ray the vertebral bodies were poorly developed, and there was anterosuperior beaking of the lower thoracic and upper lumbar vertebrae. There may be progressive impairment of gallbladder function [7].

Treatment and Prognosis

In the first reported family both children developed decerebrate rigidity; one died at 3 years 9 months and the other at 5 years 2 months. Similar neurologic deterioration was observed in the two other patients, who were alive at the time they were reported [3,5,6].

Genetics

Autosomal recessive inheritance is postulated. Prenatal diagnosis is possible, but has not been reported.

Differential Diagnosis

1. Fucosidosis is distinguished from mucopolysaccharidosis I (Hurler's syndrome) by the absence of corneal clouding, by the fact that the facial, skeletal, and visceral changes are not as severe, and by the normal urinary polysaccharide levels (see page 38).
2. In mucopolysaccharidosis II (Hunter's syndrome) and mucopolysaccharidosis III (Sanfilippo syndrome) neurologic deterioration is not as marked as in fucosidosis, and urinary polysaccharide levels are increased (see page 38).
3. Mannosidosis (see page 34) and I-cell disease (see page 28) can be distinguished by specific laboratory studies.

References

1. Durand, P., Borrone, C., and Della Cella, G. A new mucopolysaccharide lipid-storage disease? *Lancet,* **2:**1313–14, 1966.
2. Durand, P., Philippart, M., Borrone, C., Della Cella, G., and Bugiani, O. Una nuova malattia da accumulo di glicolipidi (ceremidi tetraesosidi). *Minerva Pediatr.* **19:**2187–96, 1967.
3. Durand, P., Borrone, C., and Della Cella, G. Fucosidosis. *J. Pediatr.* **75:**665–74, 1969.
4. Van Hoof, F., and Hers, H. G. Mucopolysaccharidosis by absence of alpha-fucosidase. *Lancet,* **1:**1198, 1968.
5. Loeb, H., Tondeur, M., Jonniaux, G., Mockel-Pohl, S., and Vamos-Hurwitz, E. Biochemical and ultrastructural studies in a case of mucopolysaccharidosis "F" (fucosidosis). *Helv. Paediatr. Acta,* **24:**519–37, 1969.
6. Spranger, J. W. Personal communication, 1970.
7. McKusick, V. A. The nosology of the mucopolysaccharidoses. *Am. J. Med.,* **47:**730–47, 1969.

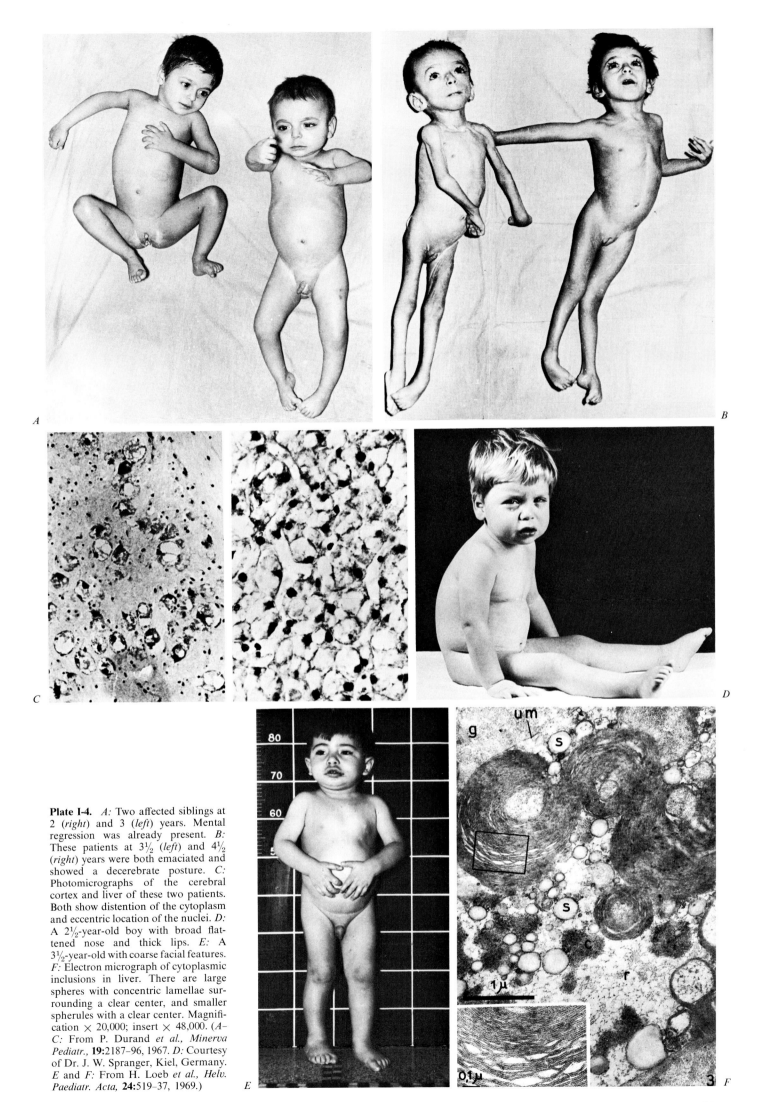

Plate I-4. *A:* Two affected siblings at 2 (*right*) and 3 (*left*) years. Mental regression was already present. *B:* These patients at 3½ (*left*) and 4½ (*right*) years were both emaciated and showed a decerebrate posture. *C:* Photomicrographs of the cerebral cortex and liver of these two patients. Both show distention of the cytoplasm and eccentric location of the nuclei. *D:* A 2½-year-old boy with broad flattened nose and thick lips. *E:* A 3½-year-old with coarse facial features. *F:* Electron micrograph of cytoplasmic inclusions in liver. There are large spheres with concentric lamellae surrounding a clear center, and smaller spherules with a clear center. Magnification × 20,000; insert × 48,000. (*A–C:* From P. Durand *et al., Minerva Pediatr.,* **19:**2187–96, 1967. *D:* Courtesy of Dr. J. W. Spranger, Kiel, Germany. *E* and *F:* From H. Loeb *et al., Helv. Paediatr. Acta,* **24:**519–37, 1969.)

13

Galactosemia

In 1908 Reuss noted galactosuria in an 8-month-old infant who had been losing weight since it was 8 weeks old. The liver and spleen were enlarged, and postmortem examination at 9 months revealed cirrhosis of the liver [1]. Galactosemia is now recognized as one of the important and, at least in part, preventable metabolic causes of mental retardation. In some parts of the world all newborns are screened for galactosemia. The incidence is estimated at 1 : 70,000 births [2,2a]. The metabolic basis is deficient activity of galactose-1-phosphate uridyl transferase (G-1-PUT), which impairs the patient's ability to metabolize galactose [3].

Physical Features

EYES: Cataracts develop within the first year in most untreated patients (*Figure B*).

ABDOMEN: Almost all untreated patients develop hepatomegaly. One quarter to one third develop ascites and enlargement of the spleen [4] (*Figures A, C, and E*).

SKIN: Jaundice develops in the first week or two of life in half of the untreated infants. A few infants have had pedal gangrene, presumably as a result of thromboses from sepsis (*Figures C and D*). Many patients are pale owing to anemia.

Nervous System

Most untreated infants are lethargic and hypotonic. Some may have increased intracranial pressure [5]. Untreated patients are usually, but not always, mentally retarded. Seizures are uncommon [4].

Pathology

In the liver the most common feature is a rosettelike arrangement of parenchymal cells about a dilated canaliculus which is frequently filled with a mass of bile pigment. Infants below 6 months of age show an active process of hepatic cell damage and repair. Older patients show evidence of inactive cirrhosis [4].

Laboratory Studies

The activity of the enzyme galactose-1-phosphate uridyl transferase is deficient in the liver, red [3] and white [6] blood cells, and cultured skin fibroblasts [7]. Untreated patients have an accumulation of galactose-1-phosphate in the erythrocytes and increased serum and urine levels of galactose. When the blood galactose level is markedly elevated, depression of blood glucose level and signs and symptoms of hypoglycemia may occur. Proteinuria, hypoproteinemia, aminoaciduria, hypoprothrombinemia, and anemia are additional findings in untreated infants [4].

Treatment and Prognosis

Untreated patients have a high death rate in infancy, and those who survive are almost always mentally retarded. Treatment consists of dietary restriction of galactose. When a child is on this diet, signs of abnormal liver and kidney function disappear and normal growth resumes. Cataracts often improve, but may persist in spite of galactose restriction. Diagnosis at birth and close dietary control in most instances are associated with nearly normal intellectual development (*Figure F*). However, even under these circumstances the intelligence may fall short of that in the parents or unaffected sibs, and there may be psychologic and social maladjustment [8].

Genetics

Autosomal recessive. There are at least two related disorders of galactose metabolism. One of these, the Duarte variant, is benign since individuals homozygous for this variant show no physical or mental abnormalities. Their red blood cell G-1-PUT activity is the same as that in the heterozygote for classic galactosemia—i.e., 50 percent of normal [9]. The second variant has been found only in Negroes. Patients with this form may develop liver disease and cataracts, and lack G-1-PUT activity in their red blood cells. However, they are able to oxidize intravenously administered galactose, presumably through an alternate metabolic pathway [10]. It is likely that classic galactosemia can be diagnosed prenatally [11].

Differential Diagnosis

1. Jaundice, anemia, hepatomegaly, and cataracts are features of some infants with congenital rubella, but they are readily distinguished by testing for urine or serum galactose or measuring the erythrocyte G-1-PUT activity (see page 118).
2. Increased intracranial pressure and jaundice associated with untreated galactosemia may lead to erroneous diagnosis of neonatal meningitis or cerebral hemorrhage.

References

1. von Reuss, A. Zuckerausscheidung im Säuglingsalter. *Wien. Med. Wochenschr.,* **58**:799–803, 1908.
2. Schwarz, V., Wells, A. R., Holzel, A., and Komrower, G. M. A study of the genetics of galactosaemia. *Ann. Hum. Genet.,* **25**:179–88, 1961.
2a. Levy, H. L. Genetic screening. In *Advances in Human Genetics,* H. Harris and K. Hirshhorn (eds.), 4th ed. Plenum Press, London, in press.
3. Kalckar, H. M., Anderson, E. P., and Isselbacher, K. J. Galactosemia, a congenital defect in a nucleotide transferase. *Biochim. Biophys. Acta.,* **20**:262–68, 1956.
4. Donnell, G. N., Bergren, W. R., and Cleland, R. S. Galactosemia. *Pediatr. Clin. North Am.,* **7**:315–32, 1960.
5. Huttenlocher, P. R., Hillman, R. E., and Hsia, Y. E. Pseudotumor cerebri in galactosemia. *J. Pediatr.,* **76**:902–905, 1970.
6. Weinberg, A. N. Detection of congenital galactosemia and the carrier state using galactose C^{14} and blood cells. *Metabolism,* **10**:728–34, 1961.
7. Krooth, R. S., and Weinberg, A. N. Studies on cell lines developed from the tissues of patients with galactosemia. *J. Exp. Med.,* **113**:1155–71, 1961.
8. Komrower, G. M., and Lee, D. H. Long-term follow-up of galactosaemia. *Arch. Dis. Child.,* **45**:367–73, 1970.
9. Beutler, E., Baluda, M. C., Sturgeon, P., and Day, R. W. The genetics of galactose-1-phosphate uridyl transferase deficiency. *J. Lab. Clin. Med.,* **68**:646–58, 1966.
10. Segal, S., Blair, A., and Roth, H. The metabolism of galactose by patients with congenital galactosemia. *Am. J. Med.,* **38**:62–70, 1965.
11. Nadler, H. L. Antenatal detection of hereditary disorders. *Pediatrics,* **42**:912–18, 1968.

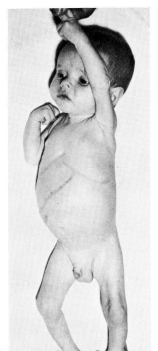

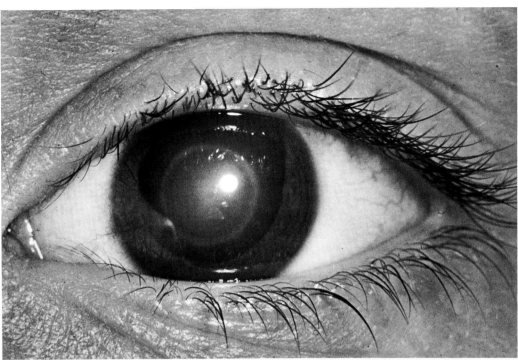

A

B

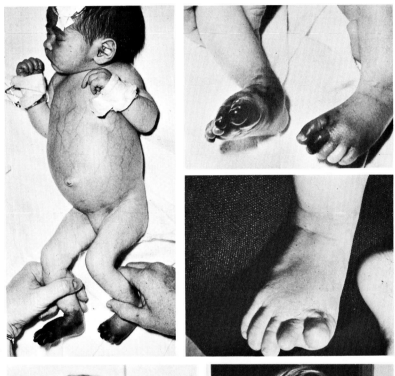

C

D

Plate I-5. *A:* An untreated 5-month-old infant with failure to thrive and liver enlargement (*outlined*). *B:* A posterior cortical cataract. This child had had an iridectomy in this eye. *C* and *D:* An untreated infant at age 3 weeks with a distended abdomen and gangrene of both feet. The close-up views show her feet at 3 weeks and later after 5 weeks of therapy with antibiotics and a lactose-free diet. She had a partial amputation of some toes, but the others healed normally. *E* and *F:* An untreated 13-month-old infant with abdominal distention and ascites before treatment and the same boy after treatment at 15 years of age. Since then he has completed high school and is gainfully employed. (*A, B,* and *D* [*bottom*]: Courtesy of Dr. G. N. Donnell, Los Angeles, Calif. *C* and *D* [*top*]: From P. J. Collipp and G. N. Donnell, *J. Pediatr.,* **54:**363–68, 1959. *E* and *F:* From G. N. Donnell *et al., Pediatr. Clin. North Am.,* **7:**315–32, 1960.)

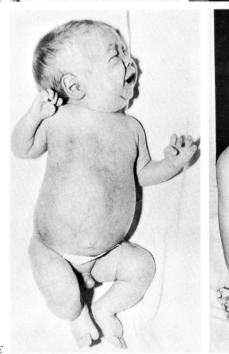

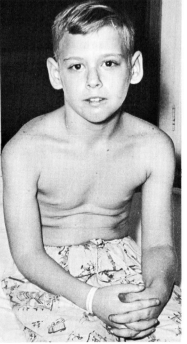

E

F

Gaucher's Disease (Cerebroside Lipidosis)

In 1882 Gaucher [1] described a patient who had died from a chronic progressive illness and had an enlarged liver and spleen associated with an accumulation of large cells which appeared to contain excess fat. Over 300 cases have subsequently been reported [2]. There are at least two forms of Gaucher's disease: the more common (noncerebral) form usually manifests in late adolescence or adulthood because of splenomegaly, abnormal bruising, or pathologic fractures [2]. In the less common (cerebral) form, hepatosplenomegaly and neurologic deterioration are usually noted during the first year of life [2]. In both forms there is accumulation of glucocerebroside due to deficient activity of glucocerebrosidase [3]. This discussion will deal only with the cerebral form of the disease, of which there are at least two genetic types affecting either infants or juveniles.

Physical Features

ABDOMEN: Enlargement of the liver and spleen develops in the first months of life (*Figures A and B*).

LYMPH NODES: Most patients develop enlargement of the peripheral lymph nodes.

Nervous System

All patients have severe impairment of psychomotor function, which is usually evident in the first months of life. Retroflexion of the head (*Figure E*), strabismus (*Figure B*), and hypertonicity are the most common neurologic manifestations. Bulbar involvement may cause bilateral facial weakness and swallowing difficulties (*Figures B and D*). In a rare juvenile variant whose onset is between 5 and 12 years of age, the neurologic symptoms are convulsions, tremor, emotional disturbances, and progressive dementia [4].

Pathology

The characteristic feature is the Gaucher cell, a large (20 to 100 microns) cell whose cytoplasm has a reticular pattern that looks like wrinkled tissue paper or crumpled silk (*Figure F*). These cells accumulate primarily in the spleen, lymph nodes, bone marrow, and liver. In the nervous system there is loss of neurons and acute nerve cell degeneration, particularly involving the cranial nerve nuclei of the midbrain, pons, and medulla. There is only slight neuronal glycolipid storage [2].

Laboratory Studies

Glucocerebroside is the main storage substance in the visceral organs. It accumulates because of deficient activity of the glucocerebroside splitting enzyme [3]. The deficiency of this enzyme can be demonstrated in both white blood cells [5] and skin fibroblasts [6]. The assay of glucocerebrosidase activity requires radioactive glucocerebroside, which is not yet generally available. White blood cells and cultured fibroblasts of patients with Gaucher's disease are also deficient in beta-glucosidase activity, an assay that utilizes a readily available nonbiologic substrate [7]. The serum acid phosphatase level is increased [8]. X-rays show a thin cortex and porous and trabeculated spongiosa in bones where storage material has accumulated [2].

Treatment and Prognosis

Most patients with cerebral Gaucher's disease die before 2 years of age. However, some have survived to adulthood [4].

Genetics

Both the cerebral and noncerebral forms are autosomal recessive traits. Only one form occurs in any given pedigree. Assay of beta-glucosidase activity in white blood cells or cultured skin fibroblasts may allow detection of the heterozygous state; however, there is some overlap with values in normal controls [7,9]. It is likely that prenatal diagnosis can be achieved by measuring glucocerebrosidase or beta-glucosidase activities in cultured amniotic fluid cells [7].

Differential Diagnosis

Hepatosplenomegaly and neurologic deterioration are also seen in infantile Niemann-Pick disease (see page 44), G_{M1} gangliosidosis (see page 22), and Wolman's disease (see page 66). In Niemann-Pick disease the child is hypotonic and listless, and the head is not retroflexed. Patients with Niemann-Pick disease may in addition have optic atrophy or a macular cherry-red spot. Patients with G_{M1} gangliosidosis often show coarse facial features and radiologic changes suggestive of the mucopolysaccharidoses. Children with Wolman's disease have calcified adrenals, which can be demonstrated by x-ray, and may have bowel obstruction.

References

1. Gaucher, P. *De l'epithelioma primitif de la rate.* Thèse de Paris, 1882.
2. Fredrickson, D. S. Cerebroside lipidosis: Gaucher's disease. In *The Metabolic Basis of Inherited Disease,* J. B. Stanbury, J. B. Wyngaarden, and D. S. Fredrickson (eds.), 2nd ed. McGraw-Hill Book Co., New York, 1966, pp. 565–85.
3. Brady, R. O., Kanfer, J. N., Bradley, R. M., and Shapiro, D. Demonstration of a deficiency of glucocerebroside-cleaving enzyme in Gaucher's disease. *J. Clin. Invest.,* **45:**1112–15, 1966.
4. Herrlin, K.-M., and Hillborg, P. O. Neurological signs in a juvenile form of Gaucher's disease. *Acta Paediatr.,* **51:**137–54, 1962.
5. Kampine, J. P., Brady, R. O., Kanfer, J. N., Feld, M., and Shapiro, D. Diagnosis of Gaucher's disease and Niemann-Pick disease with small samples of venous blood. *Science,* **155:**86–88, 1967.
6. Brady, R. O. Genetics and the sphingolipidoses. *Med. Clin. North Am.,* **53:**827–38, 1969.
7. Beutler, E., Kuhl, W., Trinidad, F., Teplitz, R., and Nadler, H. Detection of Gaucher's disease and its carrier state from fibroblast cultures. *Lancet,* **2:**369, 1970.
8. Tuchman, L. R., Goldstein, G., and Clyman, M. Studies on the nature of the increased serum acid phosphatase in Gaucher's disease. *Am. J. Med.,* **27:**959–62, 1959.
9. Beutler, E., and Kuhl, W. Detection of the defect of Gaucher's disease and its carrier state in peripheral-blood leucocytes. *Lancet,* **1:**612–13, 1970.

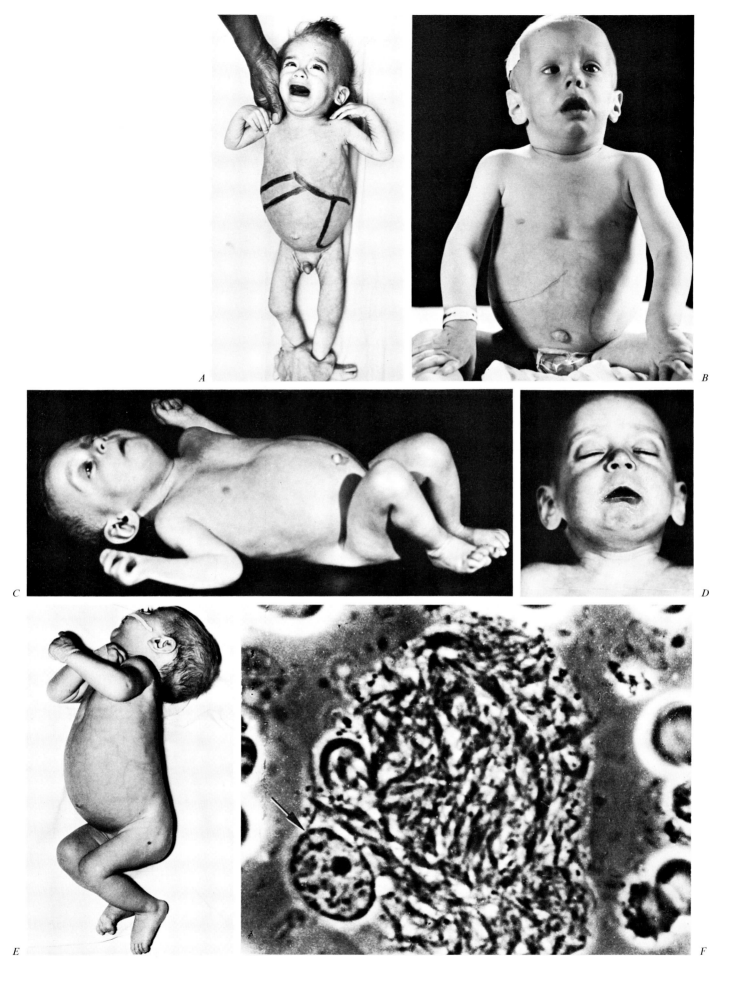

Plate I-6. *A:* Shows a 12-month-old infant with a protuberant abdomen, decorticate posture, retroflexion of his head, and strabismus. The enlarged liver and spleen are outlined. *B:* An 18-month-old child with a masklike face, strabismus, and hepatosplenomegaly. *C* and *D:* A 9-month-old child with retroflexion of the head and weakness of the facial muscles. *E:* An 8-month-old child with a protuberant abdomen and hyperextended neck. A nasogastric feeding tube is in place. *F:* A Gaucher cell with the nucleus pushed to the edge (*arrow*) and distended cytoplasm containing material that has a reticular pattern. (*A* and *F:* From Cerebroside lipidosis: Gaucher's disease, by D. S. Fredrickson, in *The Metabolic Basis of Inherited Disease,* J. B. Stanbury *et al.* [eds.], 2nd ed. McGraw-Hill, New York, 1966, pp. 565–85. Used with permission of McGraw-Hill Book Company. *B:* Courtesy of Dr. P. R. Dodge, St. Louis, Mo. *C* and *D:* Courtesy of Dr. A. C. Crocker, Boston, Mass. *E:* Courtesy of Dr. B. Hagberg, Uppsala, Sweden.)

Globoid Cell Leukodystrophy (Krabbe's Disease)

In 1916 Krabbe [1] described a brother and sister who were normal until they were 4 months old, when they developed severe tonic spasms and rapid neurologic deterioration which led to their death by the second year. Neuropathologic studies showed a severe leukodystrophy characterized by the accumulation of multinucleated globoid cells. By 1969 at least 60 cases had been reported, and the incidence of the disorder in Sweden was estimated as 1.9 per 100,000 births [2]. The biochemical basis for this disorder is deficient activity of the enzyme galactocerebroside beta-galactosidase [3,4].

Physical Features

Other than the abnormal posture there are no abnormal physical signs.

Nervous System

The infants seem healthy and have normal psychomotor development during their first months of life. Based on studies in 32 patients, the subsequent neurologic deterioration has been divided into three clinical stages [2]. In stage I, which begins at about 4 months, the child is irritable. Light or noise may provoke violent tonic spasms (*Figure A*). There may be periods of fever without signs of infection. Stage II begins 1 to 4 months later and is characterized by rapid and severe motor deterioration. There may be an opisthotonic posture; the arms often are flexed and the legs extended (*Figures B, C, and D*). Episodes of high fever and intense sweating are more frequent. There is excessive salivation and hypersecretion from the lungs, and pneumonia is a frequent complication. More than half of the patients have irregular jerks of the arms and legs, hypertonic fits, and atypical seizures. In stage III the patients have no voluntary movements, are unresponsive, and have a decerebrate posture. There is severe optic atrophy and the pupils may be unresponsive to light.

Pathology

The brain is markedly atrophied, due entirely to severe shrinkage of the white matter; myelin may be nearly totally absent (*Figure E*). The pathognomonic feature is the accumulation of large multinucleated globoid cells, which contain galactocerebroside (*Figure F*). Peripheral nerves show segmental demyelination [5].

Laboratory Studies

A profound deficiency of the enzyme galactocerebroside beta-galactosidase can be demonstrated in brain, liver, spleen [3], serum, and white blood cells [6,7] of affected patients. In most cases the cerebrospinal fluid protein content is increased to over 100 mg percent [2]. The conduction velocity in peripheral nerves is reduced, and peripheral nerve biopsy shows evidence of active and healed segmental demyelination [2].

Treatment and Prognosis

The neurologic deterioration is rapidly progressive. Death is usually due to pneumonia or aspiration. In a series of 32 cases the mean age at death was 1.2 years, with the range from $5\frac{1}{2}$ months to $2\frac{3}{4}$ years [2].

Genetics

Autosomal recessive [2]. Prenatal diagnosis has been achieved [8].

Differential Diagnosis

1. Neurologic deterioration in the first months of life occurs in patients with spongy degeneration of the central nervous system. They usually have an enlarged head (see page 112).
2. Neurologic deterioration in the first months of life also occurs in patients with Tay-Sachs disease, but they also have a cherry-red spot in the macula and diminished serum hexosaminidase A activity (see page 62).

References

1. Krabbe, K. A new familial infantile form of diffuse sclerosis. *Brain,* **39**:74–114, 1916.
2. Hagberg, B., Kollberg, H., Sourander, P., and Åkesson, H. O. Infantile globoid cell leucodystrophy (Krabbe's disease). A clinical and genetic study of 32 Swedish cases 1953–1967. *Neuropädiatrie,* **1**:74–88, 1969.
3. Suzuki, K., and Suzuki, Y. Globoid cell leucodystrophy (Krabbe's disease): deficiency of galactocerebroside beta-galactosidase. *Proc. Natl. Acad. Sci. USA,* **66**:302–309, 1970.
4. Austin, J., Suzuki, K., Armstrong, D., Brady, R., Bachhawat, B. K., Schlanker, J., and Stumpf, D. Studies in globoid (Krabbe) leukodystrophy (GLD) V. Controlled enzymic studies in ten human cases. *Arch. Neurol.,* **23**:502–12, 1970.
5. Hogan, G., Gutmann, L., and Chou, S. M. The peripheral neuropathy of Krabbe's globoid leukodystrophy. *Neurology (Minneap.),* **19**:1094–1100, 1969.
6. Malone, M. J. Deficiency in a degradative enzyme system in globoid leucodystrophy. *Trans. Am. Soc. Neurochem.,* **1**:56, 1970.
7. Suzuki, Y., and Suzuki, K. Krabbe's globoid cell leukodystrophy: deficiency of galactocerebrosidase in serum, leukocytes, and fibroblasts. *Science,* **171**:73–75, 1971.
8. Suzuki, K., Schneider, E. L., and Epstein, C. J. In utero diagnosis of globoid cell leukodystrophy (Krabbe's disease). *Biochem. Biophys. Res. Commun.,* **45**:1363–66, 1971.

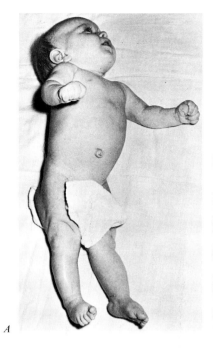

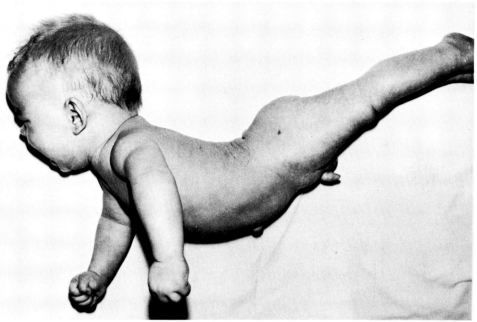

A

B

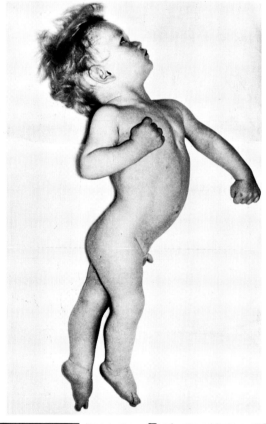

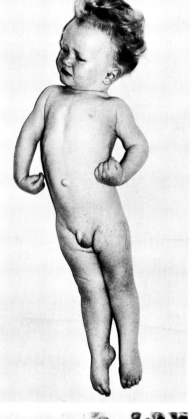

Plate I-7. *A:* A 5-month-old infant with sustained tonic decorticate posture. *B:* A crying infant with stage II of this disease, showing extension of the neck and legs and flexion of the arms. *C* and *D:* Two views of another infant in stage II with similar posture. *E:* Shows in a cross section of one hemisphere from each of two patients the marked decrease in the size of the brain of a patient with globoid cell leukodystrophy (*right,* aged 23 months), as compared with normal (*left,* aged 34 months). *F:* Typical globoid cell (*arrow*). (*A* and *E:* From J. Austin, in *Medical Aspects of Mental Retardation,* C. H. Carter [ed.], 1965, pp. 813–44. Courtesy of Charles C Thomas, Publisher, Springfield, Ill. *B* and *C:* Courtesy of Dr. B. Hagberg, Uppsala, Sweden. *D:* From B. Hagberg *et al., Neuropädiatrie,* **1:**74–88, 1969. *F:* Courtesy of Dr. E. P. Richardson, Jr., Boston, Mass.)

C

D

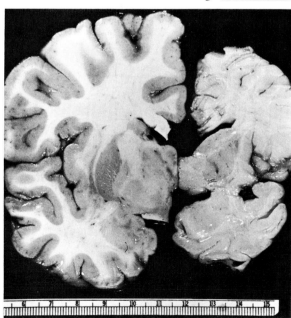

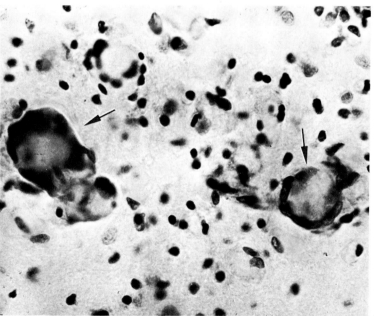

E

F

Glycogenosis, Type II (Pompe's Disease)

In 1932 Pompe [1], Bischoff [2], and Putschar [3] each independently described infants who had died with an enlarged heart and deposition of glycogen in cardiac muscle and nearly all other organs. This disorder is now referred to as type II glycogenosis, and over 100 patients have been described [4]. Clinical manifestations may involve the skeletal muscle, the heart, and the nervous system. In a rare muscular form, so far described in approximately 10 patients, only the skeletal muscle involvement causes symptoms [5,6]. However, most patients have in addition clinical evidence of heart disease (the cardiac form of the disease) or of both the heart and central nervous system (the generalized form of the disease). In all forms the activity of alpha-1,4-glucosidase (acid maltase) is deficient, at least in some tissues.

Physical Features

MOUTH: The tongue is enlarged and protrudes (*Figures A, C, and E*).

CHEST: Patients with the cardiac and generalized forms have enlarged hearts.

ABDOMEN: The liver is either of normal size or moderately enlarged.

LIMBS: The muscles often are firm and enlarged even though they are markedly hypotonic (*Figure B*), and there is marked and progressive muscular weakness. Patients with the muscular variant may have atrophied muscles in the latter stages of the disease (*Figure F*).

Nervous System

In some infants, symptoms begin at birth with feeding difficulties. Other infants develop normally for 2 to 3 months and then lose motor skills which they had attained. Deep tendon reflexes are absent. Muscular weakness is progressive and eventually approaches paralysis, and there is loss of sphincter control. Facial palsy, ptosis, a weak cry, and poor suck are usually present (*Figures A, C, and E*). Mild mental retardation has been noted in patients with the muscular form, the only form in which intelligence can be readily tested.

Pathology

Skeletal muscle fibers show displacement and destruction of myofibrils by granular glycogen deposits. In the cardiac and generalized variants the heart is round, globular, and enormously enlarged. The walls of the ventricles are thickened and massively infiltrated with glycogen [7]. There is storage of glycogen in the motor neurons of the brainstem and spinal cord.

Laboratory Studies

Glycogen levels are increased in all organs. The accumulated glycogen usually has a normal structure [4]. The accumulation probably is the result of deficient activity of the enzyme alpha-1,4-glucosidase (acid maltase). Acid maltase deficiency has been demonstrated in liver, skeletal muscle, cardiac muscle [8], leukocytes, cultured skin fibroblasts, and amniotic cells [9]. Patients with the muscular variant have a deficiency of acid maltase in muscle but not in leukocytes

[6]. The electromyogram is abnormal, and the pattern may be of value for diagnosis [7]. In the electrocardiogram a shortened P-R interval, a wide amplitude QRS, and left axis deviation are of diagnostic significance [10]. The chest x-ray shows a large, globular heart in infants with the generalized and cardiac variants (*Figure D*) and a mild to moderate increase in heart size in patients with the muscular variant [6].

Treatment and Prognosis

There is no specific treatment. Patients with both the generalized and cardiac forms usually die in the first year of life. Most patients with the muscular type have died between 1 and 4 years of age, but one as old as 15 years was reported [5]. The cause of death is pneumonia or cardiac failure.

Genetics

Autosomal recessive [4]. Diagnosis of the heterozygous state has been achieved by assay of acid maltase in lymphocytes stimulated by phytohemagglutinin [11]. Prenatal diagnosis has been achieved [9].

Differential Diagnosis

1. A protruding tongue and hypotonia are also features of patients with cretinism (see page 10) and trisomy 21 (Down's syndrome) (see page 150). Marked hypotonia in infancy is also a feature of patients with Werdnig-Hoffman disease, the Prader-Labhart-Willi syndrome (see page 48), the cerebrohepatorenal syndrome (see page 270) and the XXXXY syndrome (see page 190).
2. The muscular form of type II glycogenosis resembles certain forms of muscular dystrophy and types III and V glycogenosis. Diagnosis depends upon the demonstration of excess glycogen and of deficient alpha-1,4-glucosidase activity in muscle biopsy specimens.

References

1. Pompe, J. C. Over idiopatische hypertrophie van het hart. *Ned. Tijdschr. Geneeskd.,* **76:**304–12, 1932.
2. Bischoff, G. Zum klinischen Bild der Glykogen-Speicherungskrankheit (glykoGenose). *Z. Kinderheilkd.,* **52:**722–26, 1932.
3. Putschar, W. Über angeborene Glykogenspeicherkrankheit des Herzens-"Thesaurismosis glycogenica" (V. Gierke). *Beitr. Pathol. Anat,* **90:**222–32, 1932.
4. Sidbury, J. B., Jr. The genetics of the glycogen storage diseases. *Progr. Med. Genet.,* **5:**32–58, 1967.
5. Zellweger, H., Brown, B. I., McCormick, W. F., and Tu, J.-B. A mild form of muscular glycogenosis in two brothers with alpha-1,4-glucosidase deficiency. *Ann. Paediatr. (Basel),* **205:**413–37, 1965.
6. Roth, J. C., and Williams, H. E. The muscular variant of Pompe's disease. *J. Pediatr.,* **71:**567–73, 1967.
7. Bordiuk, J. M., Legato, M. J., Lovelace, R. E., and Blumenthal, S. Pompe's disease: electromyographic, electron microscopic, and cardiovascular aspects. *Arch. Neurol.,* **23:**113–19, 1970.
8. Hers, H. G. Alpha-glucosidase deficiency in generalized glycogen storage disease (Pompe's disease). *Biochem. J.,* **86:**11–16, 1963.
9. Nadler, H. L., and Messina, A. M. In-utero detection of type-II glycogenosis (Pompe's disease). *Lancet,* **2:**1277–78, 1969.
10. Nihill, M. R., Wilson, D. S., and Hugh-Jones, K. Generalized glycogenosis type II (Pompe's disease). *Arch. Dis. Child,* **45:**122–29, 1970.
11. Hirschhorn, K., Nadler, H. L., Waithe, W. I., Brown, B. I., and Hirschhorn, R. Pompe's disease: detection of heterozygotes by lymphocyte stimulation. *Science,* **166:**1632–33, 1969.

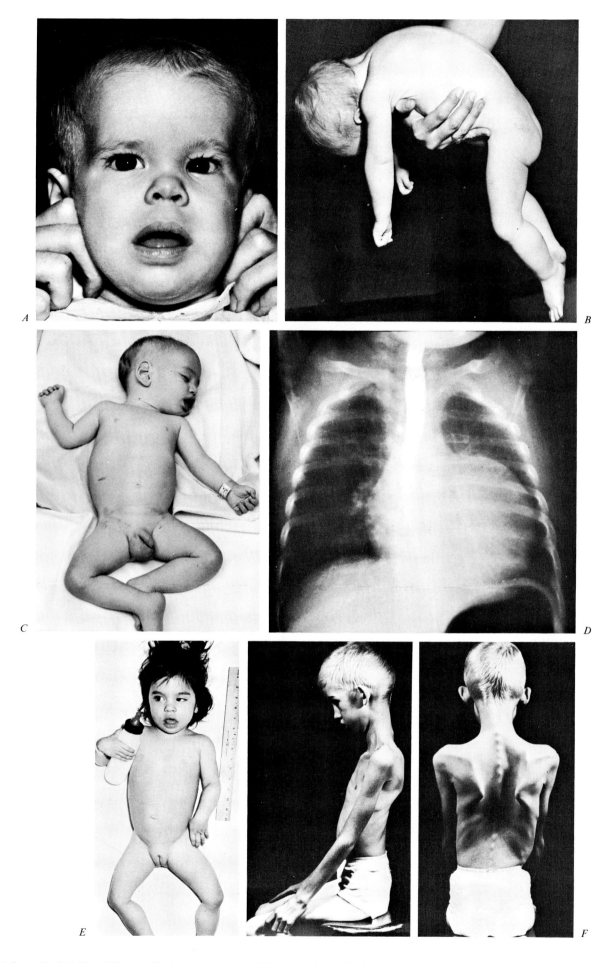

Plate I-8. *A* and *B:* A 9-month-old infant with generalized glycogenosis. She had an open mouth due to bilateral facial palsy and marked muscle hypotonia. *C* and *D:* Another infant aged 6½ months with the generalized form of this disease. He also had bilateral facial weakness, a protruding tongue, hypotonia, and large, firm muscles in the extremities. The x-ray with barium swallow shows marked cardiac enlargement and elevation of the left border of the heart due to left ventricular hypertrophy. *E:* A 14-month-old infant with the muscular variant. She had marked weakness and firmness of the skeletal muscles, ptosis, strabismus, and a protruding tongue. *F:* A 10-year-old boy with the muscular variant. He had marked muscle wasting and weakness, and at this age was unable to walk. He had developed contractures of the hips and knees. (*A* and *B:* Courtesy of Dr. P. R. Dodge, St. Louis, Mo. *C:* Courtesy of Dr. G. R. Hogan, Boston, Mass. *D:* From G. R. Hogan *et al., Neurology* [*Minneap.*], **19:**894–900, 1969. *E:* From J. C. Roth and H. E. Williams, *J. Pediatr.,* **71:**567–73, 1967. *F* [*left*]: From J. Smith *et al., Neurology* [*Minneap.*], **17:**537–49, 1967. *F* [*right*]: Courtesy of Dr. H. Zellweger, Iowa City, Iowa.)

G_{M1} Gangliosidosis (Generalized Gangliosidosis, Late Infantile Systemic Lipidosis, Familial Neurovisceral Lipidosis)

In 1959 Norman, Urich, Tingey, and Goodbody [1] described a patient who had the features of Tay-Sachs disease, but who also showed accumulation of lipid-laden histiocytes in the liver, spleen, and other organs. In the same year Craig, Clarke, and Banker [2] described a patient with the clinical and radiologic features of mucopolysaccharidosis I (Hurler's syndrome) and histiocytosis in the viscera. Since then it has become clear that these two patients with such disparate clinical features suffered from the same disorder, G_{M1} gangliosidosis. At least 20 more cases have been reported [3,3a].

The disorder is characterized by the accumulation of G_{M1} ganglioside in the brain and of the mucopolysaccharide keratan sulfate in the viscera [4], both due to deficient activity of the lysosomal enzyme beta-galactosidase [5]. There appear to be two types of G_{M1} gangliosidosis. Hepatosplenomegaly, coarse facies, and skeletal abnormalities are seen in type I, but they are absent in type II [3,6].

Physical Features

FACE: Infants with type I G_{M1} gangliosidosis have coarse facial features. The brow is prominent, the bridge of the nose is depressed, and there may be downy hirsutism on the forehead (*Figures A and C*).

EYES: Cherry-red spots in the macular region were present in 5 out of 12 patients [3].

MOUTH: The tongue is often mildly to moderately enlarged. The gums are hypertrophied.

ABDOMEN: In type I G_{M1} gangliosidosis the liver and spleen are palpable after the first 6 months.

LYMPH NODES: Minor enlargement of the lymph nodes may be present.

BACK: Dorsolumbar kyphoscoliosis is usually present, often in the first months of life.

LIMBS: In type I the hands are broad and the fingers short and stubby. There are flexion contractures of the fingers, elbows, and knees. There is hard, nontender enlargement of the wrist and ankle joints (*Figure A*).

Nervous System

Mental retardation is evident in the first year of life. The deep tendon reflexes are hyperactive. Muscle strength is poor. An exaggerated acousticomotor response has also been reported. After the first year neurologic deterioration is rapid. Tonic-clonic convulsions frequently occur. Swallowing becomes ineffective and tube feeding is necessary. Gradually blindness, deafness, decerebrate rigidity, and marked flexion contractures develop [3].

Pathology

The most striking features are visceral histiocytosis, neuronal lipidosis, and vacuoles in renal glomerular epithelial cells [3] (*Figure B*). Mucopolysaccharide storage in the cornea and ganglioside storage in retinal ganglion cells were noted in one child [3a].

Laboratory Studies

The brain contains about ten times the normal concentration of G_{M1} ganglioside (*Figure F*). The mucopolysaccha-ride keratan sulfate accumulates in the liver and spleen [4]. The accumulation of both of these substances appears to be due to deficient activity of the enzyme beta-galactosidase. This enzyme defect has been demonstrated in the brain, liver, spleen, kidney [5], and white blood cells [7] and in cultured skin fibroblasts [8]. The mucopolysaccharide levels in the urine as measured by usual techniques are normal or slightly increased [3]. However, by special techniques a marked increase of an undersulfated keratan sulfate is demonstrable [5]. The radiologic changes resemble those seen in the mucopoly-saccharidoses (*Figures D and E*).

Treatment and Prognosis

Most patients have died before 2 years of age from bronchopneumonia.

Genetics

Autosomal recessive. The heterozygous state may be detected by demonstrating a partial deficiency of beta-galactosidase in white blood cells [7] or in cultured skin fibroblasts [6]. G_{M1} beta-galactosidase activity has been demonstrated in cultured normal amniotic fluid cells [8]. Antenatal diagnosis of G_{M1} gangliosidosis should therefore be possible.

Differential Diagnosis

1. Coarse facial features, hepatosplenomegaly and a gibbus deformity are features of patients with mucopolysaccharidosis I (Hurler's syndrome) (see page 38). These patients have corneal opacities and increased polysaccharide levels in the urine.

2. A cherry-red spot in the macula and neurologic deterioration are features of patients with Tay-Sachs disease, but they do not have coarse facial features, hepatosplenomegaly, or skeletal changes (see page 62).

References

1. Norman, R. M., Urich, H., Tingey, A. H., and Goodbody, R. A.   Tay-Sachs' disease with visceral involvement and its relationship to Niemann-Pick's disease. *J. Pathol. Bact.*, **78**:409–21, 1959.
2. Craig, J. M., Clarke, J. T., and Banker, B. Q.   Metabolic neurovisceral disorder with accumulation of an unidentified substance: variant of Hurler's syndrome? *Am. J. Dis. Child.*, **98**:577, 1959.
3. O'Brien, J.   Generalized gangliosidosis. *J. Pediatr.*, **75**:167–86, 1969.
3a. Emery, J. M., Green, W. R., Wyllie, R. G., and Howell, R. R. G_{M1}-gangliosidosis. Ocular and pathological manifestations. *Arch. Ophthalmol.*, **85**:177–87, 1971.
4. Suzuki, K., Suzuki, K., and Kamoshita, S.   Chemical pathology of G_{M1}-gangliosidosis (generalized gangliosidosis). *J. Neuropath. Exp. Neurol.*, **28**:25–73, 1969.
5. Okada, S., and O'Brien, J. S.   Generalized gangliosidosis: beta-galactosidase deficiency. *Science*, **160**:1002–1004, 1968.
6. Wolfe, L. S., Callahan, J., Fawcett, J. S., Andermann, F., and Scriver, C. R. G_{M1}-gangliosidosis without chrondrodystrophy or visceromegaly. *Neurology (Minneap.)*, **20**:23–44, 1970.
7. Singer, H. S., and Schafer, I. A.   White-cell beta-galactosidase activity. *N. Engl. J. Med.*, **282**:571, 1970.
8. Sloan, H. R., Uhlendorf, B. W., Jacobsen, C. B., and Fredrickson, D. S.   Beta-galactosidase in tissue cultures derived from human skin and bone marrow: enzyme defect in G_{M1} gangliosidosis. *Pediatr. Res.*, **3**:532–37, 1969.

Plate I-9. *A:* A 2-week-old infant with coarse facial features, a depressed nasal bridge, flexion contractures of both knees, and metaphyseal swelling at the wrists and ankles. *B:* Shows a renal glomerulus of this child with swollen epithelial cells (*arrows*). Periodic acid–Schiff and hematoxylin stains ($\times$ 324). *C–D:* A 20-month-old child with a broad nasal bridge, a gibbus deformity, and swelling of his wrists. His lower thoracic and lumbar vertebrae show marked anterior beaking, especially the second lumbar vertebra (*arrow*). The medullary spaces of the tubular bones of his forearm and hands are wide, and the reticular pattern is coarse. *F:* A thin-layer chromatogram of brain gangliosides, showing the patterns in normal individuals and in patients with G_{M1} gangliosidosis, mucopolysaccharidosis I (Hurler), and Tay-Sachs disease (T-S). (*A* and *B:* From C. R. Scott *et al., J. Pediatr.* **71**:357–66, 1967. *C:* Courtesy of Dr. H. Grossman, New York, New York. *D* and *E:* From H. Grossman and B. S. Danes, Neurovisceral storage disease. *Am. J. Roentgenol. Radium Ther. Nuc. Med.,* **103**:149–53, 1968. Courtesy of Charles C Thomas, Publisher, Springfield, Ill. *F:* Courtesy of Dr. K. Suzuki, Philadelphia, Pa.)

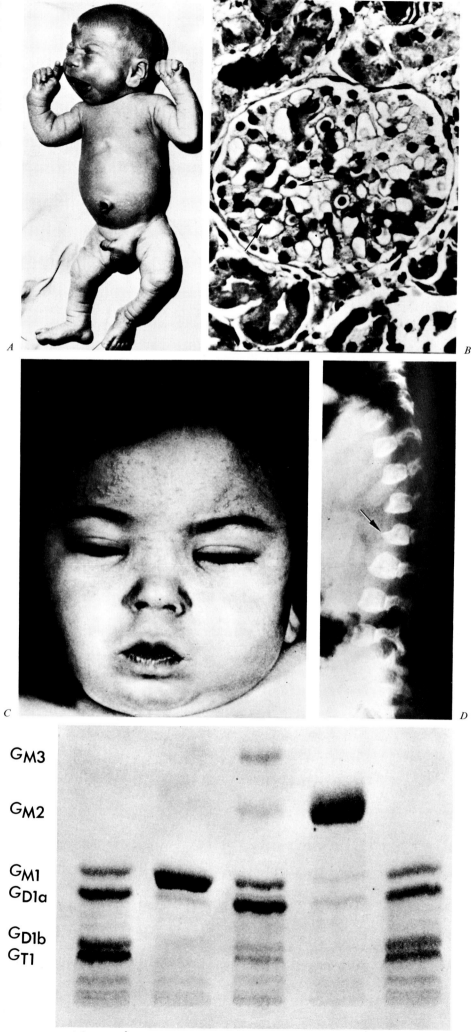

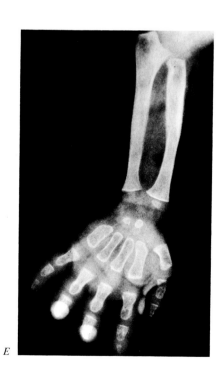

23

Hartnup Disease

In 1956 Baron, Dent, Harris, Hart, and Jepson described three siblings with a pellagralike skin rash, intermittent cerebellar ataxia, and a constant renal hyperaminoaciduria. Two of the children were also mentally retarded. A fourth sibling also had the aminoaciduria, but was otherwise healthy. The hyperaminoaciduria in these patients involved a group of monoamino-monocarboxylic (neutral) acids. Subsequent studies on these and other patients have shown that the basic abnormality in Hartnup disease is a defect of amino acid transport across the epithelial cells of the small intestine and the proximal renal tubules [2–4]. Judging from the 29 reported patients [1–7] it is evident that the ataxia, skin rash, and mental retardation are variable features, with the hyperaminoaciduria the uniform diagnostic criterion. Screening of a large number of newborns in Massachusetts has shown the incidence of Hartnup disease to be 1:20,000; none of the 16 cases detected in this way has had a skin rash or ataxia or was retarded [8].

Physical Features

SKIN: Twenty-one of 29 reported cases had a photosensitive skin eruption, which most commonly involved the exposed areas of the face and neck, and the limbs in a symmetric glove and stocking distribution (*Figures A, B, C, and D*). The rash first appeared when the children were 10 years old or younger [5]. In the acute stages of the rash the lesions are inflamed and exudative (*Figures E and F*). When it heals, a dirty brown pigmentation remains. The skin lesions tend to appear in the summer and heal in the winter. Among the precipitating factors are exposure to sunlight, infections, and poor nutrition [5].

Nervous System

Eight of 29 reported patients [1–7] were mildly to moderately retarded. Other neurologic signs and symptoms were quite variable, but when present they occurred in association with a skin rash. Emotional lability and psychotic reactions have been reported. Intermittent ataxia occurred in 12 of the 29 patients. In addition to the ataxia, some of them had vertical and horizontal nystagmus, tremor, involuntary choreiform movements, ptosis, and poor convergence. The deep tendon reflexes may be hyperactive and there may be ankle clonus. Usually the plantar responses are flexor. Several patients have had fainting spells. Convulsions have been reported but are uncommon.

Pathology

Biopsies of the skin lesions have shown hyperkeratosis, epidermal atrophy, and hyperpigmentation of the basal cell layer [6–7].

Laboratory Studies

The basic abnormality is a defect of amino acid transport across the epithelial cells of the small intestine and the proximal renal tubules [2–4]. Because of this, there is an increased urinary and fecal excretion (5 to 10 times normal) of the following free amino acids: alanine, serine, theonine, asparagine, glutamine, valine, leucine, isoleucine, phenylalanine, tyrosine, tryptophan, histidine, and citrulline. Taurine, glycine, cysteine, aspartic acid, glutamic acid, and lysine are excreted in normal or moderately increased amounts. Proline, hydroxyproline, methionine, and arginine are excreted either not at all or in very small amounts. The deficient intestinal transport of tryptophan results in an increase in the urinary excretion of indole acetic acid and indican. This occurs because intestinal bacteria convert the unabsorbed tryptophan to these indole derivatives [5].

Treatment and Prognosis

Because tryptophan in mammals is converted to nicotinic acid, it has been suggested that these patients with deficient tryptophan absorption have a deficiency of nicotinic acid. Oral nicotinamide therapy (40 to 200 mg per day) has led to marked improvement of the rash and the neurologic symptoms. This seems most effective in patients who have been malnourished [1,7]. However, it has also been noted that some patients improve without treatment. In general, the disease ameliorates spontaneously with age [5] and there is no decrease in life expectancy.

Genetics

Autosomal recessive [5].

Differential Diagnosis

1. Hyperaminoaciduria is a feature of many other diseases, such as galactosemia (see page 14) and Wilson's disease (see page 64), but in these there is a generalized increase in all amino acids and not the specific pattern found in patients with Hartnup disease.
2. A skin rash in sun-exposed areas is a feature of patients with Cockayne's syndrome, but they also have a progressive neurologic impairment (see page 82).
3. Ataxia and a facial skin rash are features of patients with ataxia-telangiectasia, but they are distinguished by their telangiectases and the absence of a hyperaminoaciduria (see page 354).

References

1. Baron, D. N., Dent, C. E., Harris, H., Hart, E. W., and Jepson, J. B. Hereditary pellagra-like skin rash with temporary cerebellar ataxia, constant renal amino-aciduria, and other bizarre biochemical features. *Lancet,* 2:421–28, 1956.
2. Milne, M. D., Crawford, M. A., Girão, C. B., and Loughridge, L. W. The metabolic disorder in Hartnup disease. *Q. J. Med.,* 29:407–21, 1960.
3. Scriver, C. R. Hartnup disease. A genetic modification of intestinal and renal transport of certain neutral alpha-amino acids. *N. Engl. J. Med.,* 273:530–32, 1965.
4. Pomeroy, J., Efron, M. L., Dayman, J., and Hoefnagel, D. Hartnup disorder in a New England family. *N. Engl. J. Med.,* 278:1214–16, 1968.
5. Jepson, J. B. Hartnup disease. In *The Metabolic Basis of Inherited Disease,* 2nd ed. Stanbury, J. B., Wyngaarden, J. B., and Fredrickson, D. S. (eds.). McGraw-Hill Book Co., New York, 1966, pp. 1283–99.
6. Nielsen, E. G., Vdesø, S., and Zimmermann-Nielsen, C. Hartnup disease in three siblings. *Dan. Med. Bull.,* 13:155–61, 1966.
7. Lopez, G. F., Velez, A. H., and Toro, G. G. Hartnup disease in two Colombian siblings. *Neurology (Minneap.),* 19:71–76, 1969.
8. Levy, H. L., Madigan, P. M., and Shih, V. E. Massachusetts metabolic disorder screening program. I. Techniques and results of urine screening. *Pediatrics* (1972, in press).

Plate I-10. *A:* A 13-year-old boy from the first reported family, with skin lesions in the sun-exposed areas. *B–D:* A 22-month-old with a similar rough, erythematous rash on her cheeks, knees, and the backs of her hands. *E* and *F:* Two brothers 5⁵/₁₂ and 13 years old. The younger boy had more marked crusting on his face and ear lobes. His intelligence was normal. The older boy had fissuring of the lips. (*A:* From D. N. Baron *et al., Lancet,* **2:**421–28, 1956. *B–D:* Courtesy of Dr. E. G. Nielsen, Odense, Denmark. *E* and *F:* From F. Lopez *et al., Neurology [Minneap.],* **19:**71–76, 1969.)

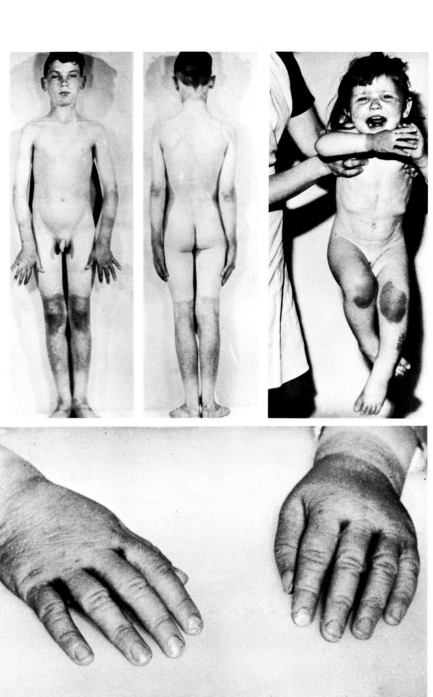

A   B

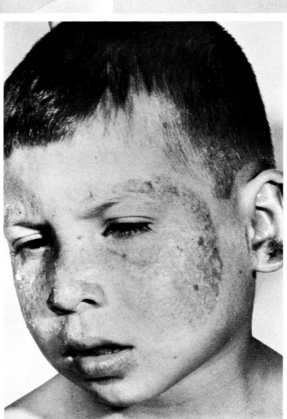
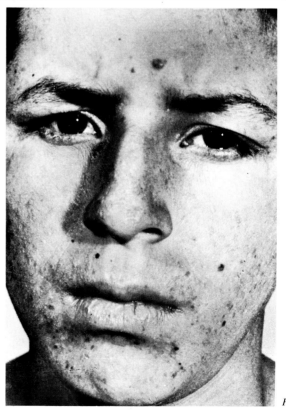

C   D

E   F

25

Homocystinuria
(Cystathionine Synthetase Deficiency)

In 1962 Field, Carson, Cusworth, Dent, and Neill [1] described a new metabolic disorder, homocystinuria, which had been detected during a survey of the urinary metabolites of mentally retarded children in Northern Ireland. In the same year Gerritsen, Vaughn, and Waisman [2] independently identified homocystine in the urine of a one-month-old child with ectopia lentis, spasticity, and multiple anomalies. Since then, more than 70 additional patients have been reported [3,4]. Deficient activity of cystathionine synthetase is the basic biochemical abnormality [5].

Physical Features

FACE: A malar flush, especially on exertion or during hot weather, is often present (*Figure B*). Prognathism is also common.

EYES: Most, if not all, patients develop dislocation lens (ectopia lentis) by the second decade. Most often the lens is partially dislocated downward (*Figures C and D*). Because of the dislocation, the iris is tremulous during eye movement, the pupil is irregular, and the anterior chamber is deep [5]. Myopia, retinal detachment, glaucoma, and cataracts [3] may develop.

MOUTH: The palate is frequently narrow and highly arched, causing the teeth to be crowded and the incisors to protrude.

CHEST: Either pectus excavatum or carinatum is often present (*Figure B*).

ABDOMEN: The liver is frequently enlarged.

BACK: Many patients develop scoliosis.

LIMBS: These patients tend to become long-limbed and knock-kneed and develop long, slender digits with increasing age (*Figures A and B*). Both flat and everted feet and pes cavus have been described [1,4].

SKIN: Livedo reticularis is often present over the limbs and chest.

HAIR: The hair is fine and fair.

Nervous System

Mental retardation is often present and varies from very mild to severe. In a survey of 38 patients, ascertained because of a dislocated lens [3], 22 were retarded. Focal neurologic signs, such as seizures or hemiplegia, may occur and are the result of thromboses. A shuffling or ducklike gait is often noted [4].

Pathology

Arterial and venous thromboses are frequent findings and may lead to brain abnormality. The liver is enlarged owing to fatty infiltration [3].

Laboratory Studies

A deficiency of the enzyme cystathionine synthetase, which catalyzes the conversion of L-homocystine to L-cystathionine, has been demonstrated in liver and brain cells [5] and cultured skin fibroblasts [6] of these patients. Excess homocystine is present in the urine and produces a positive result in the cyanide nitroprusside test [7]. Radiologic abnormalities are present [4] (*Figures E and F*).

Treatment and Prognosis

Several patients have died at an early age as a result of arterial or venous thromboses. Therapeutic approaches include maintenance of infants on a low methionine diet supplemented with cystine and a "methyl donor" such as choline [8]. Administration of pyridoxine hydrochloride can at least partially reverse the metabolic abnormalities [4,9].

Genetics

Autosomal recessive. Since normal amniotic fluid cells have been shown to have cystathionine synthetase activity, prenatal diagnosis of homocystinuria should be possible [6].

Differential Diagnosis

Dislocated lens, arachnodactyly, scoliosis, and long limbs are features of the dominantly inherited Marfan's syndrome, but these patients do not have a malar flush, stiff joints, homocystinuria, or mental retardation [3].

References

1. Field, C. M. B., Carson, N. A. J., Cusworth, D. C., Dent, C. E., and Neill, D. W. Homocystinuria. A new disorder of metabolism. (Abstract) *Xth Int. Congr. Pediatr.*, Lisbon, Spain, 1962, p. 274.
2. Gerritsen, T., Vaughn, J. G., and Waisman, H. A. The identification of homocystine in the urine. *Biochem. Biophys. Res. Commun.*, **9**:493–96, 1962.
3. Schimke, R. N., McKusick, V. A., Huang, T., and Pollack, A. D. Homocystinuria. Studies of 20 families with 38 affected members. *J.A.M.A.*, **193**:711–19, 1965.
4. Cusworth, D. C., and Dent, C. E. Homocystinuria. *Br. Med. Bull.*, **25**:42–47, 1969.
5. Laster, L. Homocystinuria due to cystathionine synthetase deficiency. *Ann. Intern. Med.*, **63**:1117–42, 1965.
6. Uhlendorf, B. W., and Mudd, S. H. Cystathionine synthetase in tissue culture derived from human skin: enzyme defect in homocystinuria. *Science*, **160**:1007–1009, 1968.
7. Carson, N. A. J., Cusworth, D. C., Dent, C. E., Field, C. M. B., Neill, D. W., and Westall, R. G. Homocystinuria: a new inborn error of metabolism associated with mental deficiency. *Arch. Dis. Child.*, **38**:425–36, 1963.
8. Perry, T. L., Hansen, S., Love, D. L., Crawford, L. E., and Tischler, B. Treatment of homocystinuria with a low-methionine diet, supplemental cystine, and a methyl donor. *Lancet*, **2**:474–78, 1968.
9. Kang, E. S., Byers, R. K., and Gerald, P. S. Homocystinuria: response to pyridoxine. *Neurology (Minneap.)*, **20**:503–507, 1970.

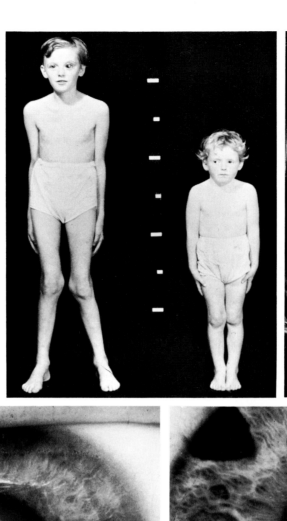

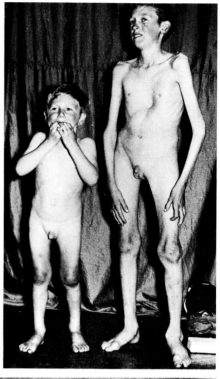

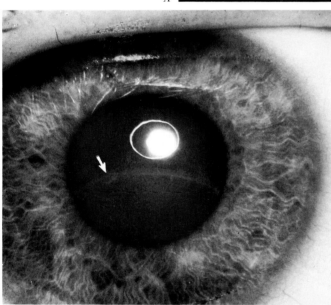

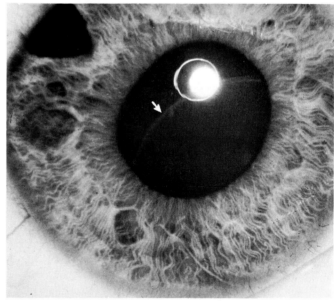

Plate I-11. *A:* Two affected sisters with light hair and dislocated lenses. The older girl had a knock-knee deformity. The younger girl had normal intelligence. *B:* Two brothers, both with a prominent malar flush. The older boy had marked pectus excavatum and long slender fingers. *C* and *D:* Close-up views of the dislocated lenses in one eye of each of two sisters. The lens is displaced (*arrows*) downward in one and laterally in the other. *E* and *F:* Lumbar spine x-rays from a 16-year-old boy showing scoliosis, osteoporosis, and enlargement of the anterior portion of the vertebral bodies. (*A:* Courtesy of Dr. N. A. J. Carson, Belfast, Ireland. *B:* From G. Turner, J. Dey, and B. Turner, *Aust. Paediat. J.,* **3:**48–53, 1967. *C* and *D:* Courtesy of Dr. D. D. Donaldson, Boston, Mass. *E* and *F:* Courtesy of Dr. P. Borns, Philadelphia, Pa.)

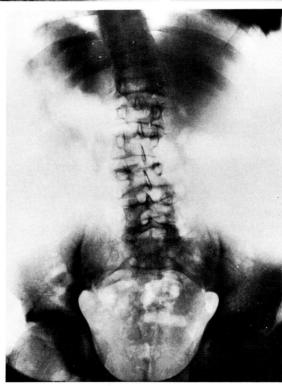

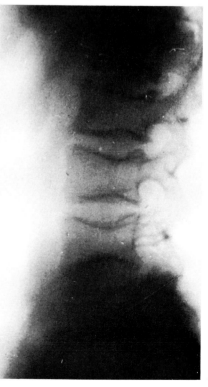

I-Cell Disease
(Leroy's Disease, Mucolipidosis II)

In 1967 Leroy and DeMars [1] reported two unrelated patients whose coarse facial features and skeletal changes suggested Hurler's disease, but whose urine did not contain increased quantities of mucopolysaccharides. Fibroblasts grown from skin biopsies of these patients contained large quantities of cytoplasmic inclusions, leading to the designation of their disease as inclusion-cell or I-cell disease. At least 19 patients have been reported to have these inclusion bodies and similar physical features [1–4,4a,4b]. However, until a specific diagnostic test is available, one cannot be certain that all of the patients have the same disorder.

Physical Features

FACE: Two patients observed over several years showed slowly progressive coarsening of their facial features. The brow was prominent. The bridge of the nose and the supra-orbital ridges were flat, and the nostrils were anteverted (*Figures A, B, and F*). The upper lip was long and thick. The gums were markedly hypertrophied [3].

EYES: The corneas are usually clear [2]. One patient had small corneal opacities [4].

ABDOMEN: The first two reported patients had mild hepatomegaly and small umbilical hernias, but the other patients have not had enlargement of either liver or spleen. The male also had an inguinal hernia and hydrocele [3].

BACK: There is thoracolumbar kyphosis (*Figure B*).

LIMBS: Joint contractures of the fingers, elbows, and shoulders were noted in early infancy [3] (*Figures A and F*).

SKIN: The skin is hard and waxy in texture.

HEIGHT: There is marked growth failure, even in the first two years of life.

Nervous System

These patients have severe psychomotor retardation.

Pathology

One autopsy failed to show an excess of lipids or abnormal mucopolysaccharides in the brain and liver [4,5]. Studies of cultured skin fibroblasts have shown numerous membrane-bound inclusions, apparently within lysosomes [6].

Laboratory Studies

The cytoplasmic inclusions in skin fibroblasts (*Figure E*) contain abundant acid phosphatase activity and are thought to be indicative of lysosomal pathology. Decreased activity of β-D-galactosidase has been observed in the liver of some, but not all, patients [2,4]. The activities of several lysosomal enzymes (β-glucuronidase, β-galactosidase, α-mannosidase, α-fucosidase, and hexosaminidase) were found to be absent or diminished in skin fibroblast cultures from a patient with I-cell disease [2]. The interpretation of this finding is still uncertain. There is no abnormality of urinary mucopolysaccharides. Peripheral lymphocytes often show vacuoles. X-rays show coarse trabeculation and broadening of metacarpals (*Figure D*). There is also slight anterior wedging of the upper border of some lumbar vertebrae [3] (*Figure C*).

Treatment and Prognosis

The progression of the physical abnormalities is evident for the first two years, but little thereafter. One death occurred at 27 months of age [4].

Genetics

Probably autosomal recessive. Cultured skin fibroblasts from two normal fathers showed the same type of inclusions as their affected children [3].

Differential Diagnosis

1. Coarse facial features, joint contractures and kyphosis occur in patients with Hurler's syndrome (mucopolysaccharidosis I), but they also have corneal opacities, more marked hepatomegaly, increased urinary mucopolysaccharides, and accelerated growth in the first year of life (see page 38).
2. Coarse facial features, stiff joints, and normal urinary mucopolysaccharides are also features of patients with G_{M1} gangliosidosis, but they are distinguished by lacking prominent inclusion bodies in fibroblasts and by having a specific deficiency of only one lysosomal enzyme, β-galactosidase, in all tissues (see page 22). By contrast, individuals with I-cell disease have prominent inclusion bodies and diminished activity of several lysosomal enzymes, including β-galactosidase, but both of these phenomena have been demonstrated only in skin fibroblasts.

References

1. Leroy, J. G., and DeMars, R. I. Mutant enzymatic and cytological phenotypes in cultured human fibroblasts. *Science,* **157**:804–806, 1967.
2. Leroy, J. G., and Spranger, J. W. I-cell disease. *N. Engl. J. Med.,* **283**:598–99, 1970.
3. Leroy, J. G., DeMars, R. I., and Opitz, J. M. I-cell disease. *Birth Defects: Original Article Series,* Vol. V, No. 4, April, 1969, pp. 174–87. Williams & Wilkins Co., Baltimore.
4. Luchsinger, U., Bühler, E. M., Mehes, K., and Hirt, H. R. I-cell disease. *N. Engl. J. Med.,* **282**:1374–75, 1970.
4a. Leroy, J. G., Spranger, J. W., Feingold, M., Opitz, J. M., and Crocker, A. C. I-cell disease: a clinical picture. *J. Pediatr.,* **79**:360–65, 1971.
4b. Tondeur, M., Vamos-Hurwitz, E., Mockel-Pohl, S., Dereume, J. P., Cremer, N., and Loeb, H. Clinical, biochemical, and ultrastructural studies in a case of chondrodystrophy presenting the I-cell phenotype in tissue culture. *J. Pediatr.,* **79**:366–78, 1971.
5. Buhler, E. M. Personal communication, 1970.
6. Hanai, J., Leroy, J., and O'Brien, J. S. Ultrastructure of cultured fibroblasts in I-cell disease. *Am. J. Dis. Child.,* **122**:34–39, 1971.

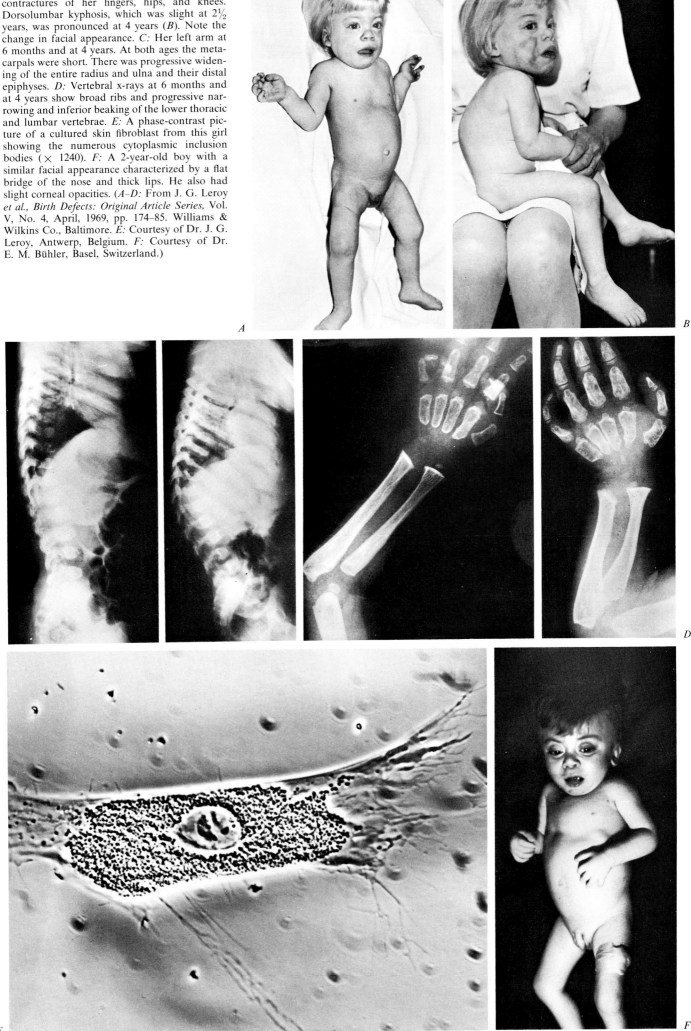

Plate I-12. *A* and *B:* One of the first two reported patients. At 2½ years (*A*) she already had flexion contractures of her fingers, hips, and knees. Dorsolumbar kyphosis, which was slight at 2½ years, was pronounced at 4 years (*B*). Note the change in facial appearance. *C:* Her left arm at 6 months and at 4 years. At both ages the metacarpals were short. There was progressive widening of the entire radius and ulna and their distal epiphyses. *D:* Vertebral x-rays at 6 months and at 4 years show broad ribs and progressive narrowing and inferior beaking of the lower thoracic and lumbar vertebrae. *E:* A phase-contrast picture of a cultured skin fibroblast from this girl showing the numerous cytoplasmic inclusion bodies (× 1240). *F:* A 2-year-old boy with a similar facial appearance characterized by a flat bridge of the nose and thick lips. He also had slight corneal opacities. (*A–D:* From J. G. Leroy *et al., Birth Defects: Original Article Series,* Vol. V, No. 4, April, 1969, pp. 174–85. Williams & Wilkins Co., Baltimore. *E:* Courtesy of Dr. J. G. Leroy, Antwerp, Belgium. *F:* Courtesy of Dr. E. M. Bühler, Basel, Switzerland.)

Lesch-Nyhan Syndrome (Hereditary Choreoathetosis, Self-Mutilation, and Hyperuricemia)

In 1964 Lesch and Nyhan [1] described two mentally retarded brothers with choreoathetosis who had a compulsive tendency to bite themselves, resulting in self-mutilation. These patients were shown to have a marked overproduction of uric acid. Later, this syndrome was shown to be associated with deficient activity of the enzyme hypoxanthine guanine phosphoribosyl transferase (HGPRT) [2]. About 150 patients with the syndrome have been detected [3].

Physical Features

FACE: At birth the face is normal. After the first or second year many patients bite their lips so severely that they cause extensive scarring and loss of tissue [4] (*Figures A and B*).

EARS: Patients over 10 years old may have uric acid tophi [4] (*Figure A*).

LIMBS: Patients may bite off the ends of fingers. Bilateral dislocation of the hips occurs as a result of spasticity of the legs. Acute gouty arthritis of the joints rarely develops.

GROWTH AND DEVELOPMENT: The height and weight are usually below the third percentile of normal.

Nervous System

All of the reported patients have been moderately or severely retarded, with IQ's below 50. Most patients have normal motor development for the first 6 to 8 months. At that time they begin to show signs of progressive generalized spastic paresis and bilateral athetosis (*Figure B*). They also develop involuntary movements, including chorea, ballismus, and tremor. The deep tendon reflexes are hyperactive and the plantar responses are extensor. The patients also have severe dysarthria and dysphagia. The most striking feature is what appears to be a compulsion to hurt or mutilate themselves. When unrestrained they often put their hands in their mouths and bite them severely. They seem to welcome the physical restraints used to prevent self-mutilation (*Figures C, D, and E*). Pain perception appears to be normal [4].

Pathology

The kidney shows extensive gouty nephropathy with urate deposits in the lumen of the tubules and in the interstitial tissue. The urate stones may cause ureteral obstruction and hydronephrosis (*Figure F*). No neuropathologic abnormalities have been consistently observed.

Laboratory Studies

A deficiency of HGPRT has been found in the brain, liver, erythrocytes [5], skin fibroblasts [2], and amniotic cells of these patients [3]. Levels of blood uric acid are usually, but not always, increased. The ratio of urinary uric acid to creatinine is increased, and measurement of this ratio is a useful screening method [6].

Treatment and Prognosis

Allopurinol has been used to lower the blood uric acid level. This is useful for the prevention and treatment of urologic complication but does not prevent the progression of the neurologic symptoms [7]. Adenine supplementation may in part reverse the biochemical abnormality, but its clinical efficacy has not been established [8]. Self-mutilation is handled with physical restraints and in some instances tooth extraction [4]. Death usually occurs before puberty because of uremia from gouty nephropathy or because of general debilitation.

Genetics

X-linked recessive. Prenatal diagnosis has been achieved [8a].

Differential Diagnosis

1. Hyperuricemia, nephrolithiasis, and mild cerebellar ataxia associated with a partial deficiency of HGPRT have been reported in two brothers [9].
2. Hyperuricemia, renal disease, spinocerebellar ataxia, and neural deafness were features of five males in one family. They had normal levels of HGPRT [10].
3. Hyperuricemia, mental retardation, and autistic behavior were features of a boy who had normal activity of HGPRT [11].

References

1. Lesch, M., and Nyhan, W. L. A familial disorder of uric acid metabolism and central nervous system function. *Am. J. Med.,* **36**:561–70, 1964.
2. Seegmiller, J. E., Rosenbloom, F. M., and Kelley, W. N. Enzyme defect associated with a sex-linked human neurological disorder and excessive purine synthesis. *Science,* **155**:1682–84, 1967.
3. Boyle, J. A., Raivio, K. O., Astrin, K. H., Schulman, J. D., Graf, M. L., Seegmiller, J. E., and Jacobsen, C. B. Lesch-Nyhan syndrome: preventive control by prenatal diagnosis. *Science,* **169**:688–89, 1970.
4. Nyhan, W. L. Clinical features of the Lesch-Nyhan syndrome. Introduction—clinical and genetic features. *Fed. Proc.,* **27**:1027–33, 1968.
5. Kelley, W. N. Hypoxanthine-guanine phosphoribosyltransferase deficiency in the Lesch-Nyhan syndrome and gout. *Fed. Proc.,* **27**:1047–52, 1968.
6. Kaufman, J. M., Greene, M. L., and Seegmiller, J. E. Urine uric acid to creatinine ratio—a screening test for inherited disorders of purine metabolism. *J. Pediatr.,* **73**:583–92, 1968.
7. Marks, J. F., Baum, J., Kay, J. L., Taylor, W., and Curry, L. Lesch-Nyhan syndrome treated from the early neonatal period. *Pediatrics,* **42**:357–61, 1968.
8. van der Zee, S. P. M., Lommen, E. J. P., Trijbels, J. M. F., and Schretlen, E. D. A. M. The influence of adenine on the clinical features and purine metabolism in the Lesch-Nyhan syndrome. *Acta Paediatr. Scand.,* **59**:259–64, 1970.
8a. Demars, R., Santo, G., and Felix, J. S. Lesch-Nyhan mutation: prenatal detection with amniotic fluid cells. *Science,* **164**:1303–1305, 1969.
9. Kelley, W. N., Rosenbloom, F. M., Henderson, J. F., and Seegmiller, V. E. A specific enzyme defect in gout associated with overproduction of uric acid. *Proc. Natl. Acad. Sci. USA,* **57**:1735–39, 1967.
10. Rosenberg, A. L., Bergstrom, L., Troost, B. T., and Bartholomew, B. A. Hyperuricemia and neuologic deficits: a family study. *N. Engl. J. Med.,* **282**:992–97, 1970.
11. Nyhan, W. L., James, J. A., Teberg, A. J., Sweetman, L., and Nelson, L. G. A new disorder of purine metabolism with behavioral manifestations. *J. Pediatr.,* **74**:20–27, 1969.

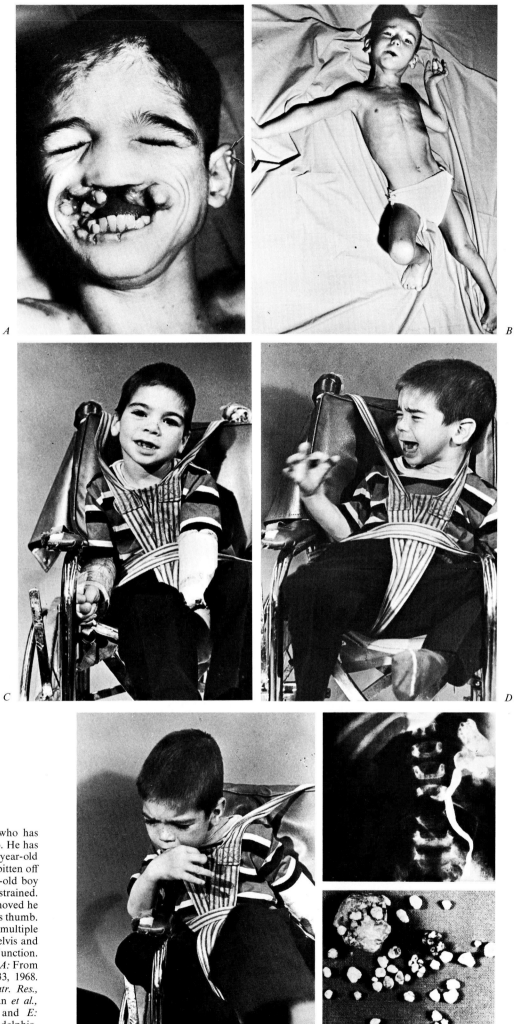

Plate I-13. *A:* A 14-year-old boy who has almost totally destroyed his upper lip. He has tophi on his left ear (*arrows*). *B:* A 5-year-old boy with athetoid posturing. He has bitten off part of his lower lip. *C–E:* A 5-year-old boy who seems happy with his arms restrained. However, when the restraints are removed he immediately begins to cry and bite his thumb. *F:* A retrograde pyelogram showing multiple translucent stones in the left renal pelvis and constriction of the left ureteropelvic junction. The stones are shown after removal. (*A:* From W. L. Nyhan, *Fed. Proc.*, **27:**1027–33, 1968. *B:* From W. L. Nyhan *et al.*, *Pediatr. Res.*, **1:**5–13, 1967. *C:* From P. H. Berman *et al.*, *Arch. Neurol.*, **20:**44–53, 1969. *D* and *E:* Courtesy of Dr. P. H. Berman, Philadelphia, Pa. *F* [*top*]: From D. S. Newcombe, *J.A.M.A.*, **198:**315–17, 1966. *F* [*bottom*]: Courtesy of Dr. D. S. Newcombe, Burlington, Vt.)

Lipodystrophy
(Lipoatrophic Diabetes Mellitus, Lipodystrophic Muscular Hypertrophy)

The absence of adipose tissue is referred to as lipodystrophy. This may be partial or complete. Patients with the partial form were described as early as 1885 [1]. This form always develops after birth, and over 200 patients have been reported. Lawrence [2] in 1946 reported the first patient with a total absence of subcutaneous fat tissue. More than 30 cases have since been reported [3-8]. This form may be congenital or acquired. The cause of lipodystrophy is not known.

Total Lipodystrophy

Physical Features

FACE: Buccal and subcutaneous fat are totally absent in both the congenital and acquired type (*Figure A*).

MOUTH: The tongue is enlarged.

ABDOMEN: Liver and spleen enlargement and umbilical hernias are common in the congenital form.

GENITALIA: The clitoris and penis are usually enlarged in the congenital form.

LIMBS: In the congenital form the hands and feet are unusually large for the chronologic age of the child. The muscle bulk is increased (*Figures B, D, and E*).

SKIN: In spite of the absence of subcutaneous fat, the skin retains normal elasticity. The superficial veins are prominent (*Figures C and F*). Hirsutism and a general increase in pigmentation are common. Localized acanthosis nigricans has also been reported [5].

HEIGHT: During the first 4 years the linear growth is far in excess of normal, but it is normal by the teen-age years.

Nervous System

Among 21 reported patients, 2 were definitely mentally retarded and 2 others were possibly retarded [3].

Pathology

Adipose tissue is absent in the subcutaneous tissues, perirenal area, epicardium, and mesentery. The liver shows marked fatty infiltration, glycogen deposition, and fibrosis. Four of 21 patients had enlarged kidneys [3]. No consistent neuropathologic abnormality has been reported.

Laboratory Studies

Serum growth hormone, insulin, triglyceride, and free fatty acid levels are usually increased [3,4,7]. All adults have had hyperglycemia, but this is present only infrequently in children [3,4]. In the congenital type, the bone age shows advanced skeletal maturation in the first years of life and there are epiphyseal hypertrophy, thickening of diaphyseal cortices, and mild metaphyseal sclerosis of the long bones [8].

Treatment and Prognosis

Therapy is directed at the management of the hyperglycemia and hyperlipemia, both of which may improve spontaneously with age.

Genetics

Autosomal recessive inheritance is likely in total congenital lipodystrophy [3].

Partial Lipodystrophy

In this disorder there is a symmetric absence of facial fat with or without disappearance of fat from the arms, chest, abdomen, and hips, and with retention of fat in the lower parts of the legs. The age of onset of the disorder has ranged from 1 to 40 years. The ratio of females to males is 3:1. In a review of 102 patients, 9 were mentally retarded, 28 had renal disease, 11 had an enlarged liver, and 3 had hyperlipemia [3].

Differential Diagnosis

1. Decreased subcutaneous fat and hirsutism are also features of patients with leprechaunism, but they do not have muscular hypertrophy or elevated serum fatty acids and insulin (see page 290).
2. A protuberant abdomen, umbilical hernia, and muscular hypertrophy may be features of patients with congenital hypothyroidism, but they do not have a deficiency of subcutaneous fat (see page 10).
3. A progressive loss of facial fat is a feature of patients with Cockayne's syndrome, but they also have progressive neurologic impairment (see page 82).

References

1. Mitchell, S. W. Singular case of absence of adipose matter in upper half of the body. *Am. J. Med. Sci.,* **90**:105-106, 1885.
2. Lawrence, R. D. Lipodystrophy and hepatomegaly with diabetes, lipaemia, and other metabolic disturbances: a case throwing new light on the action of insulin. *Lancet,* 1:724-31, 1946.
3. Senior, B., and Gellis, S. S. The syndromes of total lipodystrophy and of partial lipodystrophy. *Pediatrics,* **33**:593-612, 1964.
4. Seip, M., and Trygstad, O. Generalized lipodystrophy. *Arch. Dis. Child.,* **38**:447-53, 1963.
5. Reed, W. B., Dexter, R., Corley, C., and Fish, C. Congenital lipodystrophic diabetes with acanthosis nigricans. *Arch. Dermatol.,* **91**:326-34, 1965.
6. Wiedemann, H. R., Spranger, J., Mogharei, M., Kubler, W., Tolksdorf, M., Bontemps, M., Drescher, J., and Gunschera, H. Uber das Syndrom Exomphalos-Makroglossie-Gigantismus, über generalisierte Muskelhypertrophie, progressive Lipodystrophie und Miescher-Syndrom im Sinne diencephaler Syndrome. *Z. Kinkerheilkd.,* **102**:1-36, 1968.
7. Senior, B., and Loridan, L. Fat cell function and insulin in a patient with generalized lipodystrophy. *J. Pediatr.* **74**:972-75, 1967.
8. Wesenberg, R. L., Gwinn, J. L., and Barnes, G. R., Jr. The roentgenographic findings in total lipodystrophy. *Am. J. Roentgenol. Radium Ther. Nucl. Med.,* **103**:154-64, 1968.

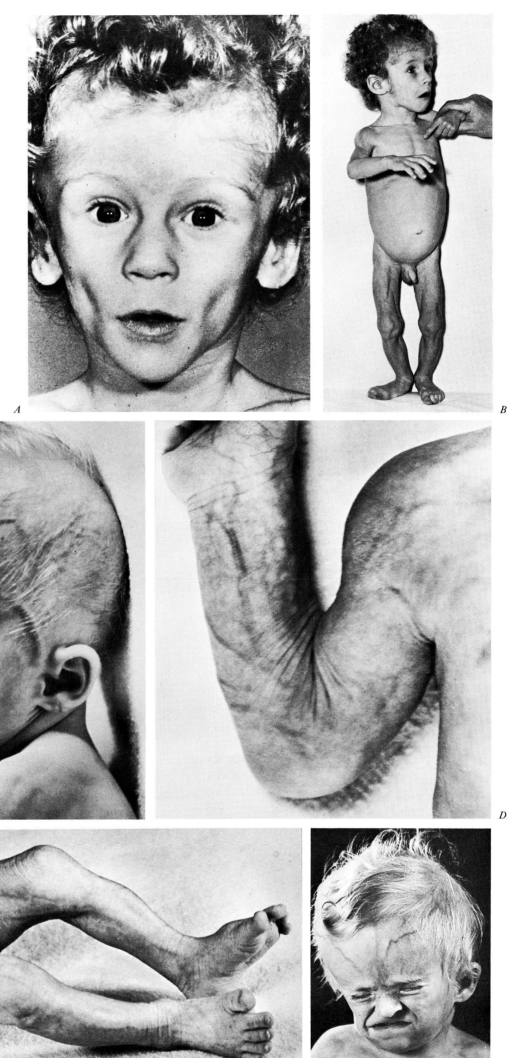

Plate I-14. *A* and *B:* An 11-month-old boy with marked lack of subcutaneous fat in the cheeks and extremities. He also had a protruding abdomen and hepatosplenomegaly. *C–E:* A 7-week-old infant with prominence of the muscles and superficial veins. *F:* The same child at age 9 months. (*A* and *B:* From M. Seip, *Acta Paediatr.*, **48:**555–74, 1959. *C–F:* From H.-R. Wiedemann *et al., Z. Kinderheilkd.,* **102:**1–36, 1968.)

A

B

C

D

E

F

Mannosidosis

In 1967 Öckerman [1] described a 4-year-old mentally retarded boy with lumbar kyphosis, an enlarged tongue, and coarse facial features resembling those of patients with the mucopolysaccharidoses. Postmortem studies showed accumulation of oligosaccharides containing mannose and glucosamine and diminished activity of the enzyme alpha-mannosidase [1–3]. Although this is the only reported case, it is likely that it represents a distinct clinical entity.

Physical Features

FACE: At 2½ years of age this patient's tongue was enlarged and his forehead prominent (*Figure A*).

EYES: The lenses contained small opacities on the anterior surface. The optic discs were gray and slightly blurred. The corneas were clear.

ABDOMEN: The liver and spleen were considered to be enlarged during the first year, but they were no longer palpable at 2½ years.

BACK: Lumbar kyphosis was first observed at 2 years, but never became severe.

HEIGHT: During the first year linear growth was unusually great, but there was practically no increase in height after age 2.

Nervous System

Motor development was slow. He could barely sit unsupported at 8 months. His peak performance was noted at 2½ years, when he could sit without support and stand with support. However, he appeared uninterested in his surroundings and did not talk. Deep tendon reflexes were hyperactive and plantar responses extensor. His muscles were hypotonic. During the last year of his life the patient suffered from unexplained attacks of violent restlessness, screaming, and vomiting which were associated with ketoacidosis. He died at 4 years 4 months during such an attack.

Pathology

The brain was slightly enlarged (1270 g). The white matter was abnormally firm and the ventricular system slightly enlarged. The cerebellum was atrophic. The neuronal cytoplasm was distended with water-soluble, periodic acid–Schiff positive material. These neuronal changes were present in many areas, including the cerebral cortex, anterior horn cells, and the myenteric plexus. In addition, there was a diffuse loss of nerve cells and gliosis. These were both particularly striking in the cerebellum, where there was widespread loss of Purkinje and granular cells. There was also diffuse loss of myelin. The spleen was moderately enlarged (170 g), as were the mediastinal and abdominal lymph nodes. The liver was not enlarged. Except for moderate enlargement of reticuloendothelial elements, the visceral organs were not remarkable.

Laboratory Studies

There was an 8- to 10-fold excess of mannose in the liver [1] and brain [3]. The abnormally accumulated material had a molecular weight of less than 5000, and was thought to represent a mannose-containing oligosaccharide derived from glycoprotein. The activity of the enzyme alpha-mannosidase in the liver, spleen, and brain gray matter was diminished to one fifth to one third of normal, while that of other lysosomal carbohydrate-cleaving enzymes was increased. These observations suggest that the disorder is due to the accumulation of certain mannose-containing oligosaccharides or of glycoprotein as a result of the deficiency of the enzyme normally responsible for their cleavage. The lymphocytes were vacuolated (*Figure B*). The patient also had hypogammaglobulinemia with a decrease of IgG, barely detectable IgM, and no detectable IgA. By x-ray the structure of the femur appeared coarsened (*Figure C*). The wrist and ankle showed mild abnormalities, resembling rickets. When the patient was 2½ years old the urinary mucopolysaccharides were increased, but at ages 3½ and 4 years they were normal.

Differential Diagnosis

Coarse facial features and recurrent infections are features of infants with mucopolysaccharidosis I (Hurler's syndrome) (see page 38), G_{M1} gangliosidosis (see page 22), and I-cell disease (see page 28), but each can be distinguished by cytologic and biochemical studies.

References

1. Öckerman, P.-A. A generalized storage disorder resembling Hurler's syndrome. *Lancet,* **2:**239–41, 1967.
2. Kjellman, B., Gamstorp, I., Brun, A., Öckerman, P.-A., and Palmgren, B. Mannosidosis: a clinical and histopathologic study. *J. Pediatr.,* **75:**366–73, 1969.
3. Öckerman, P.-A. Mannosidosis: Isolation of oligosaccharide storage material from brain. *J. Pediatr.,* **75:**360–65, 1969.

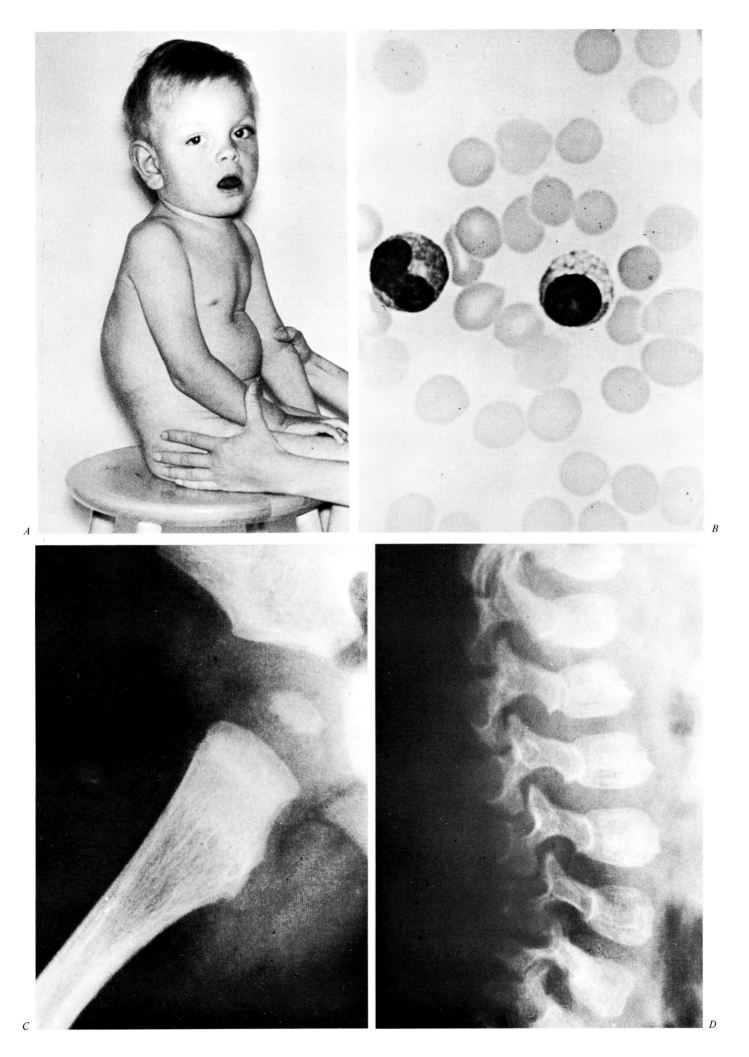

A

B

C

D

Plate I-15. *A:* The only reported patient, at 2½ years, showing an enlarged tongue and kyphosis. *B:* Shows lymphocytes with large vacuoles in the cytoplasm. *C:* Shows trabeculation in the femur at 5 months. *D:* The vertebrae were normal at 2 years 4 months. (*A–D:* From B. Kjellman *et al., J. Pediatr.,* **75:**366–73, 1969.)

Metachromatic Leukodystrophy
(Sulfatide Lipidosis)

In 1921 Witte described extensive degeneration of the white matter of the brain of a 42-year-old vagabond. He also noted extensive deposits of material which stained violet or red with basic aniline dyes such as toluidine blue. This type of staining reaction is referred to as metachromasia [3]. Metachromatic deposits were also present in the kidney and certain other organs [1]. What was later recognized as the much more common childhood form of this disease was first described by Scholz in 1925 [2]. Over 100 cases of this disorder have been described [3]. The metachromatic deposits have been identified as sulfatides [3]. This lipid accumulates due to deficient activity of the enzyme cerebroside sulfatase [4]. Recent studies in Sweden have shown the incidence to be 1:40,000 births [4a].

Physical Features

For the most part there are no abnormal physical features. The retina may show a gray discoloration of the macula with a red spot in the center. Like the cherry-red spot in Tay-Sachs disease, this change is due to the accumulation of lipids within retinal ganglion cells. The abnormality, however, is much more subtle than in Tay-Sachs disease [3]. Genu recurvatum is seen frequently in the later stages of the disease.

Nervous System

The child's development is normal until some time after the first year. The initial symptom is difficulty in walking or standing. The legs often are hypotonic and their movement ataxic, and the deep tendon reflexes diminished. Later there are incoordination of the arms, progressive difficulty in articulation and swallowing, and loss of mental function. In the final stages the patient has a decerebrate or decorticate posture and appears out of contact with his surroundings. The deep tendon reflexes often are diminished or absent (*Figures A, B, C, and E*).

Pathology

There is extensive loss of myelin in both the central and the peripheral nervous system, and accumulation of metachromatic lipids within macrophages, glial cells, and Schwann cells. Metachromatic lipids also accumulate within the proximal convoluted tubules of the kidney, and they may form polypoid masses which protrude into the lumen of the gallbladder [3].

Laboratory Studies

The main abnormality is a 5- to 100-fold excess of sulfatides in the nervous system, visceral organs [3], and urine [3]. This results from the deficiency of a normal degradative enzyme, cerebroside sulfatase [4]. Cerebroside sulfatase has two components, one heat-stable and one heat-labile. The heat-labile component appears to be identical with a well-known enzyme, arylsulfatase A, for which convenient assay methods have been developed. All patients with metachromatic leukodystrophy have deficient arylsulfatase A activity in a variety of tissues and in white blood cells [5], urine [6], and cultured skin fibroblasts [3]. Immunologic studies of the abnormal sulfatase A have shown that the enzyme is present, but functionally abnormal [6a]. Biopsy of a peripheral nerve, usually the sural nerve, permits demonstration of characteristic metachromatic inclusions. Other abnormal laboratory findings include the progressive inability of the gallbladder to concentrate radiopaque test substances, a diminished motor nerve conduction velocity, and increased protein levels in the cerebrospinal fluid [3].

Treatment and Prognosis

Metachromatic leukodystrophy usually leads to death between 3 and 6 years of age. Patients with onset of symptoms in late childhood or early adolescence have been described (*Figure E*), and they may survive until the late teens. In a rare adult form of the disease, symptoms usually do not begin before the late teens or early twenties; some of these patients have survived until the seventh decade [3].

Genetics

Autosomal recessive. The heterozygous state can be detected by measuring the arylsulfatase A activity of cultured skin fibroblasts. Prenatal diagnosis has been achieved [6b]. However, it must be kept in mind that arylsulfatase A normally develops relatively late in fetal life [7], which may make it difficult to distinguish between the heterozygous and homozygous fetus.

Variant Form

There is a rare form of metachromatic leukodystrophy associated with multiple sulfatase deficiencies. In this form there may be hepatosplenomegaly, Alder-Reilly granules in white blood cells, and certain skeletal changes resembling those in the mucopolysaccharidoses. Mucopolysaccharide levels are increased in the tissues and, usually, in the urine. There is deficient activity of arylsulfatases A, B, and C and of steroid sulfatase [3] (*Figure D*).

Differential Diagnosis

1. The early stage of metachromatic leukodystrophy may be confused with a peripheral neuropathy or a cerebellar tumor. Cerebrospinal fluid protein levels are increased in all three disorders, and the mental changes associated with metachromatic leukodystrophy may be slight or absent at this stage. Specific diagnosis depends upon laboratory procedures just described.

2. Later stages may be confused with static defects such as "cerebral palsy" due to perinatal brain injury. In metachromatic leukodystrophy careful inquiry will reveal achievement of normal developmental milestones during the first 12 to 18 months, and deep tendon reflexes usually are diminished.

References

1. Witte, F.   Ueber pathologische Abbauvorgänge im Zentralnerven-system. *Munch. Med. Wochenschr.,* **68**:69, 1921.
2. Scholz, W.   Klinische, pathologisch-anatomische und erbbiologische Untersuchungen bei familiärer, diffuser Hirnsklerose im Kindesalter. *Z. Ges. Neurol. Psychiat.,* **99**:651–717, 1925.
3. Moser, H. W.   Sulfatide lipidosis (metachromatic leukodystrophy). In *The Metabolic Basis of Inherited Disease,* J. B. Stanbury, J. B. Wyngaarden, and D. S. Fredrickson (eds.), 3rd ed. McGraw-Hill Book Co., New York, 1971.
4. Jatzkewitz, H., and Mehl, E.   Cerebroside-sulphatase and arylsulphatase A deficiency in metachromatic leukodystrophy. *J. Neurochem.,* **16**:19–28, 1969.
4a. Gustavson, K.-H., and Hagberg, B.   The incidence and genetics of metachromatic leucodystrophy in Northern Sweden. *Acta Paediatr. Scand.,* **60**:585–90, 1971.
5. Percy, A. K., and Brady, R. O.   Metachromatic leukodystrophy: diagnosis with samples of venous blood. *Science,* **161**:594–95, 1968.
6. Austin, J., Armstrong, D., Shearer, L., and McAfee, D.   Metachromatic form of diffuse cerebral sclerosis. VI. A rapid test for the sulfatase A deficiency in metachromatic leukodystrophy (MLD) urine. *Arch. Neurol.,* **14**:259–69, 1966.
6a. Stumpf, D., Neuwelt, E., Austin, J., and Kohler, P.   Metachromatic leukodystrophy (MLD). X. Immunological studies of the abnormal sulfatase A. *Arch. Neurol.,* **25**:427–31, 1971.
6b. Nadler, H. L., and Gerbie, A. B.   Role of amniocentesis in the intrauterine detection of genetic disorders. *N. Engl. J. Med.,* **282**:596–99, 1970.
7. Kaback, M. M., and Howell, R. R.   Infantile metachromatic leukodystrophy: heterozygote detection in skin fibroblasts and possible applications to intrauterine diagnosis. *N. Engl. J. Med.,* **282**:1336–40, 1970.

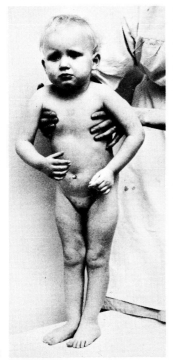

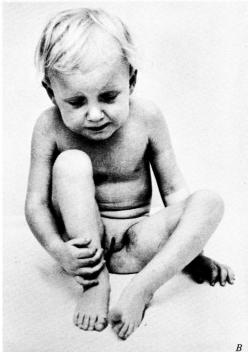

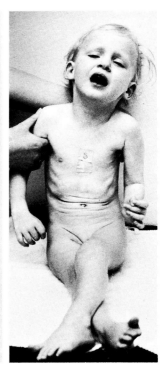

A

B

C

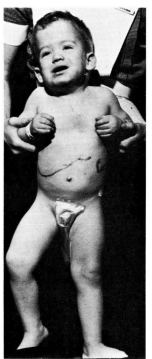

D

Plate I-16. *A–C:* Metachromatic leukodystrophy in late infancy, the age at which the disease occurs most commonly. *A:* The child needs to be supported when standing. *B:* She can no longer stand, even with support. *C:* Late stage of disease. Patient no longer able to sit, general debility, foot plantar-flexed. *D:* Variant with multiple sulfatase deficiencies. Child is 26 months old. Note enlarged liver and spleen, pectus excavatum, and in-curved little finger. *E:* Metachromatic leukodystrophy in later childhood. *Left,* 5½ years, one year before onset of symptoms: child is entirely normal. *Center,* 6 years 11 months: increasing gait difficulty, unable to stand without support. *Right,* 8 years 10 months: bedridden, requiring tube feeding. He is no longer able to speak, but recognizes family and shows pleasure when people pay attention to him. (*A* and *B:* From B. Hagberg and L. Svennerholm, *Am. J. Dis. Child.,* **104:**644–56, 1962. *C:* From B. Hagberg, Clinical symptoms, signs and tests in metachromatic leucodystrophy, in J. Folch-Pi and H. Bauer [eds.]. *Brain Lipids and Lipoproteins and the Leucodystrophies.* Elseiver, Amsterdam, 1963.)

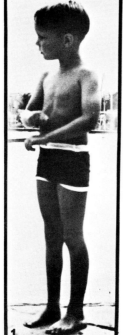

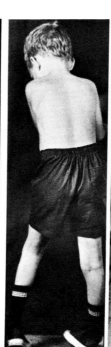

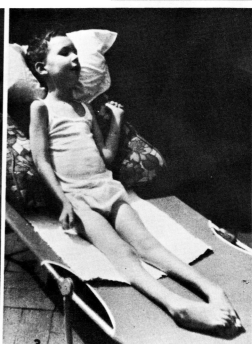

E

1

2

3

F

Mucopolysaccharidoses

In 1917 Hunter described two brothers aged 8 and 10 who had stiff joints, claw hands, a protuberant abdomen with enlargement of the liver, a short neck, noisy respirations, and deafness. One had an aortic murmur [1]. Photographs of these two patients which have been subsequently published [2] also showed abnormally coarse facial features. In 1919 Hurler described a mentally retarded boy and girl who had corneal clouding and skeletal abnormalities [3]. They had coarse facial features, which caused them to look alike even though they were unrelated. Hundreds of patients with abnormalities similar to these four children's have since been reported [2].

In 1952 the tissues of such patients were shown to contain an excess of mucopolysaccharide [4]. (Biochemists have proposed that the term *glycosaminoglycan* be substituted for the word *mucopolysaccharide*. The prefix "muco" has little meaning in modern terms. In line with present clinical usage we will refer to these substances as either polysaccharides or mucopolysaccharides.) Disorders associated with mucopolysaccharide accumulation are now referred to as the mucopolysaccharidoses. On the basis of genetic, clinical, and biochemical differences the mucopolysaccharidoses have been divided into six subclasses, MPS I through MPS VI [2,23]. We shall discuss the three mucopolysaccharidoses which are associated with mental retardation.

The cases described by Hurler are examples of MPS I. This is the most disabling and most rapidly progressive mucopolysaccharidosis, and is inherited as an autosomal recessive trait. MPS II (Hunter's syndrome) has an X-linked mode of inheritance. Even though MPS III (Sanfilippo syndrome) was first described as recently as 1961 [5], more than 50 cases are now known [6].

MPS I
(Hurler's Syndrome, Gargoylism)

Physical Features

HEAD: The head is large and the scalp veins may be prominent in young children. The anteroposterior diameter is often increased because of premature closure of the sagittal and metopic sutures.

FACE: The brow is prominent. The bridge of the nose is flattened and the tip is broad with wide nostrils. Because of narrowing of the air passages, there is often a nasal discharge. As the child becomes older the lips become larger and patulous, the mouth is held open, and the tongue becomes larger and protrudes [7] (*Figures A and B*).

EYES: Progressive clouding of the cornea is evident in the early months of life. There may also be retinal degeneration.

NECK: The neck is short.

ABDOMEN: Most males have bilateral inguinal hernias by 5 months of age. Umbilical hernias are also common. All patients have an enlarged spleen and liver by 6 to 18 months of age [7] (*Figures A and B*).

BACK: Nearly all patients develop a gibbus in the lower thoracic or lumbar spine.

LIMBS: The hands are broad and stubby. By the age of 1 year flexion contractures of the elbows and the fingers are present. Hip dislocation and foot abnormalities are also frequent findings.

SKIN: Increased body hair is common after the first 1 to 2 years.

HEIGHT: Most patients have increased linear growth in the first year, but are below the third percentile of normal by 3 years of age (*Figure A*).

Nervous System

During the first few months development may be normal; thereafter it lags progressively. Thus, while there may be only a moderate delay in achieving the ability to sit up, the ability to walk without support is either considerably delayed or never achieved. Toilet training is rarely achieved. Hearing loss

is often present. Most children slowly learn to use words, but do not form sentences. By 2 years a learning plateau is reached. Seizures are not usually observed. The deep tendon reflexes are normal [2,7].

Pathology

Distended cells and swollen collagen fibers are found in cartilage, fascia, tendons, meninges, heart valves, and blood vessels. The meninges are thickened in the region of the basal cisterns [2] (*Figure F*). Subarachnoid cysts may form, leading to communicating hydrocephalus [8]. The cytoplasm of nerve cells is distended with lipids, which consist mainly of gangliosides G_{M1}, G_{M2}, G_{M3} [9] (see *Figure 1-9F*, page 23).

Laboratory Studies

Mucopolysaccharide levels in many tissues and in the urine are more than ten times normal. In most tissues [10] and in the urine [11] the levels of the polysaccharides dermatan sulfate (formerly known as chondroitin sulfate B) and heparan sulfate (formerly known as heparitin sulfate) are equally elevated. However, in cultured skin fibroblasts only dermatan sulfate is present in excess [10]. The reason for the polysaccharide accumulation is not certain. Kinetic studies in cultured skin fibroblasts suggest that polysaccharide degradation is impaired [12]. The degradative defect demonstrable in cultured fibroblasts can be corrected by the addition of extracts of normal cultured skin fibroblasts [12] or of urine [13], and also by similar extracts prepared from patients with MPS II or MPS III [14].

These extracts have the properties of an acid hydrolase [13]—i.e., the type of enzyme that might normally function to degrade mucopolysaccharides. There is as yet no information as to which enzyme is involved. A partial deficiency of activity of the acid hydrolase beta-galactosidase has been demonstrated in the brain, liver, kidney, and spleen [15]. The physiologic significance of the beta-galactosidase deficiency is not established. Beta-galactosidase does not appear to act on the polysaccharides accumulated in MPS I [16], and the corrective factors in the extracts referred to above do not have beta-galactosidase activity [13]. For these reasons it is doubted that a deficiency of this enzyme is the primary defect.

The urinary polysaccharide excess can be detected by screening tests [17], and confirmed and quantitated by more elaborate biochemical assays [11]. Blood cells often contain abnormal granules [2]. Abnormal metachromasia [18] and excess polysaccharide can be demonstrated in cultured skin fibroblasts [10].

An omega-shaped sella turcica is a frequent x-ray finding [6] (*Figure D*). The bodies of T_{12} and L_1 vertebrae are hooklike because of underdevelopment of the superior portion (*Figure C*). The ribs are spatulate. The shafts of long bones are short, with dilatation of the medullary cavity and thinning of the cortex. The terminal phalanges are often hypoplastic. The metacarpals are broad and taper proximally (*Figure E*). Coxa valga and a deformed, poorly mineralized head of the femur are common [2].

Treatment and Prognosis

Recently infusions of plasma have been proposed as a treatment. Whether or not this will prove generally effective and have long-term benefit is not yet known [18a]. Repair of hernias and hydroceles may be necessary in males. A ventriculoatrial shunt may help correct the communicating hydrocephalus, which otherwise can cause blindness and further mental deterioration. These children usually die of respiratory infection or cardiac failure before 10 years of age [2].

Genetics

Autosomal recessive. The heterozygous state can in many cases be detected by demonstrating abnormal metachromasia [18] or excess dermatan sulfate [10] in cultured skin fibroblasts. Prenatal diagnosis has been achieved by demonstrating

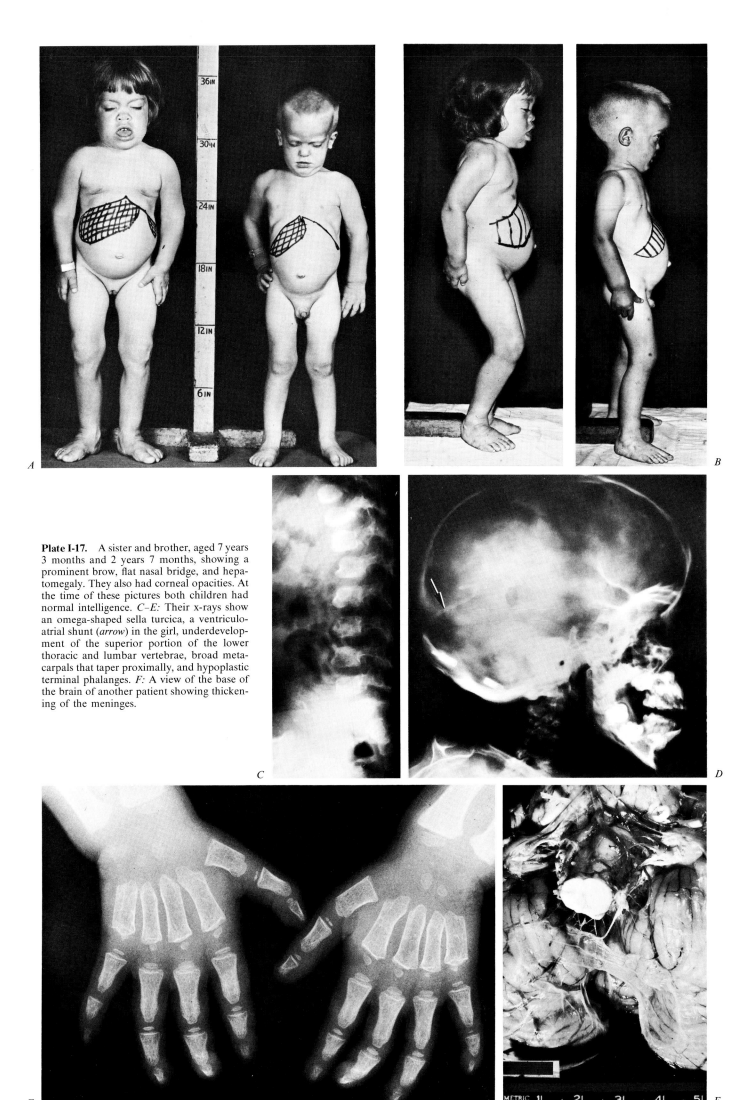

A

B

Plate I-17. A sister and brother, aged 7 years 3 months and 2 years 7 months, showing a prominent brow, flat nasal bridge, and hepatomegaly. They also had corneal opacities. At the time of these pictures both children had normal intelligence. *C–E:* Their x-rays show an omega-shaped sella turcica, a ventriculoatrial shunt (*arrow*) in the girl, underdevelopment of the superior portion of the lower thoracic and lumbar vertebrae, broad metacarpals that taper proximally, and hypoplastic terminal phalanges. *F:* A view of the base of the brain of another patient showing thickening of the meninges.

C

D

E

F

excessive quantities of *N*-sulfated polysaccharides, such as heparan sulfate, which contain sulfate linked to an amino group, in amniotic fluid samples [19], or by demonstrating abnormal polysaccharide kinetics in cultured amniotic fluid cells [20]. However, reliance on studies of the amniotic fluid alone has not always been successful [20a].

Differential Diagnosis of the Mucopolysaccharidoses

A. Disorders without increased urinary polysaccharides: In fucosidosis (see page 12), mannosidosis (see page 34), G_{M1} gangliosidosis (see page 22), and I-cell disease (see page 28), the patient's appearance and the x-ray abnormalities may resemble those in the mucopolysaccharidoses. However, in all these disorders the urinary mucopolysaccharide levels are normal.

B. Differentiation among the mucopolysaccharidoses:
   1. Corneal clouding occurs in MPS I, but not in MPS II or III.
   2. Mental retardation is a feature of MPS I, II, and III but not of MPS IV, V, VI [2,23].
   3. MPS II is X-linked. All the other mucopolysaccharidoses are inherited as autosomal recessive traits.
   4. Appearance, corneal clouding, and x-ray changes may be indistinguishable in patients with MPS I and those with MPS VI (the Maroteaux-Lamy syndrome). However, patients with MPS VI have normal intelligence, and their urine contains an excess of dermatan sulfate only. Patients with MPS I excrete both dermatan sulfate and heparan sulfate [2].
   5. In the most common mucopolysaccharidoses (MPS I and II) there is an excess of both heparan sulfate and dermatan sulfate in the urine; these disorders thus cannot be differentiated by the study of urine. The pattern of mucopolysacchariduria is of greatest diagnostic value in MPS III (in which only heparan sulfate is excreted in excess) and MPS VI (only dermatan sulfate is in excess) [2,11].
   6. The "tissue culture typing" techniques [14,23a] promise to provide a differentiation of these disorders at the enzymatic level. However, they are not now generally available.

MPS II
(Hunter's Syndrome)

Physical Features

HEAD: The head is often enlarged. The forehead and the sagittal suture are prominent.

FACE: The facial abnormalities resemble those in MPS I, but are not as severe. The bridge of the nose is broad and flat (*Figures A, B, C, D, and E*). Patients usually have a chronic nasal discharge because of narrow air passages. Some have thickened lips, but this is not evident for several years (*Figure E*). The tongue may be enlarged, but usually only after the age of 5 years [7].

EYES: In contrast to MPS I, there is no corneal clouding. Two patients with symptoms of night blindness had clumping of pigment in the peripheral fundus [21].

NECK: The neck is short.

ABDOMEN: In a study [7] of 19 patients, 7 had inguinal hernias and hydroceles. Small umbilical hernias were also common. Enlargement of the liver and spleen was consistently present by 1 to 2 years (*Figures A and B*).

BACK: Lumbar kyphosis is only occasionally noted. When kyphosis is present, the lower back has a rounded shape which is evident by 1 to 5 years of age.

LIMBS: Limited joint extension is usually evident by 2 years (*Figures D, E, and F*).

SKIN: The body hair is increased after 2 to 4 years.

HEIGHT: Linear growth is either increased or normal at first. It becomes subnormal by 3 to 6 years.

Nervous System

The period of normal development is longer than in MPS I, so that mental retardation usually is not noted until the second year. Most patients learn how to use words and some sentences, and toilet training may be achieved. A clumsy and broad-based gait and hyperkinetic behavior are common between 2 and 6 years, but after 5 to 6 years physical activity slows down. Deep tendon reflexes are normal. In a study of 19 patients, 6 had hearing loss. Seizures occur, especially in older patients [7].

Pathology

See MPS I.

Laboratory Studies

See MPS I. Except for the fact that the degradative defect in cultured skin fibroblasts from MPS II patients can be corrected by extracts from MPS I tissue cultures or urine, most laboratory studies in MPS II patients yield results similar to those in MPS I. The x-ray changes also resemble those in MPS I but are usually not as severe.

Treatment and Prognosis

Recently infusions of leukocytes [18b] and plasma [18a] have been suggested as a treatment. However, it is not known at this time whether either or both substances will be generally effective and have long-term benefit. Surgery is indicated for the hernias.

Death often occurs at age 8 to 15 years, usually from pulmonary infection or as a complication of seizures and neurologic deterioration. In certain pedigrees patients have survived until the fifth decade. Such patients may have normal intelligence [2].

Genetics

X-linked recessive. The female carrier shows metachromasia in some, but not all, of her skin fibroblasts; this mosaicism is a reflection of her heterozygous state [18]. Prenatal diagnosis of the affected male fetus has been reported [20].

Differential Diagnosis

See above.

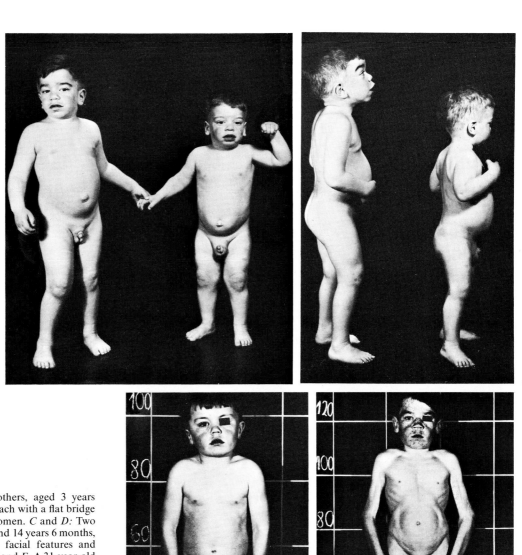

Plate I-18. *A* and *B:* Two brothers, aged 3 years 7 months and 2 years 2 months, each with a flat bridge of the nose and protuberant abdomen. *C* and *D:* Two brothers, aged 5 years 6 months and 14 years 6 months, the older showing more coarse facial features and limited extension of his elbows. *E* and *F:* A 31-year-old man with a broad nasal bridge, thick lips, flexed elbows, marked hirsutism, and short stature. (*A* and *B:* Courtesy of Dr. A. C. Crocker, Boston, Mass. *C* and *D:* Courtesy of Dr. W. M. Teller, Ulm, Germany. *E* and *F:* From J. P. Gills *et al., Arch. Ophthalmol.,* **74:**596–603, 1965.)

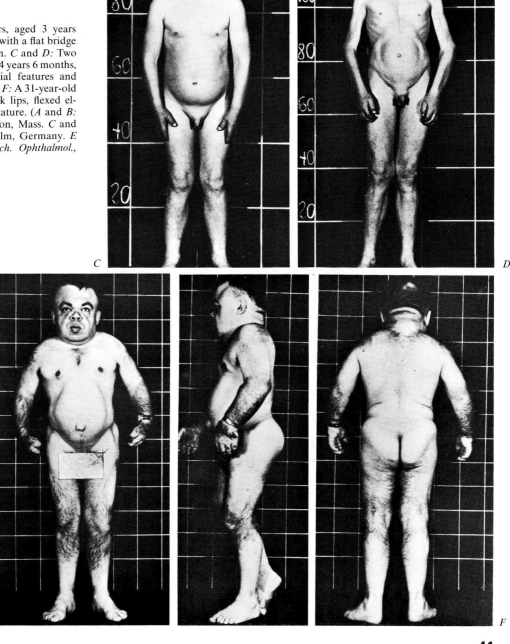

MPS III
(Sanfilippo Syndrome, Polydystrophic Oligophrenia, Heparitinuria)

Physical Features

HEAD: The head is normal or slightly enlarged.

FACE: The bridge of the nose is slightly flattened. The lips and tongue are occasionally thick and enlarged, but this is only evident after 5 years of age [4] (*Figures B and D*). In infancy the facial features are normal (*Figure A*) and in some patients they remain so (*Figure E*).

EYES: Clinically evident corneal clouding has not been present in any cases.

NECK: The neck may be short (*Figure C*).

ABDOMEN: The liver is moderately enlarged in 70 to 80 percent of patients, the spleen palpable in about 20 percent [6] (*Figure B*).

BACK: A gibbus deformity does not develop.

LIMBS: Moderate joint contractures may develop by 4 to 6 years of age (*Figure F*). Most common are mild flexion contractures of the elbow and fingers. There may also be a genu valgum deformity [6].

Nervous System

Early mental development appears to be normal (*Figure A*); mental regression is first noted between 1 and 4 years. The child becomes difficult to control, and speech deteriorates and is later lost altogether. The gait becomes awkward and broad-based after the first 2 to 3 years. Drooling is common. Ultimately these children are bedridden and demented [6,7].

Pathology

The brain weight is diminished and both the cerebral and cerebellar cortices appear atrophic. In two patients [22] there was a moderate loss of neurons in the cerebral cortex.

Laboratory Studies

Total urinary polysaccharide excretion is 2 to 10 times normal; only heparan sulfate is increased [6]. Skin fibroblasts cultured from patients with MPS III contain a factor that can correct the degradative defect in fibroblasts cultured from patients with MPS I or II [14,23a]. Biochemical heterogeneity of MPS III has been suggested [23a]. Radiologic abnormalities are mild in comparison with those in MPS I and II [6] (*Figure F*).

Treatment and Prognosis

The most distressing feature is the progressive intellectual deterioration, which is profound by the time the patients are 10 years old. How long they will live is not known. Most were alive when reported, the oldest live one being 17 years old [6]. Others have died from intercurrent infections at age 2 to 18 years [6]. There is no specific treatment.

Genetics

Autosomal recessive. It is likely that the techniques for heterozygote detection described for MPS I are applicable to MPS III. Prenatal diagnosis has not been reported. The diagnostic method which depends upon abnormal kinetics [23a] in cultured amniotic fluid cells appears promising.

Differential Diagnosis
See page 40.

References

1. Hunter, C. A rare disease in two brothers. *Proc. R. Soc. Med.,* **10**:104–16, 1917.
2. McKusick, V. A. *Heritable Disorders of Connective Tissue,* 3rd ed. C. V. Mosby Co., St. Louis, 1966, pp. 325–99.
3. Hurler, G. Über eine Typ multipler Abartungen, vorwiegend am Skelettsystem. *Z. Kinderheilkd.,* **24**:220–34, 1919.
4. Brante, G. Gargoylism: a mucopolysaccharidosis. *Scand. J. Clin. Lab. Invest.,* **4**:43–46, 1952.
5. Harris, R. C. Mucopolysaccharide disorder: a possible new genotype of Hurler's syndrome. *Am. J. Dis. Child.,* **102**:741–42, 1961.
6. Rampini, S. Das Sanfilippo-Syndrom (polydystrophe Oligophrenie, HS-Mukopolysaccharidose). Bericht über 8 Fälle und Literatur übersicht. *Helv. Paediatr. Acta,* **24**:55–91, 1969.
7. Leroy, J. G., and Crocker, A. C. Clinical definition of the Hurler-Hunter phenotypes. A review of 50 patients. *Am. J. Dis. Child.,* **112**:518–30, 1966.
8. Neuhauser, E. B. D., Griscom, N. T., Gilles, F. H., and Crocker, A. C. Arachnoid cyst in the Hurler-Hunter syndrome. *Ann. Radiol. (Paris),* **11**:1–17, 1967.
9. Gonatas, N. K., and Gonatas, J. Ultrastructural and biochemical observations on a case of systemic late infantile lipidosis and its relationship to Tay-Sachs disease and gargoylism. *J. Neuropathol. Exp. Neurol.,* **24**:318–40, 1965.
10. Dorfman, A., and Matalon, R. The Hurler and Hunter syndrome. *Am. J. Med.,* **47**:691–707, 1969.
11. Kaplan, D. Classification of the mucopolysaccharidoses based on the pattern of mucopolysacchariduria. *Am. J. Med.,* **47**:721–29, 1969.
12. Fratantoni, J. C., Hall, C. W., and Neufeld, E. F. The defect in Hurler's and Hunter's syndromes: faulty degradation of mucopolysaccharide. *Proc. Natl. Acad. Sci. USA,* **60**:699–706, 1968.
13. Neufeld, E. F. Personal communication, 1970.
14. Fratantoni, J. C., Hall, C. W., and Neufeld, E. F. Hurler and Hunter syndromes: mutual correction of defect in cultured fibroblasts. *Science,* **162**:570–72, 1968.
15. MacBrinn, M., Okada, S., Woollacott, M., Patel, V., Ho, M. W., Tappel, A. L., and O'Brien, J. S. Beta-galactosidase deficiency in the Hurler syndrome. *N. Engl. J. Med.,* **281**:338–43, 1969.
16. Muir, H. The structure and metabolism of mucopolysaccharides (glycosaminoglycans) and the problem of the mucopolysaccharidoses. *Am. J. Med.,* **47**:673–90, 1969.
17. Carter, C. H., Wan, A. T., and Carpenter, D. G. Commonly used tests in the detection of Hurler's syndrome. *J. Pediatr.,* **73**:217–21, 1968.
18. Danes, B. S., and Bearn, A. G. Hurler's syndrome: demonstration of an inherited disorder of connective tissue in cell culture. *Science,* **149**:987–89, 1965.
18a. DiFerrante, N., Nichols, B. L., Donnelly, P. V., Neri, G., Hrgovcic, R., and Berglund, R. K. Induced degradation of glycosaminoglycans in Hurler's and Hunter's syndromes by plasma infusion. *Proc. Natl. Acad. Sci. U.S.A.,* **68**:303–307, 1971.
18b. Knudson, A. G., DiFerrante, N., and Curtis, J. E. Effect of leukocyte transfusion in a child with type II mucopolysaccharidosis. *Proc. Natl. Acad. Sci. U.S.A.,* **68**:1738–41, 1971.
19. Matalon, R., Dorfman, A., Nadler, H. L., and Jacobson, C. B. A chemical method for the antenatal diagnosis of mucopolysaccharidoses. *Lancet,* **1**:83–84, 1970.
20. Fratantoni, J. C., Neufeld, E. F., Uhlendorf, B. W., and Jacobson, C. B. Intrauterine diagnosis of the Hurler and Hunter syndromes. *N. Engl. J. Med.,* **280**:686–88, 1969.
20a. Brock, D. J. H., Gordon, H., Seligman, S., and Lobo, E. de H. Antenatal detection of Hurler's syndrome. *Lancet,* **2**:1324–25, 1971.
21. Gills, J. P., Hobson, R., Hanley, W. B., and McKusick, V. A. Electroretinography and fundus oculi findings in Hurler's disease and allied mucopolysaccharidoses. *Arch. Ophthalmol.,* **74**:596–603, 1965.
22. Wallace, B. J., Kaplan, D., Adachi, M., Schneck, L., and Volk, B. W. Mucopolysaccharidosis type III. Morphologic and biochemical studies of two siblings with Sanfilippo syndrome. *Arch. Pathol.,* **82**:462–73, 1966.
23. McKusick, V. A. The nosology of the mucopolysaccharidoses. *Am. J. Med.,* **47**:730–47, 1969.
23a. Kresse, H., Wiesmann, U., Cantz, M., Hall, C. W., and Neufeld, E. F. Biochemical heterogeneity of the Sanfilippo syndrome: preliminary characterization of two deficient factors. *Biochem. Biophys. Res. Commun.,* **42**:892–98, 1971.

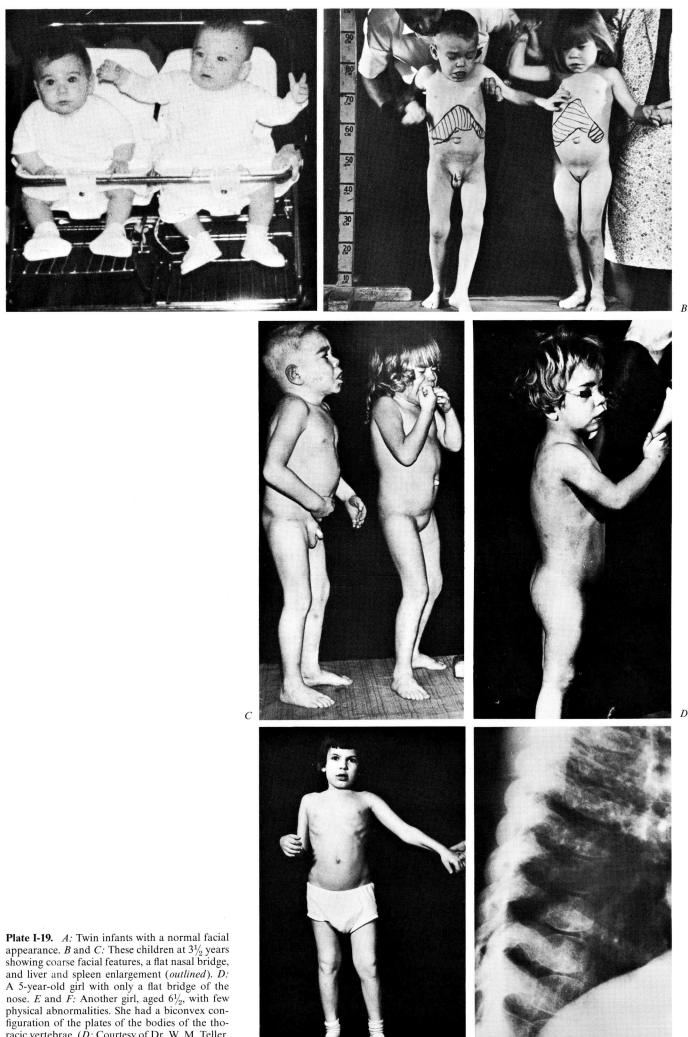

Plate I-19. *A:* Twin infants with a normal facial appearance. *B* and *C:* These children at 3½ years showing coarse facial features, a flat nasal bridge, and liver and spleen enlargement (*outlined*). *D:* A 5-year-old girl with only a flat bridge of the nose. *E* and *F:* Another girl, aged 6½, with few physical abnormalities. She had a biconvex configuration of the plates of the bodies of the thoracic vertebrae. (*D:* Courtesy of Dr. W. M. Teller, Ulm, Germany. *E* and *F:* From L. Langer, *Ann. Radio.* [*Paris*], **7:**315–25, 1964.)

Niemann-Pick Disease
(Sphingomyelin Lipidosis)

In 1914 Niemann [1] reported an 18-month-old infant who had died of a progressive illness associated with hepatosplenomegaly and whose organs were filled with foam cells. In 1927 the entity was more clearly delineated by Pick [2]. At present, all lipid storage diseases associated with sphingomyelin accumulation are included in this category. Recently 165 cases have been reviewed [3]. There are at least four types of Niemann-Pick disease [4], the most common of which is the acute infantile form originally described by Niemann and Pick (type A). Some, but not all, types are associated with deficient activity of the enzyme sphingomyelinase [5,9a]. This suggests that the underlying genetic abnormalities are quite different.

Type A

Physical Features and Nervous System

This type is rapidly progressive, with death usually occurring before 2 years of age. During the first few months of life the child feeds poorly and fails to acquire the normal early motor skills. Hypotonia and listlessness gradually become more marked (*Figure A*). Petechiae may develop due to thrombocytopenia caused by the splenomegaly. About half of the patients have generalized lymph node enlargement. A cherry-red spot in the macula is present in over half of the patients, but it may not be evident until late in the illness. The optic disc is initially normal but becomes pale; the children are always blind in the late stages of their illness. A few patients have developed skin xanthomas.

Laboratory Studies and Pathology

An absence of activity of the enzyme sphingomyelinase has been demonstrated in the spleen [5], white blood cells [6], skin fibroblasts [7] and amniotic cells [8]. As a result of the enzymatic defect sphingomyelin accumulates in the visceral organs and cerebral gray matter. For unknown reasons cholesterol also accumulates [3]. The lipids accumulate mainly within so-called Niemann-Pick cells [9], which in usual histologic preparations look like large foam cells (*Figure F*). They are found in the spleen, lymphoid tissue, liver, bone marrow, and lungs, and to a lesser extent the endocrine glands and renal glomeruli and tubules [9].

Treatment and Prognosis

Patients usually die before 3 years.

Genetics

Autosomal recessive. Between one half and one third of the patients are Jewish. Prenatal diagnosis has been achieved [8].

Differential Diagnosis

The differential diagnosis includes Tay-Sachs disease (see page 62), Gaucher's disease (see page 16), G_{M1} gangliosidosis (see page 22) and Wolman's disease (see page 66). The first three can now be differentiated with specific enzymatic assays. Patients with Tay-Sachs disease do not have hepatosplenomegaly and those with Wolman's disease have calcified adrenal glands.

Type B

Patients with this type of Niemann-Pick disease have spleen enlargement, usually between 2 and 6 years of age, as the first sign of illness [3] (*Figure B*). Enlargement of the liver and pulmonary infiltrates appear later. The mental and neurologic status remain normal. The activity of sphingomyelinase in the spleen [5] and cultured fibroblasts [7] is 1 to 5 percent of normal. Niemann-Pick cells are found in the bone marrow. Splenectomy may be necessary because of the effects of hypersplenism.

Type C

Signs of the illness usually appear between 2 and 4 years of age (*Figures C and D*). The neurologic signs are striking, and include spasticity and seizures, particularly myoclonic jerks. Macular degeneration and the presence of a cherry-red spot have been described. There is sphingomyelin excess in the viscera but not in the brain [10]. The activity of the sphingomyelin cleaving enzyme in liver and skin fibroblasts is normal [9a].

Type D

All the patients in this group have originated from Yarmouth County in Nova Scotia. Many had neonatal jaundice which persisted for 3 to 6 months. The neurologic symptoms are prominent and include school failure, cerebellar ataxia, athetosis, a masklike face, exaggerated deep tendon reflexes, and seizures. The spleen is markedly enlarged (*Figure E*); its removal may be necessary because of hypersplenism. This illness usually leads to death in adolescence or early adulthood. Sphingomyelin is increased in liver [9a], but not brain [4]. The activity of the sphingomyelin cleaving enzyme is normal in liver and skin fibroblasts [9].

References

1. Niemann, A. Ein unbekanntes Krankheitsbild. *Jahrb. Kinderheilk.,* **79**:1–10, 1914.
2. Pick, L. Über die lipoidzellige Splenohepatomegalie Typus Niemann-Pick als Stoffwechselerkrankung. *Med. Klin.,* **23**:1483–1888, 1927.
3. Fredrickson, D. S. Sphingomyelin lipidosis: Niemann-Pick disease. In *The Metabolic Basis of Inherited Disease,* 2nd ed. Stanbury, J. B., Wyngaarden, J. B., and Fredrickson, D. S. (eds.), McGraw-Hill Book Co., New York, 1966, pp. 586–617.
4. Crocker, A. C. The cerebral defect in Tay-Sachs disease and Niemann-Pick disease. *J. Neurochem.,* **7**:69–80, 1961.
5. Schneider, P. B., and Kennedy, E. P. Sphingomyelinase in normal spleens and in spleens from subjects with Niemann-Pick disease. *J. Lipid Res.,* **8**:202–209, 1967.
6. Kampine, J. P., Brady, R. O., Kanfer, J. N., Feld, M., and Shapiro, D. Diagnosis of Gaucher's disease and Niemann-Pick disease with small samples of venous blood. *Science,* **155**:86–88, 1967.
7. Sloan, H. R., Uhlendorf, B. W., Kanfer, J. N., Brady, R. O., and Fredrickson, D. S. Deficiency of sphingomyelin-cleaving enzyme activity in tissue cultures derived from patients with Niemann-Pick disease. *Biochem. Biophys. Res. Commun.,* **34**:582–88, 1969.
8. Epstein, C. J., Brady, R. O., Schneider, E. L., Brady, R. M., and Shapiro, E. In utero diagnosis of Niemann-Pick disease. *Am. J. Hum. Genet.,* **23**:533–35, 1971.
9. Crocker, A. C., and Farber, S. Niemann-Pick disease: a review of eighteen patients. *Medicine (Baltimore),* **37**:1–95, 1958.
9a. Sloan, H. R., and Fredrickson, D. S. The heterogeneity of sphingomyelin lipidoses (Niemann-Pick disease). (Abstract.) Society for Pediatric Research, Atlantic City, N.J., 1971, p. 11.
10. Philippart, M., Martin, L., Martin, J. J., and Menkes, J. H. Niemann-Pick disease. Morphologic and biochemical studies in the visceral form with late central nervous system involvement (Crocker's Group C). *Arch. Neurol.,* **20**:227–38, 1969.

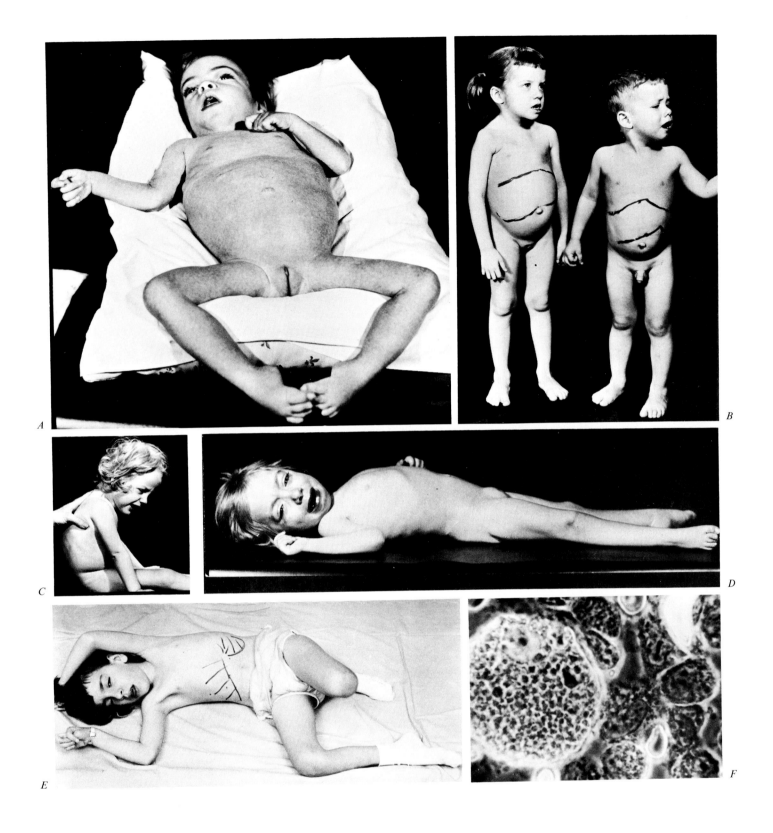

Plate I-20. *A:* An infant with type A Niemann-Pick disease who has a protuberant abdomen and flexion contractures of her legs. *B:* A sister and brother with type B disease. Their marked liver and spleen enlargement is indicated. They had no neurologic abnormalities. *C:* A girl with type C showing drooling and an inability to sit without support. *D:* Another child with type C and marked neurologic deficits. *E:* A child with type D, showing an expressionless face, protruding tongue, enlarged liver and spleen, and athetoid posturing of her hand. *F:* A Niemann-Pick cell with "foamy" cytoplasm. (*A–D:* Courtesy of Dr. A. C. Crocker, Boston, Mass. *E:* Courtesy of Dr. D. S. Fredrickson, Bethesda, Md. *F:* From Sphingomyelin lipidosis: Neimann-Pick disease, by D. S. Fredrickson, in *The Metabolic Basis of Inherited Disease,* J. B. Stanbury *et al.* [eds.], 2nd ed. McGraw-Hill Book Co., New York, 1966, pp. 586–617. Used with permission of McGraw-Hill Book Co.)

Phenylketonuria (PKU)

In 1934 Fölling [1] described ten patients who excreted phenylpyruvic acid and were mentally deficient. Later, Jervis showed that the basic metabolic defect was the inability to oxidize phenylalanine to tyrosine [2]. This entity is now referred to as classical phenylketonuria. Subsequent experience with screening of newborns for elevated serum phenylalanine has shown that several other disorders can cause an elevation of this amino acid in newborns. These include atypical phenylketonuria, transient hyperphenylalaninemia, and neonatal tyrosinemia [3]. In several surveys the incidence of phenylketonuria has been found to be 1:14,000 and 1:20,000 [3,12].

Physical Features

General appearance is normal (*Figure D*).

HEAD: Microcephaly occurs in about half of the untreated individuals [4].

EYES: Iris pigmentation is lighter than in unaffected siblings [4].

SKIN: Eczema has been noted in about a third of the untreated individuals [4] (*Figure A*). It begins in infancy and may persist to adolescence and adulthood.

HAIR: Untreated patients have lighter-colored hair and a lighter complexion than other members of their families (*Figure C*).

Nervous System

Most untreated persons with phenylketonuria have an IQ of less than 20; less than 2 percent have an IQ above 60. The severely retarded patients usually learn to walk, but only a third learn to talk. Two thirds of the untreated patients have hyperactive deep tendon reflexes; ankle and patella clonus is also common [4]. Approximately a quarter of the patients have seizures [4].

Pathology

The brain weight of most untreated patients is diminished. There is a slight to moderate deficiency of myelin [4]. In addition, a diminution of axonal-dendritic synapses has recently been demonstrated with special staining techniques [5] (*Figure E*).

Laboratory Studies

The basic abnormality is a deficiency of the enzyme phenylalanine hydroxylase, which converts phenylalanine to tyrosine and is normally present in the liver. A presumptive diagnosis is made in the newborn who is on regular protein-containing formula if the plasma phenylalanine is above 20 mg percent (normal 2–4 mg percent) and if tyrosinemia is ruled out by virtue of a tyrosine level of less than 5 mg percent [3]. In older children or adults, elevated blood phenylalanine levels can be demonstrated by bacterial inhibition [6] or fluorometric assay [7]. A diminished concentration of several tryptophan metabolites, especially serotonin and 5-hydroxy-indole-acetic acid, has also been observed [8]. The urine contains many phenylalanine metabolites, the most important of which is phenylpyruvic acid. This substance is responsible for the positive ferric chloride test, which was the main screening test prior to the development of convenient blood phenylalanine assays.

Treatment and Prognosis

A carefully controlled oral intake of phenylalanine begun before the infant is 2 months old will prevent severe mental defect [3] (*Figure B*). However, some patients who received early and well-controlled dietary treatment have shown subtle neurologic defects [9]. The diet must be controlled with great care. Excessive phenylalanine restriction can be harmful. Individuals whose serum phenylalanine levels become subnormal due to excessive restriction of phenylalanine intake have poor neurologic development, weight loss, an eczematous rash, and feeding difficulties [10]. Intrauterine and postnatal growth retardation, microcephaly, and mental retardation are frequently observed features of infants born to normal or mildly retarded phenylketonuric mothers [11] (*Figure F*). These infants do not have a deficiency of phenylalanine hydroxylase, but are presumably damaged by the elevated phenylalanine level of their mothers. It is likely that brain damage can be prevented in her child if the phenylketonuric woman is maintained on a controlled phenylalanine intake during pregnancy.

Genetics

Autosomal recessive. The heterozygous state cannot be consistently identified, although most parents of phenylketonuric children have a diminished tolerance for phenylalanine [4].

Differential Diagnosis

Untreated phenylketonuria may present as "failure to thrive," autism, or mental retardation. Since the clinical manifestations are not distinctive, diagnosis depends upon laboratory tests.

References

1. Fölling, A. Über Ausscheidung von Phenylbrenztraubensäure in den Harn als Stoffwechselanomalie in Verbindung mit Imbezillität. *Z. Physiol. Chem.*, **227**:169–76, 1934.
2. Jervis, G. A. Phenylpyruvic oligophrenia: deficiency of phenylalanine-oxidizing system. *Proc. Soc. Exp. Biol. Med.*, **82**:514–15, 1953.
3. Berman, J. L., Cunningham, G. C., Day, R. W., Ford, R., and Hsia, D. Y.-Y. Causes of high phenylalanine with normal tyrosine in newborn screening programs. *Am. J. Dis. Child.*, **117**:54–65, 1969.
4. Knox, W. E. Phenylketonuria. In *The Metabolic Basis of Inherited Disease*, J. B. Stanbury, J. B. Wyngaarden, and D. S. Fredrickson (eds.), 2nd ed. McGraw-Hill Book Co., New York, 1966, pp. 258–94.
5. Kemper, T. Personal communication, 1970.
6. Guthrie, R., and Susi, A. A simple phenylalanine method for detecting phenylketonuria in large populations of newborn infants. *Pediatrics*, **32**:338–43, 1963.
7. McCaman, M. W., and Robins, E. Fluorimetric method for the determination of phenylalanine in serum. *J. Lab. Clin. Med.*, **59**:885, 1962.
8. Hsia, D. Y.-Y. Phenylketonuria: a study of human biochemical genetics. *Pediatrics*, **38**:173–84, 1966.
9. Hackney, I. M., Hanley, W. B., Davidson, W., and Lindsao, L. Phenylketonuria: mental development, behavior and termination of low phenylalanine diet. *J. Pediatr.*, **72**:646–55, 1968.
10. Rouse, B. M. Phenylalanine deficiency syndrome. *J. Pediatr.*, **69**:246–49, 1966.
11. Yu, J. S., and O'Halloran, M. T. Children of mothers with phenylketonuria. *Lancet*, **1**:210–12, 1970.
12. Levy, H. L., Madigan, P. M., and Shih, V. E. Massachusetts metabolic disorder screening program. I. Techniques and results of urine screening. *Pediatrics* (1972, in press).

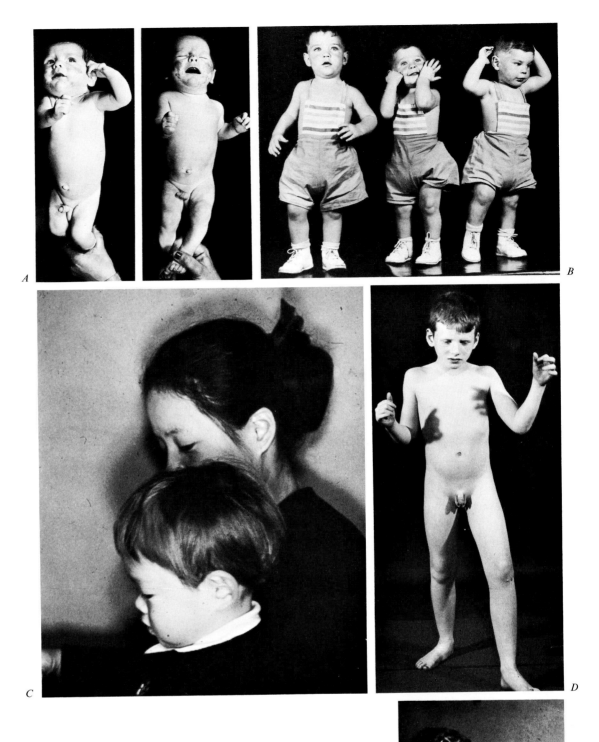

Plate I-21. *A:* Two-month-old untreated infants with facial eczema. *B:* These infants (middle and right) are shown at 19 months of age after treatment with their normal brother of the same age. These three children were triplets, but only the two with PKU were monozygous. *C:* An untreated Oriental child whose hair is slightly lighter than his mother's. *D:* A red-haired 10-year-old boy who has had no dietary treatment. He is hyperactive and frequently assumes peculiar postures. *E:* Camera lucida drawing of a cerebral cortical neuron from a 60-year-old man with untreated PKU (**1**) and a normal two-year-old child (**2**), stained by the Golgi-Cox method, which reveals the cell bodies, dendrites, and synaptic "thorns" (labeled "th"). The latter represent the site of axo-dendritic synapse. Growth and development of nerve cells is characterized by an increase in the number of synaptic "thorns." Note that in the PKU material these are few in comparison to the normal, and the cell is smaller than the 2-year-old's. The difference would have been even more striking if a nerve cell from a normal adult had been used for comparison. *F:* An untreated woman with elevated serum phenylalanine shown here with two microcephalic children. She has also had several spontaneous abortions. (*A* and *B:* Courtesy of Dr. E. S. Kang, Boston, Massachusetts. *C:* Courtesy of Dr. T. B. Fitzpatrick, Boston, Massachusetts. *E:* Courtesy of Dr. T. Kemper, Waverley, Massachusetts. *F:* Courtesy of Drs. R. E. Stevenson and C. C. Huntley, Baltimore, Maryland.)

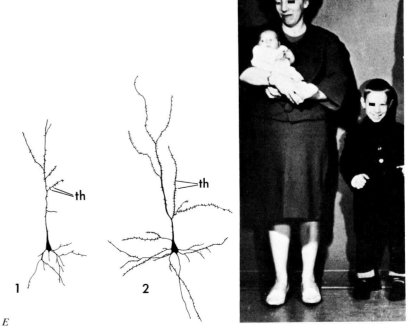

Prader-Labhart-Willi Syndrome

In 1956 Prader, Labhart, and Willi [1] described a syndrome of obesity, short stature, cryptorchidism, and mental retardation with an amyotonialike condition in the neonatal period. Since then more than 100 cases have been reported [2–5].

Physical Features

FACE: Many of these patients resemble each other because of nonspecific features, such as excessive fat and an open mouth with down-turned corners (*Figures B, C, D, and E*).

MOUTH: Severe dental caries often develop shortly after teeth have erupted. The saliva is quite thick and sticks to the lips [6].

GENITALIA: Most males have a small penis and an atrophic or nonrugated scrotum; the testes are small and either undescended or palpable in the inguinal canal (*Figure F*). A few females have had small labia majora and minora [2].

BACK: A few patients have scoliosis.

LIMBS: The hands and feet often appear to be small. This is most noticeable in the older, more obese patients.

SKIN: The skin is thick and insensitive. Often there is erythema around the hair follicles, especially on the arms where there is evidence of intense scratching and scars from previously infected scratches [6].

HEIGHT: Stature is usually normal in the first 10 years of life. However, the growth rate slows in the second decade and the adolescent growth spurt is notably lacking. The ultimate adult height is usually less than 5 feet (153 cm) [6].

WEIGHT: The mean birth weight of 44 term newborns was 3000 g, which is slightly below the normal average [2]. Because of the poor ability to suck, initial weight gain is slow. However, an excessive appetite becomes evident within the first year and weight gain rapidly increases. Most patients are clearly obese by the age of 2 years. The weight gain continues unless caloric restriction is vigorously enforced. By the teenage years these patients are markedly overweight, and quite inactive as a result. The excessive fat accumulates over the entire body, but may be quite remarkable in the lower legs, with cuffs of fat around the ankles (*Figure E*).

GROWTH AND DEVELOPMENT: Most adult-age males and females have very little axillary and pubic hair. Some females have regular menses at the expected age, but most have either irregular menses or none at all. Most adult males do not develop a beard or a masculine voice and do not have normal penis enlargement (*Figure F*).

Nervous System

Some mothers have reported that there was little fetal activity. All patients have shown marked muscular hypotonia in infancy (*Figure A*) and a delay in their developmental milestones. Most learn to walk by the age of 3 or 4 years, but their gait often remains broad-based and insecure. Speech development may be more delayed than motor development, with the vocabulary limited and articulation defective in many patients. Intelligence quotients have ranged between 20 and 90; most have an IQ between 40 and 60 [2] and are generally pleasant and cooperative, but they often have outbursts of anger when food demands are not met. They devise ingenious ways of getting food, and may resort to stealing or to eating garbage. They will eat until food is removed and seem unconcerned about the quality of the food [6].

Pathology

In the few autopsies that have been performed, no brain or muscle abnormalities have been found. Testis biopsies in adults have shown either tubular atrophy or absence of spermatogenesis [3].

Laboratory Studies

Some patients have mild diabetes mellitus with an abnormal glucose tolerance test, but acetonemia and acetonuria seldom occur. The plasma insulin response to intravenous glucose and tolbutamide is quite variable. There has been no evidence of resistance to exogenous insulin. At the age of expected puberty the excretion of 17-ketosteroids in the urine is low; females have an immature vaginal epithelium. Urinary gonadotropin levels have been low in some patients and elevated in others. In one study [7] subcutaneous fat biopsies showed elevated palmitoleic acid levels, which was suggestive of hyperlipogenesis. Serum lipid analysis has shown no abnormalities. Serial x-rays show that epiphyseal fusion progresses at a near normal rate in most patients. Almost all patients have had normal chromosomes, and the few reported abnormalities are probably unrelated to the associated Prader-Willi syndrome [2].

Treatment and Prognosis

The patients with hyperglycemia and glucosuria usually respond to oral antidiabetic agents. The life expectancy is thought to be limited by the severe obesity. Several have died of respiratory insufficiency with the Pickwickian syndrome. Accidents and pneumonia have been other causes of death [6]. There is no effective treatment of the hyperphagia.

Genetics

A predominance of males has been reported, but this is probably because the diagnosis is easier to make in the male. Almost none of the patients has another affected family member or parental consanguinity [2].

Differential Diagnosis

1. Severe neonatal hypotonia may occur in patients with the cerebrohepatorenal syndrome (see page 270), the oculocerebrorenal syndrome of Lowe (see page 248), neonatal myasthenia gravis, and Werdnig-Hoffmann's disease. The first is differentiated by associated craniofacial anomalies, flexion contractures, and stippled epiphyses; the second by aminoaciduria, cataracts, and glaucoma; the third by an edrophonium chloride test; and the fourth by electromyography and a muscle biopsy.
2. Obesity, hypogonadism, and mental retardation are features of the Laurence-Moon syndrome, but these patients often have polydactyly and retinal degeneration (see page 288).
3. Obesity, hypogonadism, and mental retardation are features of the syndrome of microcephaly, hypogonadism, and mental deficiency (Börjeson-Forssman-Lehmann syndrome), but this rare disorder is presumably X-linked (see page 58).

References

1. Prader, A., Labhart, A., and Willi, H.   Ein Syndrom von Adipositas, Kleinwuchs, Kryptorchismus and Oligophrenie nach myatonieartigem Zustand im Neugeborenenalter. *Schweiz. Med. Wochenschr.,* **86:**1260–61, 1956.
2. Zellweger, H., and Schneider, H. J.   Syndrome of hypotonia-hypomentia-hypogonadism-obesity (HHHO) or Prader-Willi syndrome. *Am. J. Dis. Child.,* **115:**588–98, 1968.
3. Steiner, H.   Das Prader-Labhart-Willi Syndrom. Eine morphologische Analyse. *Virchows Arch. (Pathol. Anat.),* **345:**205–27, 1968.
4. Gabilan, J.-C., and Royer, P.   Le syndrome de Prader, Labhart et Willi. *Arch. Fr. Pediatr.,* **25:**121–49, 1968.
5. Dunn, H. G.   The Prader-Labhart-Willi syndrome; review of the literature and report of nine cases. *Acta Paediatr. Scand.,* Supplement 186, pp. 1–38, 1968.
6. Crawford, J. D.   Personal communication, 1970.
7. Johnsen, S., Crawford, J. D., and Haessler, H. A.   Fasting hyperlipogenesis: an inborn error of energy metabolism in Prader-Willi syndrome. (Abstract.) American Pediatric Society, Atlantic City, N.J., 1967.

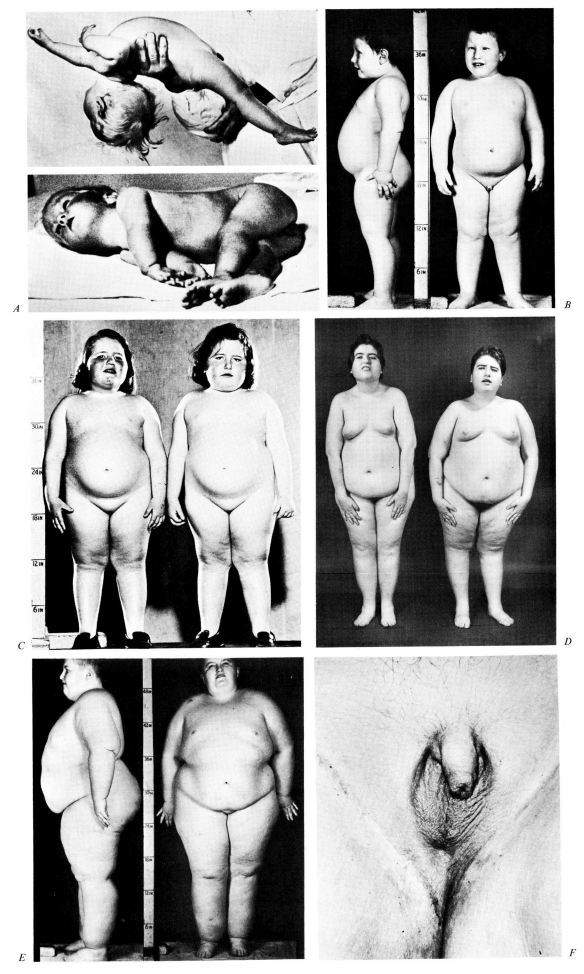

Plate I-22. *A:* Shows marked muscle hypotonia in a 10-month-old child. *B:* A 4½-year-old boy with generalized obesity and small genitalia. He weighed 64 pounds and was 40 inches tall. *C* and *D:* Twin sisters at 5 and at 29 years of age, showing their increasingly severe obesity. The relative smallness of their hands became more striking as they grew. Neither girl had any glandular breast tissue. At 29 years they were both 54 inches tall and weighed 210 pounds. *E* and *F:* A 19-year-old boy who weighed 230 pounds and was 55½ inches tall. He had cuffs of sagging fat around his ankles, and his hands appeared small. His penis was small, his testes undescended, and his pubic hair sparse. (*A* [*top*]: From A. Prader and H. Willi, *Proceedings of the Second International Congress on Mental Retardation,* Part I, S. Karger, Basel, Switzerland, 1963, pp. 353–57. *A* [*bottom*]: Courtesy of Dr. A. Prader, Zurich, Switzerland. *B, C,* and *E:* Courtesy of Dr. J. D. Crawford, Boston, Mass. *F:* From D. Hoefnagel *et al., J. Ment. Defic. Res.,* **11:**1–11, 1967.)

Pseudohypoparathyroidism
(Albright's Hereditary Osteodystrophy)

In 1942 Albright, Burnett, Smith, and Parson [1] described three patients with a peculiar physiognomy characterized by a round face and a rather thick-set figure. Like patients with hypoparathyroidism, they had hypocalcemia and hyperphosphatemia, but they were different in that they did not respond to parathyroid hormone. Therefore, their disorder was called pseudohypoparathyroidism, and it was postulated that the hypocalcemia was the result of end-organ resistance to parathyroid hormone.

In 1952 Albright, Forbes, and Henneman [2] used the term *pseudo-pseudohypoparathyroidism* to describe a young woman with the same physiognomy as patients with pseudohypoparathyroidism but normal serum levels of calcium and phosphorus. Subsequent studies have shown that the serum calcium levels in patients such as this woman may vary over the course of time so that the diagnosis changes back and forth between pseudo- and pseudo-pseudohypoparathyroidism. Family studies have shown that both disorders may exist in the same family, further suggesting that they are the same disorder. To replace both terms, the alternate of *Albright's hereditary osteodystrophy* has been proposed [3].

Recent studies [4,5] have shown that patients with pseudohypoparathyroidism have normal secretion of hormone from the parathyroid glands, but a genetic defect in the receptor tissues such that there is little or no response to the hormone.

Physical Features

FACE: Many of these patients have a round face and a prominent forehead (*Figures A, B, C, G, and J*).

EYES: Patients who have experienced chronic hypocalcemia often have cataracts.

MOUTH: Poorly developed enamel is a common finding in both the deciduous and permanent teeth and has been attributed to chronic hypocalcemia. Therefore, extensive caries are often present. Also, the crowns are small and the roots are often short with blunt ends [6].

LIMBS: A short, stocky physique is often described. Most affected children have short, stubby fingers and toes; with increasing age relative shortness of some of the metacarpals and metatarsals develops as a result of premature epiphyseal closure. The fourth digit is most often involved; the first and fifth are also frequently short (*Figures E, F, G, H, and I*). This physical sign is best demonstrated by making a fist. The

shortened metacarpal will make no knuckle (*Figure E*). The short toe may be the cause of severe foot pain (*Figure H*). The nails are often short and broad (*Figure K*).

DERMATOGLYPHICS: In one study [7] it was noted that these patients have a high incidence of distal triradii, hypothenar patterns, and tall, vertically aligned digit loops.

SKIN: Areas of subcutaneous ossification often give rise to shallow depressions of the skin of the abdomen beneath which the calcium is easily felt. Ossification is frequently palpable in the Achilles tendons and the tendons at the wrist. These areas are more easily seen radiographically than they are detected by palpation (*Figure D*).

HEIGHT: The average adult height is 56 inches (143 cm) [8].

WEIGHT: Obesity is common in patients of all ages. Their obesity is often very striking in infancy [8].

Nervous System

Most patients are mildly to moderately retarded. Impairment of olfaction and of the tastes of sour and bitter have been reported [9].

Pathology

The parathyroid and thyroid glands have been normal if the patient's serum calcium was normal, but have been hyperplastic in appearance if the patient's serum calcium was below normal [1,3].

Laboratory Studies

The plasma level of parathyroid hormone is elevated when the serum calcium level is subnormal. An excessive amount of thyrocalcitonin is present in the thyroid gland, but this is thought to be due to storage, since with prolonged hypocalcemia there is no call for its secretion [4]. There is a defective phosphaturic response to intravenous parathyroid hormone. However, this response does not always clearly differentiate these patients from normal individuals. Good differentiation is provided by the decreased urinary excretion of cyclic 3′,5′-AMP following the infusion of parathyroid hormone. This is a reflection of the patients' poor response to the hormone, which is normally mediated through activation of adenyl cyclase [5]. X-rays often show calcification of basal ganglia and soft tissues (*Figures D and L*). The metacarpals, metatarsals, and phalanges are broad and shortened owing to premature closure of the epiphyses (*Figures H and I*).

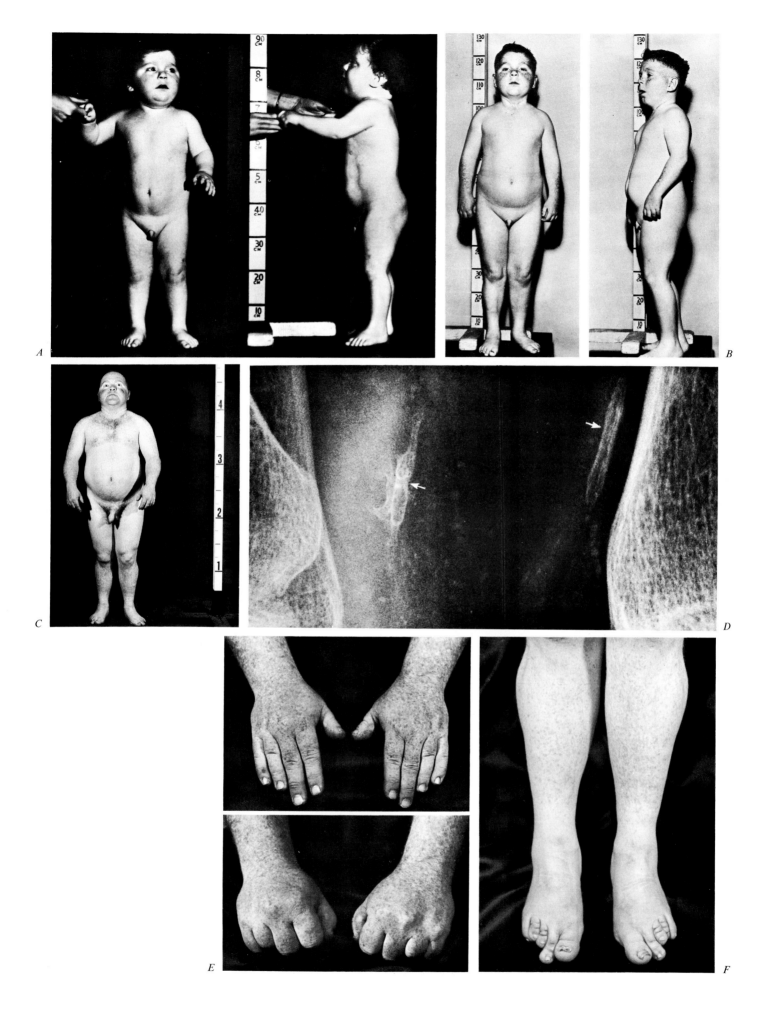

Plate I-23. *A–F:* This man was case 3 in the original report by Albright and coworkers [1]. He is shown at 3 years 3 months of age, at 9 years, and 30 years. At each age he had a round face and was moderately obese. The tracheotomy scar resulted from emergency surgery for laryngospasm; this occurred before his hypocalcemia had been recognized. The shortness of his thumb, fourth finger, and third and fourth toes became more evident as he grew older. Note in *E*

(*bottom*) the absence of the knuckle for the ring fingers. The x-rays show two views of an area of subcutaneous ossification (*arrows*). In the x-ray on the right it is shown in front of the lower end of the tibia and fibula. Note the trabecular pattern in this area of ectopic ossification. (*A* [*left*]: From F. Albright *et al., Endocrinology,* **30**:922–32, 1942. *D:* Courtesy of Dr. S. M. Krane, Boston, Mass.)

Treatment and Prognosis

Patients with hypocalcemia may have seizures, tetany, and laryngospasm. A normal serum calcium can be maintained in most patients by treatment with high doses of vitamin D and calcium supplements. Thyroidectomy does not improve, and may aggravate, the hypocalcemia [4].

Genetics

X-linked dominant inheritance has usually been postulated. However, autosomal dominant inheritance has also been suggested [10].

Differential Diagnosis

1. Brachydactyly with shortening of both the phalanges and metacarpals, obesity, and a round face are features of patients with type E brachydactyly, but they do not have cataracts, mental retardation, or subcutaneous ossification [11].
2. Hypoparathyroidism, basal ganglia calcifications, and cataracts are features of patients with the syndrome of multiple endocrine deficiencies, pernicious anemia, and moniliasis (candidiasis), but they also have moniliasis and adrenal insufficiency [12].
3. A short fourth metacarpal and short stature are features of females with Turner's (45,X) syndrome, but they also have associated anomalies, such as pterygium colli and streak gonads, as well as the chromosome abnormality (see page 178).
4. Short stature and digits, dental caries, and mental retardation are features of patients with pycnodysostosis, but they have increased bone density, multiple fractures, and small facial bones (see page 266).

5. Calcification of the basal ganglions alone can occur as an autosomal dominant disorder. These patients have no known endocrine abnormalities; their response to parathormone is normal [13].

References

1. Albright, F., Burnett, C. H., Smith, P. H., and Parson, W. Pseudo-hypoparathyroidism—an example of "Seabright-bantam syndrome": report of three cases. *Endocrinology,* **30:**922–32, 1942.
2. Albright, F., Forbes, A. P., and Henneman, P. H. Pseudo-pseudohypoparathyroidism. *Trans. Assoc. Am. Physicians,* **65:**337–50, 1952.
3. Mann, J. B., Alterman, S., and Hills, A. G. Albright's hereditary osteodystrophy comprising pseudohypoparathyroidism and pseudo-pseudohypoparathyroidism. *Ann. Intern. Med.,* **56:**315–42, 1962.
4. Lee, J. B., Tashjian, A. H., Jr., Streeto, J. M., and Frantz, A. G. Familial pseudohypoparathyroidism. Role of parathyroid hormone and thyrocalcitonin. *N. Engl. J. Med.,* **279:**1179–84, 1968.
5. Chase, L. R., Melson, G. L., and Aurbach, G. D. Pseudohypoparathyroidism: defective excretion of 3',5'-AMP in response to parathyroid hormone. *J. Clin. Invest.,* **48:**1832–44, 1969.
6. Ritchie, G. M. Dental manifestations of pseudohypoparathyroidism. *Arch. Dis. Child.,* **40:**565–72, 1965.
7. Forbes, A. P. Fingerprints and palm prints (dermatoglyphics) and palmar-flexion creases in gonadal dysgenesis, pseudohypoparathyroidism and Klinefelter's syndrome. *N. Engl. J. Med.,* **270:**1268–77, 1964.
8. Forbes, A. P. Données récentes sur le pseudohypoparathyroidisme, in *Problèmes Actuels d'Endocrinologie et de Nutrition,* No. 6, H. P. Klotz and J. Tremolieres (eds.), L'Expansion Scientifique Français, 1962, p. 111.
9. Henkin, R. I. Impairment of olfaction and of the tastes of sour and bitter in pseudohypoparathyroidism. *J. Clin. Endocrinol. Metab.,* **28:**624–28, 1968.
10. Weinberg, A. G., and Stone, R. T. Autosomal dominant inheritance in Albright's hereditary osteodystrophy. *J. Pediatr.,* **79:**996–99, 1971.
11. McKusick, V. A., and Milch, R. A. The clinical behavior of genetic disease: selected aspects. *Clin. Orthop.,* **33:**22–39, 1964.
12. Morse, W. I., Cochrane, W. A., and Landrigan, P. L. Familial hypoparathyroidism with pernicious anemia, steatorrhea and adrenocortical insufficiency. A variant of mucoviscidosis. *N. Engl. J. Med.,* **264:**1021–26, 1961.
13. Moskowitz, M. A., Winickoff, R. V., and Heinz, E. R. Familial calcification of the basal ganglions. A metabolic and genetic study. *N. Engl. J. Med.,* **285:**72–77, 1971.

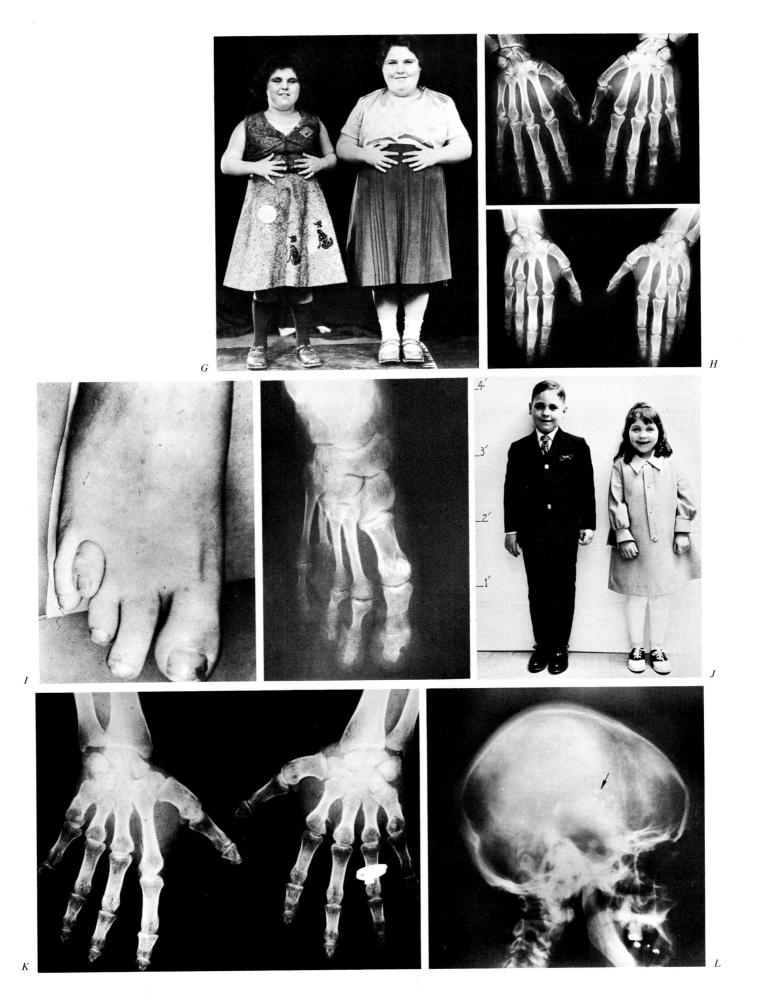

Plate I-23. *G–I:* Two sisters, 10 and 13 years old. Both were short, obese, and had a round face. The younger (*left*) had marked shortening of her fourth metatarsal and proximal placement of the fourth toe, which was quite painful and was removed. Their hand x-rays as adults show marked differences in the amount of shortening of the metacarpals, which was more extensive in the older girl. For many years only the older girl was hypocalcemic; later, her sister also developed hypocalcemia. *J:* A brother and sister with round faces, short fingers, hypocalcemia, ectopic calcifications of soft tissues, and mental retardation. *K:* An x-ray of the hands of the mother of these two children, showing shortening of all metacarpals and phalanges. She also had pseudohypoparathyroidism. *L:* Shows calcification of the basal ganglia (*arrow*), which may be present in patients with either hypoparathyroidism or pseudohypoparathyroidism. (*G:* Courtesy of Dr. J. D. Crawford, Boston, Mass. *J* and *K:* From J. B. Lee *et al.*, *N. Engl. J. Med.,* **279:**1179–84, 1968.)

Syndrome of Hypercalcemia, Elfin Facies, Supravalvular Aortic Stenosis, and Mental Retardation

In 1952 several investigators described infants with a syndrome characterized by failure to thrive, hypercalcemia, and an elfinlike facial appearance [1]. In 1961 the syndrome of an elfin face, supravalvular aortic stenosis, and mental retardation was first reported [2]. Soon patients with features of both syndromes were described and it appeared that they were in fact a single disorder [3]. Experience has shown that this syndrome may be either quite mild and hard to recognize or severe and easily identified. Experimental studies have suggested that the craniofacial and cardiovascular malformations may be related to a derangement in vitamin D metabolism during pregnancy [4]. More than 250 patients have been reported [5].

Physical Features

HEAD: A few patients with the severe form of infantile hypercalcemia have a small head as a result of premature closure of several sutures.

FACE: The elfin facies is striking and memorable, but difficult to describe. Among the features are a short, upturned nose, widely spaced eyes, epicanthic folds, full cheeks, a wide mouth, and a small chin [6] (*Figures A, C, E, and F*).

EARS: The ears tend to be low-set, and stand out from the head. The upper helix may be somewhat pointed.

MOUTH: The teeth may be small and the enamel hypoplastic. Often the lateral incisors and second premolars are absent. The mandible is hypoplastic and malocclusion is common [6].

CHEST: Systolic murmurs are frequently heard over the aortic area and throughout the lung fields.

GENITALIA: Males often have undescended testes.

HEIGHT: The more severely affected patients usually have subnormal height.

WEIGHT: The birth weight of severely affected infants is below the mean for their gestational age [1]. Failure to thrive in infancy is common.

Nervous System

As the classification of patients based on the severity of the disease suggests, some have normal intelligence and others are severely retarded. In general, the patients with the severe form are mildly to moderately retarded with IQ's between 40 and 70 [1]. Muscular hypotonia in infancy has been described in several patients.

Pathology

The most common cardiac anomalies are supravalvular aortic stenosis (*Figure D*) and peripheral pulmonary artery stenosis. Aortic hypoplasia, mitral insufficiency, and renal artery stenosis have also been described [6,7].

Laboratory Studies

In patients with the mild form of infantile hypercalcemia the only x-ray finding may be transverse bands of increased density in the metaphyses. In severely affected children there may be an increase in density at the metaphyses of the long bones, at the base of the skull (*Figure B*), and in the orbital regions. Deposits of calcium may be present in the kidneys, brain, blood vessels, and bronchi. Occasionally craniosynostosis and osteoporosis of the metaphyses are present [1]. An inability to concentrate the urine is often associated with hypercalcemia and may be severe enough to suggest vasopressin-insensitive diabetes insipidus.

Genetics

No affected siblings or parents have been reported.

Treatment and Prognosis

The hypercalcemia may last a few months or even years, but always disappears eventually without treatment. Patients with the severe form often die in the first years of life, usually from renal insufficiency [1].

Differential Diagnosis

Supravalvular aortic stenosis occurs in sporadic cases and sometimes is also transmitted as an autosomal dominant trait. While the associated vascular lesions are similar to those of this syndrome, there is no hypercalcemia, mental retardation, or elfin facies [8].

References

1. Fraser, D., Kidd, B. S. L., Kooh, S. W., and Paunier, L. A new look at infantile hypercalcemia. *Pediatr. Clin. North Am.,* **13**:503–25, 1966.
2. Williams, J. C. P., Barratt-Boyes, B. G., and Lowe, J. B. Supravalvular aortic stenosis. *Circulation,* **24**:1311–18, 1961.
3. Black, J. A., and Bonham Carter, R. E. Association between aortic stenosis and facies of severe infantile hypercalcemia. *Lancet,* **2**:745–49, 1963.
4. Friedman, W. F., and Mills, L. F. The relationship between vitamin D and the craniofacial and dental anomalies of the supravalvular aortic stenosis syndrome. *Pediatrics,* **43**:12–18, 1969.
5. Ebeling, J., Bette, L., and Schiefer, I. Ein weiterer Beitrag zu den kardiovaskulären Veränderungen und der Klinik defektgeheilter infantiler Hyperkalzämien (Williams-Beuren-Syndrom). *Arch. Kinderheilkd.,* **180**:1–14, 1969.
6. Beuren, A. J., Schulze, C., Eberle, P., Harmjanz, D., and Apitz, J. The syndrome of supravalvular aortic stenosis, peripheral pulmonary stenosis, mental retardation and similar facial appearance. *Am. J. Cardiol.,* **13**:471–83, 1964.
7. Vazquez, A. M., Zuberbuhler, J. S., and Kenny, F. M. Mitral insufficiency in association with the syndrome of idiopathic hypercalcemia of infancy. *J. Pediatr.,* **73**:907–10, 1968.
8. McCue, C. M., Spicuzza, T. J., Robertson, L. W., and Mauck, H. P., Jr. Familial supravalvular aortic stenosis. *J. Pediatr.,* **73**:889–95, 1968.

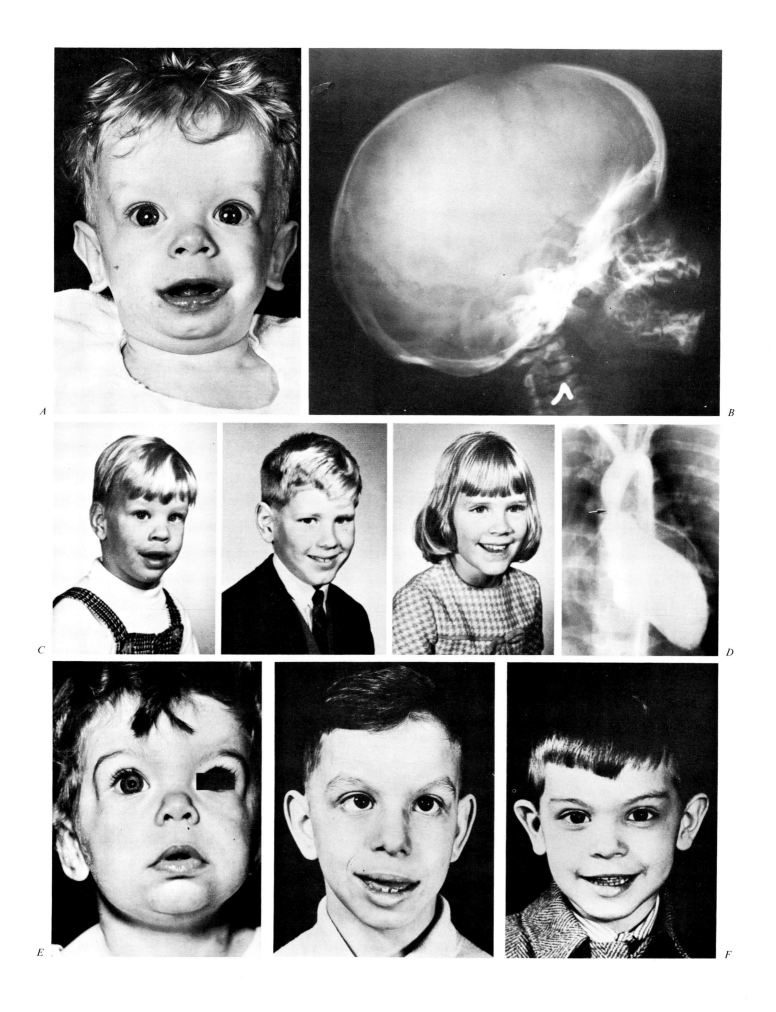

Plate I-24. *A* and *B:* An 11-month-old infant with an "elfin face" characterized by prominent brow, eyes and ears, a flat nasal bridge, and small chin. His skull x-ray shows basal sclerosis. *C* and *D:* The 6-year-old boy on the left has facial features which are similar to other patients with the hypercalcemia syndrome, in contrast to his normal brother (9 years) and sister (8 years), both of whom have normal intelligence. The x-ray during cardiac catheterization shows the area of supravalvular aortic stenosis (*arrow*) in this boy. *E:* An infant with an "elfin face" and hypercalcemia. *F:* This 7-year-old boy (*left*) has widely spaced eyes, strabismus, a broad mouth, and left facial weakness; he also had hypercalcemia and hyperostosis of his skull and long bones. He is shown with his normal younger brother. (*A* and *B:* From N. J. David *et al., Am. J. Med.,* **33:**88–110, 1962. *E:* Courtesy of Dr. J. D. Crawford, Boston, Mass. *F* [*left*]: From A. M. Vazquez *et al., J. Pediatr.,* **73:**907–10, 1968, *F* [*right*]: Courtesy of Dr. F. M. Kenny, Pittsburgh, Pa.)

Syndrome of Macroglossia, Omphalocele, Visceromegaly, and Neonatal Hypoglycemia (Beckwith-Wiedemann Syndrome)

In 1963 Beckwith [1] reported three infants with a syndrome that consisted of omphalocele, macroglossia, hyperplasia of several organs, and hypoglycemia. Wiedemann [2] described three siblings with the same syndrome in 1964. Subsequently, more than 60 patients have been reported, and several have been identified in the earlier medical literature [3–9,9a,9b].

Physical Features

HEAD: Fifteen of 59 reported patients were microcephalic [9a]. Others have had a normal head size and a prominent occiput [6,8].

FACE: A facial resemblance has been noted [6] and consists of midfacial recession, slight exophthalmos, and ridges in the frontal bone (*Figures B and D*).

EARS: One or two linear indentations are often present on the earlobe [4,6] (*Figure E*).

MOUTH: Most patients have muscular enlargement of the tongue at birth (*Figures A and C*), which may be large enough to cause respiratory obstruction. Postnatal growth of the mouth usually compensates at least partially for the large tongue. Older children may have prognathism and malocclusion.

ABDOMEN: An omphalocele or occasionally an umbilical hernia and marked enlargement of the kidneys are usually present at birth (*Figure A*). Enlargement of the liver has also been reported.

GENITALIA: Males are often cryptorchid. A few females have had a large clitoris [8].

LIMBS: A few reported patients had hypertrophy of a limb or an entire half of the body [8].

SKIN: Most newborns have a ruddy, red color because of polycythemia. Many patients have a flame nevus often in the center of the forehead and on the upper eyelids.

HEIGHT AND WEIGHT: At birth the body length is normal, but the weight is usually above average [3]. The subsequent body size is usually above the 90th percentile of normal [6,8,9].

Nervous System

A mild to moderate degree of mental retardation has been a feature of some patients [3,5,9], while others have had normal intelligence [6,8]. Both the retardation and microcephaly may be secondary to neonatal hypoglycemia.

Pathology

Adrenal cortex cytomegaly and renal medullary dysplasia, characterized by a relative increase in stroma and immature, widely separated ducts, are two principal features. Another common finding is hyperplasia of several endocrine organs with involvement of pancreatic acinar and islet cells, gonad interstitial cells, pituitary amphophil cells, and paraganglion cells. A few patients had associated malignancies, such as a Wilms' tumor and adrenal carcinoma [3].

Laboratory Studies

Severe, prolonged neonatal hypoglycemia has been noted in several patients [3,5,7]. A few have also had hypocalcemia [5]. Infants with hypoglycemia may also have hyperinsulinism; older patients usually do not have either hypoglycemia or hyperinsulinism [1,5,8]. Hyperlipemia has also been reported [10]. Posterior eventration of the diaphragm was present in 3 of 11 patients in one study [6] (*Figure F*).

Treatment and Prognosis

The recognition and treatment of hypoglycemia in infants seem to be important determinants of ultimate intelligence. The persistent muscular macroglossia in some older children requires surgical resection.

Genetics

The fact that affected siblings have been reported [2,6] (*Figure B*) suggests that this disease is genetically determined, probably autosomal recessive.

Differential Diagnosis

1. Macroglossia, a depressed nasal bridge, and an umbilical hernia are features of patients with congenital hypothyroidism, but this is usually ruled out by the absence of hypotonia, mottling and constipation, and a normal thyroxine level (see page 10).
2. Hemihypertrophy is a feature of the Silver-Russell syndrome (see page 310) and neurofibromatosis (see page 366), but each is easily differentiated by other associated physical features.
3. A ruddy color, increased birth weight, and hypoglycemia are features of infants of diabetic mothers, but they do not have either macroglossia or omphalocele.

References

1. Beckwith, J. B.   Extreme cytomegaly of the adrenal fetal cortex, omphalocele, hyperplasia of kidneys and pancreas, and Leydig-cell hyperplasia: another syndrome? Presented at Annual Meeting of Western Society for Pediatric Research, Los Angeles, California, November 11, 1963.
2. Wiedemann, H.-R.   Complexe malformatif familial avec hernie ombilicale et macroglossie. Un "syndrome nouveau"? *J. Genet. Hum.,* **13**:223–32, 1964.
3. Beckwith, J. B.   Macroglossia, omphalocele, adrenal cytomegaly, gigantism, and hyperplastic visceromegaly. *Birth Defects: Original Article Series,* Vol. V, No. 2, February, 1969, pp. 188–96. Williams & Wilkins Co., Baltimore.
4. Wiedemann, H.-R.   Das EMG-Syndrom: Exomphalos, Makroglossie, Gigantismus und Kohlenhydratstoffwechsel-Störung. *Z. Kinderheilkd.,* **106**:171–85, 1969.
5. Combs, J. T., Grunt, J. A., and Brandt, I. K.   New syndrome of neonatal hypoglycemia. Association with visceromegaly, macroglossia, microcephaly and abnormal umbilicus. *N. Engl. J. Med.,* **275**:236–43, 1966.
6. Irving, I. M.   Exomphalos with macroglossia: a study of eleven cases. *J. Pediatr. Surg.,* **2**:499–507, 1967.
7. Mariani, R., Unal, D., Spriet, A., Carcassonne, M., and Bernard, R.   Hypoglycémie du nouveau-né avec microcéphalie, macroglossie et mégalosplanchnie. *Arch. Fr. Pediatr.,* **26**:337–45, 1969.
8. Filippi, G., and McKusick, V. A.   The Beckwith-Wiedemann syndrome (the exomphalos-macroglossia-gigantism syndrome). Report of two cases and review of the literature. *Medicine (Baltimore),* **49**:279–98, 1970.
9. Sotelo-Avila, C., and Singer, D. B.   Syndrome of hyperplastic fetal visceromegaly and neonatal hypoglycemia (Beckwith's syndrome). *Pediatrics,* **46**:240–51, 1970.
9a. Cohen, M. M., Jr., Gorlin, R. J., Feingold, M., and ten Bensel, R. W.   The Beckwith-Wiedemann syndrome. Seven new cases. *Am. J. Dis. Child.,* **122**:515–19, 1971.
9b. Eaton, A. P., and Maurer, W. F.   The Beckwith-Wiedemann syndrome. *Am. J. Dis. Child.,* **122**:520–25, 1971.
10. Wiedemann, H.-R.   E.M.G. syndrome and carbohydrate metabolism. *Lancet,* **2**:104–105, 1968.

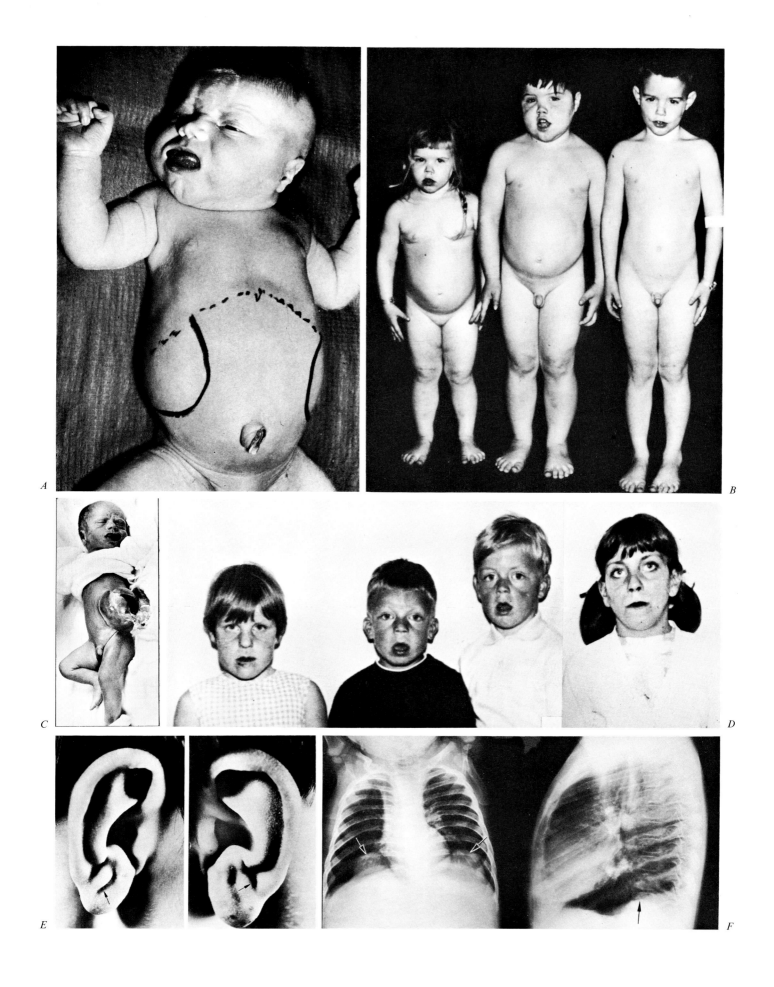

Plate I-25. *A* and *B:* A 2-day-old infant with a large protruding tongue, large kidneys outlined on his abdomen, and a small umbilical hernia. He is also shown at 4 years standing between his affected 2-year-old sister and unaffected 5-year-old brother. Both the boy and the girl are large for their ages and have a round face with a prominent skin fold from the nose to the upper portion of the cheeks. All three children have normal intelligence. *C:* An infant with a protruding tongue and omphalocele. *D:* Four unrelated children, aged 4 to 8½ years, with a similar facial appearance. They also had a midfrontal ridge. These four children are all of normal intelligence. *E:* Shows the linear indentations in the earlobes (*arrows*). *F:* Anteroposterior and right lateral chest x-ray showing the domelike eventration of the diaphragm (*arrows*). (*A* and *B:* Courtesy of Dr. J. P. Connelly, Boston, Mass. *C:* From H.–R. Wiedemann *et al., Z. Kinderheilkd.,* **102:**1–36, 1968. *D:* From H.–R. Wiedemann, *M. Kinderheilkd.,* **117:**239–42, 1969. *E* and *F:* From I. M. Irving, *J. Pediatr. Surg.,* **2:**499–507, 1967.)

Syndrome of Microcephaly, Hypogonadism, and Mental Deficiency (Börjeson-Forssman-Lehmann Syndrome)

In 1961 and 1962 Börjeson, Forssman, and Lehmann [1,2] described three related men with a syndrome characterized by microcephaly, hypogonadism, short stature, and severe mental deficiency. In 1965 Baar and Galindo [3] described one patient whom they considered to have the same syndrome.

Physical Features

HEAD: All of the patients were microcephalic.

FACE: They had excessive subcutaneous fat on the face and narrow palpebral fissures (*Figures A, B, and C*).

EARS: The ears were large (*Figures A and D*).

CHEST: The breasts were enlarged, presumably due to the accumulation of fat (*Figures B and E*).

ABDOMEN: Each of the adult patients had a marked abundance of abdominal fat (*Figure B*).

GENITALIA: Each had a very small penis. The testes were palpable in only two of the four patients and were soft and very small.

BACK: One patient had marked kyphoscoliosis [3].

LIMBS: All had a genu valgum deformity.

SKIN: There was little or no pubic and axillary hair.

HEIGHT: The heights at ages 16 to 39 years ranged from 136 to 156 cm.

Nervous System

All four patients were severely retarded, with the intelligence quotients of three of them estimated to be between 20 and 40 [1,3]. All had seizures throughout their lives.

Pathology

Two patients had postmortem examinations. In one no gross brain deformity was observed. However, gliosis was observed in the cortex and white matter, and the number of ganglion cells in the cortex was diminished [2]. The patient reported by Baar and Galindo [3] had an asymmetric skull and brain. The smaller left side of the brain showed atrophy of the central gray matter and dilatation of the lateral ventricle. Extensive demyelinization and loss of neurons was noted in both hemispheres. His breasts consisted of fibrous tissue and scattered lactiferous ducts. The testes showed many seminiferous tubules that were completely hyalinized and some that contained only Sertoli cells. The interstitial tissue contained few Leydig cells.

Laboratory Studies

Two patients had low urinary 17-ketosteroid and gonadotropin levels [2]. Protein-bound iodine, radioactive iodine uptakes, chromosome analyses, and urinary amino acid patterns were normal [2,3].

Treatment and Prognosis

One patient died at age 20 years of bronchopneumonia [2], and another [3] died suddenly at age 39 years, presumably of aspiration during a seizure.

Genetics

The three males in one family were all related through female members, two being half-brothers and the third their maternal uncle. Three females in this family had moderate mental deficiency (*Figure F*). It was suggested that this syndrome is due to an X-linked recessive mutant gene [1,2].

Differential Diagnosis

1. Hypogonadism, gynecomastia, and mental retardation are features of patients with Klinefelter's (XXY) syndrome (see page 184), the XXXXY syndrome (see page 190), and the syndrome of testicular deficiency and mental retardation (see page 60). Each of these can be differentiated by either the associated physical features or chromosome analysis.
2. Hypogonadism and mental retardation are features of the Laurence-Moon syndrome (see page 288), the syndrome of ichthyosis and hypogonadism (see page 378), and myotonic dystrophy (see page 106).

References

1. Börjeson, M., Forssman, H., and Lehmann, O. Combination of idiocy, epilepsy, hypogonadism, dwarfism, hypometabolism and morphologic peculiarities inherited as an X-linked recessive syndrome. *Proc. 2nd Int. Congr. Ment. Retard.,* Vienna (1961), Part I, pp. 188–92, 1963.
2. Börjeson, M., Forssman, H., and Lehmann, O. An X-linked, recessively inherited syndrome characterized by grave mental deficiency, epilepsy and endocrine disorder. *Acta Med. Scand.,* **171**:13–21, 1962.
3. Baar, H. S., and Galindo, J. The Borjeson-Forssman-Lehmann syndrome. *J. Ment. Defic. Res.,* **9**:125–30, 1965.

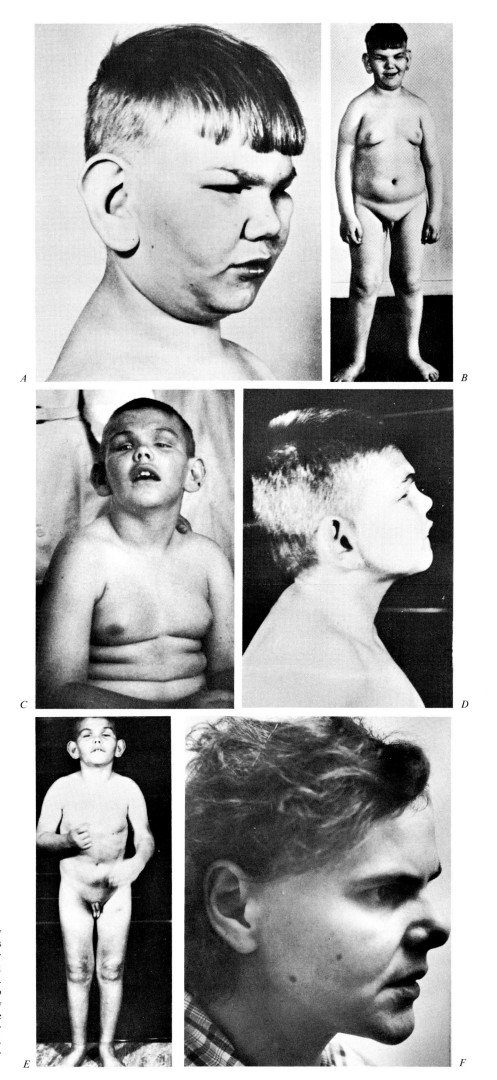

Plate I-26. *A* and *B:* A 16-year-old obese boy with prominent subcutaneous tissue under his eyes, small penis, and undescended testes. *C–E:* The 18-year-old half-brother of the first patient; they had the same mother, but different fathers. He had similar physical features and had no signs of sexual maturation. *F:* The moderately retarded maternal aunt of these two boys. She had no physical abnormalities. (*A, B, D–F:* From M. Börjeson *et al., Acta Med. Scand.,* **171:**13–21, 1962. *C:* Courtesy of Dr. H. Forssman, St. Jörgen, Sweden.)

Syndrome of Testicular Deficiency and Mental Retardation (Sohval-Soffer Syndrome)

In 1953 Sohval and Soffer [1] reported two brothers with hypogonadism, diabetes mellitus, skeletal anomalies, and mental retardation. They were considered to represent a new syndrome.

Physical Features

THROAT: One had a masculine voice; the other's voice was in the contralto range.

CHEST: Both men had enlarged breasts, part of which was attributed to glandular tissue (*Figures A and D*).

GENITALIA: The penis was small. The testes were soft and small, measuring 1.5 cm in their largest dimension.

LIMBS: One brother had cubitus valgus (*Figure A*).

SKIN: The facial and pubic hair was sparse.

HEIGHT: Their heights as adults were $63\frac{1}{2}$ and 68 inches (163 and 174 cm) with arm spans of $63\frac{1}{4}$ and $66\frac{1}{4}$ inches (162 and 170 cm), respectively.

Nervous System

Both men had poor scholastic records. When studied as adults, they were psychotic and had subnormal intelligence. One had a full-scale IQ of 56. Neither man had anosmia.

Pathology

Bilateral testicular biopsies in both patients showed small hyalinized seminiferous tubules and larger tubules with germinal aplasia (*Figures B, C, E, and F*). One man also had areas of tubular fibrosis. His brother had striking accumulations of Leydig cells (*Figure E*).

Laboratory Studies

Both men had a marked elevation of chorionic gonadotropins in the urine. Sperm analysis could not be performed, because neither man was able to ejaculate. The 17-ketosteroid levels in the urine were normal (11.1 mg per 24 hours) in one man and below normal (2.9 mg per 24 hours) in the other. Both had hyperglycemia and glucosuria. Both had bilateral cervical ribs. In addition, one had multiple anomalies of the cervical vertebrae, including atlantooccipital fusion and partial fusion of the spinous processes and posterior articulations of the second and third vertebrae. Both men had a chromatin-negative buccal smear [2].

Genetics

It is presumed that this syndrome is hereditary. A maternal aunt and three maternal cousins of these two patients were mentally deficient.

Differential Diagnosis

1. Hypogonadism, gynecomastia, and mental deficiency are also features of patients with Klinefelter's syndrome, but they have 47,XXY karyotype, hyalinized seminiferous tubules, increased height, and less severe mental deficiency (see page 184).
2. Hypogonadism and mental retardation are also features of the XXXXY syndrome (see page 190), the Laurence-Moon syndrome (see page 288), myotonic dystrophy (see page 106), the syndrome of ichthyosis and hypogonadism (see page 378) and the syndrome of microcephaly, hypogonadism, and mental deficiency (Börjeson-Forssman-Lehmann syndrome, see page 58), but each of these diseases can usually be distinguished by the other associated physical features.
3. Several familial syndromes with primary hypogonadism in phenotypic males have been described, but each can be distinguished by the associated physical features and the testicular tubule changes [3].

References

1. Sohval, A. R., and Soffer, L. J. Congenital familial testicular deficiency. *Am. J. Med.*, **14**:328–48, 1953.
2. Sohval, A. R. Personal communication, 1970.
3. Weinstein, R. L., Kliman, B., and Scully, R. E. Familial syndrome of primary testicular insufficiency with normal virilization, blindness, deafness and metabolic abnormalities. *N. Engl. J. Med.*, **281**:969–77, 1969.

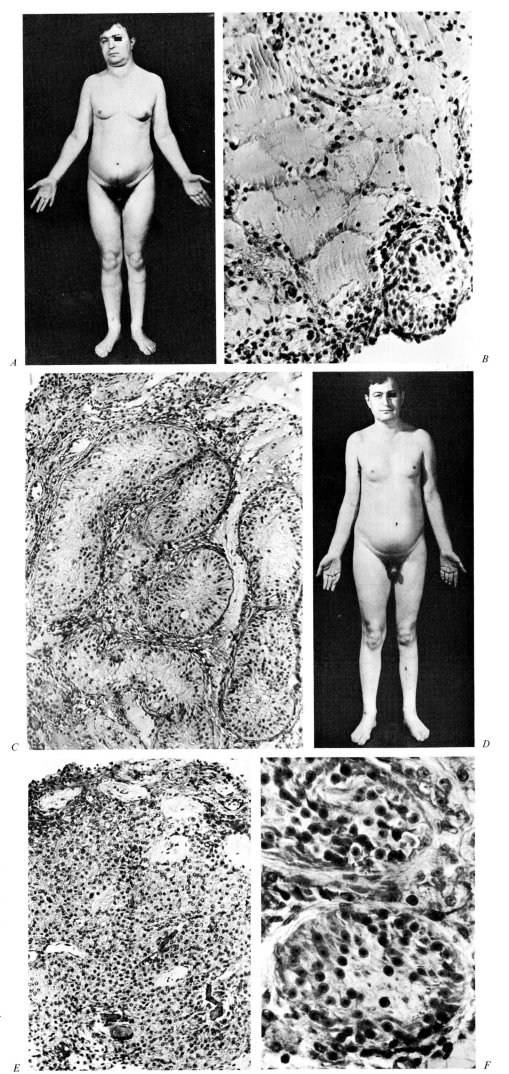

Plate I-27. *A:* A 36-year-old man with gynecomastia, cubitus valgus, and feminine pattern of pubic hair. He also had a small penis and testes. *B:* A photomicrograph of his testes biopsy showing "ghost tubules" with solid, fibrotic, and hyalinized remnants of former tubules in the center. The lower area shows tubules which contain only Sertoli cells (× 180). *C:* Shows another area of the testis biopsy with small seminiferous tubules containing only Sertoli cells (× 109). *D:* The 47-year-old brother of the first patient, with gynecomastia and a similar pubic hair pattern. *E:* Photomicrograph of the testis biopsy of the second patient showing aggregates of Leydig cells and several "ghost tubules" (× 156). *F:* A close-up view of two tubules showing that they contain only Sertoli cells (× 255). (*A–F:* From A. R. Sohval and L. J. Soffer, *Am. J. Med.,* **14:**328–48, 1953.)

Tay-Sachs Disease (G_{M2} Gangliosidosis, Familial Amaurotic Idiocy)

In 1881 Tay [1] described a 12-month-old child who had difficulty holding up its head and moving its extremities. He also noted in the macula a large white patch with a brownish-red spot in its center. Six years later Sachs [2] reported a 2-year-old girl with similar findings. It is now recognized that this disorder is associated with deficient activity of the enzyme hexosaminidase A [3]. The majority of cases occur in Jews. Among Jews in the United States the incidence is $1:6000$ births [4].

Physical Features

HEAD: Initially the head size is normal. Infants who survive for 2 years or longer have generalized head enlargement.

EYES: A cherry-red macular spot can first be detected at about $2\frac{1}{2}$ months of age (*Figure A*). In almost all cases it is fully developed between 6 and 12 months of age. Vision is preserved up to 9 to 11 months, but it deteriorates rapidly thereafter, and usually by 15 months of age the children no longer follow light. Atrophy of the optic nerve head usually develops after the first year [5].

Nervous System

Motor development is usually normal until 5 months of age. Almost always from the sixth month on there is progressive failure to acquire new skills, and loss of previously acquired skills (*Figures B and C*). A frequent finding is an exaggerated motor response to sound, consisting of an initial upward extension of the arms with flexion and/or extension of the legs, a startled facial appearance, and occasionally a shrill cry. Excessive drooling and brief bouts of unmotivated laughter occur. There are focal or generalized convulsions in almost all patients after the first year. The muscles are initially hypotonic, and the deep tendon reflexes are normal. After the first two years spasticity and rigidity are present and the reflexes are usually hyperactive [5].

Pathology

During the first 14 months of life the brain is either normal or slightly atrophic in appearance. Thereafter, the brain becomes progressively larger, owing mainly to edema and gliosis of the white matter (*Figure D*). Microscopically, the most striking feature is distention of neuronal cytoplasm due to lipid accumulation (*Figure E*). With the electron microscope concentrically laminated bodies are demonstrable within the neurons [5] (*Figure F*).

Laboratory Studies

There is a 3- to 10-fold excess of total gangliosides and sialic acid in all tissues. Ninety percent of the ganglioside in Tay-Sachs brain is G_{M2} ganglioside, which is normally present only in trace amounts. (*See Figure I-9F*, page 23). In patients with Tay-Sachs disease one of two components of the degradative enzyme hexosaminidase, component A, is absent in brain, liver, kidney, skin, plasma, and leukocytes [3].

Treatment and Prognosis

The disease is invariably progressive, with most children dying between 2 and 4 years of age. Those who survive beyond 2 years remain in an essentially vegetative state. Death is often the result of aspiration pneumonia [5].

Genetics

Autosomal recessive. It has been estimated that 1 in 40 Ashkenazi Jews (i.e., Jews of central or eastern European origin) is heterozygous for the gene that causes Tay-Sachs disease. Among non-Ashkenazi Jews and all others in the United States, about 1 in 380 is heterozygous for the gene [4]. The serum hexosaminidase A level in heterozygotes is intermediate between that of affected children and normal controls [3]. Prenatal diagnosis of Tay-Sachs disease has been reported [6].

Differential Diagnosis

1. Several children with the clinical appearance of Tay-Sachs disease have been reported who show a complete deficiency of hexosaminidase. As in the classic form of the disease, these patients have an accumulation of G_{M2} ganglioside in the central nervous system, but in addition there is storage of globoside within visceral organs. These differences, as well as the non-Jewish heritage of these patients, allow them to be separated from the classic form of this disease [7].

2. G_{M2} ganglioside accumulation may also occur in children with a partial deficiency of hexosaminidase A and a later onset of symptoms. They show ataxia and signs of progressive psychomotor retardation at 2 to 5 years of age and die at 5 to 15. They do not develop a cherry-red spot or megalencephaly [8].

3. A macular cherry-red spot may also be present in G_{M1} gangliosidosis (see page 22) and Niemann-Pick disease (see page 44).

References

1. Tay, W. Symmetrical changes in the region of the yellow spot in each eye of an infant. *Trans. Ophthalmol. Soc. U.K.*, **1**:55–57, 1881.
2. Sachs, B. On arrested cerebral development with special reference to its cortical pathology. *J. Nerv. Ment. Dis.*, **14**:541–53, 1887.
3. O'Brien, J. S., Okada, S., Chen, A., and Fillerup, D. L. Tay-Sachs disease. Detection of heterozygotes and homozygotes by serum hexosaminidase assay. *N. Engl. J. Med.*, **283**:15–20, 1970.
4. Myrianthopoulos, N. C., and Aronson, S. M. Population dynamics of Tay-Sachs disease. I. Reproductive fitness and selection. *Am. J. Hum. Genet.*, **18**:313–27, 1966.
5. *Tay-Sachs' Disease*, Volk, B. W. (ed.). Grune & Stratton, New York, 1964.
6. Schneck, L., Friedland, J., Valenti, C., Adachi, M., Amsterdam, D., and Volk, B. W. Prenatal diagnosis of Tay-Sachs disease. *Lancet*, **1**:582–84, 1970.
7. Sandhoff, K., Andreae, U., and Jatzkewitz, H. Deficient hexosaminidase activity in an exceptional case of Tay-Sachs disease with additional storage of kidney globoside in visceral organs. *Pathol. Eur.*, **3**:278–85, 1968.
8. Suzuki, K., Suzuki, K., Rapin, I., Suzuki, Y., and Ishii, N. Juvenile G_{M2}-gangliosidosis. Clinical variant of Tay-Sachs disease or a new disease. *Neurology (Minneap.)*, **20**:190–204, 1970.

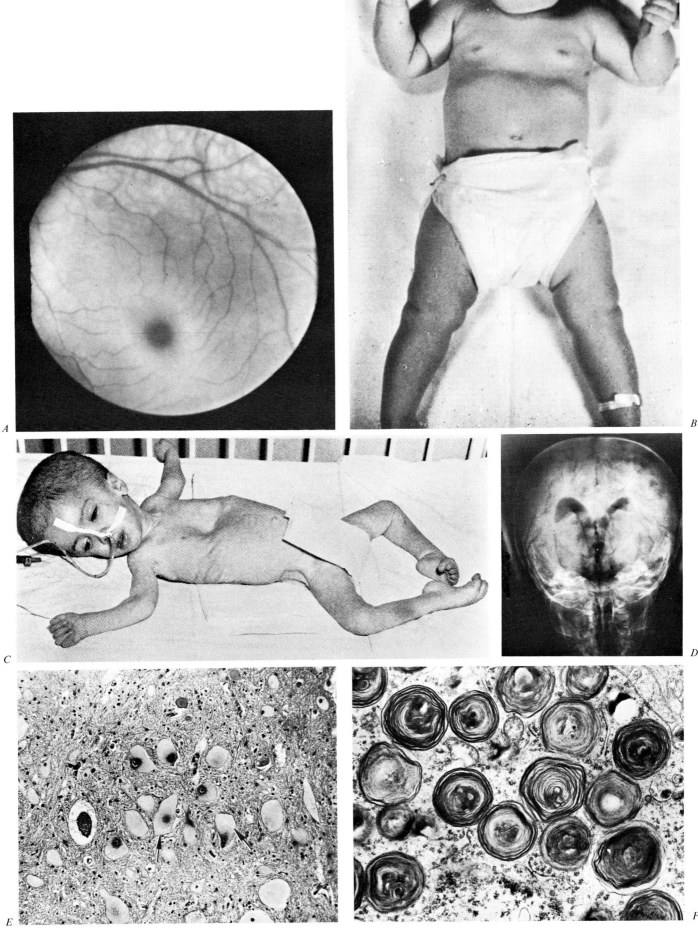

Plate I-28. *A:* The macular spot in the center of a large white patch. *B:* An 11-month-old child with motor retardation. *C:* A 3-year-old child with a large head and flaccid arms and legs. *D:* Pneumoencephalogram shows the increased thickness of the cerebral cortex and normal-size ventricles. *E:* A section of medulla showing distended neurons (*arrows*) with the nuclei displaced to the edge. *F:* Electronmicrograph showing the laminated membranous cytoplasmic bodies. (*A:* Courtesy of Dr. W. F. Hoyt, San Francisco, Calif. *B:* Courtesy of Dr. E. H. Kolodny, Waverley, Mass. *C* and *D:* From L. Schneck, in *Tay-Sachs Disease,* B. W. Volk [ed.], Grune & Stratton, New York, 1964. *E* and *F:* Courtesy of Dr. B. W. Volk, Brooklyn, N.Y.)

Wilson's Disease
(Progressive Hepatolenticular
Degeneration)

In 1912 Wilson [1] described six patients who suffered from progressive tremor, dysarthria, drooling, and rigidity. Pathologic examination revealed degeneration of the lenticular nucleus in the brain and cirrhosis of the liver. Later, pigmentation of the cornea was shown to be an important feature of the disease, and increased urinary excretion of copper and excessive amounts of copper in nervous system tissues were observed [2].

Physical Features

EYES: The Kayser-Fleischer ring of cornea pigment is the single most important diagnostic finding and when present is sufficient evidence for the diagnosis of Wilson's disease [2]. It consists of greenish-yellow or greenish-brown pigment on the undersurface of the cornea near its limbus (*Figure E*). The ring is not always complete, and is usually more marked on the superior and inferior aspects of the cornea than on the sides. It can usually be seen with the naked eye, but its presence cannot be excluded without slit lamp examination [3]. Although the Kayser-Fleischer ring is considered pathognomonic of Wilson's disease, its absence does not exclude this diagnosis [3a].

ABDOMEN: Cirrhosis of the liver is often the first manifestation of the disease, especially in children [3a]. In a series of 25 cases, 11 presented with either jaundice or hepatosplenomegaly [4]. Hemolytic anemia, bleeding, and easy bruising due to deficiencies of several clotting factors may occur. Signs of portal hypertension are frequently present.

Nervous System

The main findings are motor abnormalities; these are generally first noted between 10 and 20 years of age. Tremulousness, dysarthria, drooling (*Figure A*), and dystonic postures (*Figure B*) are common. A set expression of the face, with open mouth and stereotyped smile, is an early sign (*Figure C*). In some patients neurologic disability is not evident until the third or fourth decade and consists primarily of tremor and dysarthria. Early mental development is entirely normal. Progressive dementia may be evident as early as the school years or not until adulthood. Bizarre and disturbing psychiatric symptoms, such as paranoid delusions, may occur either early or late in the course of the illness [2,3].

Pathology

The putamen, and to a lesser extent the globus pallidus and caudate nucleus, are shrunken and discolored (*Figure D*). There are loss of neurons, glial overgrowth, and spongy degeneration in the cerebral cortex [4]. Cirrhosis of the liver is almost always present [3].

Laboratory Studies

The concentration of copper in several organs, particularly the liver, brain, and cornea, is 10 to 100 times normal [2]. Because of the importance of identifying the presymptomatic homozygous state, the laboratory diagnosis of Wilson's disease has been under intense investigation. The serum ceruloplasmin level is always below 20 mg per 100 ml, but this may also be found in individuals who never develop the disease. However, if, in an individual more than 6 months old, low serum ceruloplasmin levels are combined with increased copper excretion in the urine (more than 100 micrograms daily) and with an hepatic copper concentration in excess of 250 micrograms per gram of dry weight, the diagnosis of Wilson's disease is nearly certain [2,7].

Treatment and Prognosis

The use of the chelating agent D-penicillamine has been shown to improve the neurologic manifestations in almost all patients [5,6] (*Figure F*). The Kayser-Fleischer ring of corneal pigmentation usually diminishes or disappears with treatment. This treatment has also been recommended for patients who are apparently healthy but have the biochemical findings of Wilson's disease [7]. In a patient who could not tolerate D-penicillamine, triethylene tetramine dihydrochloride, which is also a chelating agent, was found to be effective [6].

Genetics

Autosomal recessive. The whole-body retention of intravenously injected ^{67}Cu is prolonged in individuals that are either heterozygous or homozygous for the gene that causes Wilson's disease, but does not distinguish between the two.

Differential Diagnosis

Wilson's disease must be distinguished from hepatitis or juvenile cirrhosis, and from neurologic or psychiatric disorders such as Hallervorden-Spatz disease (see page 94), dystonia musculorum deformans, multiple sclerosis, and schizophrenia. The Kayser-Fleischer ring is an important diagnostic clue, since almost all Wilson's disease patients who have had neurologic changes for over a year develop this abnormality.

References

1. Wilson, S. A. K. Progressive lenticular degeneration: a familial nervous disease associated with cirrhosis of the liver. *Brain,* **34**:295–509, 1912.
2. Scheinberg, I. H., and Sternlieb, I. Wilson's disease. *Annu. Rev. Med.,* **16**:119–34, 1965.
3. Bearn, A. G. Wilson's disease. In *The Metabolic Basis of Inherited Disease,* Stanbury, J. B., Wyngaarden, J. B., and Fredrickson, D. S. (eds.), 2nd ed. McGraw-Hill Book Co., New York, 1966, pp. 761–79.
3a. Slovis, T. L., Dubois, R. S., Rodgerson, D. O., and Silverman, A. The varied manifestations of Wilson's disease. *J. Pediatr.,* **78**:578–84, 1971.
4. Shiraki, H. Comparative neuropathologic study of Wilson's disease and other types of hepatocerebral disease. *Birth Defects: Original Article Series,* Vol. IV, No. 2, April, 1968, pp. 64–73, Williams & Wilkins Co., Baltimore.
5. Walshe, J. M. The physiology of copper in man and its relation to Wilson's disease. *Brain,* **90**:149–76, 1967.
6. Walshe, J. M. Management of penicillamine nephropathy in Wilson's disease: a new chelating agent. *Lancet,* **2**:1401–1402, 1969.
7. Sternlieb, I., and Scheinberg, I. H. Prevention of Wilson's disease in asymptomatic patients. *N. Engl. J. Med.,* **278**:352–59, 1968.
8. O'Reilly, S., Weber, P. M., Pollycove, M., and Shipley, L. Detection of the carrier of Wilson's disease. *Neurology (Minneap.),* **20**:1133–38, 1970.

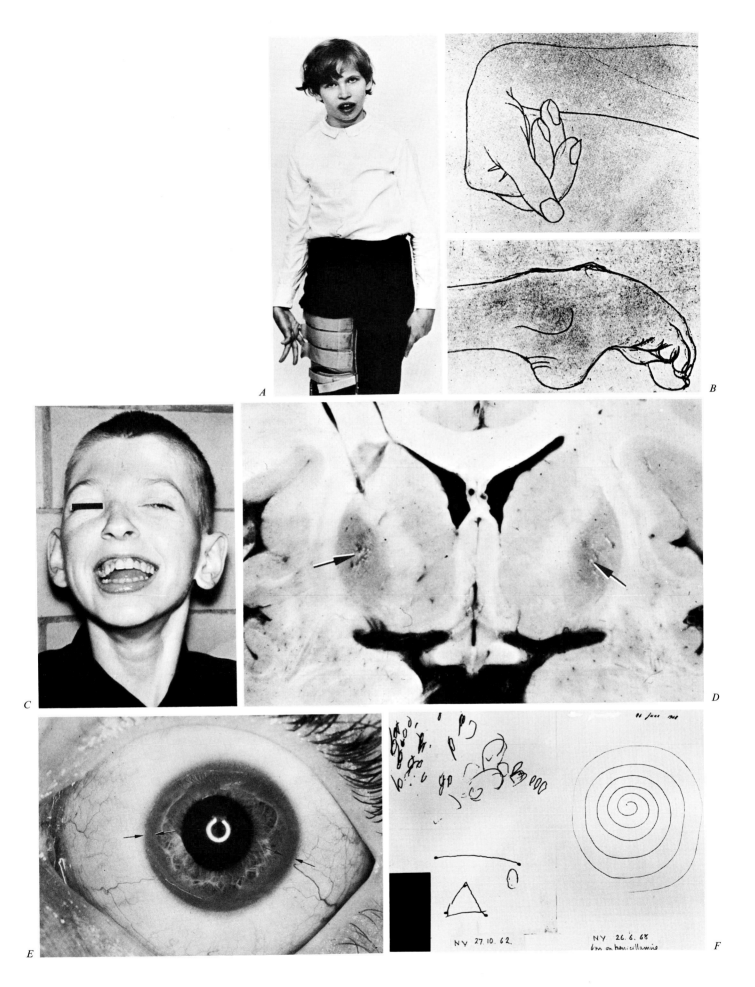

Plate I-29. *A:* A 15-year-old girl with drooling, a rigid facial expression, severe hyperextension and rigidity of the fingers of her right hand, and forced adduction of her left arm. The leg brace was used in an attempt to assist her in walking. *B:* The original drawings of Wilson, showing the characteristic hand and foot posture. *C:* A 12-year-old boy with a wide smile and athetoid hand posturing. He has the typical retraction of the upper lip, protrusion of the upper teeth, and deepening of the nasolabial folds. *D:* A section through the basal ganglia of another patient, showing the darkening of the putamen and globus pallidus (*arrows*). *E:* The brown Kayser-Fleischer ring (*arrows*) is evident even in this black-and-white print. The ring of pigment is heavier on the top and bottom of the iris. *F:* Shows the improvement in drawing in a patient before (*left*) and after (*right*) 6 years of treatment with penicillamine. (*A* and *E:* Courtesy of Drs. I. H. Scheinberg and I. Sternlieb, and Mr. M. Kurtz, Bronx, N.Y. *B:* From S. A. K. Wilson, *Brain,* **34:**295–509, 1912. *C* and *D:* Courtesy of Dr. G. R. Hogan, Boston, Mass. *F:* Courtesy of Dr. J. M. Walshe, Cambridge, England.)

65

Wolman's Disease
(Primary Familial Xanthomatosis
with Adrenal Involvement,
Acid Lipase Deficiency)

In 1956 Abramov, Schorr, and Wolman [1] described a 2-month-old infant who died with massive abdominal distention, hepatosplenomegaly, and large calcified adrenal glands. They identified the disorder as a lipidosis. Since then, 2 affected siblings of the first patient have been reported [2], as well as at least 20 other patients [3–5]. The metabolic basis of the disease has been clarified recently. The predominant accumulated lipids are fatty acid esters of cholesterol and triglycerides, and there is deficient activity of an acid lipase which normally cleaves these substances [8–10].

Physical Features

ABDOMEN: Most reported patients were first evaluated at 2 to 8 weeks of age because of vomiting, diarrhea, abdominal distention, and enlargement of the liver and spleen (*Figures A, B, and C*). They were acutely ill, and often dehydrated and in shock. In a mildly affected 8-year-old patient a moderately enlarged liver was the only abnormality [9].

SKIN: In the severely affected infants subcutaneous fat is virtually absent. They are quite pale because of severe anemia.

Nervous System

The psychomotor development of severely affected infants appears delayed. However, the infants are so debilitated and acutely ill that the presence of mental retardation cannot be clearly established. In the mildly affected 8-year-old patient mental function appeared normal [9].

Pathology

A striking feature is the symmetric enlargement of the adrenals due to a great excess of neutral fats in the adrenal cortex; secondary necrosis and calcification are also present (*Figures D and F*). The entire mucosa of the small bowel has a bright yellow, greasy, granular appearance [6]. Foam cells filled with cholesterol esters and triglycerides are present in the liver, spleen, kidney, lung, bone marrow, thymus, and lymph nodes. Assays of the cholesterol content in these organs have shown it to be 15 to 20 times normal. There are only mild pathologic changes in the brain; cholesterol levels in the gray matter are slightly elevated, and myelinization is fair to poor [3]. Brainstem, sympathetic chain, and intestinal ganglia involvement were noted in one patient [4]. Biochemical studies have shown the accumulated lipids are fatty acid esters of cholesterol [7,10] and to a lesser extent triglycerides [10]. There also appears to be accumulation of ceroid, an insoluble substance which has been only partially characterized but apparently results when unsaturated fatty acids polymerize [10]. The accumulated lipids appear to be located in lysosomes [8].

Laboratory Studies

There is deficient activity of an acid lipase which normally hydrolyzes cholesterol esters and triglycerides. The deficiency has been demonstrated in liver, spleen, and white blood cells [8,9]. By x-ray the adrenal glands are greatly enlarged, but they maintain their usual shape and position [4] (*Figure D*). Symmetrical adrenal calcifications with this appearance that are present at birth are considered almost pathognomonic of Wolman's disease. The bone marrow contains foam cells, and

the peripheral lymphocytes contain vacuoles; both of these findings are similar to those seen in Niemann-Pick disease [3,4].

Treatment and Prognosis

The severely affected infants have a steady increase in the severity of their symptoms. Initially, they vomit intermittently and have loose bowel movements. Within a few weeks they have intestinal obstruction and are debilitated and moribund. Milder forms of the disease have recently been demonstrated. The sister of a typically affected patient was normal at 8 years except for the presence of moderate hepatomegaly. No acid lipase activity was demonstrable in her white blood cells or in a liver biopsy specimen [9]. There is no specific therapy for Wolman's disease. In view of the recently described enzyme defect, a low-fat diet has been used [9].

Genetics

Autosomal recessive. In one family the heterozygotes had reduced acid lipase activity in white blood cells. Prenatal diagnosis is anticipated, but has not yet been possible [10].

Differential Diagnosis

1. Hepatosplenomegaly in early infancy, foam cells in the bone marrow, and vacuolated peripheral lymphocytes are also features of patients with the classic form of Niemann-Pick disease. However, these patients do not have adrenal calcification, and their foam cells accumulate sphingomyelin as a result of a deficiency of the enzyme sphingomyelinase (see page 44).
2. Malabsorption, vomiting, intestinal obstruction, and failure to thrive are features of some infants with cystic fibrosis, but they do not have calcified adrenal glands and do have elevated sweat sodium.

References

1. Abramov, A., Schorr, S., and Wolman, M. Generalized xanthomatosis with calcified adrenals. *Am. J. Dis. Child.,* **91**:282–86, 1956.
2. Wolman, M., Sterk, V. V., Gatt, S., and Frenkel, M. Primary familial xanthomatosis with involvement and calcification of the adrenals. *Pediatrics,* **28**:742–57, 1961.
3. Crocker, A. C., Vawter, G. F., Neuhauser, E. B. D., and Rosowsky, A. Wolman's disease: three new patients with a recently described lipidosis. *Pediatrics,* **35**:627–40, 1965.
4. Kahana, D., Berant, M., and Wolman, M. Primary familial xanthomatosis with adrenal involvement (Wolman's disease). *Pediatrics,* **42**:70–76, 1968.
5. Marshall, W. C., Ockenden, B. G., Fosbrooke, A. S., and Cumings, J. N. Wolman's disease. A rare lipidosis with adrenal calcification. *Arch. Dis. Child.,* **44**:331–41, 1969.
6. Kamoshita, S., and Landing, B. H. Distribution of lesions in myenteric plexus and gastrointestinal mucosa in lipidoses and other neurologic disorders of children. *Am. J. Clin. Pathol.,* **49**:312–18, 1968.
7. Rosowsky, A., Crocker, A. C., Trites, D. H., and Modest, E. J. Gas-liquid chromatographic analysis of the tissue sterol fraction in Wolman's disease and related lipidoses. *Biochim. Biophys. Acta,* **98**:617–23, 1965.
8. Lake, B. D., and Patrick, A. D. Wolman's disease: deficiency of E600-resistant acid esterase activity with storage of lipids in lysosomes. *J. Pediatr.,* **76**:262–66, 1970.
9. Young, E. P., and Patrick, A. E. Deficiency of acid esterase activity in Wolman's disease. *Arch. Dis. Child.,* **45**:664–68, 1970.
10. Lowden, J. A., Barson, A. J., and Wentworth, P. Wolman's disease: a microscopic and biochemical study showing accumulation of ceroid and esterified cholesterol. *Can. Med. Assoc. J.,* **102**:402–405, 1970.

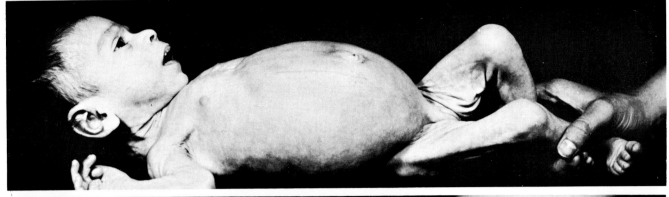

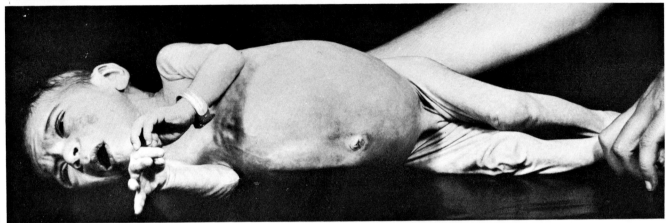

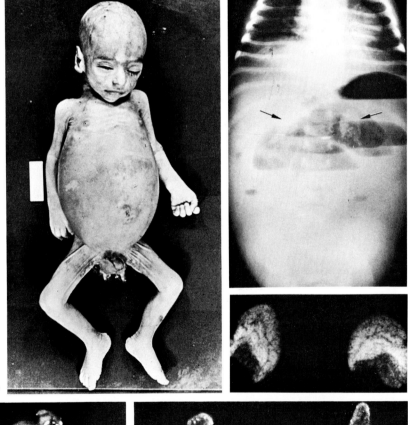

Plate I-30. *A* and *B:* A 3-month-old girl with a protuberant abdomen and wasting of the subcutaneous tissues. She weighed only 7 pounds 9 ounces at this time, while at birth she had weighed 8 pounds 3 ounces. *C–F:* A deceased infant with a grossly protuberant abdomen, lack of subcutaneous fat, and wrinkling of the skin. *D:* Abdominal x-ray shows generalized haziness, dilated loops of bowel, and calcified adrenal glands (*arrows*). The close-up view is a postmortem x-ray of both adrenal glands. *E:* Shows a section of mesentery with enlarged lymph nodes, which were golden yellow in appearance. *F:* Shows the cut surfaces of the adrenals; the cortex was also golden yellow. (*A:* From A. C. Crocker *et al., Pediatrics,* **35:**627–40, 1965. *B:* Courtesy of Dr. A. C. Crocker, Boston, Mass. *C–F:* Courtesy of Drs. D. Kahana and M. Berant, Hadera, Israel.)

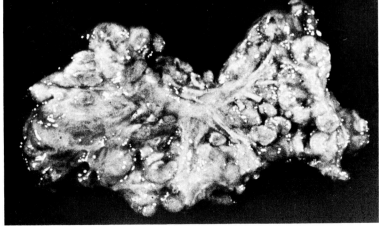

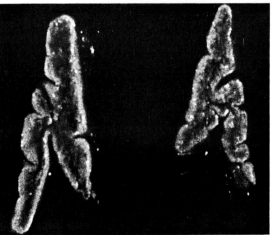

Chapter II
Progressive Diseases of Unknown Cause

Introduction

The disorders covered in this chapter are among the most difficult problems in medicine. Almost all are inherited and progressive; that is, the degree of disability increases with time. The rate of progression may be rapid, as in spongy degeneration of the white matter, or slow, as in Huntington's chorea and myotonic dystrophy. The current state of knowledge about the majority of these diseases is at stage 2 (see page 5); that is, the clinical features and mendelian pattern of inheritance have been delineated, but the biochemical basis of the disorder is obscure.

It is likely that as knowledge increases most of these disorders will be shown to be inborn errors of metabolism such as those included in Chapter I. Knowledge about cerebrotendinous xanthomatosis is in a state of transition. Here the accumulation of dihydrocholesterol (cholestanol) has recently been demonstrated, and this is almost certainly responsible for the pathologic changes. However, the biochemical basis of the cholestanol accumulation has not been determined.

The clinical manifestations of some of these disorders (Duchenne dystrophy, Friedreich's ataxia, Huntington's chorea) have been known for many years, and on this basis they can be diagnosed with considerable certainty. Other disorders, such as Farber's lipogranulomatosis and infantile neuroaxonal dystrophy, have been delineated only recently, but the phenotype is sufficiently defined to permit diagnosis. Included also are disorders for which the clinical delineations are tentative. Among these are Alper's disease, the neuronal lipidoses without sphingolipid accumulation, and Pelizaeus-Merzbacher disease.

Three of the disorders are X-linked (kinky hair disease, Duchenne dystrophy, and the syndrome of adrenocortical atrophy and diffuse cerebral sclerosis), and in three others there is an autosomal dominant mode of inheritance (Huntington's chorea, myotonic dystrophy, one form of Friedreich's ataxia). For most of the others an autosomal recessive mode of inheritance is either established or probable. The neuropathic type of arthrogryposis multiplex congenita does not appear to be genetically determined. In addition, this, as well as the other types of arthrogryposis multiplex congenita, is probably nonprogressive. Present knowledge about arthrogryposis multiplex congenita is rudimentary; it is likely that this syndrome includes several distinct entities. It is possible that at least some of the forms of arthrogryposis multiplex will in the future be classified with the congenital malformations or infectious diseases.

In many of the disorders mental retardation is a constant feature. In others, such as Friedreich's ataxia and muscular dystrophy, intellectual function more often than not is normal. These disorders have been included because available reports indicate that mental retardation occurs more frequently than in the general population. However, in some instances information on this point is conflicting. Thus, one study of patients with Friedreich's ataxia indicates that their intelligence does not vary significantly from that of the general population.

Alexander's Disease (Megalencephaly Associated with Hyaline Panneuropathy)

In 1949 Alexander described a boy who at the age of 7 months was noted to have an enlarged head and psychomotor retardation; he died at 15 months of age of a febrile illness. At postmortem examination the brain was large, and the white matter contained many eosinophilic bodies, which appeared to be degeneration products of fibrillar astrocytes [1]. Since then, at least seven additional cases have been reported [2–8].

Physical Features

HEAD: Progressive enlargement of the head is usually noted within the first year of life (*Figure A*).

Nervous System

Most of the patients showed severe psychomotor retardation within the first 6 months of life. Some never were able to raise their heads. Three patients had generalized seizures. The psychomotor deficit was progressive, and most patients developed spastic quadriparesis. Most did not develop speech. One older patient had an entirely different clinical course. She was considered normal until the age of 7 years, when she developed a left hemiparesis. Later she lost the use of her right side. The illness was slowly progressive and she died at 15 years of age. She had an IQ of 125 [5]. Even though at postmortem examination this older patient's brain showed the leukodystrophy and eosinophilic deposits in the white matter which are considered characteristic of Alexander's disease, the clinical differences from the other cases are so marked that one cannot be certain that this represents the same disease.

Pathology

Two features are essential for the diagnosis of Alexander's disease: a severe deficiency of myelin and the accumulation of numerous eosinophilic bodies in the white matter. Even on gross examination a striking softening and disintegration of white matter are evident (*Figures B and D*). Microscopic study shows a severe deficiency of myelin (*Figure C*) and the accumulation of myriads of drop-shaped eosinophilic deposits, mainly in the white matter (*Figure E*). There is considerable evidence that this material is located in fibrillar astrocytes [7]. Material with similar histochemical properties and appearance under the electron microscope is present within enlarged astrocyte processes found in certain low-grade glial tumors or glial scars. Such enlarged processes are referred to as Rosenthal fibers (*Figure F*). The abnormal material in Rosenthal fibers, and by implication that which accumulates in Alexander's disease, is thought to be derived in some way from the cytoplasm of the fibrillar astrocyte. Its chemical structure is not known. The white matter disease in some way causes an increase in brain mass, and this is responsible for the enlarged head noted clinically. Two patients, in addition, had hydrocephalus. In one of these this was shown to be due to partial obstruction of the aqueduct by hypertrophied fibrillar astrocytes [8].

Treatment and Prognosis

The affected children died between 5 and 33 months of age, except for one who lived 7 years and one 15 years [2,5].

Genetics

In one family four children (three males, one female) died of similar illnesses; however, neuropathologic studies were done on only one [4]. No other familial cases have been reported.

Differential Diagnosis

1. Most commonly head enlargement is due to hydrocephalus—i.e., an accumulation of cerebrospinal fluid within the ventricular system, most often due to obstruction. In Alexander's disease head enlargement is due mainly to megalencephaly—i.e., an increase in the brain mass. Special radiologic studies such as pneumoencephalography or ventriculography may be required to distinguish between hydrocephalus and megalencephaly. In hydrocephalus the head enlargement often shows a more rapid rate of increase, and is of greater severity, than in megalencephaly. Furthermore, many patients with hydrocephalus show better motor and mental function than patients with megalencephaly with comparable degrees of head enlargement, since the brain is not itself diseased.
2. Severe psychomotor retardation and megalencephaly are also features of patients with spongy degeneration of the central nervous system (Canavan's disease) (see page 112) and Tay-Sachs disease (see page 62). It is doubtful that Canavan's disease and Alexander's disease can be distinguished clinically. Tay-Sachs disease can be differentiated by the associated retinal lesion and the fact that megalencephaly is not evident until the second or third year.

References

1. Alexander, W. S. Progressive fibrinoid degeneration of fibrillary astrocytes associated with mental retardation in a hydrocephalic infant. *Brain*, **72**:373–81, 1949.
2. Stevenson, L. D., and Vogel, F. S. A case of macroencephaly associated with feeblemindedness and encephalopathy with peculiar deposits throughout the brain and spinal cord. *Cientia (Mex.)*, **12**:71–74, 1952.
3. Crome, L. Megalencephaly associated with hyaline pan-neuropathy. *Brain*, **76**:215–28, 1953.
4. Wohwill, F. J., Bernstein, J., and Yakovlev, P. I. Dysmyelinogenic leukodystrophy. *J. Neuropathol. Exp. Neurol.*, **18**:359–83, 1959.
5. Vogel, F. S., and Hallervorden, J. Leukodystrophy with diffuse Rosenthal fiber formation. *Acta Neuropathol. (Berl.)*, **2**:126–43, 1962.
6. Friede, R. L. Alexander's disease. *Arch. Neurol.*, **11**:414–22, 1964.
7. Schochet, S. S., Lampert, P. W., and Earle, K. M. Alexander's disease. A case report with electron microscopic observations. *Neurology (Minneap.)*, **18**:543–49, 1968.
8. Sherwin, R. M., and Berthrong, M. Alexander's disease with sudanophilic leukodystrophy. *Arch. Pathol.*, **89**:321–28, 1970.

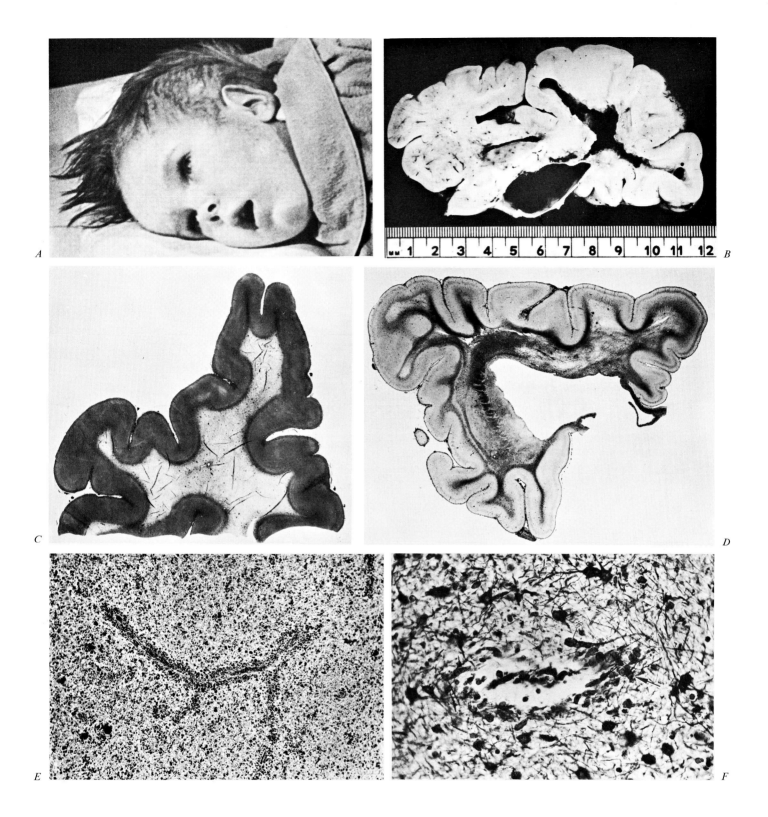

Plate II-1. *A–C:* A 2-year-old boy with head enlargement (circumference 53.7 cm). Coronal section of the brain at the level of the basal ganglia (*B*) shows the white matter completely destroyed in the centrum semiovale and outside the striate body. Histologic section of the frontal lobe (*C*) shows a severe loss of myelinated fibers. *D–F:* Parts of brain of a 2½-year-old child with severe mental retardation and seizures. The head circumference was 54 cm and the brain weight was 1180 g. The coronal section of the brain through the anterior horns of the lateral ventricles has been stained for myelin and shows extreme pallor in the central white matter due to myelin loss. Flattening of the cortex is due to postmortem distortion. Low-power photomicrograph (*E*) of white matter with phosphotungatic acid–hematoxylin stain shows glial fibers. Scattered throughout are hyalin bodies of varying size, which are most densely aggregated around the small blood vessel in the center. High-power photomicrograph (× 224) (*F*) shows dense gliosis as indicated by the interlacing fibrils. Numerous irregular structures identical with Rosenthal fibers (*arrows*) are present around the blood vessel and among the other fibers. One of these fibers (*asterisk*) is in direct continuity with a glial fibril. (*A:* Courtesy of Dr. L. Crome, Carshalton, Surrey, England. *B* and *C:* From L. Crome, *Brain,* **76:**215–28, 1953. *D–F:* Courtesy of Dr. E. P. Richardson, Jr., Boston, Mass.)

Alpers' Disease
(Progressive Degeneration of the Cerebral Cortex in Infancy, Diffuse Progressive Degeneration of the Gray Matter of the Cerebrum, Poliodystrophia Cerebri Progressiva [Infantilis])

In 1931 Alpers [1] described an infant who was apparently well until 3 months of age, when she began to have seizures and neurologic deterioration. The child died within a few weeks and at autopsy was shown to have extensive degeneration of the cerebral cortex. Subsequently several infants with similar histories and neuropathologic findings have been described [2–5]. The designation *Alpers' disease* is often used to refer to a progressive neurologic disorder which begins in infancy and is associated with a striking and diffuse neuronal loss that is most severe in the cerebral cortex. However, there has been considerable variation in the patients reported to have Alpers' disease, and it is quite possible that several disorders of different causation have been reported as examples of this syndrome. With this limitation in mind, the features of 15 reported patients [1–5] are presented.

Physical Features

HEAD: Microcephaly is present either at birth or within the first few months of life (*Figures A and B*).

Nervous System

The infants are usually normal at birth and for several weeks. The first symptoms in the reported cases were slow psychomotor development, noted between 2 and 12 months of life, or convulsions. The convulsions are usually severe and generalized; often there are myoclonic jerks. However, in six of the patients seizures were slight or absent [2,4]. As the neurologic deterioration progresses the child becomes inattentive and later unresponsive. Hyperreflexia and spasticity develop, and finally the child assumes a decerebrate posture. In some patients the pupillary light reflex is lost.

Pathology

The striking feature is diffuse and profound cerebral atrophy, which may reduce the brain weight to one fifth of normal (*Figures C and D*). There are loss of neurons and a concomitant proliferation of astrocytes in all parts of the cerebral cortex. In some cases these changes have been confined to the cerebral cortex [2,4]. In others, the cerebellum, basal ganglia, and thalamus have also been involved [1,3]. In contrast to the severe changes in the gray matter, the white matter is relatively intact, and the changes that are present are considered secondary to the neuronal loss. There is no storage of lipids in neurons.

Laboratory Studies

Air encephalography shows diffuse enlargement of the ventricular system with marked cortical atrophy and no evidence of obstruction (*Figures E and F*). Electroencephalography shows spikes and seizure patterns, but the changes are nonspecific. The cerebrospinal fluid is normal.

Genetics

Probably autosomal recessive [3–5].

Treatment and Prognosis

The neurologic deterioration is progressive. The age at death has ranged between 4 months and 5 years.

Differential Diagnosis

1. Progressive neurologic deterioration associated with brain atrophy and seizures occurs in the various types of hyperammonemia [6] and globoid cell leukodystrophy (see page 18), but each can be ruled out by clinical history and specific laboratory tests.
2. Progressive neurologic deterioration occurs in infants with Tay-Sachs disease, but they have a characteristic retinal lesion and a specific lysosomal enzyme deficiency (see page 62).

References

1. Alpers, B. J. Diffuse progressive degeneration of the gray matter of the cerebrum. *Arch. Neurol. Psychiat.,* **25**:469–505, 1931.
2. Christensen, E., and Krabbe, K. H. Poliodystrophia cerebri progressiva (infantilis). *Arch. Neurol. Psychiat.,* **61**:28–43, 1949.
3. Blackwood, W., Buxton, P. H., Cumings, J. N., Robertson, D. J., and Tucker, S. M. Diffuse cerebral degeneration in infancy (Alpers' disease). *Arch. Dis. Child.,* **38**:193–204, 1963.
4. Laurence, K. M., and Cavanagh, J. B. Progressive degeneration of the cerebral cortex in infancy. *Brain,* **91**:261–80, 1968.
5. Palinsky, M., Kozinn, P. J., and Zahtz, H. Acute familial infantile heredo-degenerative disorder of the central nervous system. *J. Pediatr.,* **45**:538–45, 1954.
6. Efron, M. L. Diseases of the urea cycle. In *The Metabolic Basis of Inherited Disease,* J. B. Stanbury, J. B. Wyngaarden, and D. S. Fredrickson, (eds.), 2nd ed. McGraw-Hill Book Co., New York, 1966, pp. 393–408.

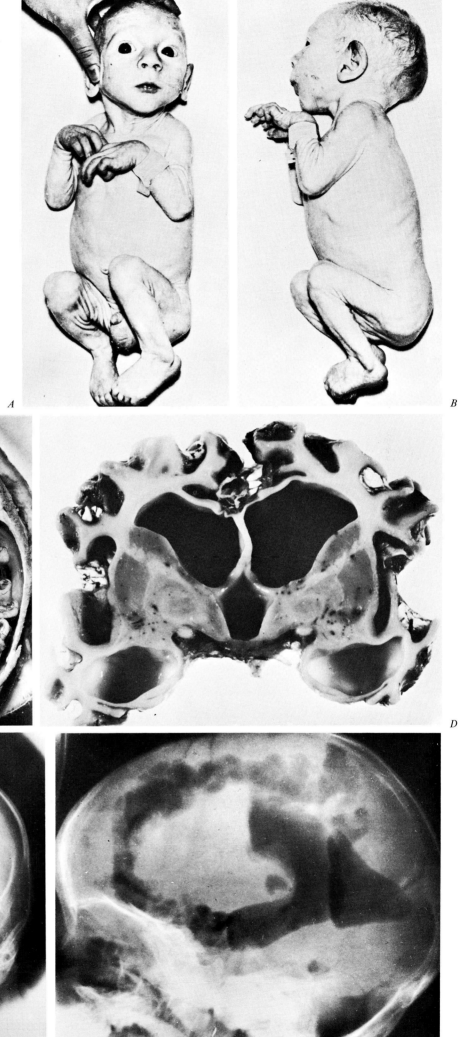

Plate II-2. *A* and *B:* An infant with marked microcephaly and wasting. He had seizures as a newborn and later had flexor spasms in all limbs and increased muscle tone. He died at 14 weeks of age. *C* and *D:* Show the marked atrophy of the cerebral cortex and large lateral ventricles in contrast to the apparently normal basal ganglia, as shown in the coronal cross section. *E* and *F:* Pneumoencephalograms showing the large lateral ventricles, thin cerebral cortex, and small cranium. (*A–C, E,* and *F:* Courtesy of Dr. K. M. Laurence, Penarth, Wales. *D:* From K. M. Laurence and J. B. Cavanagh, *Brain,* **91:**261–80, 1968.)

75

Arthrogryposis Multiplex Congenita

The term *arthrogryposis* means "curved joint." Curved joints, or flexion contractures, can occur in many disease states. In most of these there are other more specific or important abnormalities, so that the joint changes are not featured in the name. However, there is one syndrome in which the congenital joint abnormalities are so striking that they represent the major clinical manifestation and source of disability. This syndrome is called arthrogryposis multiplex congenita. So far, four types have been defined, and these will be described separately. Children with all of these types share several physical and neurologic features. Often there are webbing of the skin and subcutaneous tissue and an absence of skin folds in the contracted joints. There is evidence of muscle wasting, and the joints have a fusiform configuration. Kyphoscoliosis often develops. These patients do not have any signs of progressive neurologic disease. Their intelligence is usually normal; the incidence of mental deficiency is not known, but is considered greater than that in the general population [1].

Early and vigorous treatment is recommended for these patients. Physical therapy, manipulation, and splinting help many of the deformities. Such nonoperatic procedures have been particularly helpful for the arm deformities. A variety of surgical procedures may be necessary to correct the leg deformities, but in most instances it has been possible to achieve the alignment and stability required for independent ambulation. Prolonged treatment using braces, casts, and splints is necessary to maintain the corrections of the joint deformities once they are obtained [1,2].

Neuropathic Type

The child with the neuropathic type of arthrogryposis multiplex congenita may have the joints fixed in almost any position. Most often the arms are rotated inward, the elbows are extended, the hands have an ulnar deviation, the hips are flexed, the knees are partly flexed or extended, and the feet are in an equinovarus position (*Figure A*). Occasionally joint subluxations are present. There is usually some motion of the joints. The muscles are small, weak, and hypotonic. Usually the deep tendon reflexes cannot be elicited.

The most important changes are in the spinal cord. The lumbosacral segments are devoid of anterior horn cells, and the anterior roots contain either very few fibers or none at all. In the other levels of the spinal cord the number of anterior horn cells is greatly reduced (*Figure B*). The muscle fibers are small and show evidence of denervation atrophy. The muscle spindles are normal, and the longitudinal and transverse striations are preserved [3,4]. Use of the electromyogram appears to be the most reliable laboratory test for distinguishing the neuropathic from the myopathic form of arthrogryposis multiplex congenita [5]. The cause is unknown, and no genetic factors have been identified. A viral infection in fetal life has been suggested as a possible cause [4].

Myopathic Type

Children with the myopathic type of arthrogryposis are severely hypotonic at birth (*Figure D, left*). There is marked muscular weakness. Contractures usually develop several months after birth and result in flexion contractures of the hip, knee, and elbow (*Figures C, D [right], and Figure E*). There is weakness of the facial, extraocular, and oropharyngeal muscles. The deep tendon reflexes are decreased or absent. The electromyogram shows polyphasic potentials, but the changes can usually be differentiated from those in the neuropathic type [5]. Nerve conduction velocities are normal. The affected muscles have lost a large fraction of their fibers, which are replaced by fat and fibrous tissue (*Figure F*). The remaining fibers show features seen in the muscular dystrophies. The anterior horn cells and peripheral nerves are normal [6,7].

The electromyographic and histopathologic studies tend to place the myopathic form of arthrogryposis multiplex among the muscular dystrophies. However, unlike the other types of muscular dystrophy, the involvement of muscle does not appear to be progressive. Half of the cases reported in the literature died before the age of 13 years [7]. The highest death rate is observed in infancy, and death is usually caused by respiratory infections. The patients who survive usually have a stationary course. In several reported families an autosomal recessive mode of inheritance was considered likely.

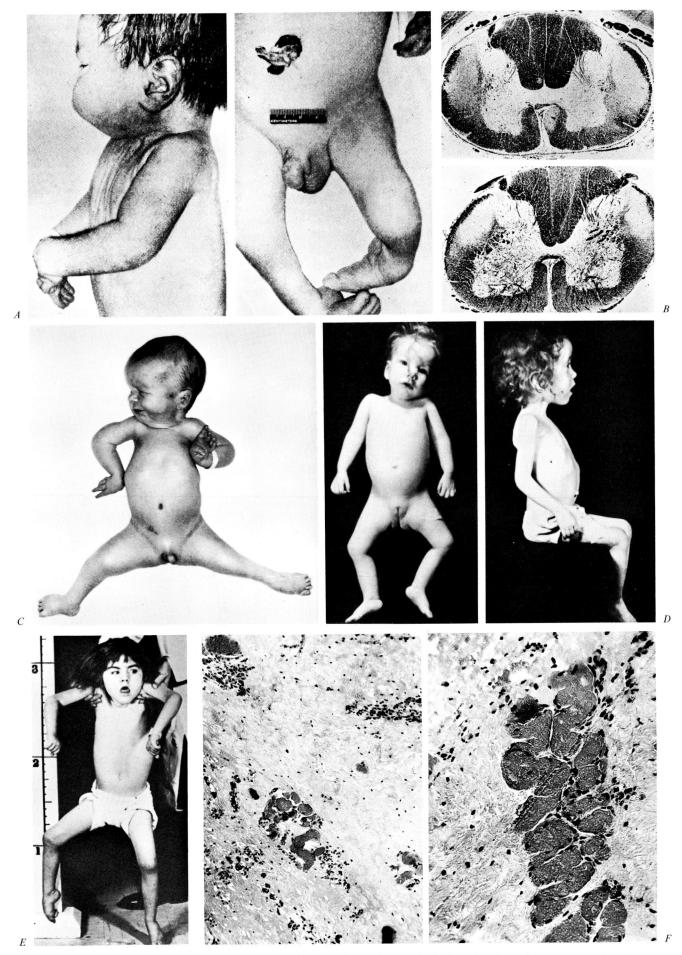

Plate II-3. *A* and *B:* A 9-day-old male infant with the neuropathic type of arthrogryposis. He had severe micrognathia, abducted shoulders, flexion contractures of the elbows, wrists, interphalangeal joints, and knees, and equinovarus deformities of both feet. There were neither cerebral nor peripheral nerve abnormalities. The spinal cord (*B, top*) was small and showed a marked diminution in the number of anterior horn cells in comparison with a normal control (*B, bottom*). *C:* An infant with multiple flexion deformities of all limbs. *D* (*left*): A 10-month-old girl with marked muscle hypotonia. At 2½ years she could walk with support and had normal intelligence. *D* (*right*): A 3-year-old girl who had developed muscle contractures. *E:* A 5-year-old girl who was hypotonic at birth and has developed contractures. *F:* Muscle biopsy from girl in *D* (*right*) at 6 years showing myofibers largely replaced by connective tissue. The remaining muscle fibers vary in size (hematoxylin and eosin; *left* × 92, *right* × 219). (*A* and *B:* From D. B. Drachman and B. Q. Banker, *Arch. Neurol.* [*Chicago*], **5:**89–93, 1961. *C:* From M. O. Tachdjian, *Pediatr. Clin. North Am.*, **14:**307–58, 1967. *D–F:* From H. Zellweger *et al.*, *Am. J. Dis. Child.*, **114:**591–602, 1967.)

Other Types of Arthrogryposis Multiplex

Two families have been described in which arthrogryposis multiplex congenita was associated with nodular fibrosis of the anterior spinal nerve roots [8,9] (*Figures K and L*). In these cases the neuronal population in the anterior horns of the spinal cord was normal. The affected children died in the first few months of life. The genetic data suggest an autosomal recessive mode of inheritance.

One of us has studied a profoundly retarded boy with arthrogryposis multiplex who died when he was 6 years old (*Figures G and H*). His brain weighed only 460 g, compared with the normal of 1150 g for this age. The ventricular system was widely dilated, encroaching on the central white matter, which nowhere exceeded 0.7 cm in width. There was only rudimentary development of the hippocampal formation and corpus callosum (*Figures I and J*). There was no obstruction to cerebrospinal fluid circulation. The spinal cord was normal. The number of anterior horn cells was not reduced. It was concluded that this represented an encephalopathic form of arthrogryposis multiplex. The cause of the brain abnormality has not been determined. It appeared to be congenital and nonprogressive. The fact that one previous sib had the same type of joint contractures suggests that it was genetically determined. Three other sibs are normal.

Differential Diagnosis

1. Some of the conditions of which arthrogryposis is a feature are as follows:
   a. Cerebrohepatorenal syndrome (see page 270).
   b. Syndrome of blepharophimosis and congenital contractures (see page 320).
   c. Dysmorphogenesis of joints, brain, and palate (see page 278).
   d. Syndrome of elbow contractures, corneal opacities, pointed nose, and mental retardation (see page 324).
   e. Syndrome of micrognathia, malformed ears, clubfoot, and flexion deformities (pseudotrisomy 18) (see page 336).
   f. Syndrome of phocomelia, flexion deformities, and facial anomalies (see page 340).
   g. Chromosome 18 trisomy (see page 156).
   h. XXXXY syndrome (see page 190).
   i. Contractural arachnodactyly [10].
   j. The popliteal pterygium syndrome [11].
   k. Diastrophic dwarfism [12].
   l. Syndrome of cryptorchidism, chest deformities, contractures, and arachnodactyly (see page 332).
   m. The Kuskokwim syndrome (an inherited form of arthrogryposis described in Alaskan Eskimos) [13].
   n. Syndrome of cataracts, microcephaly, kyphosis, and joint contractures [14].

2. Clinical differentiation of the various types of arthrogryposis multiplex congenita is difficult. The pattern of joint contracture does not allow differentiation [5]. The electromyographic changes appear to be the most reliable method: in the neuropathic form there are action potentials of abnormally large amplitude, as well as certain other changes [5]. The abnormalities on muscle biopsy must be interpreted with caution, since some neuropathic cases show changes that are usually associated with myopathy. Only a small portion of the myopathic cases have shown increased serum creatine phosphokinase and aldolase activities [5,7].

3. Lethal syndrome of microcephaly, cerebral anomalies, hypertelorism, and flexion deformities [15].

References

1. Friedlander, H. L., Westin, G. W., and Wood, W. L., Jr. Arthrogryposis multiplex congenita. A review of forty-five cases. *J. Bone Joint Surg. (Br.),* **50-A**:89–112, 1968.
2. Fisher, R. L., Johnstone, W. T., Fisher, W. H. Jr., and Goldkamp, O. G. Arthrogryposis multiplex congenita: a clinical investigation. *J. Pediatr.,* **76**:255–61, 1970.
3. Adams, R. D., Denny-Brown, D., and Pearson, C. M. *Diseases of Muscle,* 2nd ed. Harper & Row, New York, 1962, pp. 310–18.
4. Drachman, D. B., and Banker, B. Q. Arthrogryposis multiplex congenita. Case due to disease of the anterior horn cells. *Arch. Neurol.,* **5**:77–93, 1961.
5. Amick, L. D., Johnson, W. W., and Smith, H. L. Electromyographic and histopathologic correlations in arthrogryposis. *Arch. Neurol.,* **16**:512–23, 1967.
6. Banker, B. Q., Victor, M., and Adams, R. D. Arthrogryposis multiplex due to congenital muscular dystrophy. *Brain,* **80**:319–34, 1957.
7. Zellweger, H., Afifi, A., McCormick, W. F., and Mergner, W. Severe congenital muscular dystrophy. *Am. J. Dis. Child.,* **114**:591–602, 1967.
8. Peña, C. E., Miller, F., Budzilovich, G. N., and Feigin, I. Arthrogryposis multiplex congenita. Report of two cases of a radicular type with familial incidence. *Neurology (Minneap.),* **18**:926–30, 1968.
9. Bargeton, E., Nezelof, C., Guran, P., and Job, J. C. Étude anatomique d'un cas d'arthrogrypose multiple congénitale et familiale. *Rev. Neurol. (Paris),* **104**:479–89, 1961.
10. Beals, R. K., and Hecht, F. Congenital contractural arachnodactyly. A heritable disorder of connective tissue. *J. Bone Joint Surg. (Br.),* **53-A**:987–93, 1971.
11. Hecht, F., and Jarvimen, J. M. Heritable dysmorphic syndrome with normal intelligence. *J. Pediatr.,* **70**:927–35, 1967.
12. Langer, L. O., Jr. Diastrophic dwarfism in early infancy. *Am. J. Roentgenol. Radium Ther. Nucl. Med.,* **93**:399–404, 1965.
13. Wright, D. G., and Aase, J. The Kuskokwim syndrome: an inherited form of arthrogryposis in the Alaskan Eskimo. *Birth Defects: Original Article Series,* Vol. V, No. 3, March, 1969, pp. 91–95, Williams & Wilkins Co., Baltimore.
14. Lowry, R. B., MacLean, R., McLean, D. M., and Tischler, B. Cataracts, microcephaly, kyphosis, and limited joint movement in two siblings: a new syndrome. *J. Pediatr.,* **79**:282–84, 1971.
15. Neu, R. L., Kajii, T., Gardner, L. I., and Nagyfy, S. F. A lethal syndrome of microcephaly with multiple congenital anomalies in three siblings. *Pediatrics,* **47**:610–12, 1971.

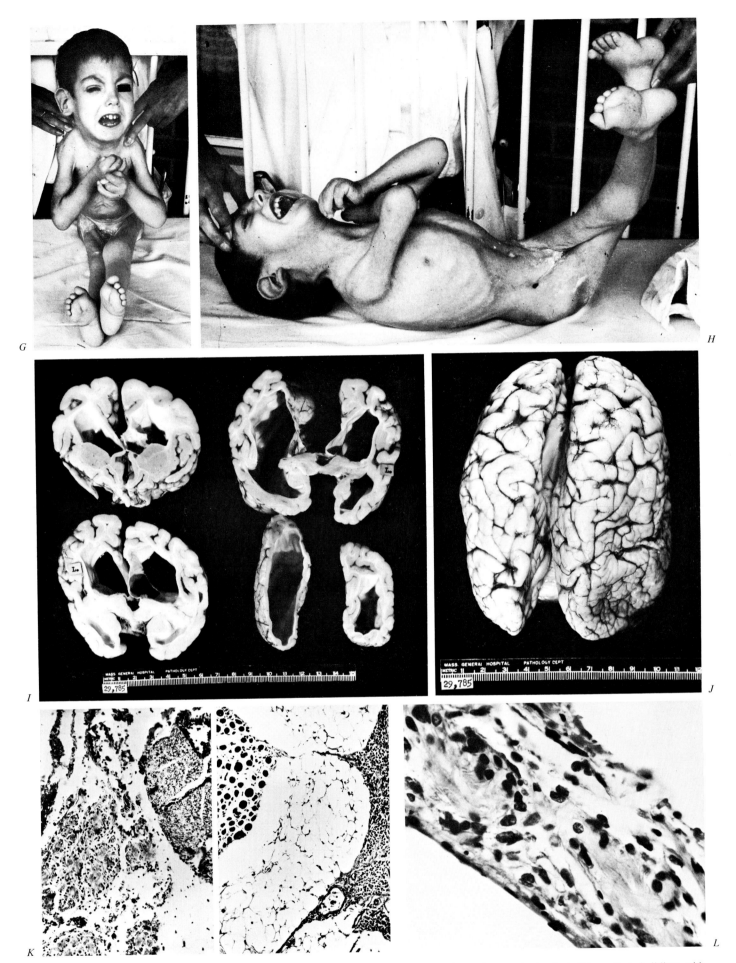

G H

I J

K L

Plate II-3. *G–J:* A 6-year-old boy with the encephalopathic type of arthrogryposis. He had communicating hydrocephalus, flexion deformities of the elbows and hips, extended legs, clubbed feet, and severe mental deficiency. The external appearance and convolutional patterns of his brain are normal, except for thinness and partial collapse of the occipital and posterior parietal portions. This is due to loss of cerebral substance and ventricular dilation, shown in the cross sections. The cerebral white matter is markedly reduced, and the corpus callosum cannot be identified. The basal ganglia and thalamus appeared normal. *K (left):* Shows obliteration with fibrosis of the normal anterior root in the first of two affected siblings with arthrogryposis due to nodular fibrosis of the anterior spinal roots. The well-preserved posterior root may be seen in the right upper corner (hematoxylin and eosin, × 90). *K (right):* Shows groups of normal-sized or slightly hypertrophied fibers at the top left, and on the right very small fibers (*arrow*) characteristic of neural atrophy. *L:* A cross section of an anterior thoracic root in the second child, showing multiple areas of fibrosis (hematoxylin and eosin, × 300). (*K* and *L:* From C. E. Peña *et al., Neurology* [*Minneap.*], **18:**926–30, 1968.)

Cerebrotendinous Xanthomatosis

In 1936 Schneider[1] reported a mentally defective epileptic patient who had developed cataracts when he was 26 years old and later showed progressive neurologic deterioration. Postmortem study showed extensive lipid deposits around the small vessels in the dentate nucleus, substantia nigra, and basal ganglia [1]. The next year van Bogaert, Scherer, and Epstein [2] described a man with a similar history and pathologic findings and noted the presence of tendon xanthomas. By 1969 more than 10 additional cases had been reported [3–6]. The main clinical features have been found to be ataxia, cataracts, and tendon xanthomas. Recently accumulation of cholestanol (dihydrocholesterol) has been demonstrated in the nervous system.

Physical Features

FACE: Two patients had symmetric xanthelasmas on the eyelids [2,5].

EYES: Most of the reported patients had cataracts. These became evident in childhood or early adulthood.

LIMBS: Eight of the 10 reported patients had tendon xanthomas [3]. The Achilles tendon is the most common site (*Figures C, E, and F*). They are first noted in childhood or early adult life.

Nervous System

The illness can be subdivided into three clinical stages. In stage I the child does not have any clearly defined physical or neurologic abnormalities, but may be mildly or moderately mentally retarded and thus be placed in special classes. The second stage may begin in adolescence, or not until the age of 40 years or more [3]. The main features are dementia, ataxia, tremor, and mild spasticity. Examination reveals a paucity of facial expression, a stiff and unsteady gait, and moderate dysmetria. Speech has an explosive quality, and becomes progressively less intelligible. There is increasing dysphagia, and there may be drooling (*Figures A and B*). Deep tendon reflexes are hyperactive and plantar responses extensor. At least two patients have shown a rhythmic tremor of the palate, a physical sign that is referred to as palatal myoclonus [6]. The patient in stage III is bedridden and almost totally helpless. His speech is only an unintelligible grunt or entirely absent. He shows progressive paralysis, atrophy of limbs, and severe swallowing difficulty.

Pathology

The most striking abnormalities are found in the cerebellum. Here there are granulomatous lesions of the white matter, extensive loss of myelin, and atrophy of adjacent cerebellar folia. In tissue sections of the cerebellum one sees many needlelike clefts which represent areas from which crystals were dissolved out in the process of preparing the section. Similar but less extensive lesions and areas of demyelination are also seen in the brainstem. The tendon xanthomas show a dense accumulation of narrow crystalline clefts within granulomatous lesions that contain many large mononuclear cells with foamy cytoplasm and multinucleated giant cells (*Figure D*).

There is an accumulation of cholestanol in the brains of affected patients [4,5,6,6a]. The ratio of cholestanol to cholesterol is 0.2 or even 0.5, compared to 0.01 or less in normal brains.

Laboratory Studies

The serum cholesterol level was normal in five out of seven patients, the others showing levels as high as 450 mg percent [3,5]. In one patient all serum lipids and lipoproteins were normal [5]. The plasma cholestanol level is usually not increased. The tendon xanthomas have shown a moderate accumulation of cholestanol, to 4 to 9 percent of cholesterol; in all tissues of normal individuals cholestanol does not exceed 1 percent of cholesterol. Roentgenograms of the ankle show enlarged and sometimes calcified soft tissue masses (*Figure F*).

Treatment and Prognosis

The first two reported patients [1,2] were severely disabled in their early twenties and incapacitated by 30 years of age. Other patients have had milder neurologic symptoms. One man did not develop any symptoms until after age 50 and was only moderately disabled when he died of a myocardial infarction at 58 years of age. His 57-year-old sister was also only mildly affected [3]. There is no specific treatment.

Genetics

Autosomal recessive [3].

Differential Diagnosis

1. Tendon xanthomas, xanthelasmas, and progressive spastic paraplegia occur in patients with hyperlipemia and/or hypercholesterolemia who develop spinal cholesterolosis. These patients do not have cataracts, ataxia, or dementia [7].

2. Patients with hereditary tendinous xanthomatosis without hyperlipemia do not have cataracts, neurologic symptoms, or mental deficiency [8].

3. A masklike facies, dementia, ataxia, tremor, and spasticity also occur in patients with Wilson's disease, but they also have the Kayser-Fleischer ring and do not have either tendon xanthomas or cataracts (see page 64).

References

1. Schneider, C. Über eine eigenartige Hirnerkrankung. *Allg. Z. Psychiat.,* **104**:144–63, 1936.
2. van Bogaert, L., Scherer, H. J., and Epstein, E. *Une forme cérébrale de la cholesterinose généralisée (Type particulier de lipidose à cholesterine).* Masson et Cie., Paris, 1937.
3. Schimschock, J. R., Alvord, E. C., and Swanson, P. D. Cerebrotendinous xanthomatosis. Clinical and pathological studies. *Arch. Neurol.,* **18**:688–98, 1968.
4. Menkes, J. H., Schimschock, J. R., and Swanson, P. D. Cerebrotendinous xanthomatosis. The storage of cholestanol within the nervous system. *Arch. Neurol.,* **19**:47–53, 1968.
5. Gardner-Medwin, D., Kishimoto, Y., Derby, B. M., and Moser, H. W. Cerebrotendinous xanthomatosis: *in vivo* labeling of cerebral sterols and sterol esters. *Trans. Am. Neurol. Assoc.,* **96**, 1971 (in press).
6. Philippart, M., and van Bogaert, L. Cholestanolosis (cerebrotendinous xanthomatosis). A follow-up study on the original family. *Arch. Neurol.,* **21**:603–10, 1969.
6a. Stahl, W. L., Sumi, S. M., and Swanson, P. D. Subcellular distribution of cerebral cholestanol in cerebrotendinous xanthomatosis. *J. Neurochem.,* **18**:403–13, 1971.
7. van Bogaert, L. Spinal cholesterolosis. *Brain,* **88**:687–96, 1965.
8. Harlan, W. R., Jr., and Still, W. J. S. Hereditary tendinous and tuberous xanthomatosis without hyperlipidemia. A new lipid-storage disorder. *N. Engl. J. Med.,* **278**:416–22, 1968.

Plate II-4. *A–D:* A 34-year-old man who had slowly become incapacitated and at this age showed a blank facial expression, had a rigid smile, and drooled. There were xanthomas of the Achilles tendons, which had gradually increased in size until age 32 years and then stopped growing. The tendon biopsy showed extensive deposits of cholesterol. *E:* Shows the characteristic hard, nontender, swollen tendons of a 57-year-old woman, more marked in the left ankle. *F:* The x-ray of this woman's 58-year-old brother shows massive soft tissue enlargement of the Achilles tendon (*outlined by arrows*). (*A–D:* Courtesy of Dr. B. M. Derby, New York, N.Y. *E* and *F:* From J. R. Schimschock *et al., Arch. Neurol.* [*Chicago*], **18:**688–98, 1968.)

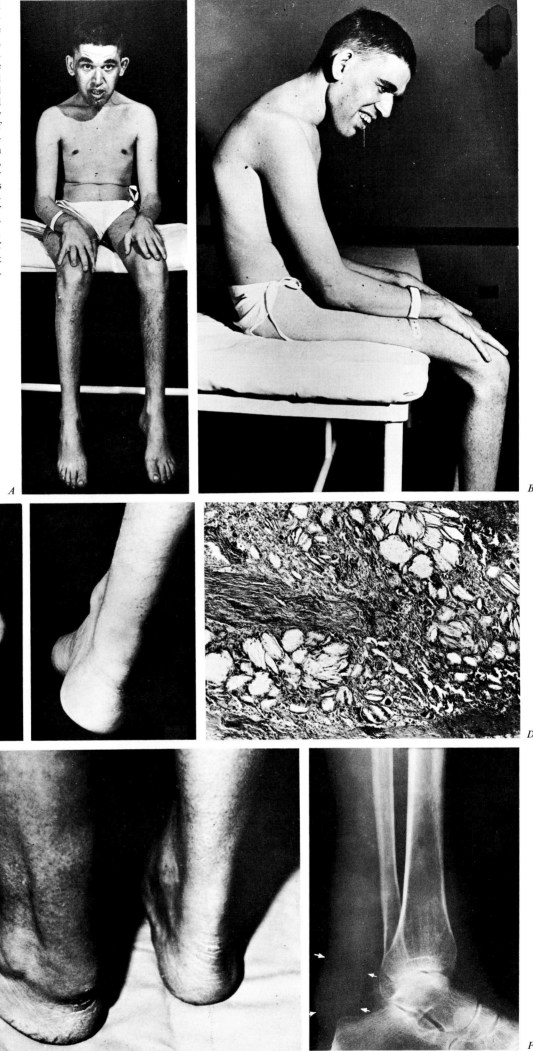

Cockayne's Syndrome (Cockayne-Neill Dwarfism)

Cockayne in 1936 [1] and again in 1946 [2] described a brother and sister with dwarfism, microcephaly, mental retardation, peculiar retinal pigmentation, optic atrophy, exposure dermatitis, and progressive neurologic deterioration. Neill and Dingwall [3] described two brothers with similar features. More than 20 patients have subsequently been described [4–9].

Physical Features

HEAD: All of the reported patients have been microcephalic.

FACE: At birth the appearance is normal. A loss of subcutaneous fat gradually develops during childhood. Older patients usually have a senile appearance with sunken eyes and prominence of the maxilla and nose (*Figures A, B, D, and E*).

EYES: The vision is initially normal. Pigmentary retinal degeneration, optic atrophy, and arterial narrowing gradually develop during childhood. Other common but less frequent eye findings are cataracts, loss of the macular reflex, nystagmus, lack of tearing, and poor response to mydriatic drugs [4].

EARS: The ears appear prominent because of the loss of subcutaneous fat in the face.

CHEST: The trunk is short and sometimes barrel-shaped.

BREASTS: At the age of expected puberty the females do not have normal breast development [2].

GENITALIA: Several of the reported males have had cryptorchidism. At puberty the penis is of normal size, but the testes remain small and the pubic hair growth often has a feminine pattern.

BACK: Some patients have a stooped posture and dorsal kyphosis.

LIMBS: The arms and legs appear to be disproportionately long in comparison to the trunk. The hands seem disproportionately large. The range of motion of the hips, knees, and ankles becomes progressively more restricted (*Figures A, B, and D*).

SKIN: A scaly, erythematous dermatitis develops after exposure to the sun, usually on the hands, legs, face, and ears. The dermatitis of the face may have a "butterfly" distribution (*Figure C*). Older patients have thickened, wrinkled skin, especially on the face.

HEIGHT: The length at birth is normal. Shortness of stature is evident in childhood. Adults are usually less than 4 feet (123 cm) tall.

WEIGHT: These patients are usually thin.

Nervous System

Early psychomotor development is slow. The mental deficiency is marked, with most IQ estimates below 50. Evidence of progressive neurologic deterioration is usually apparent in the second decade. The muscle power diminishes and the gait becomes awkward. Nystagmus, ataxia, an intention tremor, and incoordination develop. Initially the deep tendon reflexes are hyperactive, later hypoactive. Most patients become blind and deaf.

Pathology

The brain is small and the cerebral cortex and cerebellum appear atrophic. There is a marked reduction in the cerebral white matter. Myelin stains show a patchy demyelinization that is often severe in the subcortical white matter (*Figure F*). Calcification may be marked; it is symmetrically distributed in the cortex, basal ganglia, and cerebellum [5]. Segmental demyelination in peripheral nerves has also been reported [6]. Renal biopsies in two patients [7] showed thickening of the mesangium and the basement membrane of the glomerulus, some collapsed capillary loops, hyalinized glomeruli, and tubular atrophy with interstitial fibrosis.

Laboratory Studies

The cerebrospinal fluid protein is usually increased. Three reported patients [7,8] had diminished glomerular function; one [8] also had azotemia and hyperchloremic acidosis. This latter patient also had type II hyperlipoproteinemia and fasting hyperinsulinemia. Another patient [9] had hyperglycemia and an increased plasma insulin level. The skeletal maturation is normal. A thickened calvarium and anterior notching of the thoracic vertebrae are sometimes present. Intracranial calcifications are often visible on the skull x-ray, especially in the region of the basal ganglia.

Treatment and Prognosis

By 20 years of age these patients are usually unable to care for themselves. Death usually occurs in late childhood or early adulthood from inanition and respiratory infections.

Genetics

Autosomal recessive.

Differential Diagnosis

1. Patients with progeria have the same prematurely senile appearance and short stature. However, they are not mentally retarded and do not have a progressive neurologic disorder [10].
2. Photosensitive dermatitis and short stature are also features of Bloom's syndrome. However, these patients are not mentally retarded and do not have a progressive neurologic disorder [11].
3. The neuropathologic changes seen in patients with Cockayne's syndrome resemble those found in the Pelizaeus-Merzbacher syndrome (see page 98).

References

1. Cockayne, E. A. Dwarfism with retinal atrophy and deafness. *Arch. Dis. Child.,* **11**:1–8, 1936.
2. Cockayne, E. A. Dwarfism with retinal atrophy and deafness. *Arch. Dis. Child.,* **21**:52–54, 1946.
3. Neill, C. A., and Dingwall, M. M. A syndrome resembling progeria: a review of two cases. *Arch. Dis. Child.,* **25**:213–21, 1950.
4. Coles, W. H. Ocular manifestations of Cockayne's syndrome. *Am. J. Ophthalmol.,* **67**:762–64, 1969.
5. Moossy, J. The neuropathology of Cockayne's syndrome. *J. Neuropathol. Exp. Neurol.,* **26**:654–60, 1967.
6. Moosa, A., and Dubowitz, V. Peripheral neuropathy in Cockayne's syndrome. *Arch. Dis. Child.,* **45**:674–77, 1970.
7. Ohno, T., and Hirooka, M. Renal lesions in Cockayne's syndrome. *Tohoku J. Exp. Med.,* **89**:151–66, 1966.
8. Fujimoto, W. Y., Greene, M. L., and Seegmiller, J. E. Cockayne's syndrome: report of a case with hyperlipoproteinemia, hyperinsulinemia, renal disease, and normal growth hormone. *J. Pediatr.,* **75**:881–84, 1969.
9. Cotton, R. B., Keats, T. E., and McCoy, E. E. Abnormal blood glucose regulation in Cockayne's syndrome. *Pediatrics,* **46**:54–60, 1970.
10. Villee, D. B., Nichols, G. Jr., and Talbot, N. B. Metabolic studies in two boys with classical progeria. *Pediatrics,* **43**:207–16, 1969.
11. Bloom, D. The syndrome of congenital telangiectatic erythema and stunted growth. *J. Pediatr.,* **68**:103–13, 1966.

Plate II-5. *A* and *B:* Brothers at two ages (11½ and 15¾ years on left and 10 years later) showing the short stature, exposure dermatitis, relatively large hands and feet, and a progressive loss of facial fat. *C:* A 7-year-old boy with redness and crusting of the face, arms, and hands. *D–F:* A 12-year-old girl who is unable to stand. She has a prominent nose and chin, pubic hair, little breast development, but normal menses. The coronal section of her cerebral hemisphere passes through the globus pallidus. The Lopez myelin stain (*left*) shows a patchy absence of myelin resulting in a mottled appearance of the white matter. The cresyl violet stain (*right*) shows deeply a large dark area of calcific deposits in the globus pallidus and putamen. (*A:* From R. M. Paddison *et al., Dermatol. Trop. Ecol. Geographica,* **2:**195–203, 1963. *B:* From W. H. Coles, *Am. J. Ophthalmol.,* **67:**762–64, 1969. *C:* Courtesy of Dr. J. Windmiller, Dallas, Tex. *E:* Courtesy of Dr. T. B. Fitzpatrick, Boston, Mass. *F:* Courtesy of Dr. E. P. Richardson, Jr., Boston, Mass.)

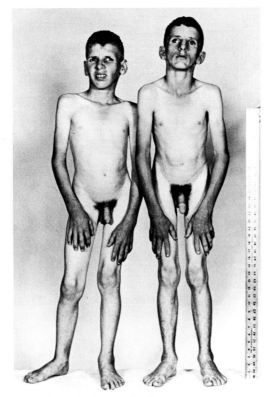
A

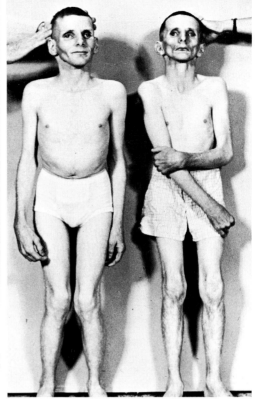
B

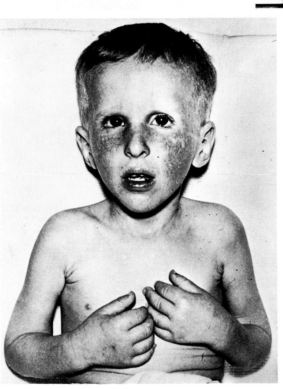
C

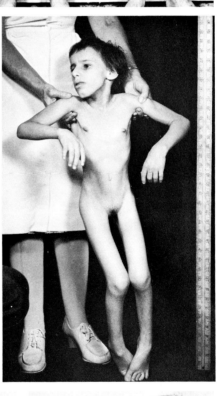
D

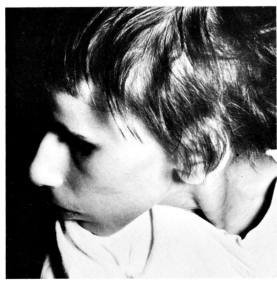
E

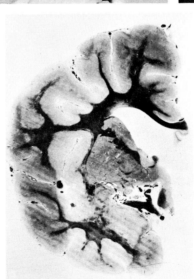

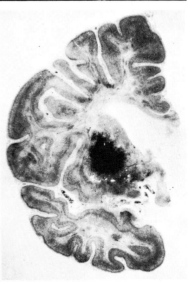
F

Familial Amyotrophic Dystonic Paraplegia

In 1964 Gilman and Horenstein [1] reported a family in which a brother and sister had progressive muscle wasting, dystonia, and spastic weakness of the limbs. Ten other family members had milder signs and symptoms. The authors considered this a new hereditary disorder.

Nervous System

The two severely affected patients had poor school performances before their muscle disease was evident. The man's intelligence quotient was 47 at age 19 years and 56 at age 37 years. The woman's intelligence quotient was 57 at age 13 years and 53 at 19 years. Their earliest symptoms were leg cramps and aching pains and difficulty in walking in the teenage years. By 19 years both had a stiff gait, increased lumbar lordosis, and stiff hips and knees. The muscle tone and strength were diminished in both the arms and the legs; the deep tendon reflexes were hyperactive. When walking, their arms were abducted, elbows flexed, and hands pronated (*Figure C*). Within a few years weakness of the neck, shoulder, elbow, and wrist muscles and distal wasting of the leg (*Figures A and B*), thenar, hypothenar, and interosseous muscles (*Figure E*) were evident. The tongue was asymmetric (*Figure D*) and dystonic. Pseudobulbar palsy and dystonia of the tongue caused severe impairment of speech. The sister at age 40 years had an inappropriate smile, bilateral facial weakness, an absent gag reflex, and slow swallowing, and was incontinent. Fasciculations were occasionally present. Sensation was always normal. Two nephews, ages 11 and 6 years, of the severely affected patients had cramping calf pain brought on by exercise and hyperactive deep tendon reflexes in the legs. Two siblings and ten other nieces and nephews of the severely affected patients were asymptomatic but had hyperactive tendon reflexes and mild extensor plantar responses.

Pathology

Serial muscle biopsies at ages 19 and 37 years in the severely affected man showed progressive motor unit atrophy. Autopsies on the severely affected brother and sister revealed a generalized loss of neurons that was more pronounced in the basal ganglia, especially in the substantia nigra. There was severe damage and loss of fibers in the anterior commissures. The spinal cord showed a loss of anterior horn cells. The skeletal muscle showed denervation atrophy. There was no storage substance and no inflammatory response [2].

Laboratory Studies

In the severely affected patients the nerve conduction velocity was normal, and the electromyogram showed fibrillation potentials suggesting anterior horn cell degeneration. Pneumoencephalography showed symmetric generalized ventricular dilatation in both patients (*Figure F*).

Treatment and Prognosis

The disease caused progressive and severe disability in two patients, rendering them unable to walk in early life and unable to care for themselves in later years. The muscle disease in the mildly affected individuals remained asymptomatic even at age 40.

Genetics

Autosomal dominant inheritance was suggested in this family with 12 affected members in three generations. However, there was no single affected ancestor of all of these patients, as would be expected for an autosomal dominant trait.

Differential Diagnosis

Slowly progressive spastic paralysis affecting mainly the legs occurs in patients with familial spastic paraplegia. However, they are not mentally retarded and do not develop dystonia or pseudobulbar palsy [3].

References

1. Gilman, S., and Horenstein, S. Familial amyotrophic dystonic paraplegia. *Brain*, **87**:51–66, 1964.
2. Romanul, F. C. A., and Maclane, D. Personal communication, 1970.
3. Schwarz, G. A. Hereditary (familial) spastic paraplegia. *Arch. Neurol. Psych.*, **68**:655–82, 1952.

Plate II-6. *A:* An obese 39-year-old woman who is smiling inappropriately and has wasting of the distal muscles of her arms and legs. *B–F:* Her severely affected brother. At 21 years of age he had a stiff gait characterized by accentuated lumbar lordosis, hyperextension of the knees, flexed elbows, and flexion and pronation of the wrists. *D:* Shows his tongue at age 21 which was asymmetric and dystonic. *E:* At 41 years he had muscle wasting similar to that of his sister, including marked wasting of the interosseous muscles of his hands. *F:* Pneumoencephalography on this man at age 41 years shows bilateral ventricular dilation; his sister had similar changes. For comparison with the normal pneumoencephalogram see page 97. (*A–F:* From F. Gilman and S. Horenstein, *Brain,* **87:**51–66, 1964.)

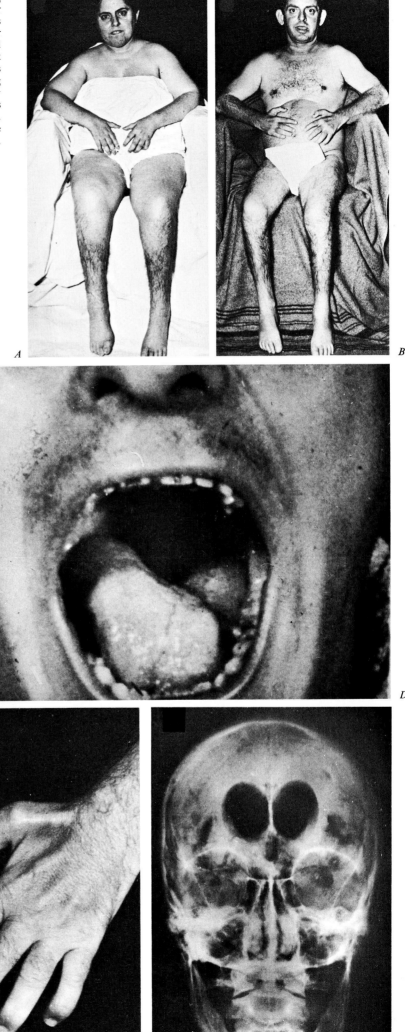

Familial Hormonal Disorder Associated with Mental Deficiency, Deaf-Mutism, and Ataxia

In 1959 Richards and Rundle [1] described five siblings with a syndrome characterized by severe mental deficiency, deaf-mutism, ataxia, and underdevelopment of secondary sex characteristics. They considered this a genetic syndrome and suggested that the two patients described by Koennicke [2] in 1919 had the same disorder.

Physical Features

BREASTS: The affected adult females had immature areolae and little or no breast tissue (*Figure B*).

GENITALIA: The external genitalia were normal, but immature in one of the two males and all three of the females.

LIMBS: Each patient had malpositioned feet, the specific deformities being pes cavus, pes planus, or talipes equinovarus (*Figures B and F*). The report did not indicate whether these deformities were present in infancy.

BACK: One patient had kyphoscoliosis (*Figure C*).

HAIR: The pubic and axillary hair was either scanty or absent (*Figures B and F*).

GROWTH AND DEVELOPMENT: The three females were considered amenorrheic, although one had had a single menstrual period.

Nervous System

The two males never learned to walk without support; the three females walked without support at 14, 15, and 24 months of age. Four of the patients were using a few single words by the second year. Mild deafness was noted in some of the patients in infancy; the hearing loss was severe by 2 to 5 years of age. At the same time those who could walk developed a staggering gait. When examined in late adolescence or adult life, all of the patients were deaf and mute. Their mental ages were estimated as between 2 and 5 years. All had horizontal nystagmus and atrophy of the distal arm and leg muscles, especially the intrinsic muscles of the hands and the muscles below the knees (*Figure D*). They could walk only with support. There was moderate ataxia of the arms and legs. The deep tendon reflexes were absent in the legs, and reduced or absent in the arms. The plantar responses were flexor in all but one instance.

Pathology

The testis biopsy in one of the males with a normal-sized penis and scanty pubic hair at age 16 years showed arrest in spermatogenesis and no evidence of Leydig cell function.

Laboratory Studies

The urinary gonadotropins, estrogen, pregnandiol, and 17-ketosteroid levels were markedly reduced.

Genetics

As the parents of these five affected siblings were second cousins, autosomal recessive inheritance of a rare mutant gene was postulated.

Treatment and Prognosis

These individuals were incapacitated by ataxia and deafness in the early years of life; they developed muscle atrophy much more slowly. None of the patients was able to care for himself or herself.

Differential Diagnosis

1. Progressive muscle weakness and ataxia are features of patients with Friedreich's ataxia, but the onset is usually between 10 and 20 years of age and there is neither deaf-mutism, hypogonadism, nor severe mental deficiency (see page 92).
2. Progressive deafness, distal muscle wasting, and mental deficiency are features of patients with the Flynn-Aird syndrome, but they also have peripheral neuritis, cataracts, and retinitis pigmentosa (see page 90).
3. Deafness, ataxia, and muscle wasting are features of patients with Refsum's disease, but they have normal intelligence, pigmentary degeneration of the retina, and a defect in phytanic acid metabolism [3].

References

1. Richards, B. W., and Rundle, A. T.   A familial hormonal disorder associated with mental deficiency, deaf mutism and ataxia. *J. Ment. Defic. Res.*, **3**:33–55, 1959.
2. Koennicke, W.   Friedreichsche Ataxie unter Taubstummheit. *Z. Ges. Neurol. Psychiat.*, **53**:161–65, 1919.
3. Steinberg, D., Vroom, F. Q., Engel, W. K., Cammermeyer, J., Mize, C. E., and Avigan, J.   Refsum's disease—a recently characterized lipidosis involving the nervous system. *Ann. Intern. Med.*, **66**:365–95, 1967.

Plate II-7. *A–D:* An affected female with small areolae and breasts, little pubic hair, clubbed feet, scoliosis, and atrophy of the intrinsic muscles of the hands. *E* and *F:* A male with normal genitalia and malpositioned feet. (*A–F:* Courtesy of Dr. B. W. Richards, Caterham, Surrey, England.)

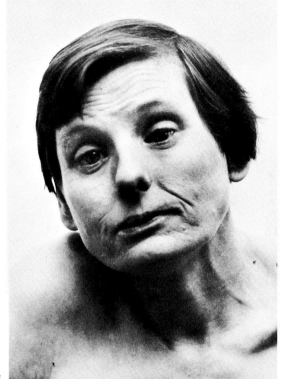

A

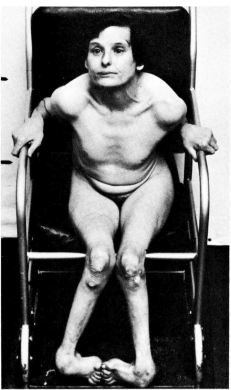

B

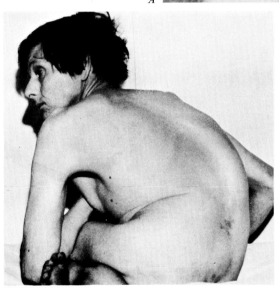

C

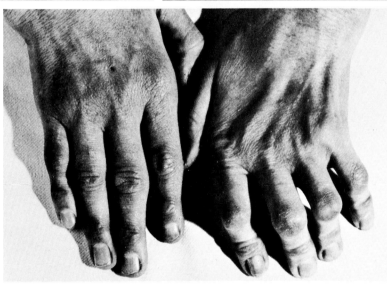

D

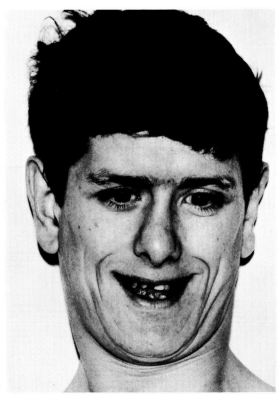

E

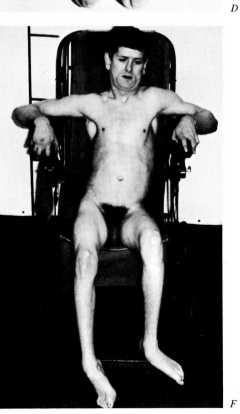

F

Farber's Lipogranulomatosis

In 1957 Farber, Cohen, and Uzman [1] described three young children who died in infancy with an illness characterized by the progressive development of tender, swollen joints, a hoarse, weak cry, and neurologic deterioration. Since then this striking combination of signs has been reported in five other patients [2,3,7]. What appears to be a milder form of the same disease has been reported in two others [4,5]. Because of the excess of free ceramide and ganglioside that were found in one patient, it has been suggested that this disease is an inborn error of lipid metabolism [3].

Physical Features

EYES: One patient at 8 months of age had a diffuse grayish opacification of the retina about the fovea with a mild cherry-red center [3,6]. One of the older and more mildly affected patients had a xanthomalike growth on the conjunctiva of one eye [4].

LARYNX: These patients develop hoarseness in the first weeks of life.

ABDOMEN: In some reported patients the liver and spleen were slightly enlarged; in others they were normal in size.

LYMPH NODES: Most patients have moderate enlargement of the lymph nodes.

LIMBS: Usually between 4 weeks and 4 months of age the interphalangeal and metacarpophalangeal joints of the hand become reddened, swollen, and tender (*Figures B, C, D, and F*). As a result of this, the infant keeps his fists tightly flexed. Subcutaneous nodules in the periarticular tissues are noted at about the same time. Ultimately the knees, wrists, and elbows also become swollen, and joint contractures develop (*Figure A*).

SKIN: Subcutaneous nodules also develop over pressure points, such as the dorsum of the spine (*Figure E*).

Nervous System

Six of the ten reported patients had neurologic abnormalities; two were normal and no mention was made of the neurologic findings in the other two [3]. Most patients had a loss of their deep tendon reflexes and mental deterioration in the terminal phase of their illness. One child had progressive paralysis, loss of deep tendon reflexes in the legs, and communicating hydrocephalus [2].

Pathology

There are two principal features: first, a proliferative and infiltrative process in the skin, subcutaneous tissue, tendons, synovia, larynx, and viscera; second, a ballooning of large neurons in the central and autonomic nervous systems. The proliferative and infiltrative process is characterized by granuloma formation, fibrosis, and a variable accumulation of foam cells distended with periodic acid–Schiff (PAS) positive material. The neurons are distended with PAS-positive cytoplasmic material; the anterior horn cells, medulla, pons, and cerebellum are most involved and the cerebral cortex least affected. The autonomic and visceral ganglia show similar changes [1,3,5]. Chemical analyses of the lymph nodes, liver, kidney, lung, and subcutaneous nodules in one child showed a 10- to 60-fold excess of free ceramide and a 5- to 10-fold excess of ganglioside [3]. In another patient ceramide levels were increased in the subcutaneous nodule and in the kidney [3a].

Laboratory Studies

The cerebrospinal fluid protein level was elevated in four patients [1–3] and normal in one patient [1]. X-rays show a nodular swelling about the peripheral joints associated with muscle atrophy and juxtaarticular bone erosion. The lungs show finely nodular parenchymal and interstitial infiltrations [7].

Treatment and Prognosis

All eight of the severely affected infants became debilitated and died between 7 and 22 months of age from inanition and infection. Treatment with steroids, radiation, antimetabolites, and alkylating agents was not helpful. One of the mildly affected patients had severe involvement of the joints, larynx, and subcutaneous tissues at 23 months of age [4], which persisted to age 12 years. He had no neurologic deficits [5]. The other mildly affected patient at 6 years of age had moderate involvement of the joints and subcutaneous tissues which appeared to be helped by chlorambucil [5].

Genetics

Autosomal recessive inheritance is postulated on the basis of an affected brother and sister in one family [1].

Differential Diagnosis

1. Swollen joints occur in the infantile form of rheumatoid arthritis, but these patients do not have hoarseness or such striking periarticular and subcutaneous nodules. The nodules in rheumatoid arthritis do not contain PAS-positive fatty macrophages.
2. Arthropathy and skin nodules occur in patients with the syndrome of lipoid dermatoarthritis or reticulohistiocytoma, but this disorder has only been described in adults [5].

References

1. Farber, S., Cohen, J., and Uzman, L. L. Lipogranulomatosis. A new lipoglyco-protein "storage" disease. *J. Mt. Sinai Hosp.,* **24:**816–37, 1957.
2. Rampini, S., and Clausen, J. Farbersche Krankheit (disseminierte Lipogranulomatose). Klinisches Bild und Zusammenfassung der chemischen Befunde. *Helv. Paediat. Acta.,* **22:**500–515, 1967.
3. Moser, H. W., Prensky, A. L., Wolfe, H. J., and Rosman, N. P. Farber's lipogranulomatosis. Report of a case and demonstration of an excess of free ceramide and ganglioside. *Am. J. Med.,* **47:**869–90, 1969.
3a. Samuelsson, K., and Zetterström, R. Ceramides in a patient with lipogranulomatosis (Farber's disease) with chronic course. *Scand. J. Clin. Lab. Invest.,* **27:**393–405, 1971.
4. Zetterström, R. Disseminated lipogranulomatosis (Farber's disease). *Acta Paediatr.,* **47:**501–10, 1958.
5. Crocker, A. C., Cohen, J., and Farber, S. The "lipogranulomatosis" syndrome; review, with report of patient showing milder involvement. In *Inborn Disorders of Sphingolipid Metabolism.* S. M. Aronson and B. W. Volk (eds.). Pergamon Press, Oxford and New York, 1966, pp. 485–503.
6. Cogan, D. G., Kuwabara, T., Moser, H., and Hazard, G. W. Retinopathy in a case of Farber's lipogranulomatosis. *Arch. Ophthalmol.,* **75:**752–57, 1966.
7. Schance, A. F., Bierman, S. M., Sopher, R. L., and O'Loughlin, B. J. Disseminated lipogranulomatosis: early roentgenographic changes. *Radiology,* **82:**675–78, 1964.

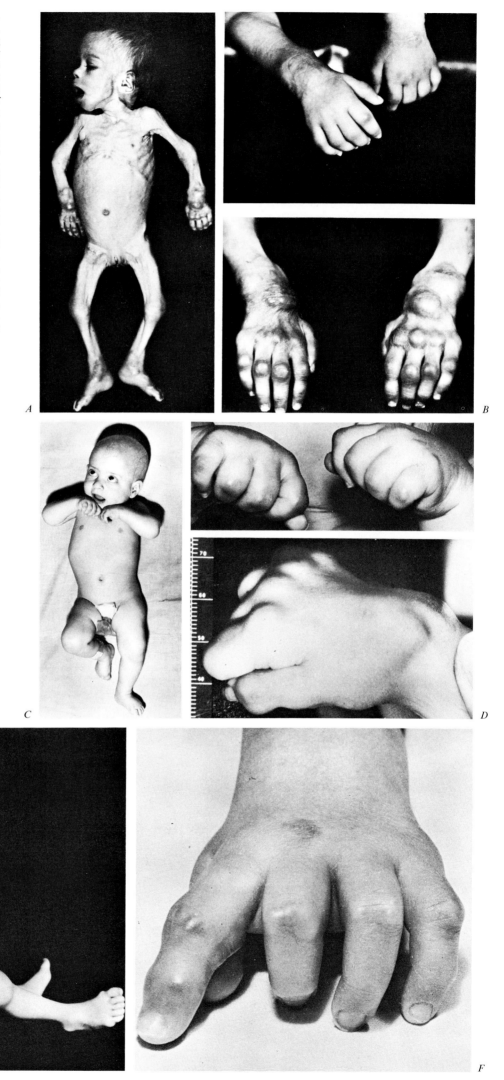

Plate II-8. *A* and *B:* A postmortem picture of one of the first reported patients. She died at 14 months of age, weighing only 7 pounds 5 ounces. Pictures of her hands show a marked progression in the soft tissue swelling and nodules over a few months time. *C* and *D:* A 4½-month-old girl with erythema and mild swelling of the interphalangeal joints. She had a hoarse voice and cried whenever she was moved. Her hands show a progression in the joint and soft tissue swelling from 4½ months (*D, top*) to 9½ months (*D, bottom*). *E* and *F:* A thin, cachectic 23-month-old boy with swollen, contracted joints and numerous soft tissue nodules over spinal processes and thorax. He had a tracheotomy cannula inserted because of laryngeal obstruction by granulomas. He had normal psychomotor development at age 15 months; he survived more than 12 years. (*A* and *B* [*top*]: Courtesy of Dr. A. C. Crocker, Boston, Massachusetts. *B* [*bottom*]: From S. Farber *et al., J. Mt. Sinai Hosp.,* **29:**816–37, 1957. *D:* From H. W. Moser *et al., Am. J. Med.,* **47:**869–90, 1969. *E* and *F:* From R. Zetterstrom, *Acta Paediatr.,* **47:**501–10, 1958.)

Flynn-Aird Syndrome

In 1965 Flynn and Aird [1] described a family in which 15 members in five generations had a disorder characterized by muscle wasting, ataxia, dementia, skin atrophy, and ocular anomalies. This was thought to be a new hereditary syndrome.

Physical Features

EYES: Fourteen patients had severe myopia, which became evident most often in the second decade of life. Eight patients had bilateral cataracts. Three had retinitis pigmentosa (*Figures D and E*); in two it was considered an atypical variety. One patient was totally blind.

MOUTH: Severe dental caries were common.

BACK: Kyphoscoliosis developed in association with the severe muscle wasting and peripheral neuritis.

SKIN: Atrophy of the skin and subcutaneous tissue over the shins and the dorsum of the feet, similar to scleroderma, was present in 13 patients (*Figure F*). Skin ulceration occurred in 5, usually on the ankles. A few patients had ichthyosis, with hyperkeratosis and lichenification primarily around the ankles (*Figure F*).

HAIR: Baldness was a late manifestation in both males (*Figures B and C*) and females.

Nervous System

All had bilateral nerve deafness, which was the earliest sign of the syndrome. Ten patients were demented. Several had seizures, characterized by episodes of expressive aphasia, blurring of vision, and numbness and paresthesias of the face and limbs. Severe muscle wasting (*Figures A, B, and F*), ataxia, intense peripheral neuritic pain, and stiffness of the joints occurred in the second decade. These changes were attributed to peripheral neuritis, which was observed in 6 patients.

Pathology

Skin biopsies showed atrophic changes and a nerve biopsy showed changes characteristic of peripheral neuritis. Three of the five brains studied were atrophic and showed changes typical of arteriosclerotic ischemia. One patient had adrenal hypertrophy and pituitary basophilic hyperplasia. Two had adrenal atrophy.

Laboratory Studies

Electroencephalographic dysrhythmias suggestive of epilepsy were found in some of the cases. In a few cases the spinal fluid protein was elevated, although in most it was normal. Two patients had diabetes mellitus, and three had cystic bone lesions.

Treatment and Prognosis

The disease did not seem to shorten life, but the handicaps caused by skeletal deformities, poor vision, and deafness resulted in severe debility early in life. The patients appeared to age prematurely.

Genetics

This syndrome appears to have been inherited in this family as an autosomal dominant trait.

Differential Diagnosis

1. Ataxia, progressive nerve deafness, atypical retinitis pigmentosa, polyneuritis with muscular weakness, and sensory changes in the extremities are features of patients with Refsum's disease, but they are not demented and do have increased phytanic acid in the blood and defective oxidation of phytanic acid [2].
2. Scleroderma, bilateral cataracts, premature aging, osteoporosis, and arteriosclerosis are features of patients with Werner's syndrome [3], but they do not have peripheral neuritis or mental deficiency and the disorder is an autosomal recessive trait.
3. Muscle weakness, cataracts, hypogonadism, and frontal balding are features of patients with myotonic dystrophy, but they have characteristic electromyographic changes and no peripheral neuritis (see page 106).
4. A dominantly inherited syndrome characterized by photic seizures, diabetes mellitus, deafness, nephropathy, and progressive cerebral degeneration has been reported [4].
5. Ataxia, atypical retinitis pigmentosa, diabetes mellitus, hypogonadism, and elevated spinal fluid protein are also features of patients with the Kearns-Sayre syndrome, which is a progressive disorder [5]. However, these patients also have ophthalmoplegia, ptosis, and cardiac arrhythmias.

References

1. Flynn, P., and Aird, R. B. A neuroectodermal syndrome of dominant inheritance. *J. Neurol. Sci.*, **2**:161–82, 1965.
2. Herndon, J. H., Steinberg, D., and Uhlendorf, B. W. Refsum's disease—defective oxidation of phytanic acid in tissue cultures derived from homozygotes and heterozygotes. *N. Engl. J. Med.*, **281**:1034–38, 1969.
3. Epstein, C. J., Martin, G. M., Schultz, A. L., and Motulsky, A. G. Werner's syndrome. A review of its symptomatology, natural history, pathologic features, genetics and relationship to the natural aging process. *Medicine (Baltimore)*, **45**:177–221, 1966.
4. Herrmann, C. Jr., Aguilar, M. J., and Sacks, O. W. Hereditary photomyoclonus associated with diabetes mellitus, deafness, nephropathy, and cerebral dysfunction. *Neurology (Minneap.)*, **14**:212–21, 1964.
5. Kearns, T. P. External ophthalmoplegia, pigmentary degeneration of the retina, and cardiomyopathy: a newly recognized syndrome. *Trans. Am. Ophthalmol. Soc.*, **63**:559–625, 1965.

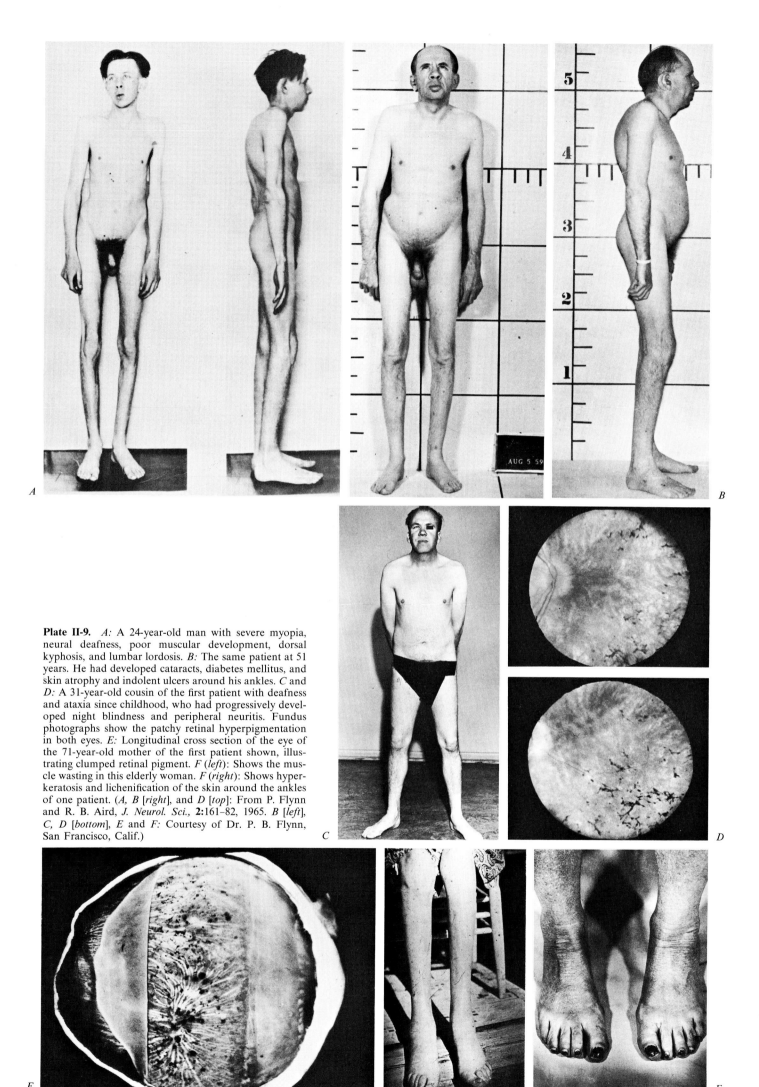

Plate II-9. *A:* A 24-year-old man with severe myopia, neural deafness, poor muscular development, dorsal kyphosis, and lumbar lordosis. *B:* The same patient at 51 years. He had developed cataracts, diabetes mellitus, and skin atrophy and indolent ulcers around his ankles. *C* and *D:* A 31-year-old cousin of the first patient with deafness and ataxia since childhood, who had progressively developed night blindness and peripheral neuritis. Fundus photographs show the patchy retinal hyperpigmentation in both eyes. *E:* Longitudinal cross section of the eye of the 71-year-old mother of the first patient shown, illustrating clumped retinal pigment. *F (left):* Shows the muscle wasting in this elderly woman. *F (right):* Shows hyperkeratosis and lichenification of the skin around the ankles of one patient. (*A, B* [*right*], and *D* [*top*]: From P. Flynn and R. B. Aird, *J. Neurol. Sci.,* **2:**161–82, 1965. *B* [*left*], *C, D* [*bottom*], *E* and *F:* Courtesy of Dr. P. B. Flynn, San Francisco, Calif.)

Friedreich's Ataxia (Hereditary Ataxia)

In 1863 Friedreich [1] described six patients with progressive ataxia and degeneration of the dorsal columns of the spinal cord. Since that time, hundreds of patients have been studied [2–7] and the entity has been defined clinically and pathologically. Affected patients usually have a combination of ataxia, speech defect, hypoactive or absent deep tendon reflexes in the legs, kyphoscoliosis, nystagmus, and foot deformity.

Physical Features

MOUTH: The palate may have a high "Gothic" arch (*Figure B*).

BACK: Scoliosis and kyphoscoliosis (*Figures A and C*), usually of a moderate degree, have been noted in 50 to 90 percent of the patients in different reports [4]. The scoliosis usually occurs in the upper thoracic region, develops late, and progresses slowly. The severity of the spinal deformity cannot be correlated with the severity of the neurologic deficit.

LIMBS: Pes cavus (*Figure D*) with retraction and flexion of the toes and sometimes inversion of the foot may be noted either before or after the neurologic deficits have become evident. In one study [5], 24 out of 31 patients had pes cavus.

Nervous System

Ataxia, the most common first neurologic symptom, is often evident at the age of 6 to 8 years. Initially the ataxia involves the legs, and a few years later the arms. Eventually the patient becomes bedridden. The muscles of the legs become flabby and eventually atrophy. The deep tendon reflexes in the legs are absent, and the plantar responses are usually extensor. Disturbances of proprioception and vibration are the most frequent sensory changes. Most patients also have a speech defect. Nystagmus is the most common eye finding. A few reported patients had a neural hearing loss [4,5]. The incidence of mental retardation is difficult to establish. In a study of 54 patients, 6 were noted to have signs of severe deterioration [2]. Out of 33 patients in another study, 3 had mental deficiency [5]. On the other hand, a careful assessment of 20 patients [6] showed that the frequency of mental deficiency was no greater than in the general population. However, 4 of the 20 patients showed evidence of dementia early in the course of the disease [6].

Pathology

The most striking histologic change is degeneration of the posterior columns, the lateral corticospinal tracts, and the dorsal and ventral spinocerebellar tracts in the spinal cord. Interstitial fibrosis is common in the myocardium of patients both with and without clinically evident heart disease [7].

Laboratory Studies

Eighteen out of 33 patients in one study showed significant cardiac abnormalities. Major electrocardiographic changes were observed in 16 and cardiac enlargement in 4 [5]. Diabetes mellitus occurred in 19 of 82 patients in one study [7] and in 2 of 33 patients in another study [5]. The cerebrospinal fluid protein concentration may be slightly increased.

Treatment and Prognosis

The mean duration of the disease has been estimated to be 16 to 24 years, and the mean age at death was 26 to 36 years [2,6]. In a study of 82 fatal cases, 60 had evidence of cardiac dysfunction and 46 died from heart failure [7].

Genetics

Two modes of inheritance have been established: autosomal recessive and autosomal dominant. The latter is much less frequently observed [2,5]. The different modes of inheritance together with the wide variation in clinical features indicate that this disorder probably represents several different genetic diseases.

Differential Diagnosis

1. Progressive ataxia, the loss of deep tendon reflexes in the limbs, and scoliosis also occur in patients with ataxia telangiectasia (see page 354). They develop telangiectases in the conjunctiva or other areas, but these are not always present when the neurologic signs are first evident.
2. Ataxia also occurs in patients with Refsum's disease [8], Hartnup's disease (see page 24), abetalipoproteinemia [9], Marinesco-Sjögren syndrome (see page 102), and metachromatic leukodystrophy (see page 36), but each can be differentiated by other clinical findings and laboratory tests.
3. Progressive ataxia can occur as an X-linked recessive disorder. However, in the families described by Shokeir [10] the age of onset was 16 to 21 years, and the ataxia was cerebellar in origin with only a mild deficiency of pyramidal function and no evidence of posterior column abnormalities, all of which features readily distinguish it from Friedreich's ataxia.

References

1. Friedreich, N. Ueber degenerative Atrophie der spinalen Hinterstränge. *Virchows Arch.*, 26:391–419, 433–59; 27:1–26, 1863.
2. Bell, J. Hereditary ataxia and spastic paraplegia. *The Treasury of Human Inheritance*, Vol. 4, Part 3, pp. 141–283, 1948. The University Press, Cambridge.
3. Greenfield, J. G. *The Spinocerebellar Degenerations*. Charles C Thomas, Springfield, Ill., 1954.
4. Heck, A. F. A study of neural and extraneural findings in a large family with Friedreich's ataxia. *J. Neurol. Sci.*, 1:226–55, 1964.
5. Boyer, S. H., Chisholm, A. W., and McKusick, V. A. Cardiac aspects of Friedreich's ataxia. *Circulation*, 25:493–505, 1962.
6. Davies, D. L. The intelligence of patients with Friedreich's ataxia. *J. Neurol. Neurosurg. Psychiatry*, 12:34–38, 1949.
7. Hewer, R. L. Study of fatal cases of Friedreich's ataxia. *Br. Med. J.*, 3:649–52, 1968.
8. Steinberg, D. Refsum's disease: a recently characterized lipidosis involving the nervous system. *Ann. Intern. Med.*, 66:365–95, 1967.
9. Farquhar, J. W., and Ways, P. Abetalipoproteinemia. In *The Metabolic Basis of Inherited Disease*, J. B. Stanbury, J. B. Wyngaarden, and D. S. Fredrickson (eds.), 2nd ed. McGraw-Hill Book Co., New York, 1966, pp. 509–22.
10. Shokeir, M. H. K. X-linked cerebellar ataxia. *Clin. Genetics*, 1:225–31, 1971.

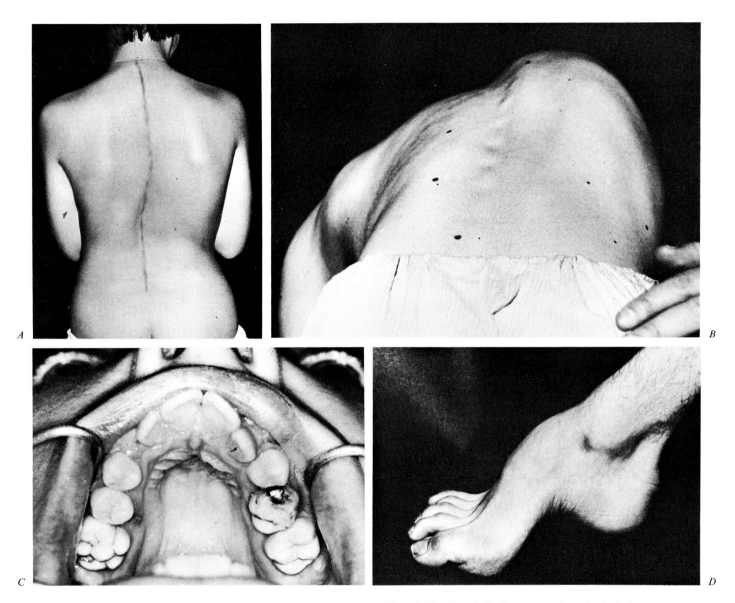

A

B

C

D

Plate II-10. *A* and *B:* Show thoracic scoliosis (spinous processes outlined with crayon) and a gothic palate in a teen-age girl who also had nystagmus, ataxia, and pes cavus. Her sister was similarly affected. *C* and *D:* Show more severe scoliosis, as well as pes cavus, in another patient. (*A:* Courtesy of Dr. A. F. Heck, Baltimore, Md. *B:* From A. F. Heck, *Neurology* [*Minneap.*], **13:**587–95, 1963. *C* and *D:* Courtesy of Dr. D. Hoefnagel, Hanover, N.H.)

Hallervorden-Spatz Disease

In 1922 Hallervorden and Spatz [1] described five siblings with a slowly progressive neurologic disease which began in late childhood. The predominant clinical features were rigidity and dementia. The striking pathologic finding was deposition of iron-containing pigment in the globus pallidus and in the substantia nigra. By 1966 more than 20 patients had been reported [2,3].

Physical Features

BACK AND LIMBS: Kyphoscoliosis and flexion contractures of the legs often develop in the late stages of the disease.

Nervous System

The patients are normal until about 7 to 9 years of age. The earliest signs are internal rotation of the ankle and an equinovarus deformity. Over the next few years the legs become increasingly rigid. Involuntary movements, such as choreoathetosis, and abnormal postures, such as torsion spasms, occur (*Figures E and F*). Speech becomes indistinct. Deterioration in mental function is evident by adolescence. Usually patients over 20 have such severe muscle rigidity in their legs that they cannot walk (*Figure B*). Subsequently, fixed flexion contractures and muscle atrophy are noted. Before contractures develop, the deep tendon reflexes and plantar responses are normal.

Pathology

The globus pallidus and substantia nigra show brown discoloration, which is evident on gross inspection of the sectioned brain. The main microscopic change is the accumulation of pigment granules, many of which appear to contain iron. In these same areas one sees swelling of the axon cylinders and a proliferation of astrocytes (*Figure C*). The changes in the other parts of the nervous system are milder. There may be a variable loss of nerve cells in the cerebral cortex and cerebellum. Occasionally there is demyelination of the posterior columns and pyramidal tracts [2].

Laboratory Studies

Despite the apparent accumulation of iron pigment in the brain, studies of iron metabolism in two patients showed no abnormalities [4].

Treatment and Prognosis

The illness is slowly progressive. Death occurs 10 to 20 years after it first becomes evident.

Genetics

Probably autosomal recessive.

Differential Diagnosis

1. The onset of rigidity at 7 to 9 years of age and dementia are features of patients with Wilson's disease. However, these patients also have a tremor, a diminished or absent serum ceruloplasmin level, and a Kayser-Fleischer ring in the cornea (see page 64).
2. Slow, nonrhythmic involuntary movements which produce bizarre postures are also features of patients with dystonia musculorum deformans. However, they do not have the same degree of generalized muscular rigidity and do not become demented.
3. Progressive involuntary movements and dementia are features of individuals with Huntington's chorea, but the age of onset is often later, the pathologic findings are different, and the mode of inheritance is autosomal dominant (see page 96).

References

1. Hallervorden, J., and Spatz, H. Eigenartige Erkrankung im extrapyramidalen System mit besonderer Beteiligung des Globus pallidus und der Substantia nigra. *Z. Ges. Neurol. Psychiat.*, **79**:254–302, 1922.
2. Kornyey, St. Die Stoffwechselstörungen bei der Hallervorden-Spatzschen Krankheit. *Arch. Psychiatr. Nervenkr.*, **205**:178–91, 1964.
3. Sacks, O. W., Aguilar, M. J., and Brown, W. J. Hallervorden-Spatz disease. Its pathogenesis and place among the axonal dystrophies. *Acta Neuropathol. (Berl.)*, **6**:164–74, 1966.
4. Szanto, J., and Gallyas, F. A study of iron metabolism in neuropsychiatric patients. Hallervorden-Spatz disease. *Arch. Neurol.*, **14**:438–42, 1966.
5. Gallyas, F., and Kornyey, St. Weiterer Beitrag zur Kenntnis der Hallervorden-Spatzschen Krankheit. *Arch. Psychiatr. Nervenkr.*, **212**:33–45, 1968.

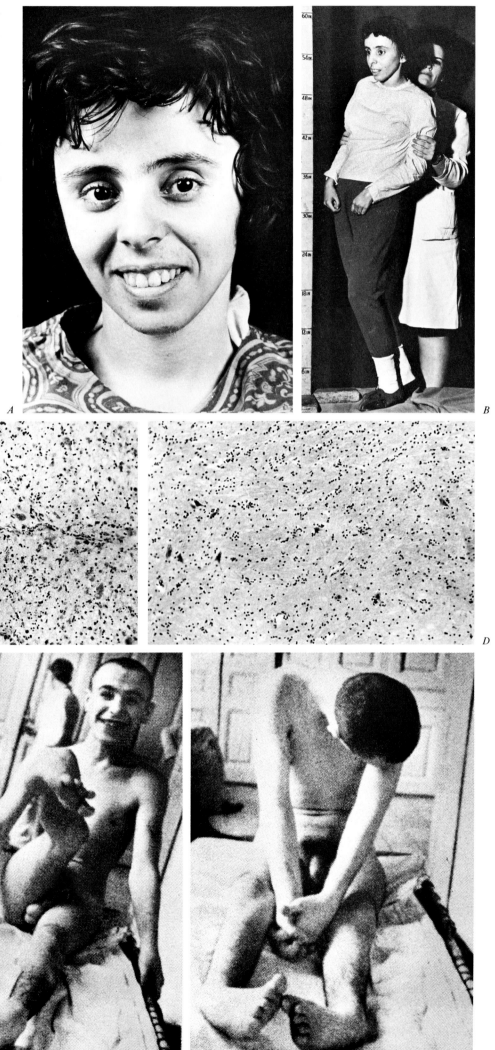

Plate II-11. *A* and *B:* A 24-year-old woman who had a staring, fixed smile, stiffness of both her arms and legs, and a tendency to fall backward. *C* and *D:* Histologic sections from the brain of the similarly affected sister of this woman (hematoxylin and eosin, × 80). *C:* Shows an affected region of the globus pallidus with pigment granules and swollen axons (*arrows*). There are no recognizable nerve cells. *D:* Unaffected region of globus pallidus. Neurons are normal in numbers and appearance. *E* and *F:* A 19-year-old, one of three affected brothers. He shows bizarre posturing, especially of his right foot. (*C* and *D:* Courtesy of Dr. E. P. Richardson, Jr., Boston, Mass. *E* and *F:* From St. Környey, *Arch. Psychiatr. Nervenkr.,* **205:**178–91, 1964.)

A

B

C

D

E

F

Huntington's Chorea

Huntington's chorea is a progressive, hereditary disease in which there are involuntary movements and dementia. Although it had been described previously, the best early description was by Huntington in 1872 [1]. Subsequently, hundreds of cases from all over the world have been reported. The prevalence in various parts of the world varies between 0.2 and 17.4 per 100,000, the highest frequency being reported in Tasmania [2]. While the average age of onset is 35 years [2], in approximately one percent of patients the disease manifests itself during the first decade.

Nervous System

In the well-known adult form of Huntington's chorea, early symptoms include changes in behavior and personality, diminished facial expression (*Figure C*), ataxia, stiff limbs, and slurred speech. Superimposed upon these nonspecific symptoms are progressive involuntary movements of the face, tongue, and limbs. Unless there is knowledge of other cases in the family, diagnosis usually is not made until these choreic movements are recognized. There is progressive dementia.

Affected children develop normally until 4 to 9 years. The first symptoms often are rigidity and a propulsive gait (*Figure B*), followed by behavior disturbances and failure in schoolwork. At that stage examination may reveal abnormal postures of the limbs and trunk, tremor, and ataxia. Deep tendon reflexes may be normal or increased, and the plantar responses flexor or extensor. Psychologic testing reveals moderate intellectual impairment. The behavioral disturbances and dementia increase in severity and there are seizures. Choreic movements are rarely observed [3] (*Figure A*). Nevertheless, the childhood disorder is classified with adult Huntington's chorea, because the affected children have had adult relatives with typical Huntington's chorea and because the neuropathologic changes in children resemble those in the adults.

Pathology

The neuropathologic changes in the adult and childhood forms resemble each other closely [4]. The essential feature is a loss of nerve cells in the caudate nucleus and putamen. These structures are reduced in size (*Figure D*), and in advanced cases loss of substance in the head of the caudate nucleus can be demonstrated with a pneumoencephalogram (*Figure E*). In the cerebral cortex there is a general reduction in the neuronal population.

Laboratory Studies

In the late stages of the disease, pneumoencephalography shows a loss of the bulge in the wall of the lateral ventricles which is normally caused by the head of the caudate nucleus (*Figures E and F*). The third ventricle is widened, but the temporal horns are not enlarged. This combination of radiologic findings is of diagnostic value [5]. Numerous biochemical and cytologic studies have been performed searching in vain for an abnormality specific for this disease [2]. While in most patients with Huntington's chorea urinary dopamine excretion is normal, it may be low in patients with the childhood form [6]. The plasma and cerebrospinal fluid levels of certain amino acids are diminished [7].

Genetics

Autosomal dominant. The childhood and adult forms occur in the same family and are presumably due to the same mutant gene. Since symptoms may not begin until the mid-thirties or later, asymptomatic young adults in affected families may not know if they themselves or their offspring are at risk. In order to help resolve this dilemma, much effort has been directed toward the development of predictive tests [2]. Among the techniques proposed are studies of the premorbid personality, electroencephalographic and electromyographic studies [2], and, recently, the administration of a test dose of levodopa, a substance that increases the involuntary movements in patients with Huntington's chorea [8].

Choreic movements are rarely seen in the childhood form of Huntington's chorea. Among the most important clues is the occurrence of chorea in other members of the family. Such an occurrence may be unknown to, or even concealed by, the family members.

Treatment and Prognosis

There is no specific treatment. In one extensive review [2] the mean duration of the typical adult form of Huntington's chorea was 13 to 16 years and that of the childhood form 7.6 to 9 years. The most common causes of death are heart disease and pneumonia, secondary to general debility. In one study, suicide was the cause of death in 7.8 percent of men and 6.8 percent of women [2].

Differential Diagnosis

1. Abnormal posture, rigidity, emotional changes, and dementia also are features of Wilson's disease (see page 64), late onset metachromatic leukodystrophy (see page 36), the neuronal lipidoses without sphingolipid accumulation (see page 110), or Hallervorden-Spatz disease (see page 94). Wilson's disease usually can be identified because of the Kayser-Fleischer ring, and metachromatic leukodystrophy by specific laboratory tests.
2. Chorea of early onset and inherited as an autosomal dominant trait was reported by Haerer *et al.* [9], but the disorder was not progressive.
3. The association of benign chorea and intention tremor with autosomal dominant inheritance was reported by Pincus and Chutorian [10].

References

1. Huntington, G. On chorea. *Med. Surg. Reptr.*, **26**:317–21, 1872. Parts reprinted in *Arch. Neurol.*, **17**:331–33, 1967.
2. Myrianthopoulos, N. C. Huntington's chorea. *J. Med. Genet.*, **3**:298–314, 1966.
3. Byers, R. K., and Dodge, J. A. Huntington's chorea in children. Report of four cases. *Neurology (Minneap.)*, **17**:587–96, 1967.
4. Jervis, G. A. Huntington's chorea in childhood. *Arch. Neurol.*, **9**:244–57, 1963.
5. Blinderman, E. E., Weidner, W., and Markham, C. H. The pneumoencephalogram in Huntington's chorea. *Neurology (Minneap.)*, **14**:601–604, 1964.
6. Barbeau, A. L-Dopa and juvenile Huntington's disease. *Lancet*, **2**:1066, 1969.
7. Perry, T. L., Hansen, S., Diamond, S., and Stedman, D. Plasma amino acid levels in Huntington's chorea. *Lancet*, **1**:806–808, 1969.
8. Klawans, H. C., Paulson, G. W., and Barbeau, A. Predictive test for Huntington's chorea. *Lancet*, **2**:1185–86, 1970.
9. Haerer, A. F., Currier, R. D., and Jackson, J. F. Hereditary nonprogressive chorea of early onset. *N. Engl. J. Med.*, **276**:1220–24, 1967.
10. Pincus, J. H., and Chutorian, A. Familial benign chorea with intention: a clinical entity. *J. Pediatr.*, **70**:724–29, 1967.

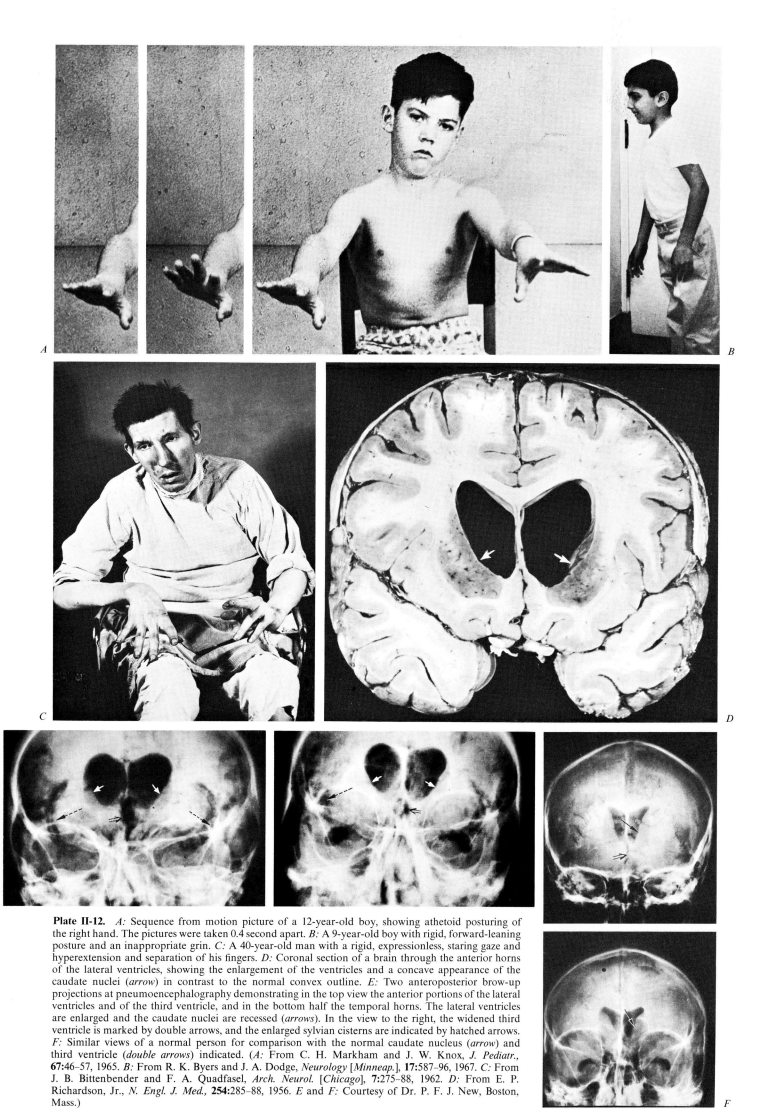

Plate II-12. *A:* Sequence from motion picture of a 12-year-old boy, showing athetoid posturing of the right hand. The pictures were taken 0.4 second apart. *B:* A 9-year-old boy with rigid, forward-leaning posture and an inappropriate grin. *C:* A 40-year-old man with a rigid, expressionless, staring gaze and hyperextension and separation of his fingers. *D:* Coronal section of a brain through the anterior horns of the lateral ventricles, showing the enlargement of the ventricles and a concave appearance of the caudate nuclei (*arrow*) in contrast to the normal convex outline. *E:* Two anteroposterior brow-up projections at pneumoencephalography demonstrating in the top view the anterior portions of the lateral ventricles and of the third ventricle, and in the bottom half the temporal horns. The lateral ventricles are enlarged and the caudate nuclei are recessed (*arrows*). In the view to the right, the widened third ventricle is marked by double arrows, and the enlarged sylvian cisterns are indicated by hatched arrows. *F:* Similar views of a normal person for comparison with the normal caudate nucleus (*arrow*) and third ventricle (*double arrows*) indicated. (*A:* From C. H. Markham and J. W. Knox, *J. Pediatr.*, **67:**46–57, 1965. *B:* From R. K. Byers and J. A. Dodge, *Neurology* [*Minneap.*], **17:**587–96, 1967. *C:* From J. B. Bittenbender and F. A. Quadfasel, *Arch. Neurol.* [*Chicago*], **7:**275–88, 1962. *D:* From E. P. Richardson, Jr., *N. Engl. J. Med.,* **254:**285–88, 1956. *E* and *F:* Courtesy of Dr. P. F. J. New, Boston, Mass.)

97

Infantile Neuroaxonal Dystrophy

In 1952 Seitelberger [1] described twin girls with a progressive disease of the nervous system. Postmortem studies showed striking swellings of the axons in the gray matter of the spinal cord and brainstem. Because of this the disease was called infantile neuroaxonal dystrophy. By 1967, 19 patients had been reported [2,3].

Nervous System

These patients have normal development until the end of the first year. Then their psychomotor development stops, and during the second and third years of life a slow regression of motor and mental functions becomes evident (*Figures A, B, and C*). A characteristic feature is the simultaneous presence of upper motor and lower motor neuron involvement. The former leads to hyperreflexia and spasticity in the arms. In the legs, signs of lower motor involvement predominate and lead to loss of reflexes and flaccidity. Diminished response to painful stimuli over the lower extremities and trunk is an early finding and of diagnostic importance. Mental function also gradually deteriorates, and the children lose their ability to speak. Optic atrophy develops late.

Pathology

The main abnormality is the presence of "spheroids" which are thought to represent focal swellings of axons (*Figure D*). There is neuronal loss, particularly in the areas where the "spheroids" are prominent. The basal ganglia, thalamus, pons medulla, and spinal cord are severely involved [1,2,3].

Laboratory Studies

Electromyography shows evidence of partial denervation of skeletal muscle, even early in the disease, but nerve conduction velocity is normal [3].

Genetics

Probably autosomal recessive [3].

Treatment and Prognosis

Most patients have died from aspiration pneumonia, usually by the age of 10 to 12 years.

Differential Diagnosis

The clinical manifestations may resemble metachromatic leukodystrophy or a primary muscle disorder. In the former there are characteristic specific biochemical abnormalities (see page 36); in the latter intelligence and sensation are normal.

References

1. Seitelberger, F. Eine unbekannte Form von infantiler lipoidspeicher Krankheit des Gehirns. *Proc. 1st Int. Congr. Neuropath.* Turin: Rosenberg & Sellier, 1952, Vol. 3, p. 323.
2. Cowen, D., and Olmstead, E. V. Infantile neuroaxonal dystrophy. *J. Neuropathol. Exp. Neurol.*, **22**:175–236, 1963.
3. Huttenlocher, P. R., and Gilles, F. H. Infantile neuroaxonal dystrophy. Clinical, pathologic, and histochemical findings in a family with 3 affected siblings. *Neurology* (*Minneap.*), **17**:1174–84, 1967.

Pelizaeus-Merzbacher Disease

In 1885 Pelizaeus [1] described five males in one family with a slowly progressive disorder characterized by nystagmus, ataxia, and spasticity. Merzbacher described in 1910 extensive loss of myelin in a male from this family. The pathologic features differ from most other white matter disorders because of the presence of "islands" of normally preserved myelin within otherwise extensively demyelinated zones [2]. While this diagnosis has been made in more than 100 reported patients [3–5], there is still considerable uncertainty whether it represents a distinct entity [2].

Physical Features

HEAD: The head circumference often is below the third percentile for age.

BACK AND LIMBS: Kyphoscoliosis and multiple joint contractures often develop in these patients after they have been bedridden for several years (*Figure E*).

HEIGHT AND WEIGHT: Linear growth and weight gain are usually below normal.

Nervous System

The infants appear normal at birth. Within the first weeks of life a side-to-side head tremor, nystagmus, and hypotonia may be evident. Over the next few months an extensor plantar response, clonus, increased deep tendon reflexes, an intention tremor, athetosis, and a hearing loss are noted. Speech is at best limited to a few words; usually only grunting sounds are made. Spasticity becomes evident, first in the legs and later in the arms. By 3 to 6 years of age many patients are immobile, with scissoring of their legs and flexed arms. Optic pallor and loss of vision develop late in the course of the disease. Dementia, a masklike facial expression, and seizures usually occur. Terminally the patients have difficulty in swallowing, vomit frequently, and are incontinent [3–5].

Pathology

There is widespread symmetric loss of myelin. A characteristic feature is the presence of islands of apparently normal myelin within large demyelinated zones. This imparts a leopard-skin pattern to tissue sections [2] (*Figure F*).

Laboratory Studies

The level of protein in the cerebrospinal fluid is normal.

Treatment and Prognosis

Most patients have died by 6 years of age, but a few have survived to adolescence or adulthood. Death is usually due to aspiration pneumonia or other complications of the debilitated state.

Genetics

While many families have exhibited X-linked recessive inheritance [3,4], other families have had affected females, suggesting autosomal recessive inheritance [5]. At this time no clinical or pathologic distinction can be made between the families showing the two types of inheritance.

Differential Diagnosis

1. Another disease with similar neurologic features has been described [6], but the patients had retinal pigment degeneration and unusual rod-shaped structures in the Schwann cell cytoplasm of sural nerve biopsies.
2. Pathologically and clinically Pelizaeus-Merzbacher disease may be difficult to distinguish from sudanophilic leukodystrophy [2,4]. The relationship between these two disorders is unclear.

References

1. Pelizaeus, Fr. Ueber eine eigenthümliche Form spastischer Lähmung mit Cerebralerscheinungen auf hereditärer Grundlage (Multiple Sklerose). *Arch. Psychiatr. Nervenkr.*, **16**:698–710, 1885.
2. Blackwood, W., McMenemey, W. H., Meyer, A., Norman, R. M., and Russell, D. S. *Greenfield's Neuropathology*, 2nd ed. Williams & Wilkins Co., Baltimore, 1963, pp. 511–12.
3. Tyler, H. R. Pelizaeus-Merzbacher disease. A clinical study. *Arch. Neurol. Psychiat.*, **80**:162–69, 1958.
4. Zeman, W., Demyer, W., and Falls, H. F. Pelizaeus-Merzbacher disease. A study of nosology. *J. Neuropathol. Exp. Neurol.*, **23**:334–54, 1964.
5. Rahn, E. K., Yanoff, M., and Tucker, S. Neuro-ocular considerations in the Pelizaeus-Merzbacher syndrome. A clinicopathologic study. *Am. J. Ophthalmol.*, **66**:1143–51, 1968.
6. Fahmy, A., Carter, T., Paulson, G., and Nance, W. E. A "new" form of hereditary cerebral sclerosis. *Arch. Neurol.*, **20**:468–78, 1969.

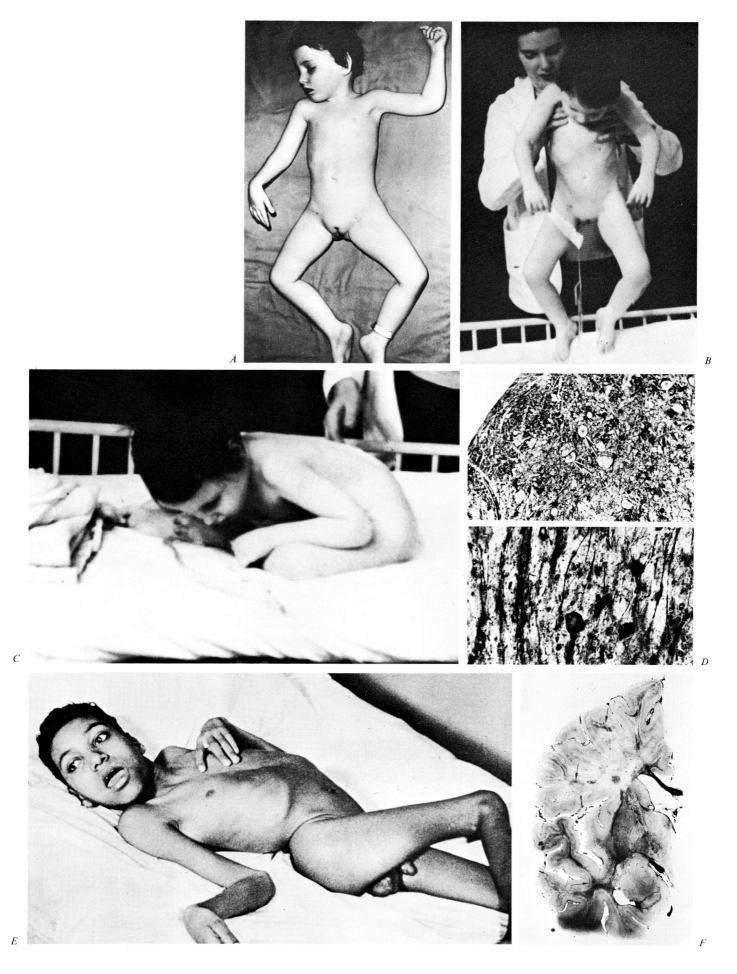

Plate II-13. *A–C:* Three sisters, ages 4, 4½, and 6 years, respectively, showing the extreme muscle weakness characteristic of infantile neuro-axonal dystrophy. The first girl also shows a tonic neck reflex position of her arms at rest, which is indicative of an upper motor neuron lesion. *D* (*top*): A section of the posterior horn of the cervical spinal cord showing multiple spheroids (*arrows*) (Bielschowsky's silver impregnation, × 80). *D* (*bottom*): A higher magnification (× 160) showing the large axonal swellings that are black due to the silver stain *E:* A 16-year-old Negro boy with Pelizaeus-Merzbacher disease. He has marked kyphoscoliosis, flexed arms and hip, small muscles, and marked hypotonia of the muscles of his wrist and fingers. *F:* Coronal section of a cerebral hemisphere showing typical irregular patches of myelin loss interspersed with islands of preserved myelin (*arrows*) (Loyez myelin stain). (*A:* From P. R. Huttenlocher and F. H. Gilles, *Neurology* [*Minneap.*], **17:**1174–84, 1967. *D:* From U. Sandbank, *Arch. Neurol.* [*Chicago*], **12:**155–59, 1965. *E:* From H. R. Tyler, *Arch. Neurol. Psychiatry,* **80:**162–69, 1958. *F:* Courtesy of Dr. E. P. Richardson, Jr., Boston, Mass.)

Kinky Hair Disease

In 1962 Menkes, Alter, Steigleder, Weakley, and Sung [1] reported a family in which five males had a disease characterized by stubby hair, neurologic deterioration in infancy, and growth retardation. Since then ten additional cases have been described [2–5,5a].

Physical Features

FACE: Several of the reported infants had micrognathia [1,5].

MOUTH: A high-arched palate was described in some of the infants.

LIMBS: Two boys had an equinovarus deformity [1,5].

HAIR: The hair is sparse, kinky, coarse, and stubby (*Figures A, C, D, and E*). It has a wiry texture when stroked. This abnormality may be evident at birth; it is clearly noticeable by the time the child is 12 weeks old. At birth the hair may be dark, but it fades to a light brown color over the next few weeks. The eyebrows may show the same changes.

HEIGHT AND WEIGHT: These patients are small for their age.

Nervous System

The infants develop normally during the first one or two months. However, soon failure of further psychomotor development and focal or generalized seizures are noted. Progressive neurologic disability then develops. The child becomes spastic, develops a decerebrate posture (*Figure B*), and appears unaware of his surroundings. Horizontal nystagmus may be present; slight pallor of the optic discs has also been noted [1–4].

Pathology

The hair shows twisting of the shafts (pili torti), fractures at regular intervals (trichorrexis nodosa), and varying diameters of the shaft (monilethrix) (*Figure F*). The brain is severely atrophied; its weight may be less than half of normal. The gyri are narrowed and the sulci are widened. The cortical gray matter is firm. The amount of cerebral white matter is reduced, and the lateral ventricles are moderately enlarged. Two patients had large subdural hematomas, presumably secondary to the cortical atrophy [1,2]. Microscopic study of the cerebral cortex shows a loss of neurons. There are scattered areas of degeneration of varying size and age, microcystic breakdown of the parenchyma, and intense proliferation of astrocytes. The cerebellum also shows marked atrophy with distortion of the normal architecture [1,2]. Changes in the spinal cord, specifically neuronal loss in the Clarke's column and degeneration of the spinocerebellar tracts, have been reported [10]. The eyes of two patients showed microcysts in the pigment epithelium of the iris, marked decrease in retinal ganglion cells, and partial atrophy of the optic nerve [4].

Laboratory Studies

Lipid analysis of brain tissue of three patients [5,6] showed a diminution of docosohexaenoic acid, particularly in the glycerophosphatide fractions. Pneumoencephalography shows marked cortical atrophy.

Treatment and Prognosis

The disease progresses relentlessly. Most patients have died between 7 months and 3½ years.

Genetics

X-linked recessive.

Differential Diagnosis

1. Abnormal hair is seen in argininosuccinic aciduria (see page 6), but these patients always excrete excess argininosuccinic acid in their urine.
2. Pili torti, a hair abnormality characteristic of kinky hair disease, occurs in two other hereditary disorders. In one of these it is associated with malformed tooth enamel [7], in the other with neural hearing loss [8]. These disorders differ from kinky hair disease since intellect is normal and there are no neurologic abnormalities.
3. Trichorrexis nodosa, pili torti, short stature, and mental retardation are also features of the syndrome reported by Tay [9] in two brothers and a sister, but they also had ichthyosiform erythroderma, a progeria-like facies, and possible autosomal recessive inheritance.

References

1. Menkes, J., Alter, M., Steigleder, G. K., Weakley, D. R., and Sung, J. H. A sex-linked recessive disorder with retardation of growth, peculiar hair, and focal cerebral and cerebellar degeneration. *Pediatrics,* **29:**764–79, 1962.
2. Aguilar, M. J., Chadwick, D. L., Okuyama, K., and Kamoshita, S. Kinky hair disease. I. Clinical and pathological features, *J. Neuropathol. Exp. Neurol.,* **25:**507–22, 1966.
3. Bray, P. F. Sex-linked neurodegenerative disease associated with monilethrix. *Pediatrics,* **36:**417–20, 1965.
4. Seelenfreund, M. H., Gartner, S., and Vingar, P. F. The ocular pathology of Menkes' disease (kinky hair disease). *Arch. Ophthalmol.,* **80:**718–20, 1968.
5. Koch, R. Personal communication, 1969.
5a. Danks, D. M., Cartwright, E., Campbell, P. E., and Mayne, V. Is Menkes' syndrome a heritable disorder of connective tissue? *Lancet,* **2:**1089, 1971.
6. O'Brien, J. S., and Sampson, E. L. Kinky hair disease. II. Biochemical studies. *J. Neuropathol. Exp. Neurol.,* **25:**523–30, 1966.
7. Appel, B., and Messina, S. J. Pili torti hereditaria. *N. Engl. J. Med.,* **226:**912–15, 1942.
8. Robinson, G. C., and Johnston, M. M. Pili torti and sensory neural hearing loss. *J. Pediatr.,* **70:**621–23, 1967.
9. Tay, C. H. Ichthyosiform erythroderma, hair shaft abnormalities, and mental and growth retardation. A new recessive disorder. *Arch. Dermatol.,* **104:**4–13, 1971.
10. Ghatak, N. R., Hirano, A., Poon, T. P., and French, J. H. Trichopoliodystrophy II. Pathological changes in skeletal muscle and nervous system. *Arch. Neurol.,* **26:**60–72, 1972.

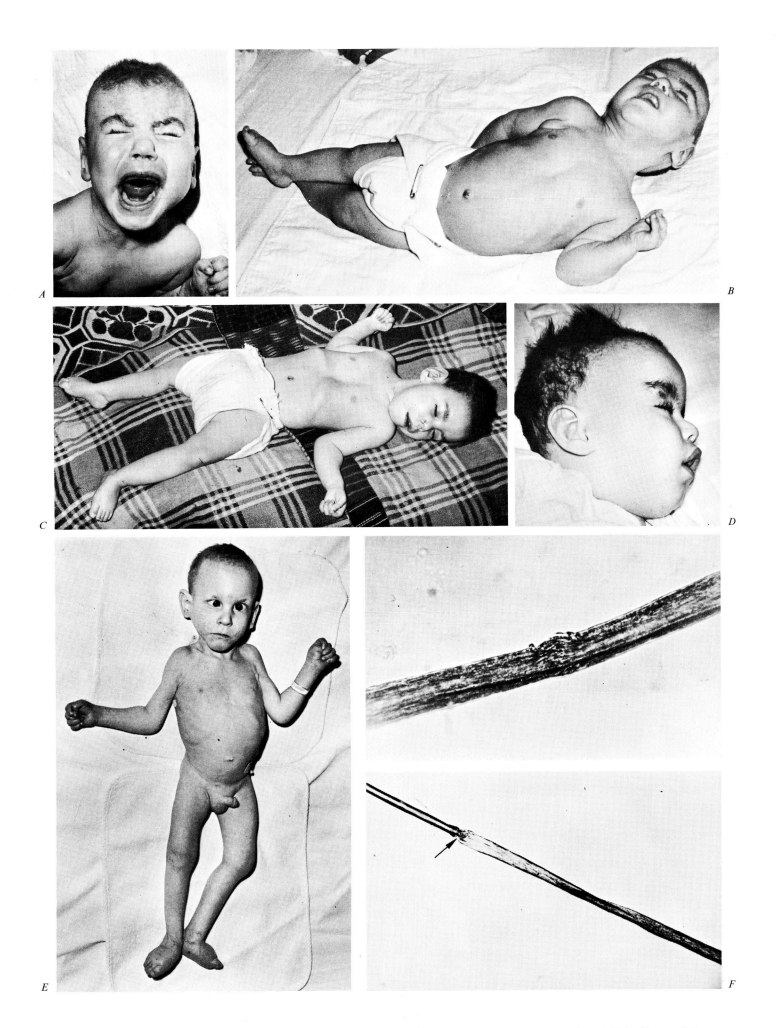

Plate II-14. *A* and *B:* A 12-month-old boy with short, stubby, kinky hair, irritability, scissoring of his legs, and opisthotonic posture. *C:* Another boy with sparse, kinky hair. He is a brother of the child shown in *A* and *B;* their mother bore 7 affected sons by 3 husbands. *D:* An infant with no motor skills, no head control, and pectus excavatum. He had intermittent seizures and recurrent pneumonia. *E:* A 3-year-old boy with short hair, strabismus, flexion contractures of his elbows, hips, and knees, and rocker-bottom feet. *F* (*left*): Shows twisting at one point near breaking point (*arrow*) of the hair shaft. *F* (*right*): Shows an area of early loss of the outer covering of a hair shaft. (*A* and *B:* From M. J. Aguilar *et al., J. Neuropathol. Exp. Neurol.,* **25:**507–22, 1966. *C:* Courtesy of Dr. C. E. Parker, Los Angeles, Calif. *D:* Courtesy of Dr. M. H. Seelenfreund, Boston, Mass. *E* and *F:* Courtesy of Dr. R. Koch, Los Angeles, Calif.)

Marinesco-Sjögren Syndrome (Hereditary Cerebellolental Degeneration with Mental Retardation)

In 1931 Marinesco, Draganesco, and Vasiliu [1] reported three sisters and a brother with a new familial disease characterized by congenital cataracts, short stature, cerebellar ataxia, and mental retardation. In 1950 Sjögren [2] reported 14 additional cases in 6 families. By 1968 at least 40 patients had been described [3–5].

Physical Features

HEAD: Some of the patients are microcephalic.

EYES: All of the reported patients have had bilateral cataracts (*Figures A and D*). The cataracts begin to develop in early infancy and by 3 to 5 years of age are sufficiently severe to markedly reduce visual acuity [5].

BACK: Several patients have had scoliosis [4].

HAIR: A few patients have had sparse hair, alopecia, or short, fine hair [3].

LIMBS: A variety of anomalies, such as clubfoot, pes planus, and short digits, have been noted in a few cases.

HEIGHT: Most patients have shortness of stature. Adults are usually less than 5 feet 6 inches (169 cm) tall [5]; some have been less than 5 feet (153 cm) tall [2].

Nervous System

The reported patients have been mildly to moderately retarded. Cerebellar ataxia is present in infancy (*Figure C*) and results in a marked delay in the development of motor skills. The patients eventually compensate for this ataxia and learn to walk. However, walking may be delayed until puberty and is never done well [5]. Dysarthric speech, strabismus, and nystagmus are also common. The deep tendon reflexes may be diminished, normal, or hyperactive. Muscle abnormalities have been noted in several patients. Mild, progressive muscle weakness may be a common feature. Some adults lose the ability to walk, which may be due to the muscle weakness. Sensation is normal [3–5].

Pathology

Very little information about the neuropathology is available. The autopsy of one child [6] showed the lesions to be almost exclusively in the cerebellum, with massive cortical atrophy that did not include the nodulus, flocculus, or paraflocculus. A 4-year-old boy (*Figure A*) had marked cerebellar atrophy (*Figure B*) with severe and uniform cell loss with marked fibrous gliosis in the cerebellar cortex, inferior olives, and pontine and vestibular nuclei [6a]. The muscle biopsy

in a patient with a mild myopathy showed a greater than normal variation in fiber size, plus increased endomyseal fibrosis and fat [5].

Treatment and Prognosis

The most important therapy is the surgical removal of cataracts. The life expectancy of these patients is unknown; one patient was 59 years old [4].

Genetics

Autosomal recessive [2].

Differential Diagnosis

1. Ataxia, scoliosis, and foot deformities are features of patients with Friedreich's ataxia, but they have normal motor development for the first 6 to 8 years of life and sensory loss in the legs, and do not have cataracts (see page 92).
2. Ataxia, cataracts, and mental retardation are features of patients with cerebrotendinous xanthomatosis, but they are distinguished by their tendon xanthomas (see page 80).
3. Cataracts, cerebellar dysplasia, and mental deficiency were features of two sisters, but they also had renal tubular necrosis and died at 4 and 8 months of age [7].
4. Three patients with cerebellar ataxia, aniridia, and mental retardation have been reported (see next section).

References

1. Marinesco, G., Draganesco, St., and Vasiliu, D. Nouvelle maladie familiale caractérisée par une cataracte congénitale et an arrêt du développement somato-neuro-psychique. *Encephale,* 26:97–109, 1931.
2. Sjögren, T. Hereditary congenital spinocerebellar ataxia accompanied by congenital cataract and oligophrenia. A genetic and clinical investigation. *Confin. Neurol.,* 10:293–308, 1950.
3. Norwood, W. F., Jr. The Marinesco-Sjögren syndrome. *J. Pediatr.,* 65:431–37, 1964.
4. Alter, M., Talbert, O. R., and Croffead, G. Cerebellar ataxia, congenital cataracts, and retarded somatic and mental maturation. *Neurology (Minneap.),* 12:836–47, 1962.
5. Alter, M., and Kennedy, W. The Marinesco-Sjögren syndrome. Hereditary cerebello-lental degeneration with mental retardation. *Minn. Med.,* 51:901–906, 1968.
6. Franceschetti, A., Klein, D., Wildi, E., and Todorov, A. Le syndrome de Marinesco-Sjögren. Première vérification anatomique. *Schweiz. Arch. neurol. Neurochir. Psychiatr.,* 97:234–40, 1966.
6a. Mahloudji, M. Personal communication, 1971.
7. Crome, L., Duckett, S., and Franklin, A. W. Congenital cataracts, renal tubular necrosis and encephalopathy in two sisters. *Arch. Dis. Child.,* 38:505–15, 1963.

Syndrome of Aniridia, Cerebellar Ataxia, and Oligophrenia

In 1965 Gillespie [1] reported a brother and sister with aniridia, cerebellar ataxia, and mental retardation. The 22-year-old girl had never been able to walk and had always had poor vision. She had dysarthric speech, small feet, and an equinovarus foot deformity. Both irides were partially absent (*Figure E*); the lenses and corneas were normal. Vision was 20/100 in both eyes. The optic discs were small, and the macular areas of the fundus appeared granular and slightly pigmented. The 19-year-old boy had similar ocular and neurologic findings (*Figure F*). His visual acuity was 20/200. He had bilateral pes planus. Both patients were considered definitely retarded, but no formal intelligence testing was performed.

In 1971 Sarsfield [2] described a 5-year-old boy with similar

features. He had partial aniridia of both eyes. His gait was ataxic and broad-based. He had gross incoordination, an intention tremor, indistinct speech, slight hypotonia in all limbs, and pes planus. His IQ was 71. A muscle biopsy and nerve conduction studies showed no abnormalities.

Skull x-rays, electroencephalograms, urine and blood amino acid screening, and chromosome karyotypes were normal in all three patients.

References

1. Gillespie, F. D. Aniridia, cerebellar ataxia, and oligophrenia in siblings. *Arch. Ophthalmol.,* 73:338–41, 1965.
2. Sarsfield, J. K. The syndrome of congenital cerebellar ataxia, aniridia and mental retardation. *Dev. Med. Child Neurol.,* 13:508–11, 1971.

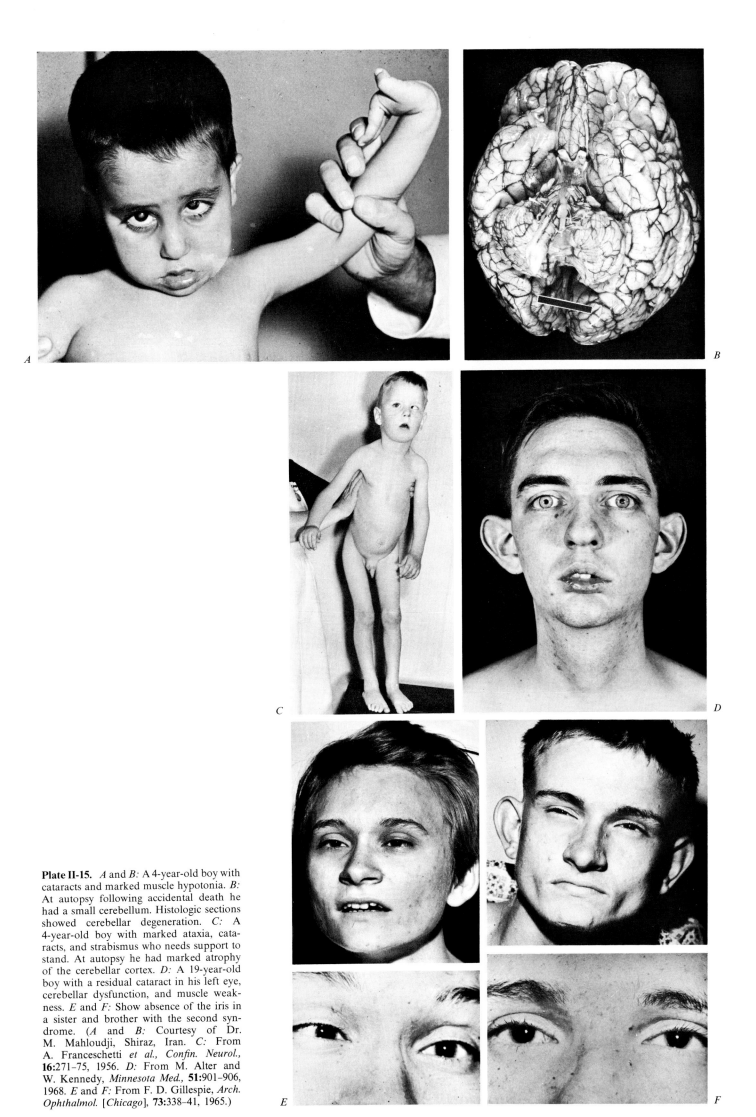

Plate II-15. *A* and *B:* A 4-year-old boy with cataracts and marked muscle hypotonia. *B:* At autopsy following accidental death he had a small cerebellum. Histologic sections showed cerebellar degeneration. *C:* A 4-year-old boy with marked ataxia, cataracts, and strabismus who needs support to stand. At autopsy he had marked atrophy of the cerebellar cortex. *D:* A 19-year-old boy with a residual cataract in his left eye, cerebellar dysfunction, and muscle weakness. *E* and *F:* Show absence of the iris in a sister and brother with the second syndrome. (*A* and *B:* Courtesy of Dr. M. Mahloudji, Shiraz, Iran. *C:* From A. Franceschetti *et al., Confin. Neurol.,* **16:**271–75, 1956. *D:* From M. Alter and W. Kennedy, *Minnesota Med.,* **51:**901–906, 1968. *E* and *F:* From F. D. Gillespie, *Arch. Ophthalmol.* [*Chicago*], **73:**338–41, 1965.)

Muscular Dystrophy, Duchenne's Pseudohypertrophic Type

The pseudohypertrophic form of muscular dystrophy was described by Duchenne [1] in 1868. This progressive disease is characterized by weakness of the trunk and proximal limb muscles, and pseudohypertrophy of certain muscle groups. It is the most common type of muscular dystrophy. Estimates of the incidence have varied from 4:100,000 in the United States [2] to 16:100,000 in northeastern England [2a].

Nervous System

The patients first show signs of involvement between 1 and 6 years of age. A waddling gait and frequent falling or clumsiness while walking and running are the most common early symptoms. About 90 percent have pseudohypertrophy of the calf muscles (*Figures A and F*). Occasionally the deltoid and triceps also show early involvement. Although the affected muscles are enlarged, they are weak and feel doughy or like rope when palpated. The hypertrophied muscles eventually atrophy over several years' time. Another early sign of the disease is weakness of the muscles of the pelvis, lumbosacral spine, and shoulder girdle. Weakness of these muscles causes the patient to have a peculiar posture and movement. When standing, he places his feet far apart and has a markedly lordotic lumbar spine (*Figures A and E*). His gait is waddling, probably because of weakness of the gluteus medius muscle. He rises from the floor by putting his hands on his knees to keep them extended and then pushes his trunk upward by working his hands up his thighs—Gower's sign (*Figures B, C, and D*). Ultimately all power over the hip, knee, shoulder, elbow, and ankle joints is lost. Atrophy spreads from the proximal to the distal muscles and the limbs become flaccid and loose. Deep tendon reflexes are lost as the muscles become involved. Shortening and contractures of muscles occur late in the disease, except for pes equinus which may be an early sign [2].

In a study [3] of 47 patients it was found that about 30 percent were mentally deficient in that they had IQ's below 75. The intellectual impairment was not progressive. The verbal and performance aspects of the IQ were equally impaired.

Pathology

The disruption of the architecture of the muscle by columns of fat cells is an early and prominent histologic feature. Later, there is an increase in the number of very small, but otherwise perfectly formed, fibers which are intermingled with large hypertrophic fibers. In the late stages of the disease there is extreme atrophy of muscle spindle cells with characteristic rows of nuclei [4]. Myocardial fibrosis and infiltration by fat occur in the advanced stages of the disease. The neuropathologic findings have not been consistent. In one study [5] cerebral abnormalities were reported in each of 3 retarded patients. However, in another study [6] (a prospective study of 21 cases), no consistent pathologic changes in the central nervous system were found.

Laboratory Studies

The serum creatinine phosphokinase level is the most useful test, for it may be markedly elevated in children less than 6 months old who have no clinical evidence of muscular dystrophy. Several other serum enzymes are elevated, but they lack specificity for muscle damage and may be elevated in other conditions, such as liver disease or myocardial infarction [2].

Treatment and Prognosis

The disease is relentlessly progressive. The rate of progression is greater the earlier the age of onset. Most patients in whom the onset is in early childhood are confined to wheelchairs by 9 to 12 years of age. Once they are unable to walk, contractures and scoliosis develop rapidly. About three fourths are dead before the age of 20 years. Exercise and activity are encouraged to the limit of tolerance; even brief periods of inactivity often produce a rapid progression of weakness.

Genetics

X-linked recessive. About 70 to 75 percent of female carriers can be identified by estimation of serum creatine kinase activity. Some of those in whom enzyme activity is normal can be recognized by means of quantitative electromyography and muscle biopsy [7]. However, when these tests reveal no abnormalities, one cannot rule out the possibility that the female relative is a carrier of the mutant gene. Prenatal diagnosis of fetal sex and the abortion of all males have been elected by some families in which the mother is a known carrier.

Differential Diagnosis

1. Three other less severe types of X-linked muscular dystrophy with similar pelvifemoral involvement have been described [8]. Each can be distinguished by the clinical course, enzyme levels, and muscle biopsy findings. None is associated with mental deficiency.
2. Pseudohypertrophy may be seen in patients with limb girdle and fascioscapular muscular dystrophy, but they are distinguished by the distribution of the muscle weakness, serum levels of muscle enzymes, and the autosomal dominant inheritance [2].
3. Hypertrophied muscles are also a feature of patients with myotonia congenita, but they have myotonia and do not have pelvifemoral muscle weakness or mental deficiency.

References

1. Duchenne, G. B. A. Recherches sur la paralysie musculaire pseudohypertrophique, ou paralysie myosclerosique. *Arch. Gen. Med.,* **11**:5–25, 179–209, 305–21, 421–43, 552–88, 1868. Parts translated and reprinted in *Arch. Neurol.,* **19**:628–36, 1968.
2. Zundel, W. S., and Tyler, F. H. The muscular dystrophies. *N. Engl. J. Med.,* **273**:537–43, 596–601, 1965.
2a. Gardner-Medwin, D. Mutation rate in Duchenne type of muscular dystrophy. *J. Med. Genet.,* **7**:334–37, 1970.
3. Prosser, E. J., Murphy, E. G., and Thompson, M. W. Intelligence and the gene for Duchenne muscular dystrophy. *Arch. Dis. Child.,* **44**:221–30, 1969.
4. Adams, R. D., Denny-Brown, D., and Pearson, C. M. *Diseases of Muscle. A Study in Pathology,* 2nd ed. Harper & Row, New York, 1962, pp. 329–31.
5. Rosman, N. P., and Kakulas, B. A. Mental deficiency associated with muscular dystrophy. A neuropathological study. *Brain,* **89**:769–88, 1966.
6. Dubowitz, V., and Crome, L. The central nervous system in Duchenne muscular dystrophy. *Brain,* **92**:805–808, 1969.
7. Walton, J. N. Carrier detection in X-linked muscular dystrophy. *J. Genet. Hum.,* **17**:497–510, 1969.
8. Mabry, C. C., Roeckel, I. E., Munich, R. L., and Robertson, D. X-linked pseudohypertrophic muscular dystrophy with a late onset and slow progression. *N. Engl. J. Med.,* **273**:1062–70, 1965.

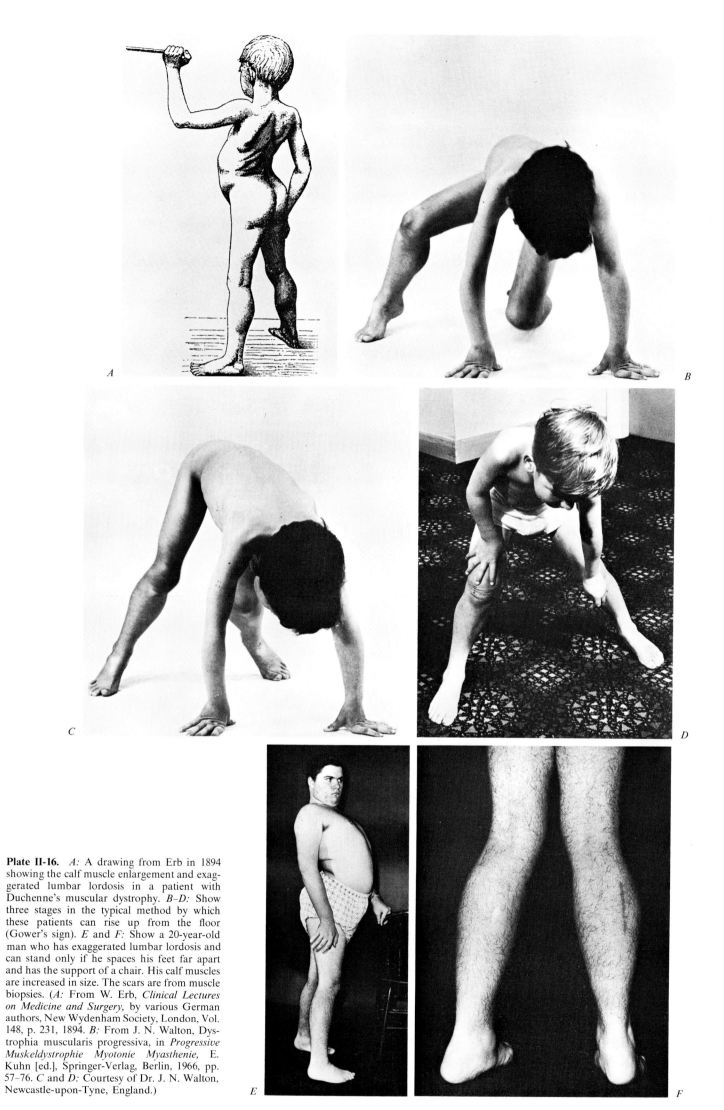

Plate II-16. *A:* A drawing from Erb in 1894 showing the calf muscle enlargement and exaggerated lumbar lordosis in a patient with Duchenne's muscular dystrophy. *B–D:* Show three stages in the typical method by which these patients can rise up from the floor (Gower's sign). *E* and *F:* Show a 20-year-old man who has exaggerated lumbar lordosis and can stand only if he spaces his feet far apart and has the support of a chair. His calf muscles are increased in size. The scars are from muscle biopsies. (*A:* From W. Erb, *Clinical Lectures on Medicine and Surgery,* by various German authors, New Wydenham Society, London, Vol. 148, p. 231, 1894. *B:* From J. N. Walton, Dystrophia muscularis progressiva, in *Progressive Muskeldystrophie Myotonie Myasthenie,* E. Kuhn [ed.], Springer-Verlag, Berlin, 1966, pp. 57–76. *C* and *D:* Courtesy of Dr. J. N. Walton, Newcastle-upon-Tyne, England.)

Myotonic Dystrophy (Dystrophia Myotonica)

In 1909 Batten and Gibb [1] and Steinert [2] independently described patients with both myotonia and muscle wasting. Subsequently hundreds of patients have been studied. It has been shown that myotonic dystrophy has an insidious onset which may be first evident in childhood or not until middle-age. The symptoms are quite variable and include cataracts, hypogonadism, immunoglobulin abnormalities, skull changes, mental retardation, and cardiac abnormalities, in addition to myotonia and widespread muscle atrophy [3–7]. The estimates of its incidence have been between 2.5 and 5 per 100,000 [3].

Physical Features

HEAD: Frontal balding is common in adults (*Figure I*) and may be present as early as the second decade. Marked under-development of the temporalis muscle may be noticeable in infancy [4].

FACE: Moderate prognathism occurs in a fourth of the patients [3].

EYES: Most patients have cataracts, which are usually peripheral, punctate, and multirefractile. Bilateral cataracts develop in most patients by adulthood (*Figure J*), but may be visible on slit-lamp examination in young children [5]. They are first visible in the anterior and posterior cortex of the lens just beneath the capsule. A stellate cataract, which may take years to develop, appears later in the posterior cortex. Elderly patients have the typical senile cataract [8].

MOUTH: A high-arched palate is often noted.

LIMBS: An equinovarus deformity is common in affected infants.

GENITALIA: Testicular atrophy occurs in many adult males.

GROWTH AND DEVELOPMENT: Males often lose their potency. Females may have no menses or abnormal menses [3].

Nervous System

Striking hypotonia may be evident in infancy. Affected children have an expressionless face due to facial diplegia, an open mouth, drooling, and difficulty with feeding (*Figures A, B, C, and G*). As they get older, dysarthria and generalized muscle weakness are more evident. Sometimes they have marked lumbar lordosis due to the weakness of trunk muscles. Atrophy of the sternocleidomastoid muscles (causing a long, thin neck; *Figures A, B, and D*), the temporalis muscles (resulting in temple hollowing; *Figure I*), and the orbicularis muscles (causing ptosis; *Figure A*) are present in many children, as well as in adults. In general, the affected adults have more evidence of muscle atrophy, especially in the distal portion of the limbs. Like the affected children, they have weak facial muscles and lack facial expression. All patients have the myotonic phenomenon, but to varying degrees.

Symptomatic myotonia is observed primarily in the hand muscles (*Figures E and F*); the patients are unable to relax their hand after a handshake. Myotonia of the orbicularis oculi is indicated by lid lag. Percussion myotonia can be elicited in the tongue (*Figure H*), thenar and deltoid muscles. Sharp tapping of these muscles causes a rapid contraction and slow recoil that produces dimpling of the muscles at the point of percussion [3–7].

Mental retardation is evident in many of the patients in all age groups. One review [5] noted that 43 out of 55 reported childhood cases were retarded. Another [6] noted that 26 of 36 cases with onset before age 16 years were mentally retarded. The intelligence quotients of the 15 tested were mostly between 50 and 60, with the range from 38 to 70. In a study [4] of 38 patients, 6 were severely retarded, 6 were mildly retarded, and 13 adults had personality disorders. In general, the degree of mental deficiency remains constant in childhood and in the adult years.

Pathology

The prominent feature in the muscle is enlargement of scattered muscle fibers with centrally placed nuclei in long rows. These changes may be seen in muscles that do not show any sign of atrophy. Another characteristic feature is the presence of a homogeneous ring of sarcoplasm around a central fascicle of myofibrils. This sarcoplasmic ring is referred to as "Ringbinden" [8]. True hypertrophy is always present. The atrophied testes show a marked decrease in the number of seminiferous tubules and either an increase or a decrease in the interstitial cells of Leydig (*Figure K*). No other specific endocrine gland changes have been consistently observed [3].

Laboratory Studies

Studies [9] on myosin prepared from myotonic dystrophic muscle suggested that its myosin ATPase is abnormally stable to alkaline pH. Electromyography shows a characteristic "dive-bomber" pattern: initially there are spontaneous bursts of fibrillationlike potentials which are of a high frequency in the beginning and then gradually decrease. Cardiac rhythm and conduction abnormalities are present in most patients; in a study [7] of 22 patients, 78 percent had either an abnormal rhythm or prolonged PR or QRS intervals. Thickening of the cranial vault (*Figure L*), large sinuses, and a small sella are often present [3,7]. In one study [10], low serum levels of IgG and an accelerated breakdown of IgG were present. In another study [7], the levels of both IgG and IgM were low. Elevated levels of insulin were noted in one study [11], but not in another [7]. Abnormally large amounts of acid muco-polysaccharides have been observed in skin fibroblasts by histochemical staining techniques [12].

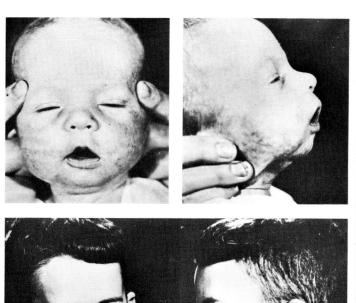

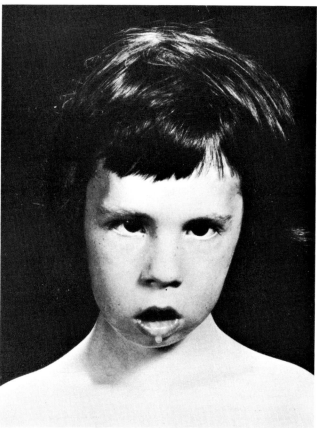

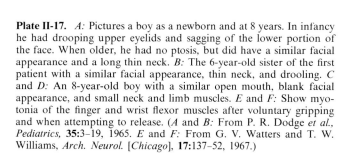

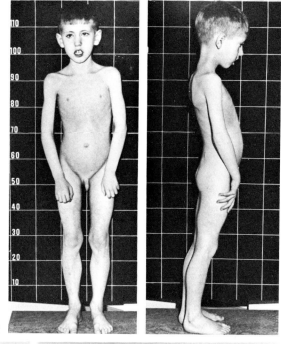

Plate II-17. *A:* Pictures a boy as a newborn and at 8 years. In infancy he had drooping upper eyelids and sagging of the lower portion of the face. When older, he had no ptosis, but did have a similar facial appearance and a long thin neck. *B:* The 6-year-old sister of the first patient with a similar facial appearance, thin neck, and drooling. *C* and *D:* An 8-year-old boy with a similar open mouth, blank facial appearance, and small neck and limb muscles. *E* and *F:* Show myotonia of the finger and wrist flexor muscles after voluntary gripping and when attempting to release. (*A* and *B:* From P. R. Dodge *et al., Pediatrics,* **35:**3–19, 1965. *E* and *F:* From G. V. Watters and T. W. Williams, *Arch. Neurol.* [*Chicago*], **17:**137–52, 1967.)

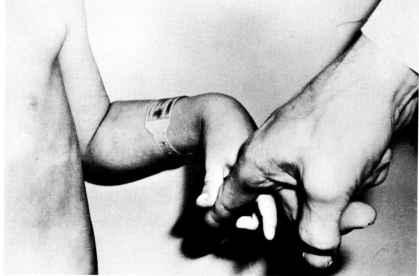

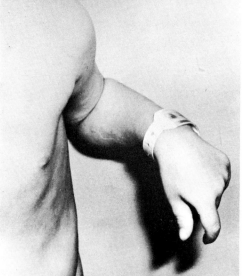

Treatment and Prognosis

Many of the problems of infants, such as feeding difficulties, ptosis, and weakness of trunk muscles, improve with age.. Quinine is sometimes helpful in relieving the myotonia. Adult patients with hypogonadism are usually sterile. The disease progresses steadily without remissions to invalidism. Pulmonary infections are a common cause of death. Few patients survive beyond the sixth decade.

Genetics

Autosomal dominant. Often the affected individual seems to have no similarly affected relatives and is initially considered to represent a spontaneous genetic mutation. However, in view of the wide variability of the clinical manifestations it is important to carefully examine all of the immediate relatives. The best means for detecting mildly affected individuals are the neurologic examination, the slit-lamp examination for cataracts, and electromyography. It has often been suggested that the disease appears earlier in subsequent generations. However, this has been disproven in many studies. The reasons for this apparent genetic anticipation are that the presence of a known affected relative prompts earlier recognition in younger patients, that the number of younger patients recognized is offset by the number of late-onset adults who are missed, and that the patients with an earlier onset of symptoms usually do not become parents [7].

The close linkage of the locus of the gene for myotonic dystrophy to that of secretor may be of value in prenatal diagnosis. In suitable families ABH secretor status of the fetus could be established from the amniotic fluid and would indicate with high probability whether or not the fetus had myotonic dystrophy [13].

Differential Diagnosis

1. Myotonia is a feature of patients with myotonia congenita, but they have normal intelligence, have no abnormality on muscle biopsy, develop muscle hypertrophy rather than atrophy, and have no endocrinologic abnormalities.
2. Myotonic dystrophy is considered a feature of Rieger's syndrome, but these patients also have aniridia, hypodontia, and several other eye and tooth anomalies [14].
3. Muscle hypotonia, ptosis, facial diplegia, and clubfoot are also features of patients with the Möbius syndrome, but they often have other cranial nerve palsies, do not have myotonia, and do not develop muscle atrophy, cataracts, and frontal balding (see page 296).

References

1. Batten, F. E., and Gibb, H. P. Myotonia atrophica. *Brain,* **32**:187–205, 1909.
2. Steinert, H. Myopathologische Beiträge. I. Über das klinische und anatomische Bild des Muskelschwunds der Myotoniker. *Dtsch. Z. Nervenheilkd.,* **37**:58–104, 1909.
3. Caughey, J. E., and Myrianthopoulos, N. C. *Dystrophia Myotonia and Related Disorders.* Charles C Thomas, Publisher, Springfield, Ill., 1963.
4. Dodge, P. R., Gamstorp, I., Byers, R. K., and Russell, P. Myotonic dystrophy in infancy and childhood. *Pediatrics,* **35**:3–19, 1965.
5. Calderon, R. Myotonic dystrophy: a neglected cause of mental retardation. *J. Pediatr.,* **68**:423–31, 1966.
6. Watters, G. V., and Williams, T. W. Early onset myotonic dystrophy. Clinical and laboratory findings in five families and a review of the literature. *Arch. Neurol.,* **17**:137–52, 1967.
7. Bundey, S., Carter, C. O., and Soothill, J. F. Early recognition of heterozygotes for the gene for dystrophia myotonica. *J. Neurol. Neurosurg. Psychiatry,* **33**:279–93, 1970.
8. Adams, R. D., Denny-Brown, D., and Pearson, C. M. *Diseases of Muscle. A Study in Pathology,* 2nd ed. Harper & Row, New York, 1962, pp. 324–84.
9. Samaha, F. J., and Gergely, J. Biochemistry of normal and myotonic dystrophic human myosin. *Arch. Neurol.,* **21**:200–207, 1969.
10. Wochner, R. Accelerated breakdown of immunoglobulin G (IgG) in myotonic dystrophy: a hereditary error of immunoglobulin catabolism. *J. Clin. Invest.,* **45**:321–29, 1966.
11. Huff, T. A., Horton, E. S., and Lebovitz, H. E. Abnormal insulin secretion in myotonic dystrophy. *N. Engl. J. Med.,* **277**:837–41, 1967.
12. Swift, M. R., and Finegold, M. J. Myotonic muscular dystrophy: abnormalities in fibroblast culture. *Science,* **165**:294–96, 1969.
13. Renwick, J. H., and Bolling, D. R. An analysis procedure illustrated on a triple linkage of use for prenatal diagnosis of myotonic dystrophy. *J. Med. Genet.,* **8**:399–406, 1971.
14. Busch, G., Weiskopf, J., and Busch, K.-T. Dysgenesis mesodermalis et ectodermalis Rieger oder Reiger'sche Krankheit. *Klin. Monatsbl. Augenheilkd.,* **136**:512–23, 1960.

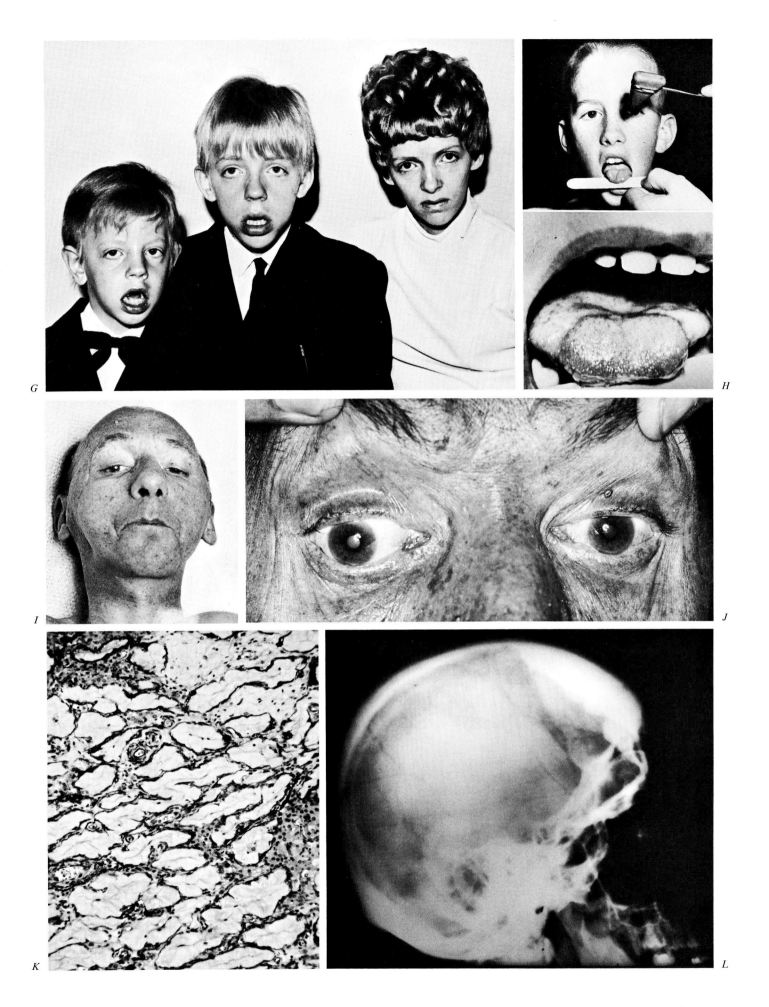

Plate II-17. *G:* An affected mother and her two affected sons. Both boys were mildly retarded, and their mother had borderline normal intelligence. *H (top):* Shows the eliciting of muscle myotonia by percussion. *H (bottom):* Shows in another patient the resulting sustained contraction of the tongue muscles with indenting of the lateral margins. *I, J, K:* A 55-year-old man with marked frontal balding, wasting of the temporal, facial, and neck muscles, and cataracts. His testes showed wavy hyalinized tubules separated by irregular aggregates of Leydig cells ($\times$ 137, elastic tissue stain). *L:* Shows hyperostosis most marked in the frontal region. (*G* and *H* [*bottom*]: From G. V. Watters and T. W. Williams, *Arch. Neurol.* [*Chicago*], **17:**137–52, 1967. *H* [*top*]: From P. R. Dodge, Neurologic history and examination, in *Pediatric Neurology,* T. W. Farmer [ed.], Hoeber Medical Division, Harper & Row, New York, 1964, pp. 1–64. *K:* Courtesy of Drs. A. Schiller and R. E. Scully, Boston, Mass. *L:* Courtesy of Dr. G. R. Hogan, Boston, Mass.)

109

Neuronal Lipidoses Without Sphingolipid Accumulation (Batten's Disease, Batten-Spielmeyer-Vogt Disease, Juvenile Amaurotic Idiocy, Bielschowsky-Jansky Disease, Kufs Disease, Myoclonic Variant of Cerebral Lipidosis)

The term *neuronal lipidosis* refers to disorders in which the neuronal cytoplasm is distended because of lipid accumulation. In all instances in which the metabolic disturbance has been defined, the accumulated lipids have been shown to contain the base sphingosine and these lipids are referred to as sphingolipids. In the disorders discussed in this section, there is a variable degree of lipid accumulation within the neuronal cytoplasm. The structure of the accumulated lipids has not been identified. However, it appears well established that there is no sphingolipid accumulation. As the large number of names suggests, the classification of this group of disorders is controversial. The first description was by Batten [1], who in 1903 described two siblings aged 8 and 13 years who had reddish-black spots in the maculae and pigmentary degeneration of the retina and suffered from convulsions and mental deterioration. Other authors have reported patients who had similar clinical features but differed as to the age of onset of their neurologic symptoms. The different eponyms reflect in part this difference in age of onset: Bielschowsky-Jansky [2], late infancy; Batten-Spielmeyer-Vogt [1,3,4], childhood and adolescence (juvenile form); Kufs [5], adulthood. The patients described by Seitelberger and coworkers [6] differed in that myoclonus and cerebellar ataxia were prominent features. The relationship among these disorders is undetermined. It has been proposed that all of these entities are variations of a single disease [7]. However, this must be considered tentative.

Physical Features

EYES: Ocular changes are common. They may be the first manifestation of disease [8], may occur after neurologic changes develop [7], or may never occur [5]. When visual disturbances are present, central vision often is first impaired, and visual acuity may be markedly reduced with little or no fundic change. In one large series, three stages of ocular changes were described [8]. In the first stage there was a narrowing of retinal vessels and slight pallor of the optic disc. In the second stage there was severe visual impairment, and small yellow lesions containing small pigmented granules were noted in the periphery of the retina. In the third stage there was marked optic atrophy, thin retinal vessels (*Figure D*), and many pigmented lesions in the periphery of the retina. In the most advanced cases these lesions covered the entire retina [8].

Nervous System

While all patients eventually develop neurologic impairment, including dementia, the age at which this occurs varies from late infancy to adulthood. Initial mental and motor development are normal. The types and sequence of neurologic symptoms vary. In Sjögren's large series, dementia and emotional lability preceded by several years the development of a parkinsonian syndrome (*Figures A and B*), and spasticity, hyperreflexia, and extensor plantar responses were present only in the final stages [8] (*Figure C*). In the Bielschowsky-Jansky type, cerebellar ataxia is a striking feature [2]. Myoclonus is prominent in another type [6].

Pathology

The brain is atrophied and the cortex is thinned. Neurons are reduced in number, and the neuronal cytoplasm contains lipid inclusions with properties similar to those of lipofuscin, a material that normally accumulates with aging. Except for this, no consistent lipid abnormalities have been found.

Laboratory Studies

Laboratory diagnosis based upon study of readily accessible tissues is difficult. Vacuoles in lymphocytes or azurophilic granules in blood polymorphonuclear cells (*Figure E*) may be present but not invariably so [9]. Rectal biopsy may show lipid storage in ganglion cells, and under the electron microscope the lipid inclusions have a characteristic "fingerprint" pattern [10] (*Figure F*), which differs from the lamellar pattern seen in the disorders associated with ganglioside storage, such as Tay-Sachs disease (see *Figure 1-28, F*, page 63). At times brain biopsy has been resorted to for diagnosis, but indications for such a procedure must be examined with great care.

Prognosis

Age at death varies from early childhood to adulthood. The interval between onset of symptoms and death varies from a few years to decades.

Genetics

Autosomal recessive.

Differential Diagnosis

Because of the lack of specificity of the clinical manifestations and laboratory studies, definitive diagnosis of these disorders is difficult, and may not be possible during life. Often, presumptive diagnosis depends upon exclusion of disorders more readily diagnosed. Among others these include Tay-Sachs disease (see page 62), G_{M1} gangliosidosis (see page 22), Niemann-Pick disease (see page 44), globoid leukodystrophy (see page 18), metachromatic leukodystrophy (see page 36), and subacute sclerosing panencephalitis [12].

References

1. Batten, F. E. Cerebral degeneration with symmetrical changes in the maculae in two members of a family. *Trans. Ophthalmol. Soc. UK*, **23**:386–90, 1903.
2. Bielschowsky, M. Über spätinfantile familiärer amaurotischer Idiotie mit Kleinhirnsymptomen. *Dtsch. Z. Nervenheilkd.*, **50**:7–29, 1913.
3. Spielmeyer, W. Weitere Mittheilung Über eine besondere Form von familiärer amaurotischer Idiotie. *Neurol. Centralblatt*, **24**:1131–32, 1905.
4. Vogt, H. Familiärer amaurotischer Idiotie, histologische und histopathologische Studien. *Arch. Kinderheilkd.*, **51**:1–35, 1909.
5. Kufs, H. Über eine Spätform der amaurotischen Idiotie und ihre heredofamiliären Grundlagen. *Z. Ges. Neurol. Psychiat.*, **95**:169–88, 1925.
6. Seitelberger, F., Jacob, H., and Schnabel, R. The myoclonic variant of cerebral lipidosis. In *Inborn Disorders of Sphingolipid Metabolism*, S. M. Aronson and B. W. Volk (eds). Pergamon Press, New York, 1967, p. 43.
7. Zeman, W., and Dyken, P. Neuronal ceroid-lipofuscinosis (Batten's disease): relationship to amaurotic family idiocy. *Pediatrics*, **44**:570–83, 1969.
8. Sjögren, T. Die Jevenile amaurotische Idiotie. Klinische und erblichkeitsmedizinische Untersuchungen. *Hereditas*, **14**:197–426, 1931.
9. Strough, J. C., Zeman, W., and Merritt, A. D. Leukocyte abnormalities in familial amaurotic idiocy. *N. Engl. J. Med.*, **274**:36–38, 1966.
10. Elsner, B., and Prensky, A. L. Ultrastructure of rectal biopsies in juvenile amaurotic idiocy. *Neurology* (*Minneap.*), **19**:834–40, 1969.
11. Herman, M. M., Rubinstein, L. J., and McKhann, G. M. Additional electron microscopic observations on two cases of Batten-Spielmeyer-Vogt disease (neuronal ceroid-lipofuscinosis). *Acta Neuropathol.* (*Berl.*), **17**:85–102, 1971.
12. Freeman, J. M. The clinical spectrum and early diagnosis of Dawson's encephalitis, with preliminary notes on treatment. *J. Pediatr.*, **75**:590–603, 1969.

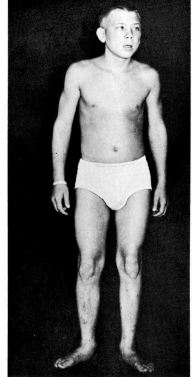
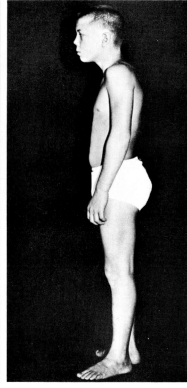

A

B

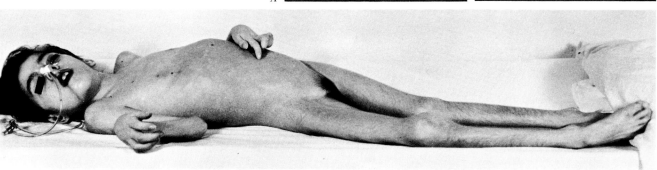

C

Plate II-18. *A* and *B:* A 15-year-old boy with stiff posture and a blank stare. He first had visual disturbances at 5 years. *C:* A comatose 7½-year-old girl with myoclonic hyperexcitability and hirsutism. Her neurologic deterioration began at 4 years. *D:* Shows typical coarse granular macular degeneration with atrophy of the retinal vessels. *E:* Shows basophilic hypergranulation of a neutrophil (*left*) and lymphocyte vacuolization (*right*). *F:* Electron micrograph of cytoplasm of a ganglion cell filled with inclusions ($\times$ 18,300). Note the fingerprint pattern. Some of the inclusions have no apparent limiting membrane (*single arrow*), and others have a visible membrane (*two arrows*). (*A–E* [*bottom*]: Courtesy of Dr. W. Zeman, Indianapolis, Ind. *E* [*top*]: From W. Zeman and J. C. Strouth, in *Inborn Errors of Sphingolipid Metabolism,* S. M. Aronson and B. W. Volk [eds.]. Pergamon Press, New York, 1966, pp. 475–84. *F:* From B. Elsner and A. L. Prensky, *Neurology* [*Minneap.*], **19**:834–40, 1969.)

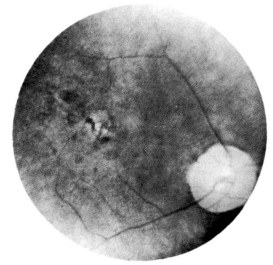

D

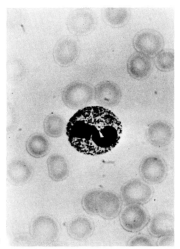
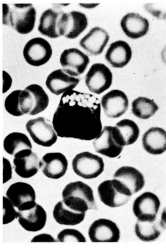
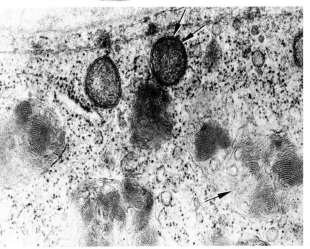

E

F

Spongy Degeneration of the Central Nervous System in Infancy (Canavan's Disease)

In 1949 van Bogaert and Bertrand [1] described three Jewish infants with a degenerative disorder of the nervous system characterized by macrocephaly and widespread demyelinization. In retrospect it was apparent that Globus and Strauss [2] in 1928 and Canavan [3] in 1931 had described patients with this same illness. Over 30 patients have now been reported [4,5].

Physical Features

HEAD: Head enlargement is usually evident by the time the infant is 6 months old (*Figures C and D*). The increase in size is slowly progressive and is often associated with frontal bossing and a tense anterior fontanel.

HAIR: It has been noted that 6 of 10 affected children had blond hair and 4 had red hair. This may be significant, since in most cases unaffected family members had dark hair [4].

Nervous System

The infants may appear normal until the second or third month of life, when it is noted that they lack head control. Certain developmental attributes, such as grasping, visual fixation and following, smiling, and cooing seemed to be acquired at the appropriate time, only to be lost subsequently. By 4 to 5 months of age all motor activity is reduced and the muscle tone is diminished. An internal strabismus was noted in 4 of 10 patients between 3 and 10 months [4]. Subsequently optic atrophy, roving eye movements, nystagmus, and blindness are evident. The limbs become spastic, the legs usually being first affected. In the late stages the patients show little responsiveness to their environment (*Figures A and B*). The limbs are held in decorticate or decerebrate postures (*Figure D*). Feeding is difficult due to pseudobulbar palsy. Tonic or "cerebellar fits," in which there is a periodic exaggeration of opisthotonic decerebrate postures in response to noise or manipulation of the limbs, are commonly present. Three of 10 patients had generalized seizures [4].

Pathology

The brain is larger and heavier than normal, and this accounts for the increase in the head circumference. The ventricular system may be enlarged, but not to the extent seen in obstructive hydrocephalus. The characteristic microscopic feature is widespread vacuolization, which has led to the name *spongy degeneration* (*Figures E and F*). This involves mainly the lower layers of cerebral cortex and the white matter. There is widespread disintegration of myelin.

Laboratory Studies

The cerebrospinal fluid protein level is usually normal [4]. The spinal fluid pressure may be increased. Chemical analyses in brain samples from four patients have shown an accumulation of water, which reduced the dry weight to one half to one third of normal. Myelin lipids were reduced. It was postulated that chronic edema of white matter was the primary

disturbance and that the loss of myelin was secondary to this [6].

Genetics

Autosomal recessive. Most cases have occurred in Jewish families who came from eastern Poland and the western Ukraine [4]. This is the same area from which most families with Tay-Sachs disease originate. In some families there were affected individuals in earlier generations, which may be a reflection of a high incidence of this rare mutant gene in this ethnic group and geographic area. One affected child was born to parents of Irish extraction [5].

Treatment and Prognosis

Death usually occurs between 7 months and 4 years [1–5]. Four exceptional patients survived until the ages of 7 to 11 years [7], and one child was alive at $13\frac{1}{2}$ years [8].

Differential Diagnosis

1. Neurologic deterioration occurs in the first months of life in patients with Tay-Sachs disease, but they also have a macular cherry-red spot and diminished activity of serum hexosaminidase A, and head enlargement does not occur until the second to fourth year (see page 62).

2. Neurologic deterioration also occurs in infants with globoid cell leukodystrophy (Krabbe's disease), but they do not have an enlarged head and usually have an increased spinal fluid protein concentration (see page 18).

3. Enlargement of the head and neurologic deterioration are also features of patients with Alexander's disease (see page 72).

4. Patients with obstructive hydrocephalus may develop head enlargement in the first months of life, but they usually do not have the severe neurologic deficits seen in patients with spongy degeneration of the central nervous system in infancy.

References

1. van Bogaert, L., and Bertrand, I. Sur une idiotie familiale avec dégénérescence spongieuse du névraxe. *Acta Neurol. Belg.*, **49:**572–87, 1949.
2. Globus, J. H., and Strauss, I. Progressive degenerative subcortical encephalopathy (Schilder's disease). *Arch. Neurol. Psychiatr.*, **20:**1190–1228, 1928.
3. Canavan, M. M. Schilder's encephalitis periaxialis diffuse. Report of a case in a child aged sixteen and one-half months. *Arch. Neurol. Psychiatr.*, **25:**299–308, 1931.
4. Banker, B. Q., Robertson, J. T., and Victor, M. Spongy degeneration of the central nervous system in infancy. *Neurology (Minneap.)*, **14:**981–1001, 1964.
5. Hogan, G. R., and Richardson, E. P. Spongy degeneration of the nervous system (Canavan's disease); report of a case in an Irish-American family. *Pediatrics*, **35:**284–94, 1965.
6. Kamoshita, S., Rapin, I., Suzuki, K., and Suzuki, K. Spongy degeneration of the brain. A chemical study of two cases including isolation and characterization of myelin. *Neurology (Minneap.)*, **18:**975–85, 1968.
7. Adachi, M., and Volk, B. W. Protracted form of spongy degeneration of the central nervous system (van Bogaert and Bertrand type). *Neurology (Minneap.)*, **18:**1084–92, 1968.
8. Hogan, G. R. Personal communication, 1970.

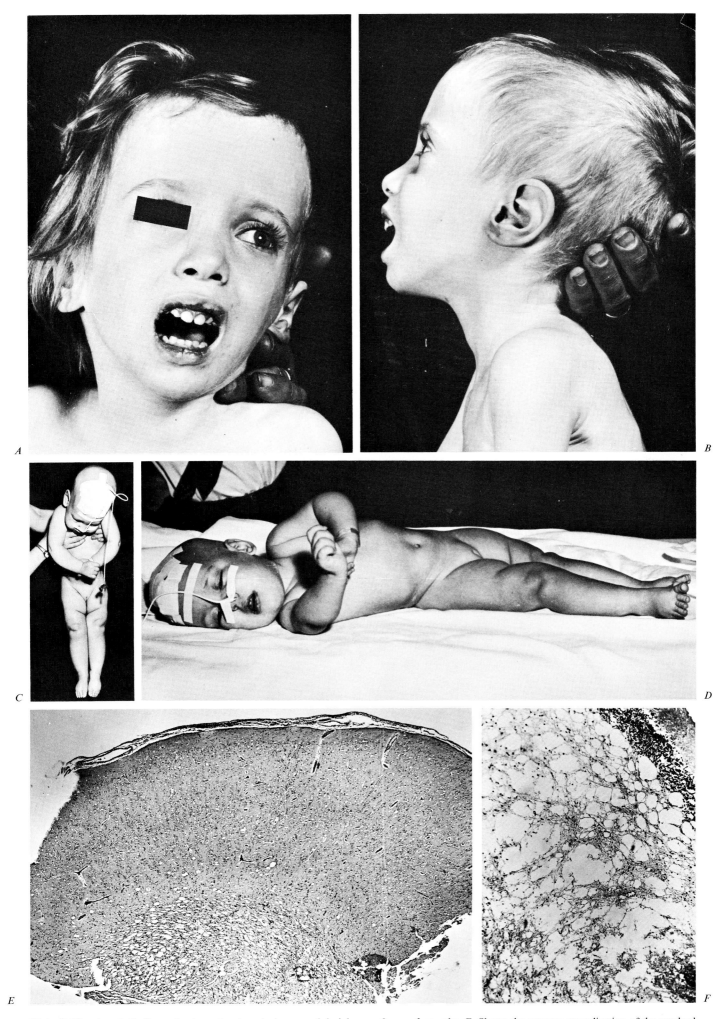

Plate II-19. *A* and *B*: Show the large head and absence of facial expression in a 4½-year-old girl who was blind and had decorticate posture. *C–F*: A 17-month-old girl with hypotonia of the neck muscles, flexed arms, and hyperextension of the legs. She also had macrocephaly and was fed by nasogastric tube. She died of pneumonia at 9 years 3 months. *E*: Shows the extreme vacuolization of the cerebral subcortex and white matter of this child. *F*: Shows extreme vacuolization of the white matter of the cerebellar folium. (*A* and *B*: Courtesy of Dr. B. Q. Banker, Cleveland, Ohio. *C–F*: From G. M. ZuRhein *et al., Neurology* [*Minneap.*], **10**:998–1005, 1960.)

Syndrome of Adrenocortical Atrophy and Diffuse Cerebral Sclerosis

In 1923 Siemerling and Creutzfeldt [1] reported a young boy who had generalized hyperpigmentation and later neurologic deterioration. At autopsy he had diffuse cerebral sclerosis and adrenal atrophy. By 1971 more than 20 additional cases had been described [2–6,6a]. The causation is not known.

Physical Features

SKIN: Dusty brown pigmentation involves the entire body, buccal mucosa, and scars (*Figures A, B, and C*). It usually develops between 3 and 10 years of age, always a few years before the onset of neurologic symptoms. However, one reported patient, a boy who died when 7 years old, did not have increased pigmentation [6].

Nervous System

The signs and symptoms of neurologic deterioration are first evident between 5 and 15 years of age. The initial symptoms are variable and include visual field defects, weakness of one or both arms or legs, or extraocular palsies. Subsequently clumsiness, indistinct speech, and mental deterioration are apparent and become progressively severe. Eventually, the patients develop blindness and spastic quadriplegia with hyperactive deep tendon reflexes and extensor plantar responses. Convulsions are uncommon [2–6].

Pathology

The neurologic disturbances result from widespread destruction of myelin in the cerebral hemispheres (*Figure D*) and brainstem (*Figure E*). As in multiple sclerosis there are perivascular infiltrates of lymphocytes and fat-laden macrophages (*Figure F*). The cerebral cortex is normal. One reported patient had no histologic abnormalities of the cerebral cortex, but biochemical studies showed abnormalities in the cortex [6a]. The adrenal cortices show severe atrophy [2]. One patient had a virtual absence of basophilic cells in the pituitary gland [6].

Laboratory Studies

The expected signs of adrenal cortex atrophy include hypoglycemia, diminished excretion of urinary hydroxy- and ketosteroids, low plasma cortisol, and a failure to respond to the administration of adrenocorticotropic hormone. Once the neurologic symptoms are present, the spinal fluid protein may be moderately increased. As in multiple sclerosis, a "first-zone" colloidal gold curve may be present, which probably reflects an increase in the cerebrospinal fluid gamma globulins.

Treatment and Prognosis

Unfortunately, the correction of the hypoadrenalism does not prevent the onset of neurologic deterioration. Death usually occurs between 6 months and 3 years after the onset of neurologic symptoms.

Genetics

Probably X-linked recessive [4].

Differential Diagnosis

The combination of adrenal insufficiency and progressive neurologic disorder is virtually pathognomonic of the syndrome of adrenocortical atrophy and diffuse cerebral sclerosis. In addition, there are two reports of Addison's disease in association with spastic paraplegia [7,8]. These cases were not studied pathologically, and their relationship to the present disorder is unclear.

References

1. Siemerling, E., and Creutzfeldt, H. G. Bronzekrankheit und sklerosierende Encephalomyelitis (Diffuse Sklerose). *Arch. Psychiatr. Nervenkr.,* **68**:217–44, 1923.
2. Turkington, R. W., and Stempfel, R. S., Jr. Adrenocortical atrophy and diffuse cerebral sclerosis (Addison-Schilder's disease). *J. Pediatr.,* **69**:406–12, 1966.
3. Aguilar, M. J., O'Brien, J. S., and Taber, P. The syndrome of familial leukodystrophy, adrenal insufficiency and cutaneous melanosis. In *Inborn Disorders of Sphingolipid Metabolism,* S. M. Aronson and B. W. Volk (eds.). Pergamon Press, New York, 1967, pp. 149–66.
4. Vick, N. A., and Moore, R. Y. Diffuse sclerosis with adrenal insufficiency. *Neurology (Minneap.),* **18**:1066–74, 1968.
5. Sotos, J. F. Personal communication, 1969.
6. Hoefnagel, D., van den Noort, S., and Ingbar, S. H. Diffuse cerebral sclerosis with endocrine abnormalities in young males. *Brain,* **85**:553–68, 1962.
6a. Forsyth, C. C., Forbes, M., and Cumings, J. N. Adrenocortical atrophy and diffuse cerebral sclerosis. *Arch. Dis. Child.,* **46**:273–84, 1971.
7. Penman, R. W. B. Addison's disease in association with spastic paraplegia. *Br. Med. J.,* **1**:402, 1960.
8. Harris-Jones, J. N., and Nixon, P. G. F. Familial Addison's disease with spastic paraplegia. *J. Clin. Endocrinol. Metab.,* **15**:739–44, 1955.

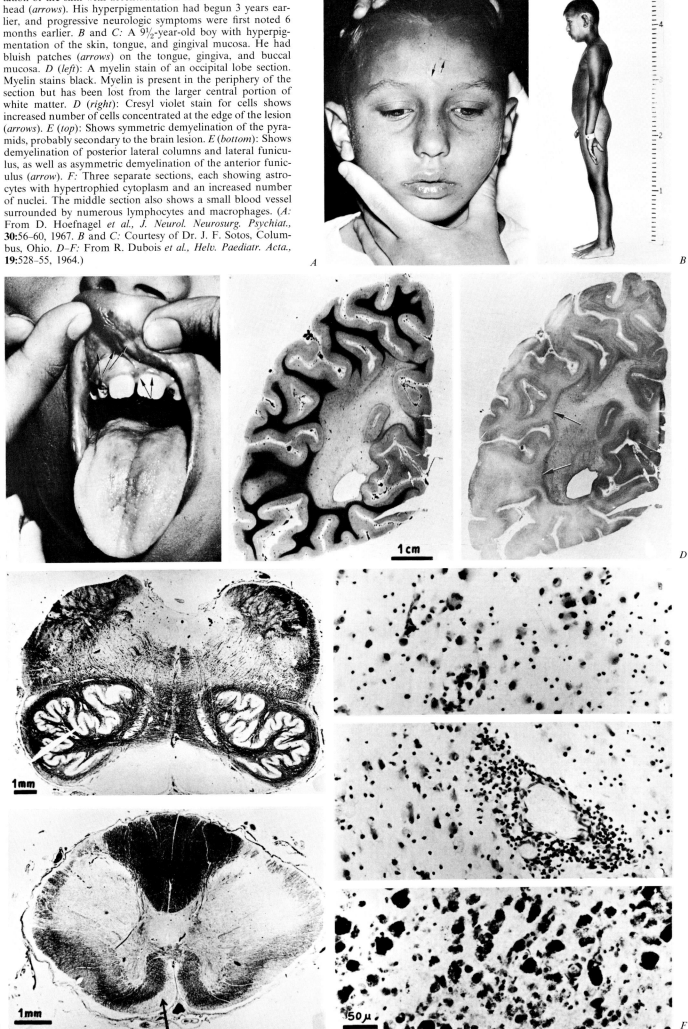

Plate II-20. *A:* A 9¼-year-old boy with diffuse hyperpigmentation of the skin with accentuation in small scars of the forehead (*arrows*). His hyperpigmentation had begun 3 years earlier, and progressive neurologic symptoms were first noted 6 months earlier. *B* and *C:* A 9½-year-old boy with hyperpigmentation of the skin, tongue, and gingival mucosa. He had bluish patches (*arrows*) on the tongue, gingiva, and buccal mucosa. *D* (*left*): A myelin stain of an occipital lobe section. Myelin stains black. Myelin is present in the periphery of the section but has been lost from the larger central portion of white matter. *D* (*right*): Cresyl violet stain for cells shows increased number of cells concentrated at the edge of the lesion (*arrows*). *E* (*top*): Shows symmetric demyelination of the pyramids, probably secondary to the brain lesion. *E* (*bottom*): Shows demyelination of posterior lateral columns and lateral funiculus, as well as asymmetric demyelination of the anterior funiculus (*arrow*). *F:* Three separate sections, each showing astrocytes with hypertrophied cytoplasm and an increased number of nuclei. The middle section also shows a small blood vessel surrounded by numerous lymphocytes and macrophages. (*A:* From D. Hoefnagel *et al., J. Neurol. Neurosurg. Psychiat.,* **30:**56–60, 1967. *B* and *C:* Courtesy of Dr. J. F. Sotos, Columbus, Ohio. *D–F:* From R. Dubois *et al., Helv. Paediatr. Acta.,* **19:**528–55, 1964.)

115

Chapter III

Acquired Conditions Associated with Mental Retardation

Introduction

Acquired conditions that cause brain damage in the fetus, newborn, and child include many common problems: prematurity, perinatal anoxia, birth trauma, maternal malnutrition, intrauterine infections, meningitis, encephalitis, teratogens, poisons, kernicterus, and head trauma. Because several of these problems may coexist in one pregnancy and delivery, and because their effects are often nonspecific, the frequency of each acquired condition as a cause of mental retardation is difficult to estimate. This chapter deals with the few conditions that have associated physical abnormalities that aid in their clinical recognition.

Infections in women during pregnancy are common. One study of 30,000 women showed that 5 percent had at least one viral infection, excluding the common cold [1]. The infections that are known to cause damage to the fetus are still only a small number. We have selected for discussion five intrauterine and perinatal infections that cause recognizable physical abnormalities in the affected newborn and infant. The responsible organisms are viruses (rubella, cytomegalovirus, and herpes), treponemata (syphilis), and protozoa (toxoplasmosis). Their effects can be quite varied. There is a general similarity in many of the effects, such as thrombocytopenia, hepatosplenomegaly, intracranial calcifications, and retinitis. However, each of these infections has shown a wide variability from infant to infant. Recognition of the breadth of the spectrum of clinical infection has been facilitated by the advent of new techniques for virus isolation and by specific macroglobulin assays. More complete ascertainment of infected infants has shown that some never show any signs of damage, others show signs at birth and recover, and others seem normal at birth but show neurologic damage a few months or years later. While much progress has been made in estimating the frequency of various intrauterine infections and their clinical manifestations, little progress has been made in treatment of the infected infants. Only for congenital syphilis is there an effective therapeutic agent.

The second group of diseases or conditions discussed in this chapter consists of teratogenic agents. One of these, thalidomide, is fortunately no longer available, but has left a large number (estimated at 7000) of affected children in its wake. The other two, aminopterin and warfarin, are rare causes of congenital malformations. A recent addition to this group is maternal phenylketonuria, which is briefly discussed in Chapter I. At least 68 children born to mothers with phenylketonuria have been reported, almost all of whom have been mentally retarded [2]. In addition, they often show growth failure and have microcephaly and congenital heart defects. It has also been suggested that the anticonvulsants trimethadione and paramethadione are teratogenic, but no consistent pattern of malformations has been observed [4]. Not included in this chapter are chemical agents that cause brain damage but no physical abnormalities. One of these, chronic lead poisoning, has caused far more brain damage than all of the teratogens just listed. Chronic lead poisoning usually occurs in 2- to 5-year-old children. Of those children who have an episode of acute lead encephalopathy and survive, 25 percent have severe permanent brain damage [3].

The last two conditions discussed in this chapter are kernicterus and the battered-child syndrome, both postnatally acquired conditions. The prospects for eliminating kernicterus have been greatly improved by new methods of managing hyperbilirubinemia and preventing Rh sensitization. The same cannot be said for the battered child. More infants and children suffering parental abuse are now being recognized. Unfortunately, the prevention of brain damage by physical abuse is fraught with problems of a magnitude equal to that posed by the untreatable intrauterine infections.

References

1. Sever, J. L., and White, L. R. Intrauterine viral infections. *Annu. Rev. Med.,* **19:**471–86, 1968.
2. Yu, J. S., and O'Halloran, M. T. Children of mothers with phenylketonuria. *Lancet,* **1:**210–12, 1970.
3. Chisholm, J. J., Jr., and Kaplan, E. Lead poisoning in childhood—comprehensive management and prevention. *J. Pediatr.,* **73:**942–50, 1968.
4. German, J., Kowal, A., and Ehlers, K. H. Trimethadione and human teratogenesis. *Teratology,* **3:**349–62, 1970.

Intrauterine and Perinatal Infections
Congenital Rubella Syndrome

In 1941 Gregg [1] first reported the high incidence of congenital defects in infants whose mothers had had a rubella infection in early pregnancy. Based on the observations of Gregg and others, the rubella syndrome was shown to include cataracts, deaf-mutism, congenital heart disease, microcephaly, and mental retardation. Studies of the 1964–1965 epidemic in the United States in which more than 30,000 infants were affected greatly extended the understanding of the effects of maternal rubella on the fetus and newborn. Careful prospective studies, including virus isolation, showed that the symptomatic newborn represents only part of a broad clinical spectrum. At one end of the spectrum, as many as 15 percent of the first trimester infections may end in spontaneous abortions [2]. At the other end, many infants have only defects not readily detected in the newborn period.

Physical Features

EYES: In a study of 376 affected children [3], cataracts (*Figure A*) were present in 108, glaucoma (*Figure C*) in 12 and retinopathy (*Figure B*) without cataracts or glaucoma in 147 patients. The cataracts, which may be unilateral or bilateral, result from the virus being in the lens. The cataracts may be visible at birth or may not be detectable for several weeks. When fully developed, they have a dense white pearly center surrounded by a zone of less dense material and a clear peripheral zone. Microphthalmia is frequently associated with cataracts (*Figure A*). The glaucoma may be present at birth or not until the child is several weeks old. The pigmentary retinopathy is most prominent in the perimacular area and consists of intermingled areas of black pigmentation and depigmentation. The retinopathy is nonprogressive and does not interfere with visual acuity.

ABDOMEN: Newborns often have a palpable liver and spleen (*Figure D*). An increased incidence of indirect inguinal hernias has been reported [4].

SKIN: Petechiae and ecchymoses (*Figures C, D, and E*) were present in 85 out of 376 newborns in one study [3]. These lesions, which are due to thrombocytopenia, appear as discrete macules on the face, trunk, and arms within 24 to 48 hours after birth. The petechiae are usually gone by 5 to 10 days of age, although the platelet count may remain low for several weeks. In general, these skin lesions occur in the more severely affected newborn, usually in association with hepatitis, jaundice, and hepatosplenomegaly. Skin dimples around the knees and elbows and mottling of the skin (*Figure F*) are occasionally present.

HEIGHT AND WEIGHT: Many newborns have a low birth weight and length for their gestation age. In general, the infants with more signs of intrauterine infection have more severe growth retardation. It has been suggested that a growth spurt occurs after the child's continuous rubella infection has terminated [5].

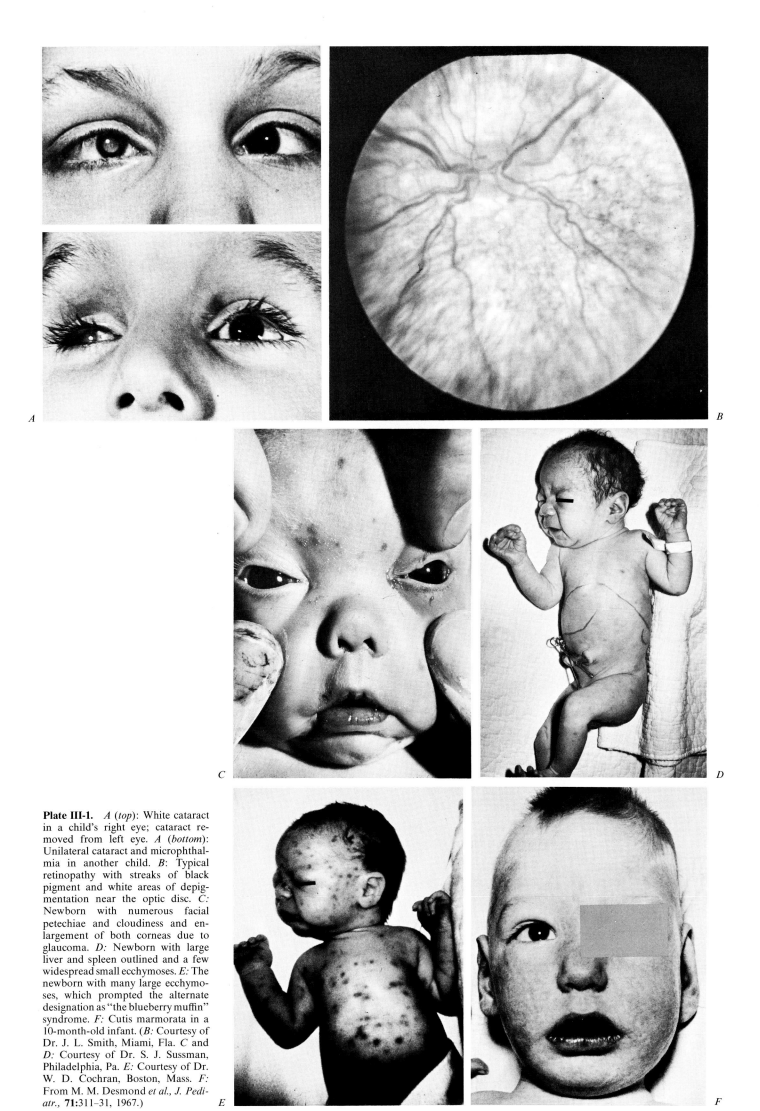

Plate III-1. *A (top):* White cataract in a child's right eye; cataract removed from left eye. *A (bottom):* Unilateral cataract and microphthalmia in another child. *B:* Typical retinopathy with streaks of black pigment and white areas of depigmentation near the optic disc. *C:* Newborn with numerous facial petechiae and cloudiness and enlargement of both corneas due to glaucoma. *D:* Newborn with large liver and spleen outlined and a few widespread small ecchymoses. *E:* The newborn with many large ecchymoses, which prompted the alternate designation as "the blueberry muffin" syndrome. *F:* Cutis marmorata in a 10-month-old infant. (*B:* Courtesy of Dr. J. L. Smith, Miami, Fla. *C* and *D:* Courtesy of Dr. S. J. Sussman, Philadelphia, Pa. *E:* Courtesy of Dr. W. D. Cochran, Boston, Mass. *F:* From M. M. Desmond *et al., J. Pediatr.,* **71:**311–31, 1967.)

119

Nervous System

Neurologic abnormalities were noted in 81 of 100 patients in one study [6]. About half had signs of encephalitis and meningitis in the neonatal period (*Figure 1*). In the study of 376 patients [3] whose mothers had rubella, 170 had psychomotor retardation, the severity of which ranged from minimal intellectual impairment to severe mental retardation with spastic quadriparesis. Sensorineural hearing loss was found in 252 of the 376 children, including 68 in whom this was the only sign of the rubella syndrome. The degree of the hearing loss and the audiometric findings vary from patient to patient. Abnormal vestibular function is a common finding, especially in children with hearing loss.

Pathology

The central nervous system pathology is quite variable. The brain weight is usually subnormal. Vasculitis, multifocal areas of parenchymal necrosis, and perivascular calcification may be widely distributed in the brain and spinal cord. Leptomeningitis may occur alone or in combination with other lesions. Degenerative changes and inflammatory reactions are often present in the cochlear duct and the organ of Corti. Developmental malformations of the nervous system are usually not present [7].

The most common major malformations involve the cardiovascular system, and are usually limited to the segment of the vascular tree formed by the pulmonary arteries, ductus arteriosus, and aortic isthmus. The most common abnormalities are patent ductus arteriosus and stenosis of the pulmonary artery and its branches. Septal defects and myocardial necrosis have been noted in several infants [8]. Other common pathologic findings are giant cell hepatitis, glomerulosclerosis, nephrocalcinosis, splenic fibrosis, and atrophy of the thymus.

Laboratory Studies

The rubella virus has been isolated from placentas and all fetal tissues and body fluids. Infected infants continue to shed the virus for several months after birth. Cultures of cataractous lenses removed at 36 months of age have yielded rubella virus.

Several tests for rubella antibodies have been developed: a neutralizing antibody test, a fluorescent antibody test, and a complement-fixation test. The neutralizing and fluorescent antibodies appear at the time of the rash and persist indefinitely, which makes these tests valuable in determining whether a woman is susceptible to rubella. For the pregnant woman exposed to rubella the most rapid and economical test for active infection is the complement-fixation test, using both acute and convalescent serum to test for the rise in antibody levels.

Children with congenital rubella may exhibit diminished delayed-type hypersensitivity [9]. Hypoplastic anemias and immunoglobulin deficiencies have often been noted. X-rays of long bones of small infants show tubular and ovoid radiolucent areas in the metaphyses of the long bones. These are interspersed between areas of increased density, and rarely persist beyond the first 4 months of life (*Figures K and L*).

Treatment and Prognosis

No antirubella agent is available. In general, the earlier the maternal infection the more severe its damaging effect on the child. While the incidence of defects is highest if the infection occurred in the first trimester, serious neurologic problems have also been observed in infants infected after the first trimester [10]. Auditory and ocular defects should be looked for as early as possible, and vigorous efforts should be made to correct these sources of sensory deprivation. Cataract removal is recommended once the eyes are of reasonable size (usually after 6 months of age) [3]. The education of the affected children requires teachers trained in the instruction of multiply handicapped children.

Prevention

Several attenuated rubella virus vaccines are being developed which are safe and immunogenic [11]. It is hoped that the widespread use of routine rubella vaccines will prevent rubella epidemics from occurring in the future.

There has been controversy over whether giving intramuscular gamma globulin to a pregnant woman prevents damage to the fetus if the mother acquires a rubella infection. It has been suggested that receiving gamma globulin may only prevent a mother from developing signs of rubella infection and thereby give her a false sense of security.

Differential Diagnosis

1. Petechiae, jaundice, and hepatomegaly in the newborn infant can also be caused by congenital toxoplasma (see page 124), syphilis (see page 126), cytomegalovirus (see page 122), herpesvirus (see page 130), and bacterial infections, and by erythroblastosis fetalis.
2. Microcephaly, spasticity, microphthalmia, and deafness may also be caused by congenital toxoplasma (see page 124) and cytomegalovirus (see page 122) infections, but these diseases usually cause chorioretinitis and rarely cataracts.
3. Congenital glaucoma and cataracts are features of patients with the oculocerebrorenal syndrome of Lowe, but they usually have severe hypotonia, and aminoaciduria, and no liver enlargement (see page 248).

References

1. Gregg, N. McA. Congenital cataract following German measles in the mother. *Trans. Ophthalmol. Soc. Aust.*, 3:35–46, 1941.
2. Cockburn, W. C. World aspects of the epidemiology of rubella. *Am. J. Dis. Child.*, 118:112–22, 1969.
3. Cooper, L. Z., Ziring, P. R., Ockerse, A. B., Fedun, B. A., Kiely, B., and Krugman, S. Rubella. Clinical manifestations and management. *Am. J. Dis. Child.*, 118:18–29, 1969.
4. Hardy, J. B., and Sever, J. L. Indirect inguinal hernia in congenital rubella. *J. Pediatr.*, 73:416–18, 1968.
5. Michaels, R. H., and Kenny, F. M. Postnatal growth retardation in congenital rubella. *Pediatrics*, 43:251–59, 1969.
6. Desmond, M. M., Wilson, G. S., Melnick, J. L., Singer, D. B., Zion, T. E., Rudolph, A. J., Pineda, R. G., Ziai, M.-H., and Blattner, R. J. Congenital rubella encephalitis. Course and early sequelae. *J. Pediatr.*, 71:311–31, 1967.
7. Tartakow, I. J. The teratogenicity of maternal rubella. *J. Pediatr.*, 66:380–91, 1965.
8. Hastreiter, A. R., Joorabchi, B., Pujatti, G., van der Horst, R. L., Patacsil, G., and Sever, J. L. Cardiovascular lesions associated with congenital rubella. *J. Pediatr.*, 71:59–65, 1967.
9. White, L. R., Leiken, S., Villavicencio, O., Abernathy, W., Avery, G., and Sever, J. L. Immune competence in congenital rubella: Lymphocyte transformation, delayed hypersensitivity, and response to vaccination. *J. Pediatr.*, 73:229–34, 1968.
10. Hardy, J. B., McCracken, G. H., Jr., Gilkeson, M. R., and Sever, J. L. Adverse fetal outcome following maternal rubella after the first trimester of pregnancy. *J.A.M.A.*, 207:2414–20, 1969.
11. Karchmer, A. W., Herrmann, K. L., Friedman, J. P., Shope, T. C., Page, E. E., Jr., Dressler, M. S., Armes, W. H., Jr., and Witte, J. J. Comparative studies of rubella vaccines. *Am. J. Dis. Child.*, 118:197–202, 1969.

Plate III-1. *G:* An 18-month-old child with marked muscular hypotonia. *H:* An 18-month-old child with extension and scissoring of the legs reflecting muscular hypertonia. *I:* A 5-month-old infant with constant opisthotonic posturing and severe growth retardation who at autopsy was shown to have leptomeningitis and extensive parenchymal necrosis. *J:* An infant who when standing with support would slowly retract his head fully due to hypotonia of the neck muscles. *K* and *L:* Radiolucent areas in the distal femora and proximal tibiae which cleared during 6 weeks and by the time the child was 2 months old. (*G–J:* From M. M. Desmond *et al., J. Pediatr.,* **71:**311–31, 1967. *K* and *L:* From A. J. Rudolph *et al., Am. J. Dis. Child.,* **110:**428–33, 1965.)

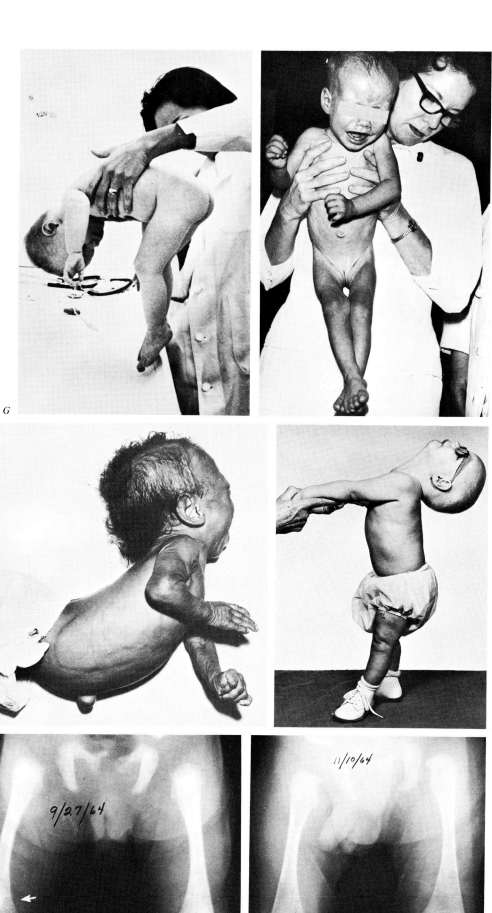

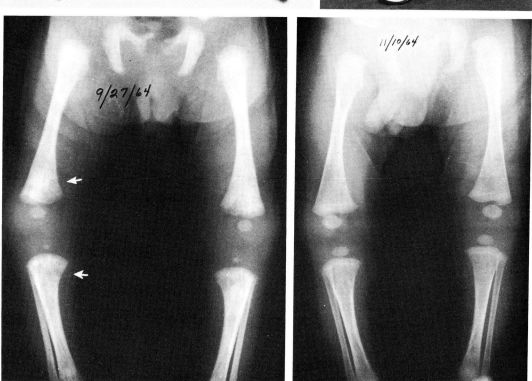

Congenital Cytomegalovirus Infection

Only during the past twenty years have intrauterine infections due to cytomegalovirus been recognized. At first the diagnosis was made when inclusion-bearing cells were found in tissues at autopsy. Since 1957 virus isolation, and thus more complete ascertainment of infants with viruria, have been possible. In three prospective studies, 0.6 to 1.2 percent of the newborns [1,2] and 3.0 percent [3] of the pregnant mothers were excreting cytomegalovirus. It seems likely that this is a primary maternal infection, not a latent infection [2]. Prospective studies have shown that the clinical spectrum of congenital cytomegalovirus infection is much broader than had been realized: many infants with viruria have no perinatal signs of infection and have normal development; some with signs of infection at birth have normal neurologic development (*Figure E*); some who appear normal at birth subsequently show signs of neurologic damage from the intrauterine infection [1,2,4].

Physical Features

HEAD: Microcephaly may be evident at birth or not apparent until the child is several months old. In a study [4] of 18 newborns with signs of intrauterine infection, microcephaly was noted in 7 during the first weeks of life and in 1 other child during the second year.

EYES: Chorioretinitis is a common finding. Microphthalmia and optic atrophy are less frequently present.

ABDOMEN: Enlargement of the liver and spleen or the spleen alone may be present at birth and persist for several weeks or months (*Figures A and B*). Indirect inguinal hernias are more common than in uninfected infants [5].

SKIN: A petechial rash due to thrombocytopenia is often present for a few hours or days after birth (*Figures A and C*). Jaundice is frequently associated with hepatomegaly.

WEIGHT: A low birth weight for gestational age and premature delivery are frequent findings. In a study of 26 infants [2] 9 had a birth weight less than 2500 g.

HEIGHT: The length at birth and subsequent linear growth are usually below average.

Nervous System

Of the 26 patients with viruria at birth, only 2 had definite neurologic abnormalities [2]. In general, infants with signs of infection may have seizures and signs of meningoencephalitis. Out of 18 newborns with signs of infection at birth, 7 subsequently had mental and motor retardation, several having hyperactivity, spasticity (*Figure D*), and seizures as well [4]. Four children were deaf. The mental retardation may be mild or severe.

Pathology

The intrauterine infection is generalized, and inclusion-bearing cells may be found in any organ. Central nervous system changes include cerebral petechiae, ventricular and subarachnoid hemorrhage, granulomatous encephalomyelitis with periventricular calcification, and scattered areas of necrosis. Both polymicrogyria and hydrocephalus have been reported. Interstitial nephritis, pneumonitis, and hepatitis are other common findings [6].

Laboratory Studies

The most specific diagnostic tests are virus isolation and the fluorescent antibody test for cytomegalovirus IgM macroglobulin. Virus excretion may persist until the child is several months old. The disadvantage of the fluorescent antibody test is that it does not always detect asymptomatic virus excretors [1,7]. The complement-fixation test is less specific than virus isolation and the fluorescent antibody test, but more widely available. A high maternal titer is suggestive of intrauterine infection, and this is confirmed by the demonstration of a rising titer in the infant during the first six months. An absent or low titer in a mother whose infant is less than 3 months old is strong evidence against an intrauterine infection. The study of urine sediment for intranuclear inclusion bodies (*Figure F*) is not a very reliable test, for many infants with viruria have not had inclusion bodies in the cells of the urine sediment.

Skull x-rays may show cerebral calcifications in several areas, especially in the periventricular region. Transient x-ray changes in the long bones, primarily lucent areas interspersed between smaller zones of sclerosis and serrated metaphyses, have been reported [8].

Treatment and Prognosis

A few infants with cytomegalovirus infection have been treated with synthetic chemotherapeutic agents, especially idoxuridine, but consistently favorable results have not been obtained [9]. While it is often stated that a mother with one infected infant is not likely to have an infected infant in a subsequent pregnancy, congenital infections in infants from two consecutive pregnancies have been observed [10].

Differential Diagnosis

1. Neonatal jaundice, hepatosplenomegaly, purpura, and petechiae may also be caused by congenital syphilis (see page 126) and herpesvirus (see page 130) infections, bacterial sepsis, and erythroblastosis fetalis.

2. Chorioretinitis, microphthalmia, microcephaly, and spasticity may also be present after intrauterine infection with toxoplasma (see page 124) or rubella (see page 118).

3. Intracranial calcifications may be present in patients with tuberous sclerosis (see page 380), Sturge-Weber syndrome (see page 372), teratomas, astrocytomas, pseudohypoparathyroidism (see page 50), and toxoplasmosis (see page 124). Although intracranial infections in patients with congenital toxoplasmosis are more widely disseminated than those in patients with cytomegalovirus infection, the x-ray findings are not a reliable means of distinguishing between these two infections.

References

1. Birnbaum, G., Lynch, J. I., Margileth, A. M., Lonergan, W. M., and Sever, J. L. Cytomegalovirus infections in newborn infants. *J. Pediatr.*, **75**:789–95, 1969.
2. Starr, J. G., Bart, R. D., Jr., and Gold, E. Inapparent congenital cytomegalovirus infection. Clinical and epidemiologic characteristics in early infancy. *N. Engl. J. Med.*, **282**:1075–78, 1970.
3. Feldman, R. A. Cytomegalovirus infection during pregnancy. A prospective study and report of six cases. *Am. J. Dis. Child.*, **117**:517–21, 1969.
4. McCracken, G. H., Jr., Shinefield, H. R., Cobb, K., Rausen, A. R., Dische, M. R., and Eichenwald, H. F. Congenital cytomegalic inclusion disease. A longitudinal study of 20 patients. *Am. J. Dis. Child.*, **117**:522–39, 1969.
5. Lang, D. J. The association of indirect inguinal hernia with congenital cytomegalic inclusion disease. *Pediatrics*, **38**:913–16, 1966.
6. Naeye, R. L. Cytomegalic inclusion disease. The fetal disorder. *Am. J. Clin. Pathol.*, **47**:738–44, 1967.
7. Hanshaw, J. B., Steinfeld, H. J., and White, C. J. Fluorescent-antibody test for cytomegalovirus macroglobulin. *N. Engl. J. Med.*, **279**:566–70, 1968.
8. Graham, C. B., Thal, A., and Wassum, C. S. Rubella-like bone changes in congenital cytomegalic inclusion disease. *Radiology*, **94**:39–43, 1970.
9. Conchie, A. F., Barton, B. W., and Tobin, J. O'H. Congenital cytomegalovirus infection treated with idoxuridine. *Br. Med. J.*, **4**:162–63, 1968.
10. Embil, J. A., Ozere, R. L., and Haldane, E. V. Congenital cytomegalovirus infection in two siblings from consecutive pregnancies. *J. Pediatr.*, **77**:417–21, 1970.

Plate III-2. *A:* A newborn infant with jaundice, hepatomegaly, and petechiae. *B:* A 14-week-old infant with marked enlargement of the liver and spleen outlined on the abdomen. *C* and *D:* One-day-old infant with petechiae and ecchymoses. The same child at 4 years of age when he had a left hemiparesis and spasticity, microcephaly, and an IQ of less than 60. *E:* A 3½-year-old boy of average intelligence who had a proven neonatal infection. *F:* The large cytomegalic inclusion body (*arrow*) within a renal tubular cell. (*A:* Courtesy of Dr. J. B. Hanshaw, Rochester, N.Y. *B* and *E:* Courtesy of Dr. D. J. Lang, Durham, N.C. *C:* From A. M. Margileth, *Pediatrics,* **15:**270–83, 1955. *D:* Courtesy of Dr. A. M. Margileth, Washington, D.C. *F:* From S. Kibrick and P. A. Taft, *Clin. Pediatr.* [*Phila.*], **3:**153–60, 1964.)

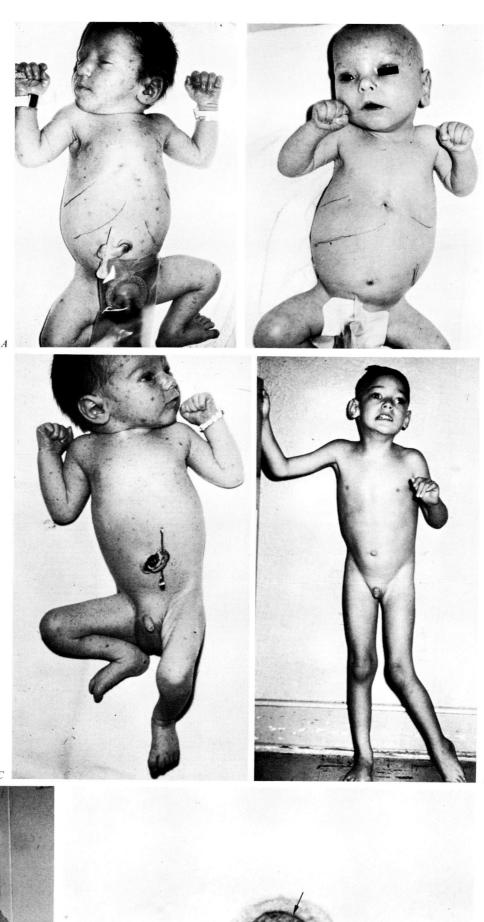

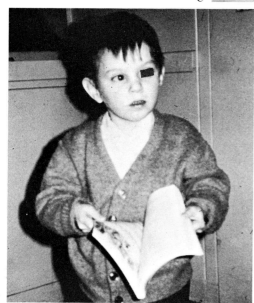

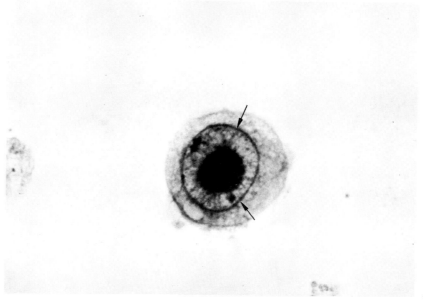

Congenital Toxoplasmosis

Toxoplasmosis as a cause of human central nervous system infection was first reported in 1939 in studies of a one-month-old infant with encephalomyelitis [1]. Subsequent studies have shown that the responsible organism is *Toxoplasma gondii,* a ubiquitous protozoan parasite. While the infection may be acquired by adults and children, it is the congenital (transplacental intrauterine) infection that usually causes brain damage and mental retardation. As with other intrauterine infections, the fetus may be aborted or stillborn, or may survive. Some infants show signs of infection at birth; others seem normal at birth but show evidence of severe brain damage a few months later [2–4]. Neither the incidence of congenital toxoplasmosis in the United States nor the frequency with which it causes mental retardation is known. In France the incidence has been estimated as about 1 affected infant per 1000 livebirths [5].

Physical Features

HEAD: In a review [5] of 300 affected infants, 26 percent had either microcephaly or hydrocephalus (*Figures D and E*).

EYES: The most common eye anomaly is chorioretinitis, which may be present at birth, develop in the first weeks of life, or in some instances not appear until the teen-age years. Seventy-six percent of the 300 infected infants had chorioretinitis [5]. This retinopathy is usually bilateral and the retinitis is present in the macula and the periphery (*Figure C*). Microphthalmia (*Figure A*) may be evident at birth. Cataracts (*Figure B*), glaucoma, and optic atrophy are less common eye findings.

ABDOMEN: Enlargement of the liver and spleen may be present at birth and persist for several days or weeks. This is often associated with signs of abnormal liver function.

SKIN: The infected newborn infant may have petechiae and purpura (due to thrombocytopenia), pallor, or jaundice.

Nervous System

Seizures are common in infected infants and older children. Spastic limbs, deafness, and mental retardation are frequent neurologic sequelae, in addition to microcephaly and hydrocephalus.

Pathology

The toxoplasma organisms produce a very destructive granulomatous inflammation throughout the body. The organisms are seen as pseudocysts in the granulomas. Large inflammatory lesions, necrosis, calcification, and cyst formation are most severe in the cerebral cortex, the basal ganglia, and the periventricular tissues. The meninges and ependyma show miliary tubercles. Hydrocephalus has been attributed to choroid damage by the periventricular inflammation and to occlusion of the aqueduct of Sylvius by ependymitis.

Laboratory Studies

The specific diagnosis of congenital toxoplasmosis can be established either by the demonstration of the organism in body tissues or by serologic means. The simplest and most specific serologic test is the IgM-fluorescent antibody test [6].

Both the neutralizing antibody test developed by Sabin and Feldman and the complement-fixing antibody test are more widely available, but they measure 7S antibodies, which may have been passively acquired from the mother. Therefore, when these tests are used active infection can only be established if the antibody titers rise in serial serum samples. The neutralizing antibodies persist for several years, a fact that is useful in attempting to diagnose congenital toxoplasmosis in a 2- or 3-year-old child. If infected *in utero,* both a child and its mother should have antibody titers of 1:256 or slightly less. If the mother has a negative or very low neutralizing antibody titer within three years of the child's birth, the child probably does not have congenital toxoplasmosis [3].

Focal cerebral calcifications visible in skull x-rays have been shown to increase in size with age [2]. They are often scattered throughout the cerebrum, although they are more common in the periventricular and basal ganglia areas (*Figure F*). Thirty-two percent of the 300 patients with congenital toxoplasmosis in one study [5] had intracranial calcifications.

Treatment and Prognosis

The only available treatment is sulfadiazine and pyrimethane, a folic acid antagonist. This therapy has not been very successful in humans, although the combination has been effective in animal studies. While most investigators state that there is no evidence of an increased risk of an infected infant in a subsequent pregnancy, this opinion has been contested [3].

Differential Diagnosis

1. Neonatal petechiae, jaundice, and hepatosplenomegaly may also be seen in infants with congenital rubella (see page 118), syphilis (see page 126), cytomegalovirus (see page 122), herpesvirus (see page 130), and bacterial infections, and in erythroblastosis fetalis.
2. Chorioretinitis, microphthalmia, microcephaly, and spasticity may also be present in infants with congenital rubella (see page 118) and cytomegalovirus (see page 122) infections.
3. Intracranial calcifications may be present in patients with herpesvirus and cytomegalovirus infections (see pages 130 and 122), tuberous sclerosis (see page 380), Sturge-Weber syndrome (see page 372), teratomas, astrocytomas, and pseudohypoparathyroidism (see page 50).

References

1. Wolf, A., Cowen, D., and Paige, B. Human toxoplasmosis: occurrence in infants as encephalomyelitis: verification by transmission to animals. *Science,* 89:226–27, 1939.
2. Sabin, A. B. Toxoplasmosis. A recently recognized disease of human beings. *Adv. Pediatr.,* 1:1–56, 1942.
3. Feldman, H. A. Toxoplasmosis, *N. Engl. J. Med.,* 279:1370–75, 1431–37, 1968.
4. Miller, M. J., Seaman, E., and Remington, J. S. The clinical spectrum of congenital toxoplasmosis: problems in recognition. *J. Pediatr.,* 70:714–23, 1967.
5. Couvreur, J., and Desmonts, G. Congenital and maternal toxoplasmosis: review of 300 congenital cases. *Dev. Med. Child Neurol.,* 4:519–30, 1962.
6. Remington, J. S., Miller, M. J., and Brownlee, I. IgM antibodies in acute toxoplasmosis. 1. Diagnostic significance in congenital cases and a method for their rapid demonstration. *Pediatrics,* 41:1082–91, 1968.

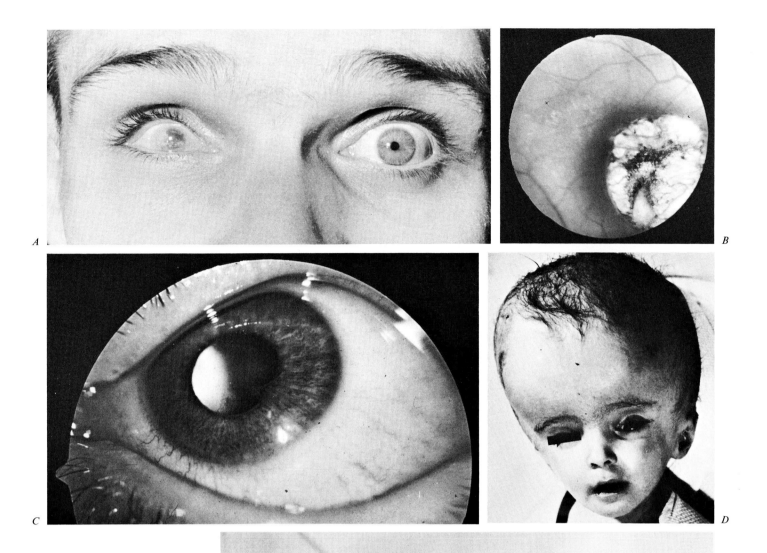

Plate III-3. *A:* Unilateral microphthalmia in a 26-year-old man with intracranial calcifications and subnormal intelligence. *B:* Shows the large retinal scar in this man's normal-size left eye. *C:* An extensive cataract and retrolental mass in a 3-year-old child. *D:* A 2½-year-old child with severe obstructive hydrocephalus from whose brain toxoplasma was isolated. *E:* A 7-year-old child with severe hydrocephalus (note the protrusion through the burr hole), growth retardation, and spasticity, who was the first serologically diagnosed case of surviving congenital toxoplasmosis. *F:* Cerebral calcifications in a 10-year-old boy. (*C:* Courtesy of Dr. M. Warburg, Copenhagen, Denmark. *D:* Courtesy of Dr. J. S. Remington, Stanford, Calif. *E:* Courtesy of Dr. A. B. Sabin, Cincinnati, Ohio. *F:* From Toxoplasmosis, by A. B. Sabin, in Volume I, *Advances in Pediatrics,* Copyright © 1942, Year Book Medical Publishers, Inc. Used by permission of Year Book Medical Publishers; reproduced by courtesy of Dr. B. Crothers and with permission of the Children's Hospital, Boston, Mass.)

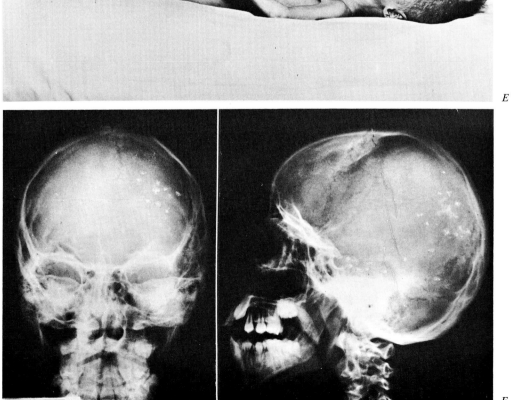

Congenital Syphilis

Syphilis as an acquired adult disease has increased in frequency in many countries in recent years. As an inevitable result, each year an increasing number of infants are born with congenital syphilis [1–5]. Unfortunately many young physicians are not familiar with the signs and symptoms of congenital syphilis.

Transmission of the treponema organism from the mother to the fetus usually does not occur until after the first 4 months of pregnancy. The chance of this occurring depends on how long the mother has been infected. The longer she has had the infection, the less likely she is to have any treponemata in her bloodstream because of protective antibodies that she has produced. Therefore, the longer a mother has had syphilis, the more likely she is to have a normal child. If the mother's infection is recent, either fetal death with stillbirth or congenital syphilis is much more likely [1]. The overall mortality of untreated congenital syphilis may be as high as 50 percent, with 25 percent of the infected fetuses dying before birth and another 25 percent shortly after birth [2]. Fortunately, the chances of an infant's survival and the eradication of the infection are good if the mother is treated during the last weeks of pregnancy or the infant is treated in the first months of life.

The physical signs of congenital syphilis are different for affected individuals of different ages. The course of the congenital infection resembles that of the secondary and late stages of acquired syphilis, except that the lesions develop more quickly in patients with the congenital infection.

Physical Features and Nervous System

INFANTS

Prematurity: The severely infected fetus is likely to be born prematurely and have a protuberant abdomen and withered skin (*Figures A and D*)

Snuffles: A mucoid nasal discharge appears at 1 to 2 weeks of age and becomes purulent or hemorrhagic (*Figures C, D, and F*)

Skin lesions: Copper-colored or red, round macules appear in the perioral and anogenital regions, especially on the buttocks and the posterior thighs (*Figure D*)

Petechiae and a purpuric skin rash due to thrombocytopenia may be seen on the first day of life

Mucous membrane or mucocutaneous fissures and condylomas

Hepatosplenomegaly (*Figure E*)
Lymphadenopathy, especially epitrochlear
Meningitis
Painful pseudoparalysis due to subepiphyseal fractures or epiphyseal dislocations; x-rays show destructive metaphyseal lesions [5a] and osteochondritis at the ends of long bones, osteitis of the phalanges, periostitis, and periosteal new bone formation (*Figure B*)

CHILDREN

Saddle nose deformity
Hypoplasia of the deciduous teeth
Mental deficiency with abnormal behavior, such as delusions or hallucinations
Organic dementia
Seizures

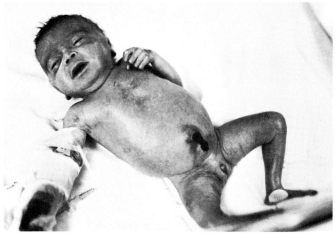

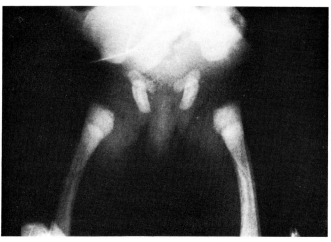

A

B

Plate III-4. *A* and *B:* A 7-day-old infant with distended abdomen and froglike position. Her x-rays show periosteal new bone formation in the mid-femur. *C:* Shows mucoid and hemorrhagic rhinorrhea and conjunctival discharge in a newborn. *D:* An infant with hemorrhagic lesions of the nose and mouth and a wasted appearance. *E:* A 1-month-old infant with hepatosplenomegaly and generalized red macules. *F:* An infant with severe snuffles whose thumb had become secondarily infected. (*A:* From J. B. Hardy *et al., J.A.M.A.,* **212:**1345–49, 1970. *B:* Courtesy of Dr. J. B. Hardy, Baltimore, Md. *C:* From Syphilis-rediscovered, by S. Olansky, in *Disease-A-Month,* Copyright © 1967, Year Book Medical Publishers, Inc. Used by permission of Year Book Medical Publishers. *D* and *F:* From A. C. Curtis and O. S. Philpott, Jr., *Med. Clin. North Am.,* **48:**707–19, 1964. By courtesy of Department of Pediatrics, Vanderbilt University School of Medicine, Nashville, Tennessee. *E:* From L. Juhlin, *Acta Derm. Venereol.* [*Stock.*], **48:**166–69, 1968.)

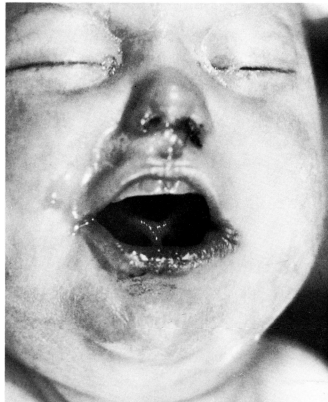

C

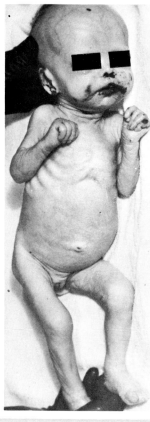

D

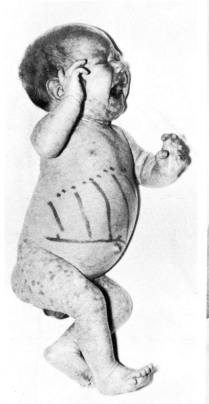

E

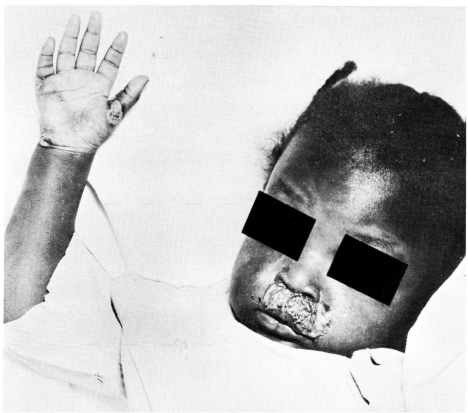

F

127

ADULTS

Frontal bossing due to skull overgrowth—the most common finding in one study [5]: present in 86.7% of 271 patients

Interstitial keratitis: Present in 8.8% in this study [5] (*Figure G*)

Pupils unequal and irregular in shape, with loss of reaction to light and preservation of reaction in accommodation (*Figure H*)

Chorioretinitis (*Figure I*)

Optic atrophy

Saddle nose: Present in 73.4% of the patients [5]

Short maxilla: Present in 83.8% [5]

High palatal arch

Prominent mandible

Rhagades, which are scars left by destructive skin lesions about the lips and cheeks (*Figure J*); present in 7.6% [5]

Neural deafness: Present in 3.3% [5]

Dental defects: Central incisor hypoplasia with notching and wide spacing (Hutchinson's teeth); present in 63.1% [5] (*Figure K*)
Small atrophic cusps on the occlusal surface of the first permanent molar (mulberry molar)

Saber shin following tibial osteitis (*Figure L*)

Hydrarthrosis due to syphilitic synovitis, especially of the knees (Clutton's joints)

Neurosyphilis: The diagnosis is usually established during the teen-age years, but may not appear until after age 50; these patients may have all of the clinical manifestations of acquired neurosyphilis, except tabes dorsalis and paresis, which are uncommon

Pathology

There is a general interstitial inflammatory cell infiltrate in the placenta and many internal organs combined with varying degree of fibrosis.

Laboratory Studies

The diagnosis can be readily made by dark-field examination of scrapings from the umbilical cord, skin lesions, or condylomas for the treponema organisms. Another specific method of diagnosis is the indirect fluorescent antibody test, which demonstrates the newborn infant's macroglobulin syphilis antibody [6]. Because the macroglobulin cannot cross the placenta, this test provides a clear differentiation of the infected newborn from infants with passively acquired positive serology. The most widely used diagnostic tests are the blood serology tests, the Hinton or VDRL. These tests identify serum reagin which can cross the placental barrier and require serial serum samples to distinguish between actively and passively acquired reagin. If the reagin in the newborn has been passively acquired, the serologic titer will fall to zero in a few weeks [6a].

Treatment and Prognosis

Treatment with one intensive course of penicillin almost always eradicates congenital syphilis from newborns. However, failures of intensive treatment of both the pregnant mother and the newborn infant have been reported [7]. Although older children and young adults may have permanent brain damage from untreated congenital syphilis, adequate treatment can produce some improvement and is always worthwhile [1].

Differential Diagnosis

1. Neonatal petechiae, purpura, and hepatosplenomegaly can also be caused by intrauterine rubella (see page 118), cytomegalovirus (see page 122), herpesvirus (see page 130), and toxoplasma (see page 124) infections, as well as bacterial sepsis and erythroblastosis fetalis.
2. Chorioretinitis is also caused by intrauterine toxoplasma (see page 124), cytomegalovirus (see page 122), herpesvirus (see page 130), and rubella (see page 118) infections.
3. Painful pseudoparalysis also occurs in patients with scurvy and the battered-child syndrome (see page 140). In both of these disorders, unlike congenital syphilis, there are periosteal hemorrhages which become calcified.

References

1. Olansky, S. Syphilis—rediscovered. *Disease-a-Month,* May 1967.
2. Curtis, A. C., and Philpott, O. S., Jr. Prenatal syphilis. *Med. Clin. North Am.,* **48:**707–19, 1964.
3. Brown, W. J., and Moore, M. B., Jr. Congenital syphilis in the United States. *Clin. Pediatr.,* **2:**220–22, 1963.
4. Woody, N. C., Sistrunk, W. F., and Platou, R. V. Congenital syphilis: a laid ghost walks. *J. Pediatr.,* **64:**63–67, 1964.
5. Fiumara, N. J., and Lessell, S. Manifestations of late congenital syphilis. An analysis of 271 patients. *Arch. Dermatol.,* **102:**78–83, 1970.
5a. Wilkinson, R. H., and Heller, R. M. Congenital syphilis: resurgence of an old problem. *Pediatrics,* **47:**27–30, 1971.
6. Alford, C. A., Jr., Polt, S. S., Cassady, G. E., Straumfjord, J. V., and Remington, J. S. γM-fluorescent treponemal antibody in the diagnosis of congenital syphilis. *N. Engl. J. Med.,* **280:**1086–91, 1969.
6a. Starling, P. F. Diagnosis and treatment of syphilis. *N. Engl. J. Med.,* **284:**642–53, 1971.
7. Hardy, J. B., Hardy, P. H., Oppenheimer, E. H., Ryan, S. J., Jr., and Sheff, R. N. Failure of penicillin in a newborn with congenital syphilis. *J.A.M.A.,* **212:**1345–49, 1970.

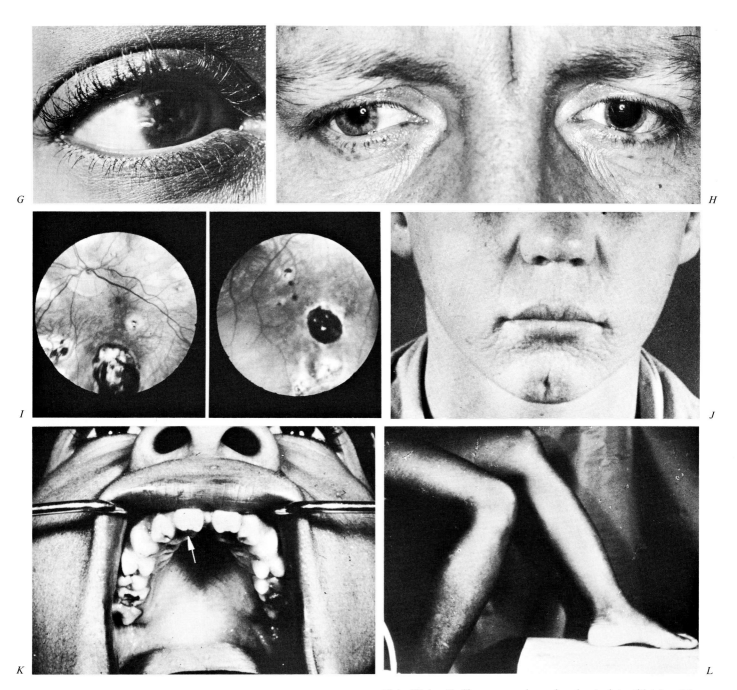

Plate III-4. *G:* Shows corneal scarring due to interstitial keratitis. *H:* Shows a dilated, unresponsive left pupil (Adie's pupil) in a 38-year-old man with chorioretinitis, optic atrophy, and blindness. *I:* Chorioretinitis in this man. *J:* Shows rhagades around the mouth and in the nasolabial folds. *K:* Shows bifid central incisors (*arrow*) in the permanent teeth of an adult. *L:* Shows the saber shin deformity. (*G, J,* and *L:* From *Syphilis, A Synopsis,* W. J. Brown [ed.], U.S. Department of Health, Education, and Welfare, Public Health Service, Publication No. 1660, U.S. Government Printing Office, 1967. *K:* From A. C. Curtis and O. S. Philpott, Jr., *Med. Clin. North Am.,* **48:**707–19, 1964.)

Perinatal Herpesvirus Infection

In the past few years it has become evident that infection of the fetus and newborn by *Herpesvirus hominis* is an important cause of neurologic damage and mental retardation [1]. The virus can be acquired in three ways: from the mother's infected genitalia (*Figure A*) by an ascending infection, during passage through an infected birth canal, or by transplacental spread [2]. Since signs of herpetic infection are not noted in most newborns until a few days after birth, the first two routes of infection appear to be the most common. The prevalence of herpetic genital infections has been estimated as 1:650 pregnant women [2]. The frequency of infected newborn infants has been estimated to be 1 in 3,500 to 1 in 30,000 [1]. The infant's infection may be either generalized or localized, and there is great variability in the severity of the illness. As with the other intrauterine infections, the infected infants may have a variety of neurologic and ocular defects or may have no physical signs of infection [1,3].

Physical Features

EYES: The eye can be the primary site of the infection or secondarily infected. One or both eyes may be affected. The most common manifestations are conjunctivitis, followed by keratitis and chorioretinitis (*Figure C*). The chorioretinitis is slow to develop and may be noted after several weeks of negative examinations. The residual ocular defects include corneal and retinal scars and cataracts (*Figure D*). A few patients are completely blind [4].

MOUTH: Herpetic gingivostomatitis is occasionally noted.

ABDOMEN: About a third of the 98 patients with disseminated disease in one review [1] had an enlarged liver. Another third had only jaundice. One tenth had both hepatomegaly and jaundice. Eleven of the 98 patients had splenomegaly.

SKIN: Vesicles (*Figure B*) are the most common skin lesions; petechiae and a generalized erythematous macular exanthem may also occur. The first vesicular lesions are usually noted at birth or within the first 2 weeks of life and may recur repeatedly up to 2 years after birth. The recurrent lesions are smaller than the original ones and tend to resolve 2 to 4 days after their appearance [1].

WEIGHT: A low birth weight for the gestational age is common in infants with disseminated infection.

Nervous System

Meningoencephalitis is the most frequent type of acute nervous system involvement. The residual neurologic defects include microcephaly (*Figure E*), hydrocephalus, porencephalic cysts, and varying degrees of psychomotor retardation [1,4].

Pathology

Evidence of the viral infection is found in every organ system. Meningoencephalitis is the most common neuropathologic finding.

Laboratory Studies

Two types of herpesvirus have been identified by their antigenic and biologic differences. Herpesvirus type 1 commonly infects the oral mucosa and type 2 the genitalia. The type 2 virus is usually isolated from infected newborns. To establish by serologic methods a diagnosis of neonatal infection, serial increases in either type 1 or type 2 antibody must be demonstrated. During the early course of the primary infection the infant's total serum IgM may increase [4a]. A specific IgM herpes antibody can be demonstrated by the indirect fluorescent antibody technique with umbilical cord blood serum or the infant's serum. The liver function test results are often abnormal even in the absence of jaundice and hepatosplenomegaly. A bleeding diathesis with decreased intravascular coagulation due to a deficiency of several clotting factors is a common finding in fatally ill infants [4a,5]. Skull x-rays may show intracranial calcification [6] (*Figure F*).

Treatment and Prognosis

Most patients with disseminated infection and nervous system involvement do not survive. Many with localized infection and nervous system involvement survive, but almost all have residual neurologic damage. Although there has been only limited experience [7,8] in the treatment of infants with intravenous 5-iodo-2'-deoxyuridine, it is recommended for patients with nervous system involvement. By contrast, infants with infection localized outside of the nervous system and those who are entirely asymptomatic almost always survive and most have no apparent sequelae [1].

Prevention

Cesarean section appears to be an effective means of preventing neonatal infection, if performed before the rupture of the membranes. Another recommended preventive measure is the administering of large doses of commercial gamma globulin to the infant, although there is no evidence that it works [1].

Differential Diagnosis

1. Neonatal jaundice, petechiae, and hepatosplenomegaly may also be caused by congenital syphilis (see page 126), toxoplasma (see page 124), cytomegalovirus (see page 122), rubella (see page 118), and bacterial infections and erythroblastosis fetalis.
2. Microcephaly, hydrocephalus, chorioretinitis, and intracranial calcifications may also be features of patients with congenital toxoplasma (see page 124) and cytomegalovirus (see page 122) infections.
3. Periventricular calcifications are often seen in patients with intrauterine cytomegalovirus infections (see page 122).

References

1. Nahmias, A. J., Alford, C. A., and Korones, S. B. Infection of the newborn with *Herpesvirus hominis*. In *Advances in Pediatrics*, Volume 17, Year Book Medical Publishers, Chicago, 1970, pp. 185–226.
2. Nahmias, A. J., Josey, W. E., and Naib, Z. M. Neonatal herpes simplex infection. Role of genital infection in mother as the source of virus in the newborn. *J.A.M.A.*, **199**:164–68, 1967.
3. Torphy, D. E., Ray, C. G., McAlister, R., and Du, J. N. H. Herpes simplex virus infection in infants: a spectrum of disease. *J. Pediatr.*, **76**:405–408, 1970.
4. Hagler, W. S., Walters, P. V., and Nahmias, A. J. Ocular involvement in neonatal herpes simplex virus infection. *Arch. Ophthalmol.*, **82**:169–76, 1969.
4a. Catalano, L. W., Jr., Safley, G. H., Museles, M., and Jarzynski, D. J. Disseminated herpesvirus infection in a newborn infant. Virologic, serologic, coagulation, and interferon studies. *J. Pediatr.*, **79**:393–400, 1971.
5. Miller, D. R., Hanshaw, J. B., O'Leary, D. S., and Hnilicka, J. V. Fatal disseminated herpes simplex virus infection and hemorrhage in the neonate. Coagulation studies in a case and a review. *J. Pediatr.*, **76**:409–15, 1970.
6. South, M. A., Tompkins, W. A. F., Morris, C. R., and Rawls, W. E. Congenital malformation of the central nervous system associated with genital type (type 2) herpesvirus. *J. Pediatr.*, **75**:13–18, 1969.
7. Partridge, J. W., and Millis, R. L. Systemic herpes simplex infection in a newborn treated with intravenous idoxuridine. *Arch. Dis. Child.*, **43**:377–81, 1968.
8. Tuffli, G. A., and Nahmias, A. J. Neonatal herpetic infection: report of two premature infants treated with systemic use of idoxuridine. *Am. J. Dis. Child.*, **118**:909–14, 1969.

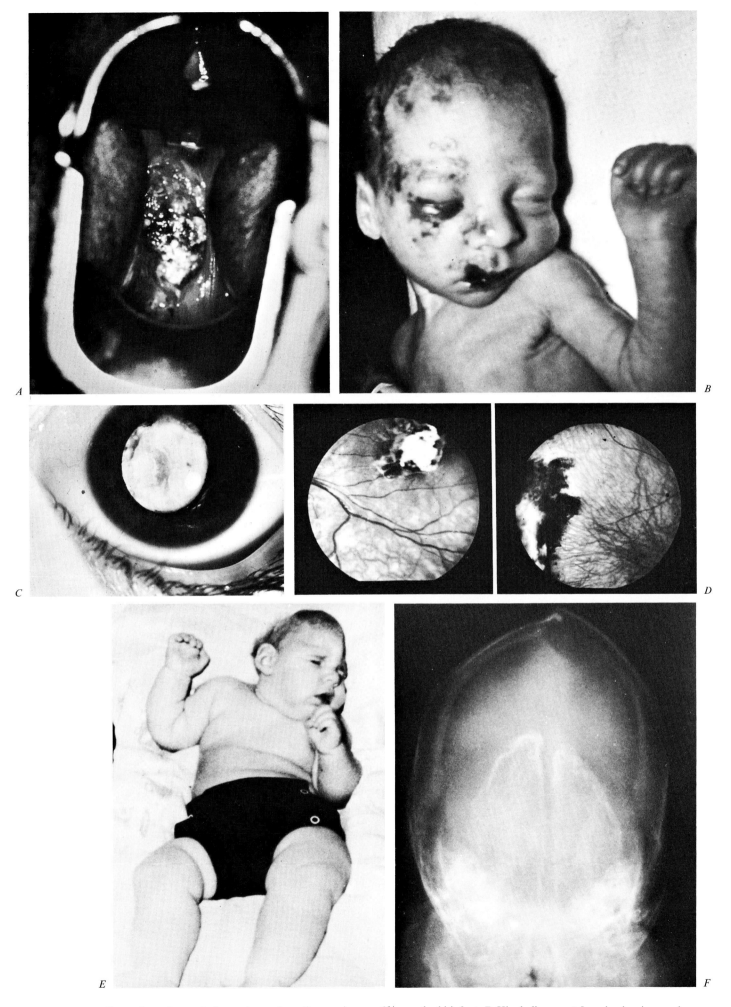

Plate III-5. *A:* Shows through a vaginal speculum a fungating cervical lesion due to herpesvirus in a mother on the day of delivery. Her infant, born by cesarean section, developed a herpes infection, including skin vesicles, on the thirteenth day of life. *B:* Herpetic skin vesicles on the face of a 16-day-old infant. *C* and *D:* A cataract and retinal scar in a child who had perinatal herpes. *E:* A microcephalic 9½-month-old infant. *F:* His skull x-ray at 5 weeks showing overlapping of the cranial bones and intracranial calcification. (*A:* From A. J. Nahmias *et al., J.A.M.A.,* **199:**132–36, 1967. *B–D:* Courtesy of Dr. A. J. Nahmias, Atlanta, Ga. *E:* From M. A. South *et al., J. Pediatr.,* **75:**13–18, 1969. *F:* Courtesy of Dr. M. A. South, Houston, Tex.)

131

Teratogens
Thalidomide

In 1960 and 1961 an outbreak of limb deformities occurred in West Germany [1] and Australia [2] that was subsequently attributed to the maternal ingestion of thalidomide. Pregnant women who took this drug between 35 and 50 days after the first day of the last menstrual period were most likely to bear affected children [3,4]. Before this drug was removed from the market more than 7000 infants in Europe, Australia, South America, and Japan were affected [5].

Physical Features

FACE: The nasal bridge is broad and flat. A midfrontal nevus flammeus is common.

EYES: In a study of 38 infants, 3 had microphthalmia, including 1 with clinical anophthalmia on the other side, 2 had colobomas of the choroid, and 4 had bilateral epiphora [6].

EARS: The external ear and auditory canal may be malformed or absent (*Figures A, B, and D*). In a review [4] of 494 infants, 87 had external ear deformities; of these, 47 had no associated limb deformities.

MOUTH: In a study of 39 children, about half (19) had enamel hypoplasia of the primary teeth and 4 were missing primary lateral incisors [5a].

LIMBS: Out of 203 patients in one survey [1,7], half had deformities only of the arms, 30 percent of both the arms and the legs, and 2 percent only of the legs. Radial forearm anomalies, such as an absent radius, triphalangism of the thumbs, and hypoplasia of the thenar eminence (*Figure C*), are the most common upper limb deformities. The arms and hands may be shortened or the long bones may be entirely absent (*Figures A, D, E, and F*). However, digits are usually present even in severe phocomelia. Shortening of the long bones is the most common lower limb anomaly. Dislocation of the hips is frequent.

Nervous System

Most patients with thalidomide embryopathy have normal intelligence; the incidence of mental retardation is low, but greater than in the normal population. Cranial nerve abnormalities, especially deafness and sixth [6] and seventh nerve palsies, are the most common neurologic abnormalities. Microcephaly and meningoencephalocele have also been reported [8].

Pathology

Cardiac defects and intestinal anomalies are the most common internal malformations. In the review of 203 patients [1,7] there were 17 cardiac and 13 intestinal anomalies, the latter including duodenal, esophageal, and anal atresia. In this group there were two patients with anencephaly and three

with microcephaly. Aplasia and hypoplasia of the inner ear have also been reported [9].

Treatment and Prognosis

An extensive rehabilitative program is under way in the countries with a large number of affected children.

Differential Diagnosis

1. Phocomelia, ear deformities, and capillary hemangiomas are features of the patients with the syndrome of phocomelia, flexion deformities, and facial anomalies, but they are distinguished by their facial appearance, contractures, scant silvery hair, corneal opacities, and an autosomal recessive mode of inheritance (see page 340).
2. Phocomelia is a feature of patients with the syndrome of tetraphocomelia, cleft lip and palate, and genital hypertrophy, but they are distinguished by having cleft lip and palate and genital hypertrophy, as well as by having more severe limb deformities (see page 344).
3. Anomalies of the radius and thumb are features of patients with Fanconi's anemia, but they are readily distinguished by also having hyperpigmentation, pancytopenia, and increased chromosome breakage (see page 282).
4. Patients with the Holt-Oram syndrome [10] usually have congenital heart disease and deformities of the radius and thumb, although some may have phocomelia. They do not have lower limb deformities or ear anomalies. This syndrome is due to an autosomal dominant mutant gene.

References

1. Lenz, W., and Knapp, K. Die Thalidomid-Embryopathie. *Dtsch. Med. Wochenschr.*, **87**:1232–42, 1962.
2. McBride, W. G. Thalidomide and congenital abnormalities. *Lancet*, **2**:1358, 1961.
3. Lenz, W. Malformations caused by drugs in pregnancy. *Am. J. Dis. Child.*, **112**:99–106, 1966.
4. Knapp, K., Lenz, W., and Nowack, E. Multiple congenital abnormalities. *Lancet*, **2**:725, 1962.
5. Mellin, G. W., and Katzenstein, M. The saga of thalidomide. *N. Engl. J. Med.*, **267**:1184–92, 1238–44, 1962.
5a. Axrup, K., d'Avignon, M., Hellgren, K., Henrikson, C.-O., Juhlin, I.-M., Larsson, K. S., Persson, G. E., and Welander, E. Children with thalidomide embryopathy: odontological observations and aspects. *Acta Odontol. Scand.*, **24**:3–21, 1966.
6. Zetterström, B. Ocular malformations caused by thalidomide. *Acta Ophthalmol.*, **44**:391–95, 1966.
7. Taussig, H. B. A study of the German outbreak of phocomelia. The thalidomide syndrome. *J.A.M.A.*, **180**:1106–14, 1962.
8. Horstmann, W. Hinweise auf zentralnervöse Schäden im Rahmen der Thalidomid-Embryopathie. *Z. Kinderheilkd.*, **96**:291–307, 1966.
9. Rosendal, T. Thalidomide and aplasia-hypoplasia of the otic labyrinth. *Lancet*, **1**:724–25, 1963.
10. Holt, M., and Oram, S. Familial heart disease with skeletal malformations. *Br. Heart J.*, **22**:236–42, 1960.

Plate III-6. *A* and *B:* A child with no left arm, phocomelia of the right arm, and small, malformed ears. The abdominal scar is from a pyloromyotomy in infancy. *C:* Bilateral distally placed, fingerlike thumbs. *D:* A child with only 3 digits on each hand, very short arms, and a malformed ear. *E* and *F:* A child with phocomelia whose x-ray showed only one rudimentary bone in the right arm, 4 metacarpals, and 4 digits. (*A* and *B:* Courtesy of Dr. F. A. Baughman, Jr., Grand Rapids, Mich. *C:* From G. W. Mellin and M. Katzenstein, *N. Engl. J. Med.*, **267:**1184–92, 1238–44, 1962. *D–F:* From M. Sulamaa, *Clin. Pediatr.* [*Phila.*], **2:**251–57, 1963.)

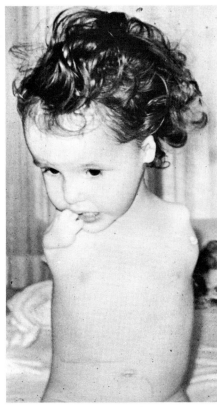
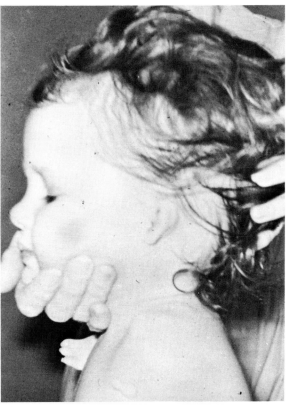

A

B

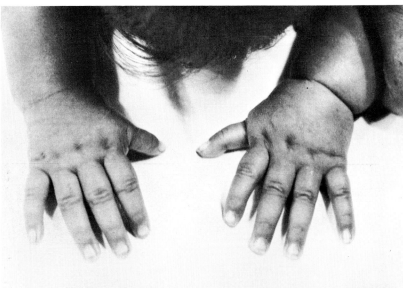
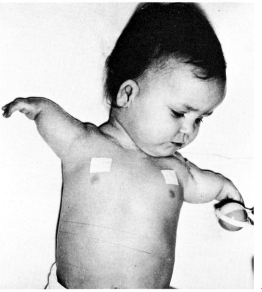

C

D

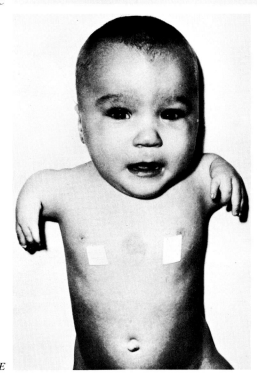
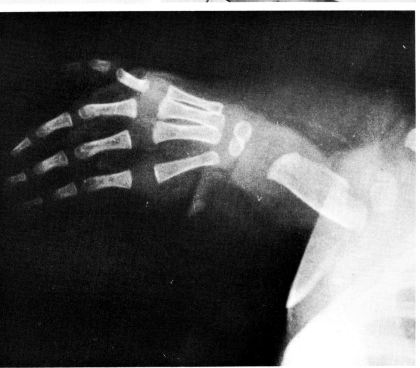

E

F

Aminopterin and Amethopterin

Folic acid antagonists used in the first trimester of pregnancy to induce abortion can cause multiple congenital anomalies in both liveborn infants and abortuses. Apparently the teratogenic effects of aminopterin and its methyl derivative, amethopterin, are similar. Nine affected fetuses and infants have been reported since 1952 [1–4].

Physical Features

HEAD: Either enlargement of the head due to hydrocephalus or skull deformity due to craniosynostosis (*Figures E and F*) has been present in most patients.

FACE: The newborn infants have had a striking appearance, with the hair swept back and prominent eyes and ears (*Figures A and B*). Hypertelorism and a flat nasal bridge have been described in the three reported patients who survived the longest (*Figure C*).

LIMBS: Three infants have had a clubfoot deformity. One child [4] had no toes on one foot and only one on the other (*Figure F*). Another infant [2] had synostosis of the hands and feet and bilateral dislocation of the hips. Shortening of the limbs, particularly the forearms, has also been reported [3] (*Figure D*).

WEIGHT: All of the infants have had a low birth weight for their gestational age.

HEIGHT: The surviving infants have been short, in one case to a marked degree [6].

Nervous System

A 4-year-old child had an IQ of 66 [3]. Another child had normal mental development at 15 months [4] and borderline normal intelligence and poor speech at 5 years [6].

Pathology

Many different cerebral anomalies, such as anencephaly, hydrocephalus, meningomyelocele formation, and cerebral hypoplasia, have been present in some of the abortuses and infants who died shortly after birth.

Laboratory Studies

Most patients have had craniosynostosis, delayed ossification, and skull defects. No chromosome abnormalities have been found.

Treatment and Prognosis

Of the 4 infants born after 35 weeks gestation, 1 lived only 29 hours and the oldest of the other 3 was 4 years old [3,4].

Differential Diagnosis

1. Craniosynostosis, skull defects, and absent digits were features of the patient reported by Herrmann and Opitz (see page 238), but he also had acrocephaly and no history of intrauterine exposure to either aminopterin or amethopterin [5].
2. Hydrocephalus and prominent eyes are features of patients with the cloverleaf skull deformity, but these patients do not have multiple limb deformities (see page 234).

References

1. Thiersch, J. B. Therapeutic abortions with a folic acid antagonist, 4-aminopteroylglutamic acid (4-amino P.G.A.) administered by the oral route. *Am. J. Obstet. Gynecol.,* **63:**1298–1304, 1952.
2. Warkany, J., Beaudry, P. H., and Hornstein, S. Attempted abortion with aminopterin (4-aminopteroylglutamic acid). *Am. J. Dis. Child.,* **97:**274–81, 1959.
3. Shaw, E. B., and Steinbach, H. L. Aminopterin-induced fetal malformation. *Am. J. Dis. Child.,* **115:**477–82, 1968.
4. Milunsky, A., Graef, J. W., and Gaynor, M. F., Jr. Methotrexate-induced congenital malformations. *J. Pediatr.,* **72:**790–95, 1968.
5. Opitz, J. M. Personal communication, 1970.
6. Milunsky, A. Personal communication, 1971.

Plate III-7. *A:* Newborn with swept-back hair, a small chin, low-set ears, and abnormal posturing of hands and feet. This infant died at 29 hours of age. *B–D:* Another child who had similar swept-back hair as a newborn. At 4½ years she had a prominent nose, hypertelorism, a small chin, and short forearms. *E* and *F:* A one-week-old infant with acrocephaly, low-set ears, hypertelorism, only one toe on one foot, and none on the other. (*A:* From J. Warkany *et al., Am. J. Dis. Child.,* **97:**274–81, 1959. *B* and *D:* From E. B. Shaw and H. L. Steinbach, *Am. J. Dis. Child.,* **115:**477–82, 1968. *C:* Courtesy of Dr. E. B. Shaw, San Francisco, Calif. *E:* Courtesy of Dr. A. Milunsky, Boston, Mass. *F:* From A. Milunsky *et al., J. Pediatr.,* **72:**790–95, 1968.)

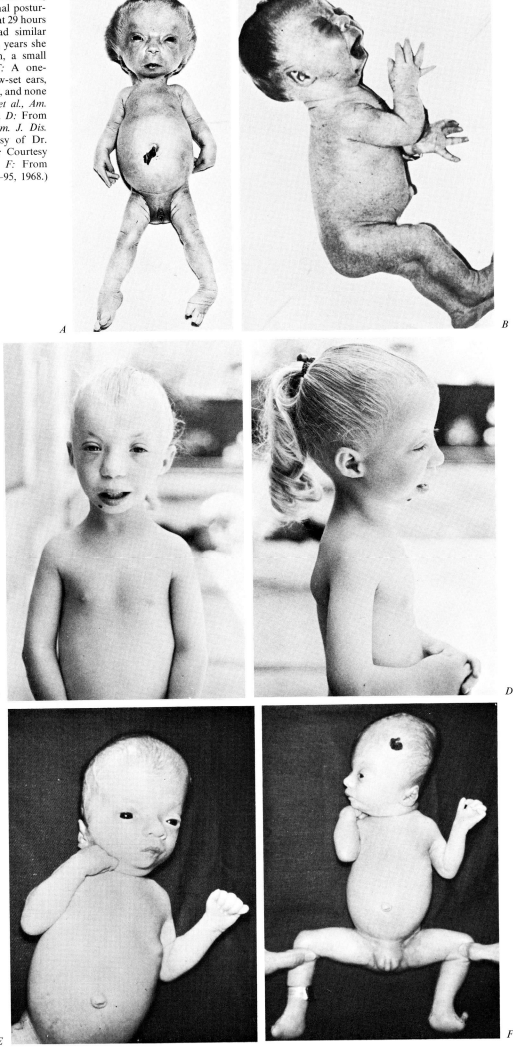

Warfarin

Two infants with similar deformities have been born to mothers with prosthetic mitral valves who took warfarin throughout the first 7 and 8 months of pregnancy [1–4]. While two other patients undergoing similar anticoagulant therapy have had normal infants [5], it has been suggested that warfarin may be a teratogenic agent. Infants whose mothers received warfarin after the first 20 weeks of pregnancy [6], or whose mothers had a mitral valve prosthesis but no anticoagulant therapy, have shown no abnormalities [7]. Obviously, more data are needed before the teratogenicity of warfarin can be established with certainty.

The first reported patient [1] was born after a pregnancy during which her mother received warfarin daily for the first 8 months and digitoxin and either sulfisoxazole or erythromycin for 9 months. At birth the child had marked hypoplasia of the nasal cartilage and bone, and nasal obstruction. Subsequent evaluation showed that she was severely retarded, had optic atrophy, and was blind. At 4 years of age [2] she had underdevelopment of the nose (*Figures A and B*) and scoliosis. X-rays in infancy showed stippling of the sacrum, a prominent occiput, and an abnormal sella turcica (*Figures C and D*).

The second patient [3] was born after a pregnancy during which her mother received warfarin daily for 7 months and digitalis daily and benzathine penicillin each month for the entire 9 months. At birth she also had markedly hypoplastic nasal structures (*Figures E and F*) and difficulty in breathing due to nasal obstruction. The child's subsequent development has been below normal and she has had seizures. She also has short limbs and clubbing of the digits [4].

References

1. DiSaia, P. J. Pregnancy and delivery of a patient with a Starr-Edwards mitral valve prosthesis. Report of a case. *Obstet. Gynecol.,* **28**:469–72, 1966.
2. Baker, S. M. Personal communication, 1969.
3. Kerber, I. J., Warr, O. S., and Richardson, C. Pregnancy in a patient with a prosthetic mitral valve associated with a fetal anomaly attributed to warfarin sodium. *J.A.M.A.,* **203**:223–25, 1968.
4. Kerber, I. J. Personal communication, 1969.
5. Johnson, A. S., Meyers, M. P., Eckhous, A. S., Bacher, B., and Limia, A. Successful pregnancies in patients with prosthetic mitral valves. *Mich. Med.,* **65**:718–19, 1966.
6. Jennings, J. A., and Hodgkinson, C. P. Anticoagulation for pulmonary embolism in pregnancy. *Obstet. Gynecol.,* **24**:85–88, 1964.
7. Ueland, K., Tatum, H. J., and Metcalfe, J. Pregnancy and prosthetic heart valves. Report of successful pregnancies in 2 patients with Starr-Edwards aortic valves. *Obstet. Gynecol.,* **27**:257–60, 1966.

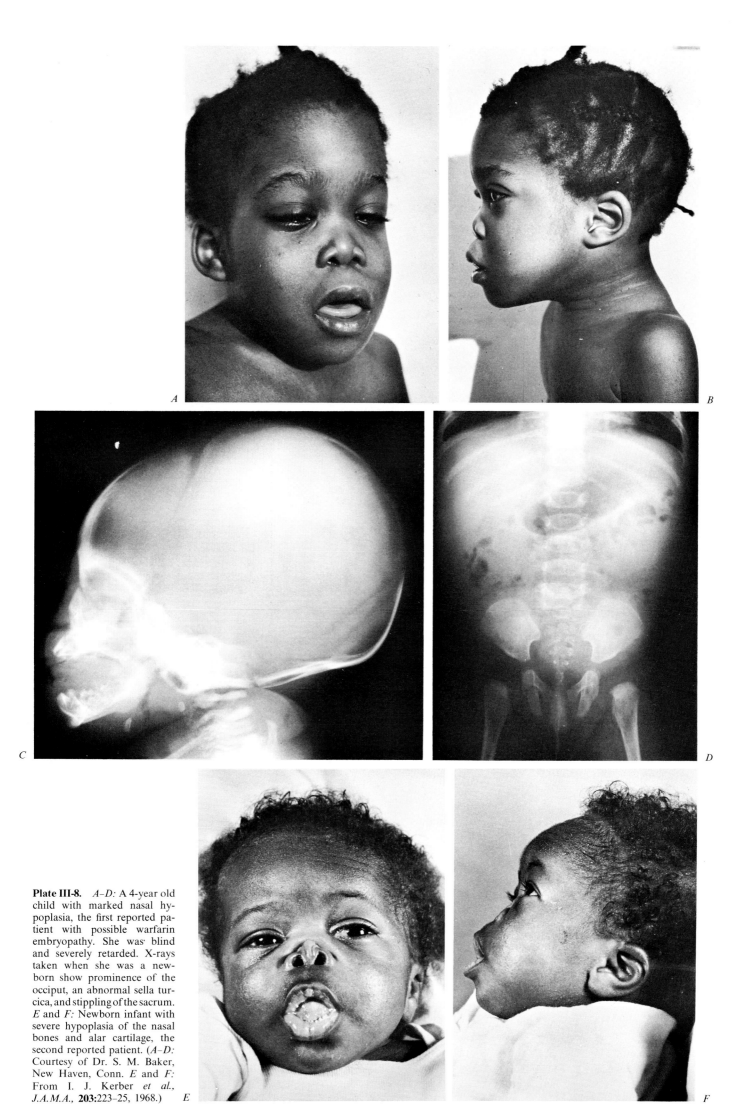

Plate III-8. *A–D:* A 4-year old child with marked nasal hypoplasia, the first reported patient with possible warfarin embryopathy. She was blind and severely retarded. X-rays taken when she was a newborn show prominence of the occiput, an abnormal sella turcica, and stippling of the sacrum. *E* and *F:* Newborn infant with severe hypoplasia of the nasal bones and alar cartilage, the second reported patient. (*A–D:* Courtesy of Dr. S. M. Baker, New Haven, Conn. *E* and *F:* From I. J. Kerber *et al.,* *J.A.M.A.,* **203:**223–25, 1968.)

Other Acquired Conditions
Kernicterus

Kernicterus, which means nuclear jaundice, occurs almost exclusively in newborn infants with unconjugated hyperbilirubinemia, the most common cause of which is hemolysis due to Rh incompatibility. The harmful bilirubin is the unconjugated form that remains unbound after the binding capacity of serum albumin has been exceeded. Being lipid-soluble, the unbound, unconjugated bilirubin readily crosses the blood-brain barrier of the newborn infant and is deposited in the brain. The neurologic deficiencies of children and adults with kernicterus have been attributed to the toxic effect of unconjugated bilirubin on cellular function [1,2].

Physical Features

MOUTH: The portions of the deciduous teeth ossifying at the time of the hyperbilirubinemia are discolored; initially they are yellow and later green. For the newborn infant this means that the ends of the central and lateral incisors, but not the molars, may be stained.

Nervous System

The affected newborn shows a definite sequence of neurologic signs in the first week of life [3]. At first the infant is lethargic and hypotonic. Later, fever, opisthotonic posturing (*Figure A*), and a high-pitched cry develop. As a third phase, the infant develops hypertonicity of the limb muscles by the end of the first week of life. Many of the infants who exhibit these signs of kernicterus do not survive. Those who do survive have immature posture patterns in the first months of life. Their motor development is retarded. They often have muscular hypotonia with hyperreflexia. Later in the preschool and in the early school years athetoid posturing and grimacing (*Figures B, C, D, E, and F*) gradually develop. Many of these patients also have a neurosensory hearing loss, which may be mild or severe. While many children with kernicterus are mentally retarded, some, even among those with severe extrapyramidal movements and deafness, have borderline or low normal intelligence [4,5].

In a prospective study [6] of 405 newborns with a bilirubin level of at least 15 mg percent, 59 patients (15 percent) developed one or more neurologic abnormalities. Sensorineural hearing loss, athetosis, and mental retardation were more likely to develop the higher the level of unconjugated bilirubin. In this same study [7] of 405 patients, 17 (4.2 percent) had a sensorineural hearing loss which varied from mild to profound. The hearing loss occurred in some patients with, and in others without, other neurologic abnormalities.

Pathology

If death occurs in the neonatal period, the brain shows intense yellow pigmentation of the globus pallidus, subthalamic nucleus, vestibular nuclei in the brainstem, and inferior olivary nuclei. Often there is less intense discoloration of other nuclei as well. The ganglion cells in the pigmented regions appear to be damaged. If the child dies a few weeks after birth, the yellow stain is no longer visible, but nerve cell loss and gliosis are present in the involved areas.

Treatment and Prognosis

Anoxia, acidosis, prematurity, sepsis, and the levels of blood sugar and serum albumin, as well as the amount of unconjugated bilirubin, are factors in the development of kernicterus [4,8]. Obviously, treatment must be intensive and individualized. Exchange transfusion remains the principal therapy. Whereas in the past serum bilirubin of 20 mg percent was indication for exchange, lower limits have been set for sick and premature infants [8] and higher limits for normal term newborns [1]. In recent years phototherapy has often been used to reduce the level of serum indirect bilirubin in premature infants [9], but the value of this for the sick premature has not been established.

Prevention

The treatment of severe erythroblastosis has expanded to include intrauterine transfusions for the fetus with severe hemolytic disease. Preventive measures have recently been introduced which should greatly reduce the incidence of Rh sensitization. Hyperimmune gamma globulin administered to an Rh-negative mother within 72 hours after the birth of an Rh-positive child will prevent the mother from becoming sensitized to this antigen and developing anti-Rh antibodies that would affect subsequent Rh-positive fetuses [10].

Differential Diagnosis

1. Spasticity and athetoid posturing also develop in children who experienced neonatal cerebral anoxia.
2. Deafness and spasticity are features of some children with the rubella syndrome, but they also may have cataracts and congenital heart defects (see page 118).
3. Choreoathetosis and mental retardation are features of patients with the Lesch-Nyhan syndrome, but they also have self-mutilation, hyperuricemia, and a defect in uric acid metabolism, and do not have neonatal hyperbilirubinemia (see page 30).

References

1. Diamond, I. Kernicterus: revised concepts of pathogenesis and management. *Pediatrics,* **38**:539–42, 1966.
2. Silberberg, D. H., Johnson, L., and Ritter, L. Factors influencing toxicity of bilirubin in cerebellum tissue culture. *J. Pediatr.,* **77**:386–96, 1970.
3. Van Praagh, R. Diagnosis of kernicterus in the neonatal period. *Pediatrics,* **28**:870–76, 1961.
4. Byers, R. K., Paine, R. S., and Crothers, B. Extrapyramidal cerebral palsy with hearing loss following erythroblastosis. *Pediatrics,* **15**:248–54, 1955.
5. Crothers, B., and Paine, R. *The Natural History of Cerebral Palsy.* Harvard University Press, Cambridge, Mass. 1959.
6. Hyman, C. B., Keaster, J., Hanson, V., Harris, I., Sedgwick, R., Wursten, H., and Wright, A. R. CNS abnormalities after neonatal hemolytic disease or hyperbilirubinemia. A prospective study of 405 patients. *Am. J. Dis. Child.,* **117**:395–405, 1969.
7. Keaster, J., Hyman, C. B., and Harris, I. Hearing problems subsequent to neonatal hemolytic disease or hyperbilirubinemia. *Am. J. Dis. Child.,* **117**:406–10, 1969.
8. Gartner, L. M., Snyder, R. N., Chabon, R. S., and Bernstein, J. Kernicterus: high incidence in premature infants with low serum bilirubin concentrations. *Pediatrics,* **45**:906–17, 1970.
9. Behrman, R. E., and Hsia, D. Y.-Y. Summary of a symposium on phototherapy for hyperbilirubinemia. *J. Pediatr.,* **75**:718–26, 1969.
10. Freda, V. J., Gorman, J. G., and Pollack, W. Rh factor: prevention of isoimmunization and clinical trial on mothers. *Science,* **151**:828–29, 1966.

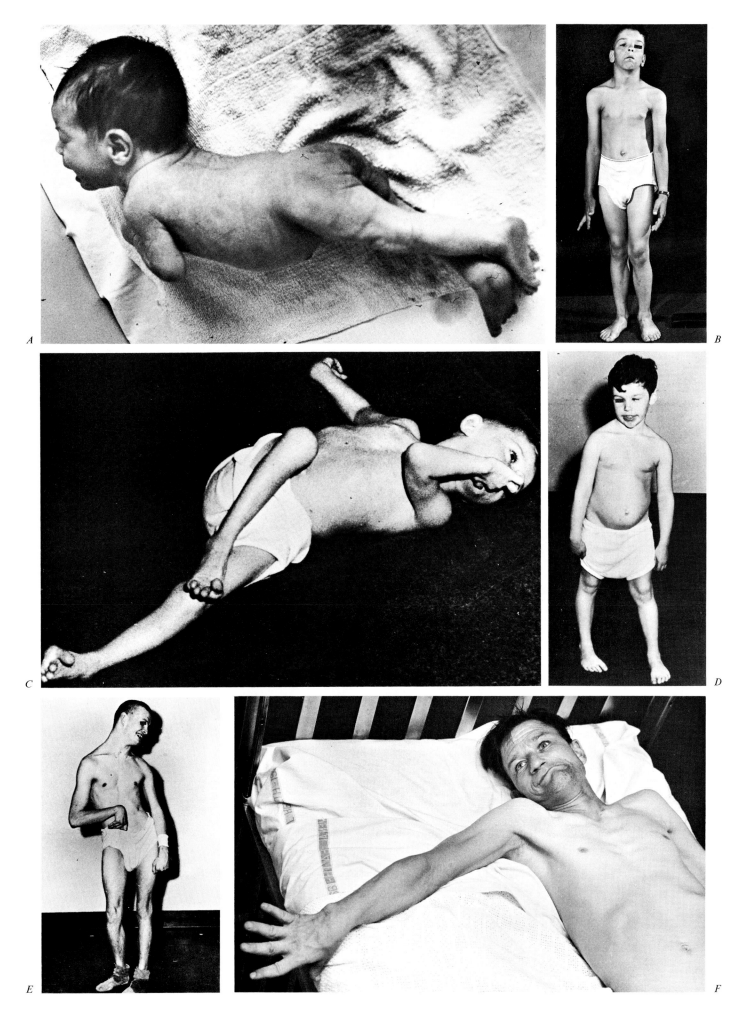

Plate III-9. *A:* A 5-month-old child with severe spasticity who had neonatal hyperbilirubinemia due to glucose-6-phosphate dehydrogenase deficiency. *B:* A 15-year-old retarded boy with grimacing and athetoid movements of one arm whose neonatal hyperbilirubinemia had been due to Rh incompatibility. *C:* A 4-year-old boy with severe athetosis and an IQ of 25 in whom kernicterus was confirmed at autopsy. *D:* A 7-year-old with an IQ of 60 whose neonatal hyperbilirubinemia was due to Rh incompatibility. *E:* A 22-year-old man with athetosis and an IQ of 30. *F:* A 41-year-old man with facial grimacing, athetoid posturing of his arm, and an IQ of 60. (*A:* Courtesy of Dr. S. Doxiadis, Athens, Greece. *C–E:* Courtesy of Dr. H. Yannet, Southbury, Conn.)

139

Battered-Child Syndrome

Physical abuse and neglect of children have always been regrettably common. Increasing concern about the problem has been generated in the United States during the past twenty years by publicity about the social, psychiatric, medical, radiologic, and pathologic results of the abuse and neglect of children. For example, a survey reported in 1962 of 71 hospitals and 77 district attorneys covering a one-year period revealed that 749 children were known to have been maltreated, resulting in 78 fatalities and 114 cases of brain damage [1]. Later studies have shown that the problem is widespread, that many children with more subtle signs of abuse are not usually recognized, and that the true incidence of fatal injuries or permanent brain damage has not been established. The term *battered-child syndrome* has been used to refer to the results of both physical abuse and emotional and nutritional neglect.

Affected children are usually toddlers or preschool-age children, with an occasional infant as young as a few weeks of age or a teen-ager. In most instances the child's general health and hygiene are poor, malnutrition is evident, and the injuries are both old and new. If the children are seen before their condition has become chronic and severe, the physician may not recognize that their injuries are parent-induced. Often the parents will bring a child to a hospital emergency room for treatment of a laceration or fracture which they say was caused by an accident. The child is too frightened to protest, and the physician is too busy to either obtain a careful history or thoroughly examine the child for other evidence of abuse [2].

The abuse of children occurs in all socioeconomic, ethnic, and religious groups. Fathers, mothers, older siblings, or babysitters may be responsible. Parents who are guilty of child abuse often give an outward impression of devotion to and concern for their children. However, more thorough evaluation of these parents reveals personality traits such as immaturity, impulsiveness, antisocial behavior, and lack of warmth toward the maltreated child, as well as more serious psychiatric disorders. The parents act as if the child exists primarily to satisfy parental needs and as if the child's needs are unimportant. The child who does not fulfill the needs and requirements of the parents deserves punishment. Therefore, the child is punished for its failures and to make the child "shape up" and perform better. The parent who is guilty of neglect, rather than physical abuse, responds to disappointments in the child's behavior by giving up and abandoning efforts to even mechanically care for the child. In many cases the abusive or neglectful parent was also raised in an atmosphere in which there was a lack of a deep sense of being cared for [3].

The mechanism of physical abuse is usually assault or the use of abnormal physical restraints. The examining physician may see many different manifestations of old and new injuries, especially skin lesions, skeletal trauma, and neurologic symptoms.

Physical Features

SKIN: The morphology of the skin lesions is similar to that of the implements used to inflict the trauma, such as belt buckles, straps, ropes, coat hangers, or burning cigarettes (*Figures A, B, C, and D*). Bleeding is usually present in the abrasions and scars and is usually purpuric (*Figure E*), almost never petechial. The lesions are concentrated in clusters on the trunk and buttocks and less frequently on the head and the proximal portions of the limbs [4]. Some children are forced to sit on hot objects or in hot water as punishment (*Figure D, bottom*).

HEIGHT AND WEIGHT: Children suffering from chronic abuse and neglect are usually subnormal in both height and weight.

Nervous System

The child who has experienced emotional deprivation, neglect, and abuse often exhibits delinquency or other types of abnormal behavior. Retardation in intellectual and social development is common [5]. Brain damage is usually the result of subdural hematomas. The residual evidence of this trauma may be skull fractures (*Figure I*), microcephaly (*Figure F*), or hydrocephalus. Spinal cord injury may result from trauma to the spine [6].

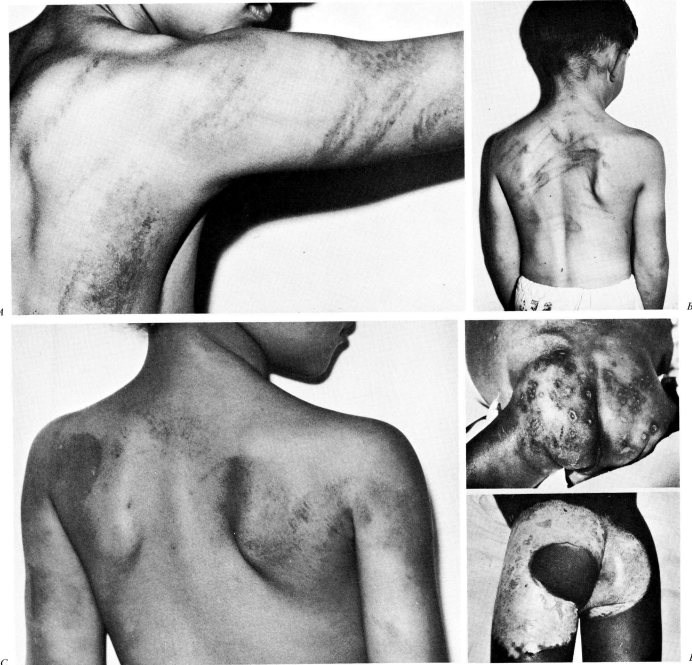

Plate III-10. *A:* Shows bruises due to rope restraints. *B:* Shows linear ecchymoses probably produced by a belt. *C:* Shows ecchymoses produced by the heel of a shoe. *D* (*top*): Small buttock scars produced by cigarette burns. *D* (*bottom*): Severe buttock burns caused by the infant being forced to sit on a radiator after having wet his diapers. *E:* Shows bruises from severe abdominal trauma which resulted in fatal intestinal and mesenteric hemorrhage. *F:* A 7-year-old boy with severe microcephaly following bilateral subdural hematomas and a broken arm at age 2 months. (*A–C:* Courtesy of Dr. S. J. Sussman, Philadelphia, Pa. *D* [*top*]: Courtesy of Dr. G. R. Hogan, Boston, Mass. *D* [*bottom*]: Courtesy of Dr. G. W. Hazard, Hyannis, Mass. *E:* From R. J. Touloukian, *Pediatrics,* **42:**642–46, 1968.)

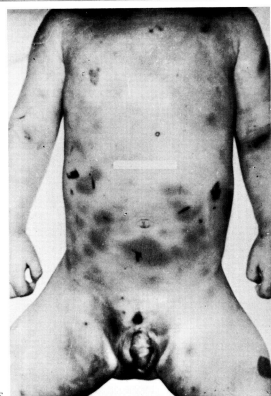

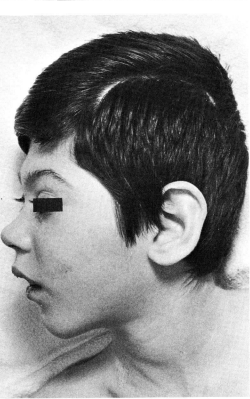

Laboratory Studies

The most common x-ray findings are injuries to the limbs. Unless gross fractures, dislocations, or epiphyseal separations are produced, no signs of bone injury are found during the first week after the specific injury. Reparative changes may first become manifest about 12 to 14 days after the injury. An abused infant may develop massive subperiosteal hematomas which elevate the active periosteum so that new bone formation takes place around and along the entire length of the shaft (*Figures G and H*) [7]. The forces applied in grasping and seizing usually involve traction and torsion, which are likely to produce epiphyseal separation and periosteal shearing. Shaft fractures result from direct blows or from bending and compression forces. Repetition of injury can produce lesions in several areas and in different stages of healing. If an injured bone is not adequately immobilized and trauma occurs repeatedly in the same area, the healing will be accompanied by an excessive local reaction and hemorrhage, and ultimately exaggerated repair.

Multiple linear skull fractures (*Figure I*) and an associated subdural hematoma (*Figure J*) may be the result of head trauma Blows to the back can produce anterior wedging of the vertebrae and associated intervertebral disk-space narrowing (*Figures K and L*) [6]. The chronically abused and neglected child often shows evidence of iron deficiency, malnutrition, and dehydration.

Prevention

Early recognition of the abused child and rehabilitative efforts for both the child and the parents are essential if further abuse is to be prevented. Most states in the United States have laws requiring the reporting of suspected cases of child abuse.

Differential Diagnosis

1. Scurvy is commonly suggested as an alternative diagnosis, since it also produces large calcifying subperiosteal hemorrhages, ecchymoses in the skin, and hematuria. However, scurvy is a generalized disease with uniform osteoporosis and widely scattered skin lesions. Scurvy is quite rare before the age of 6 months.

2. Congenital syphilis can cause similar lesions in the periosteal and metaphyseal areas. However, other skin manifestations of congenital syphilis, the tendency to symmetric distribution of the bone lesions, and a persistently positive serologic test should clearly distinguish this disease from the battered-child syndrome (see page 140).

3. Infants with osteogenesis imperfecta may have skull and limb fractures, a mosaic ossification pattern of the cranial vault, and shaft fractures. The abused child's fractures usually are limited to the metaphyseal regions of the long bones or appear as discrete linear skull fractures in an otherwise normal cranium.

4. Children with congenital indifference to pain can have multiple fractures and excessive callus formation as a consequence of inadequate immobilization. However, they should be readily distinguished by their sensory deficit (see page 254).

References

1. Kempe, C. H., Silverman, F. N., Steele, B. F., Droegemueller, W., and Silver, H. K.   The battered-child syndrome. *J.A.M.A.*, **181**:17–24, 1962.
2. Holter, J. C., and Friedman, S. B.   Child abuse: early case finding in the emergency department. *Pediatrics*, **42**:128–38, 1968.
3. Helfer, R. E., and Kempe, C. H. (eds.).   *The Battered Child.* University of Chicago Press, Chicago, 1968.
4. Sussman, S. J.   Skin manifestations of the battered-child syndrome. *J. Pediatr.*, **72**:99–101, 1968.
5. Elmer, E., and Gregg, G. S.   Developmental characteristics of abused children. *Pediatrics*, **40**:596–602, 1967.
6. Swischuk, L. E.   Spine and spinal cord trauma in the battered child syndrome. *Radiology*, **92**:733–38, 1969.
7. Fontana, V. J., Donovan, D., and Wong, R. J.   The "maltreatment syndrome" in children. *N. Engl. J. Med.*, **269**:1389–94, 1963.

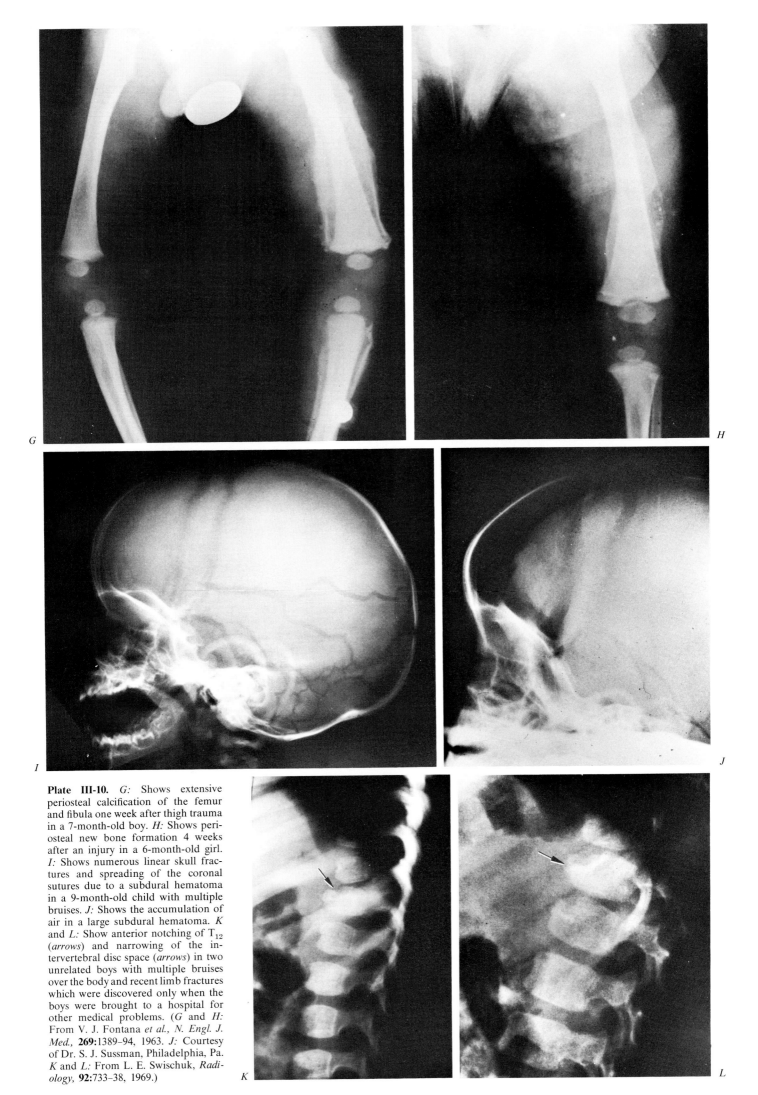

Plate III-10. *G:* Shows extensive periosteal calcification of the femur and fibula one week after thigh trauma in a 7-month-old boy. *H:* Shows periosteal new bone formation 4 weeks after an injury in a 6-month-old girl. *I:* Shows numerous linear skull fractures and spreading of the coronal sutures due to a subdural hematoma in a 9-month-old child with multiple bruises. *J:* Shows the accumulation of air in a large subdural hematoma. *K* and *L:* Show anterior notching of T$_{12}$ (*arrows*) and narrowing of the intervertebral disc space (*arrows*) in two unrelated boys with multiple bruises over the body and recent limb fractures which were discovered only when the boys were brought to a hospital for other medical problems. (*G* and *H:* From V. J. Fontana *et al., N. Engl. J. Med.,* **269:**1389–94, 1963. *J:* Courtesy of Dr. S. J. Sussman, Philadelphia, Pa. *K* and *L:* From L. E. Swischuk, *Radiology,* **92:**733–38, 1969.)

Chapter IV
Chromosomal Abnormalities

Introduction

In 1959 Lejeune, Gautier, and Turpin [1] described the first abnormality of human chromosomes, the association of 47 chromosomes with Down's syndrome. Since then, chromosome analysis has been used extensively in the evaluation of retarded children and adults. In an effort to establish the overall frequency of chromosomal abnormalities, both consecutive liveborn infants and aborted fetuses have been studied. The prevalence of chromosomal abnormalities in liveborn infants is about 1 : 200. This means that each year in the United States about 20,000 infants are born with chromosomal abnormalities [2]. The overall frequency of these abnormalities is even higher if one considers all fetuses. About 4 percent of all fetuses carry a chromosomal abnormality; over 90 percent of these fetuses are eliminated as spontaneous abortions. Of those who are liveborn, half have autosomal abnormalities and the other half have sex chromosomal abnormalities [3]. The prevalence of the most common chromosomal abnormalities in liveborn infants is estimated as follows:

21 trisomy	1 : 500–1 : 800	[4]
XYY syndrome	1 : 1000	[5]
XXX syndrome	1 : 1000	[6]
XXY (Klinefelter's) syndrome	1 : 1400	[5]
XO (Turner's) syndrome	1 : 3300	[6]
18 trisomy	1 : 6800	[7]
13 trisomy	1 : 7600	[7]

*For the autosomal syndromes only the karyotypes of affected females are indicated, although males can also be affected.

As more abnormalities have been described, the nomenclature for the human chromosome complement has become more complex. According to the Denver classification (1960) the autosomes are divided into seven groups and are numbered from 1 to 22 based as nearly as possible in order of descending length. Designating the groups as A to G, the 22 pairs of autosomes are divided in this way: pairs 1–3 are group A, 4 and 5 are group B, 6–12 are group C, 13–15 are group D, 16–18 are group E, 19 and 20 are group F, and 21 and 22 are group G. The X chromosome is in group C, and the Y chromosome is in group G. At the Chicago conference in 1966, an expanded system of nomenclature was introduced [8]. Modifications of this nomenclature were added at the Paris conference in 1971 [11]. The presence of one additional chromosome (trisomy) is indicated by a plus (+) followed by the letter or number identifying the chromosome, and absence of one chromosome by a minus (−). For example, 47,XY, +21 indicates a male with trisomy 21, and 45,XX, − 13 indicates a female missing chromosome 13. The long arm of a chromosome is designated by the letter "q" and the short arm by the letter "p." Therefore, 46,XX,4p− indicates a female with deletion of the short arm of one chromosome in pair number 4. A ring chromosome is designated by the letter "r"; 46,XY,r13 means a male with a ring chromosome 13.

Early work with chromosome analysis focused on patients with multiple deformities, endocrine abnormalities, and mental retardation, in the expectation that they would be most likely to have chromosomal abnormalities. With the extension of chromosome analyses to consecutive newborns and less severely handicapped individuals, two facts have emerged. First, it is evident that many of the children with chromosomal abnormalities cannot be detected clinically in infancy because they do not have any distinguishing physical characteristics. Only one fourth of the infants with chromosomal abnormalities in one study [2] could have been detected by their physical features. The infants with the 47,XYY, 47,XXY, and 47,XXX syndromes would not have been detected, but the infants with autosomal trisomies 21, 18, and 13 had recognizable features. Second, as more patients with the same chromosomal abnormalities have been detected, it has been evident that wide phenotypic variability is the rule, not the exception. To identify and differentiate the various syndromes by clinical examination the physician must look carefully for minor congenital anomalies, which are a common feature of patients with these syndromes. This awareness has introduced new terms in the description of patients that do not always mean the same thing to each examiner: triangular face, carp-shaped mouth, beaklike nose, high-arched palate, long philtrum, relative prognathism, micrognathia, posteriorly rotated ears, short neck, widely spaced nipples, and hypoplastic nails. Two examples of this enthusiasm for anatomic detail are the new interest in dermatoglyphics and the elaborate descriptions of ear deformities. Because of this emphasis we have included a special section on dermatoglyphics in this chapter. Out of respect for the fact that many clinicians cannot remember the anatomic regions of the external ear, a diagram is included:

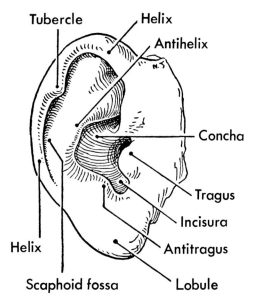

(From J. C. B. Grant, *A Method of Anatomy: Descriptive and Deductive,* 6th ed. Williams & Wilkins Co., Baltimore, 1958.)

While the recognition of anomalies in the identification of chromosomal abnormality syndromes has gained new importance, it must be emphasized that no single anomaly is pathognomonic of any syndrome. For example, cleft lip, epicanthic folds, hypertelorism, webbing of the neck, ptosis, a small chin, small and malformed ears, a single transverse palmar crease, hypogenitalism, lymphedema, and clinodactyly are each associated with several syndromes. It is the total pattern of anomalies, rather than a single anomaly, which may indicate the correct clinical diagnosis of a specific chromosomal abnormality syndrome.

The understanding of the chromosomal abnormality syndromes is being rapidly extended. Nevertheless, some of the newly recognized syndromes, such as G monosomy, 18p−, 18q−, 13q−, 4p−, extra small acrocentric, XXYY, XXXY, XXXX, and XXXXX, have been observed in so few individuals that phenotypic correlations are very tentative. In the case of some disorders, such as the XXXXY syndrome, the affected individuals have been ascertained with a bias toward those with mental retardation and skeletal and genital anomalies. Still others, such as the XXX and XYY syndromes, have no definite associated physical abnormalities [9,10]. Continued experience, especially with the screening of consecutive newborns, will certainly make the phenotype-karyotype correlations more accurate.

An unknown, but possibly substantial, degree of refinement in the clinical delineation of chromosomal abnormalities will result from the use of the new chromosome staining techniques. The first was the quinacrine fluorescent method [12], which provides the ability to distinguish between chromosomes 21 and 22 and to identify the distal segment of the long arms of the Y chromosome, among other attributes. Three more methods, namely, the constitutive heterochromatin, Giemsa, and reverse Giemsa, have recently been developed [11]. Each stain has unique advantages. Together they allow identification of each pair of chromosomes. Furthermore, they will provide new insight into both minor variations in chromosome structure and small, but significant, deletions.

References

1. Lejeune, J., Gautier, M., and Turpin, R. Les chromosomes humains en culture de tissus. *C. R. Acad. Sci. (D) (Paris),* **248:**602–603, 1959.
2. Lubs, H. A., and Ruddle, F. H. Chromosomal abnormalities in the human population: estimation of rates based on New Haven newborn study. *Science,* **169:**495–97, 1970.
3. Polani, P. E. Autosomal imbalance and its syndromes, excluding Down's. *Br. Med. Bull.,* **25:**81–92, 1969.
4. Lejeune, J. The 21-trisomy—current stage of chromosomal research. *Progr. Med. Genet.,* **3:**144–77, 1964.
5. Ratcliffe, S. G., Stewart, A. L., Melville, M. M., and Jacobs, P. A. Chromosomes studies on 3500 newborn male infants. *Lancet,* **1:**121–22, 1970.
6. Court Brown, W. M. Sex chromosome aneuploidy in man and its frequency with special reference to mental subnormality and criminal behavior. *Int. Rev. Exp. Pathol.,* **7:**31–97, 1969.
7. Taylor, A. I. Autosomal trisomy syndromes: a detailed study of 27 cases of Edwards' syndrome and 27 cases of Patau's syndrome. *J. Med. Genet.,* **5:**227–52, 1968.
8. Summitt, R. L. Chromosome nomenclature. *J. Pediatr.,* **76:**314–23, 1970.
9. Kohn, G., Winter, J. S. D., and Mellman, W. J. Trisomy X in three children. *J. Pediatr.,* **72:**248–52, 1968.
10. Court Brown, W. M. Males with an XYY sex chromosome complement. *J. Med. Genet.,* **5:**341–49, 1968.
11. Hecht, F., Wyandt, H. E., and Erbe, R. W. Revolutionary cytogenetics. *N. Engl. J. Med.,* **285:**1482–84, 1971.
12. Caspersson, T., Lomakka, G., and Zech, L. The 24 fluorescence patterns of the human metaphase chromosomes—distinguishing characters and variability. *Hereditas,* **67:**89–102, 1971.

Dermatoglyphics

The analysis of dermatoglyphics has blossomed as a clinical science in the enthusiasm for describing chromosomal abnormalities. The term *dermatoglyphics,* which literally means "skin carvings," is used to refer to the configurations formed by the epidermal ridges on the palms, soles, and digits of all primates. By custom the palmar and digital flexion creases are also included, although these are not true epidermal patterns. The dermal ridges develop between the thirteenth and nineteenth gestational weeks and are thought to reflect the shape of the fetal hand during that time [1,2]. The primary cause of the abnormal shape of the hand may be a chromosomal abnormality, a teratogen, or a mutant gene. While almost all individuals with chromosomal abnormalities have abnormal dermal patterns, a particular pattern is never a specific feature of any syndrome [3]. However, the dermal patterns, like minor congenital anomalies, are often helpful in identifying the child with a possible chromosomal abnormality [3–5].

The three basic patterns on the tips of the fingers and toes are the arch, the loop, and the whorl, which differ in the number of triradii present. A triradius is the point formed by the meeting of three different ridge fields. A simple arch has no triradius and is composed of a succession of gently curving ridges (*Figure A*). A loop has one triradius and may be designated as ulnar or radial, depending on the direction of the loop (*Figure A*); an ulnar loop opens toward the ulnar margin of the hand and has the triradius on the radial side. Whorls have two triradii and are of two general types—either concentric ridges around a single center (*Figure A*) or a double-loop pattern. The ridge count refers to the number of ridges intersecting a line drawn from the center of a loop to the center of a triradius; in whorls, one counts only the larger of the two numbers. The distribution of fingerprint patterns varies among different populations and for each digit. In general, ulnar loops are the most common pattern and arches the least common [5].

The palm is divided into three main areas. The hypothenar area is on the ulnar side. The thenar area is at the base of the thumb. The four interdigital areas are at the bases of and between the digits. The axial triradius is usually located near the proximal margin of the palm between the thenar and hypothenar eminences (*Figures B and C*). When patterns are present in either of these areas, they are usually loops or whorls. In a number of chromosomal abnormality syndromes the axial triradius is displaced distally and associated with hypothenar patterns (*Plate IV-2, H,* page 153).

The dermal ridges of the sole are similar to those of the palm in that there are major areas and patterns, such as arches, loops, and whorls. The areas are the hallucal, the hypothenar, the thenar, the interdigital (*Figure E*), and the calcar, which is on the heel. The hallucal area is the most useful for the study of plantar patterns and may be the only area on the sole that has a truly unique pattern suggestive of a medical disorder. Whereas the loop distal pattern is the most frequent in the normal population, the arch tibial pattern occurs in about half of the patients with trisomy 21 [4] (*Plate IV-2, J,* page 153).

The flexion creases on the palms represent the places where the skin is attached to underlying structures. There are usually three flexion creases (*Figures C and D*). If the two distal creases are fused, the single line formed is called a simian line or transverse palmar crease (*Plate IV-2, H,* page 153). If the two distal creases on the palm do not fuse, but are joined by a third small crease, it is called a transitional simian crease. Most people have two flexion creases on all fingers, except their thumbs. A single flexion crease on the fifth finger is usually associated with clinodactyly. While a simian crease occurs in about 5 percent of the normal population, and clinodactyly is associated with many disorders, the presence of both a simian crease and a single fifth finger crease often is a feature of individuals with Down's syndrome (*Plate IV-2, G and H,* page 153). However, these features also occur in association with other chromosome abnormalities, such as 49,XXXXY.

References

1. Cummins, H., and Midlo, C. *Finger Prints, Palms and Soles: An Introduction to Dermatoglyphics,* Dover Publications, New York, 1961.
2. Mulvihill, J. J., and Smith, D. W. The genesis of dermatoglyphics. *J. Pediatr.,* **75**:579–89, 1969.
3. Penrose, L. S. Finger-prints, palms and chromosomes. *Nature,* **197**:933–38, 1963.
4. Holt, S. B. *The Genetics of Dermal Ridges.* Charles C Thomas Publisher, Springfield, Ill., 1968.
5. Stough, T. R., and Seely, J. R. Dermatoglyphics in medicine. *Clin. Pediatr.,* **8**:32–41, 1969.

Plate IV-1. *A:* Fingertips (*above*) from which fingerprints (*below*) have been made, illustrating left to right simple arch, loop, and whorl. *B* and *C:* Normal palm and palm print showing the main topographic areas. *D* and *E:* Normal sole and sole print showing the main topographic areas. (*A–E:* From J. R. Miller and J. Giroux, *J. Pediatr.,* **69:**302–12, 1966.)

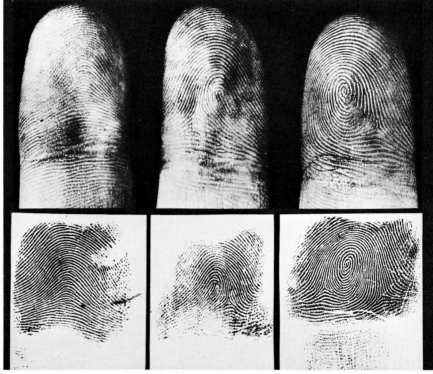

A

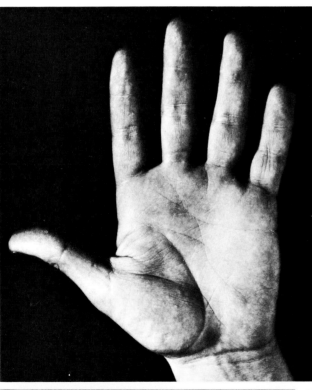

B

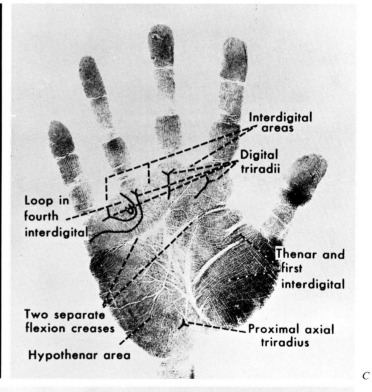

Interdigital areas

Digital triradii

Loop in fourth interdigital

Thenar and first interdigital

Two separate flexion creases

Proximal axial triradius

Hypothenar area

C

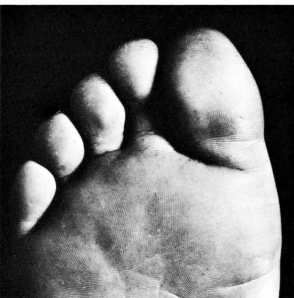

D

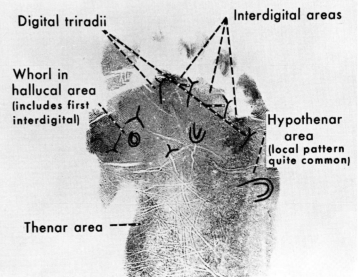

Digital triradii

Interdigital areas

Whorl in hallucal area (includes first interdigital)

Hypothenar area (local pattern quite common)

Thenar area

E

Autosomal Syndromes
Chromosome 21 Trisomy
(Down's Syndrome; 47,XX,+21)

Since the clinical description by Langdon Down in 1866 [1], mongolism, or to use the preferred term, *Down's syndrome,* has become a familiar clinical syndrome. In 1959 LeJeune, Gautier, and Turpin [2] first identified its association with an extra chromosome in the 21–22 group, which by custom is referred to as a number 21. Subsequent studies have shown Down's syndrome to be the most common autosomal abnormality, with a frequency of about 1:700 newborns [3].

Physical Features

HEAD: The outstanding feature is brachycephaly with prominence of the forehead, shortening of the anteroposterior diameter, and flattening of the occiput (*Figure C*). The cranial capacity is below normal.

FACE: The round, flat face is characterized by a flat nasal bridge, epicanthic folds, and palpebral fissures that slant upward (*Figures A and B*). In a study [5] of 93 children under 10 years of age with Down's syndrome epicanthic folds were present in 60 percent (controls, 20 percent), and the upward palpebral slant occurred in 91 percent (controls, 14 percent). The nose is considered small in about half of the cases; the nasal bones are underdeveloped and there is a tendency for the nares to point forward instead of down [4]. Rhinitis is common.

EYES: The most common findings are two iris anomalies, hypoplasia of the iris stroma and Brushfield spots. The latter are white, elevated aggregates of stromal fibers in the pupillary margin of the iris (*Figure E*). In the study [5] of 216 patients with Down's syndrome, 70 percent had Brushfield spots (controls, 12 percent). Iris hypoplasia was present in 48 percent of the patients and 17 percent of the controls.

EARS: The ears are usually small and simple in appearance, often having an overfolded upper helix, poor antihelix development, and a small lobe (*Figure C*).

MOUTH: Protrusion of the tongue is common in newborns (*Figure A*) and is attributed to the small mouth. The tongue is otherwise normal in appearance at birth, but in older patients there are hypertrophy of the vallate papillae and a furrowed appearance (*Figure F*). The palate is normal in height, narrow, and short [6]. The teeth often erupt late and are misshapen and small. Congenital absence of both deciduous and permanent teeth is common, especially the third molars, second premolars, and lateral incisors [6a].

NECK: The neck is short and broad and the hairline reaches farther down the back than normal. Infants have looseness of the skin over the neck and shoulders, but webbing of the neck is rare.

BREASTS: During puberty the breasts remain small, but in adults they may be of normal size. At all ages the nipples are small, the areolae are indistinct, and little glandular tissue is palpable [4,7].

ABDOMEN: In children the abdomen is usually protuberant, and diastasis recti and umbilical hernia are common.

GENITALIA: Males often have a small penis, scrotum, and testes. Females have large labia majora [4,7].

LIMBS: The hands, feet, and digits are broad and shortened. Clinodactyly of the fifth finger (*Figure G*) and a wide space between the first and second toes (*Figure I*) are present in the majority of the patients. The joints in the upper and lower limbs are usually hyperextensible, especially in infants and young children. Clubfeet were observed in 1.1 percent of the children in one study [8].

DERMATOGLYPHICS: The most common features are a transverse palmar crease ("simian crease"), a single flexion crease of the fifth finger in association with clinodactyly, a distal axial triradius on the palms (*Figure H*), ulnar loops on all fingers, and a tibial arch in the hallucal area of the soles (*Figure J*).

SKIN: The hands and feet often have a mottled, and sometimes cyanotic, appearance in infants and adults. The cheeks of infants are usually red and scaly. Generalized rough, dry skin becomes increasingly frequent with advancing age [7].

HAIR: Beards tend to be slight. The axillary and pubic hair in adults is scanty and straight. Scalp hair is smooth and soft in children and more sparse and rough in older patients [7]. Recurrent focal alopecia is a common problem in adults (*Figure C*).

HEIGHT: The length at birth is below average, and height is below the normal range at all ages.

GROWTH AND DEVELOPMENT: There have been a few instances of females becoming pregnant, about half of whom bore infants with 21 trisomy [9]. There are no reports of proven fertility in males.

Plate IV-2. *A:* A newborn infant showing the flat, round face, epicanthic folds, upward palpebral slant, and slight tongue protrusion. *B* and *C:* A 17-year-old boy with focal alopecia, flat occiput, small ears with an overfolded helix, and an open-mouthed expression. *D:* Shows extensive facial wrinkling and frontal balding in an edentulous 53-year-old man. *E:* Close-up view of an eye illustrating Brushfield spots, the white clumps in the periphery of the iris stroma. *F:* Furrowing of the tongue in a 13-year-old boy. (*A:* Courtesy of Dr. C. R. Scott, Seattle, Wash. *E:* From D. D. Donaldson, *Arch. Ophthalmol.* [*Chicago*], **65:**26–31, 1961.)

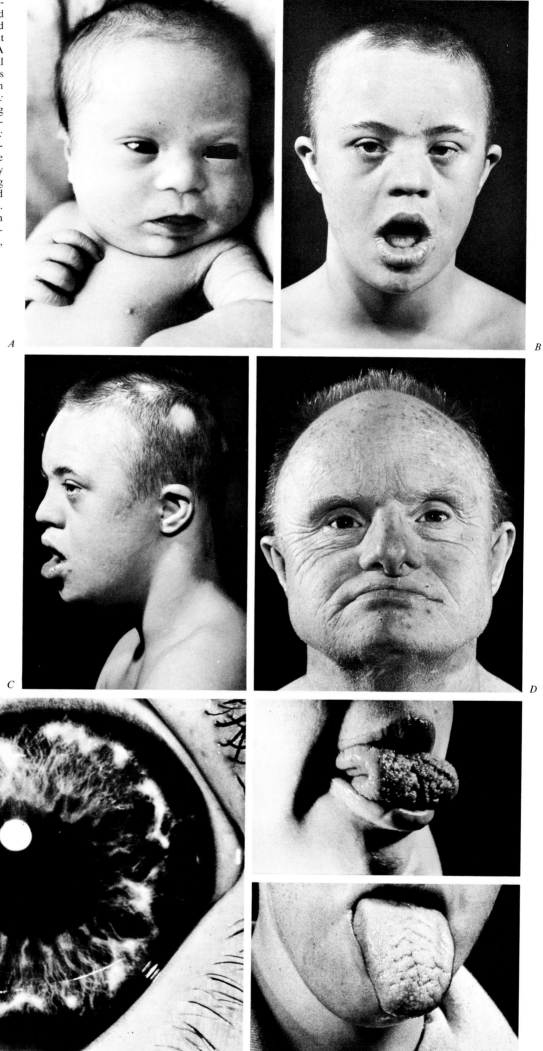

Nervous System

The level of intelligence ranges from mild to severe retardation. Serial studies in the first 4 years show that these children usually have slow, steady development [10]. These patients usually have a docile and happy demeanor, both as children and as adults. However, they can also be emotionally disturbed, as suggested by a study of 86 patients under 8 years of age, of whom 11 had emotional problems [11]. Generalized muscular hypotonia is characteristic of newborns and infants, but it becomes less pronounced with increasing age. In general, movements are slow, clumsy, and poorly coordinated. The gait in adults may be unsteady and the feet are kept wide apart [3].

Pathology

No abnormality of the brain has been consistently observed, although the brain size and weight are usually below average. Several adult patients have been reported to have progressive mental deterioration and the neuropathologic changes of Alzheimer's disease [12]. Acute leukemia is more common than in the normal population. The common internal anomalies are congenital heart disease, duodenal atresia, and Hirschsprung's disease. In a study of 2421 patients [8], 29 percent had congenital heart disease and 2.6 percent had duodenal obstruction due to either atresia or annular pancreas. In this study 23 patients had developed leukemia.

Laboratory Studies

X-rays of the pelvis in most patients show narrow acetabular and iliac angles, slender ischial rami, and coxa valga. Endocrine disorders, such as diabetes mellitus [13], hypothyroidism, and precocious puberty, have been observed in several patients, but the frequency is not known. Many different tests of thyroid function have been reported as abnormal by some investigators and normal by others [4]. Hyperuricemia, which may be due to overproduction of uric acid, has been observed in all age groups [14]. Elevations of several red and white blood cell enzymes, such as alkaline phosphatase, galactose-1-phosphate uridyl transferase and glucose-6-phosphate dehydrogenase, have been reported. A persistent elevation of hemoglobins F and A_2 was observed during the first few months of life in 11 out of 12 infants studied [15]. Many different types of bone marrow dysfunction, such as polycythemia, leukocytosis, and thrombocythemia, have been reported [16].

Treatment and Prognosis

About 25 to 30 percent die during the first year of life and about 50 percent during the first 5 years. The most frequent causes of death are respiratory infections and congenital heart disease [17]. Control studies are in progress to evaluate the value of 5-hydroxytryptophan in improving muscle tone [18]. Although some improvement in muscle tone and activity has been noted, one study [18a] showed that this treatment seemed to induce a seizure disorder in 15 percent of the patients.

Genetics

Ninety-five percent of the patients with Down's syndrome have 47 chromosomes with an extra number 21 chromosome (*Figure K*). Most of the remainder have 46 chromosomes with translocation of the long arm of an extra number 21 either to a D group or to another G group chromosome [4,7]. Mosaicism for trisomy 21 and a normal cell line is relatively rare. In general, the incidence of trisomy 21 increases with increasing maternal age, whereas translocation Down's syndrome occurs independent of maternal age. The incidence of Down's syndrome is about 1:1600 in mothers less than 20 years old and 1:75 for mothers over 40 [3]. For women who have already had one child with 21 trisomy, the risk of having a second affected child is between 1 and 2 percent for women below age 30; no increased risk has been documented for the woman who had her first affected child after the age of 30 [20]. Translocation Down's syndrome has special significance for the entire family. In one study [19] the risk of a female D/21 translocation carrier (*Figure L*) having a child with Down's syndrome was about 9 percent; for a male D/21 translocation carrier the risk was about 4 percent. Based on only 6 families the recurrence risk for a 21/22 translocation carrier was 5 percent. If the parent is a 21/21 translocation carrier, his or her chance of having an affected child is 100 percent. The differentiation of a 21/22 from a 21/21 translocation can now be made by quinacrine fluorescent studies [21].

Differential Diagnosis

1. Muscular hypotonia, a flat bridge of the nose, epicanthal folds, clinodactyly, and simian crease are also features of patients with the 49,XXXXY syndrome, but they often have vertebral anomalies and prognathism (see page 190).
2. Children with congenital hypothyroidism have muscular hypotonia and a protruding tongue (see page 10).
3. Hypotonia and a flat, round face with an upward eye slant and a flat nasal bridge are features of patients with the cerebrohepatorenal syndrome (see page 270).
4. Hypotonia, epicanthic folds, and simple but large ears are features of infants with the 5p− syndrome, but they also have hypertelorism, a downward palpebral slant, and a catlike cry (see page 170).

References

1. Down, J. L. H.   Observations on an ethnic classification of idiots. *Clin. Lect. Rep. Lond. Hosp.,* **3**:259–62, 1866.
2. Lejeune, J., Gautier, M., and Turpin, R.   Les chromosomes humains en culture de tissus. *C. R. Acad. Sci.* (*D*) (*Paris*), **248**:602–603, 1959.
3. Fabia, J.   Illegitimacy and Down's syndrome. *Nature,* **221**:1157–58, 1969.
4. Penrose, L. S., and Smith, G. F.   *Down's Anomaly.* Little, Brown & Co., Boston, 1967.
5. Solomons, G., Zellweger, H., Jahnke, P. G., and Opitz, E.   Four common eye signs in mongolism. *Am. J. Dis. Child.,* **110**:46–50, 1965.
6. Shapiro, B. L., Gorlin, R. J., Redman, R. S., and Bruhl, H. H.   The palate and Down's syndrome. *N. Engl. J. Med.,* **276**:1460–63, 1967.
6a. Cohen, M. M., Sr., and Cohen, M. M., Jr.   The oral manifestations of trisomy G (Down syndrome). *Birth Defects: Original Article Series,* Vol. VIII, No. 7, June, 1971, pp. 241–51. Williams & Wilkins Co., Baltimore.
7. Gustavson, K.-H.   *Down's Syndrome: A Clinical and Cytogenetical Investigation.* Almquist & Wiksells, Uppsala, 1964.
8. Fabia, J., and Drolette, M.   Malformations and leukemia in children with Down's syndrome. *Pediatrics,* **45**:60–70, 1970.
9. Finley, W. H., Finley, S. C., Hardy, J. P., and McKinnon, T.   Down's syndrome in mother and child. *Obstet. Gynecol.,* **32**:200–203, 1968.
10. Koch, R., Share, J., Webb, A., and Graliker, B. V.   The predictability of Gesell developmental scales in mongolism. *J. Pediatr.,* **62**:93–97, 1963.
11. Menolascino, F. J.   Psychiatric aspects of mongolism. *Am. J. Ment. Defic.,* **69**:653–60, 1965.
12. Olson, M. I., and Shaw, C.-M.   Presenile dementia and Alzheimer's disease in mongolism. *Brain,* **92**:147–56, 1969.
13. Milunsky, A., and Neurath, P. W.   Diabetes mellitus in Down's syndrome. *Arch. Environ. Health,* **17**:372–76, 1968.
14. Pant, S. S., Moser, H. W., and Krane, S. M.   Hyperuricemia in Down's syndrome. *J. Clin. Endocrinol. Metab.,* **28**:472–78, 1968.
15. Wilson, M. G., Schroeder, W. A., and Graves, D. A.   Postnatal change of hemoglobins F and A_2 in infants with Down's syndrome (G trisomy). *Pediatrics,* **42**:349–53, 1968.
16. Weinberger, M. M., and Oleinick, A.   Congenital marrow dysfunction in Down's syndrome. *J. Pediatr.,* **77**:273–79, 1970.
17. Lilienfeld, A. J.   *Epidemiology of Mongolism.* Johns Hopkins Press, Baltimore, 1969, pp. 104–105.
18. Bazelon, M., Barnet, A., Lodge, A., and Shelburne, S. A., Jr.   The effect of high doses of 5-hydroxytryptophan on a patient with trisomy 21. *Brain Res.,* **11**:397–411, 1968.
18a. Coleman, M.   Infantile spasms associated with 5-hydroxytryptophan administration in patients with Down's syndrome. *Neurology* (*Minneap.*), **21**:911–19, 1971.
19. Hamerton, J. L.   Fetal sex. *Lancet,* **1**:516–17, 1970.
20. Mikkelsen, M.   Down's syndrome. Current stage of cytogenetic research. *Humangenetik,* **12**:1–28, 1971.
21. Caspersson, T., Hultén, M., Lindsten, J., Therkelsen, A. J., and Zech, L. Identification of different Robertsonian translocations in man by quinacrine mustard fluorescence analysis. *Hereditas,* **67**:213–20, 1971.

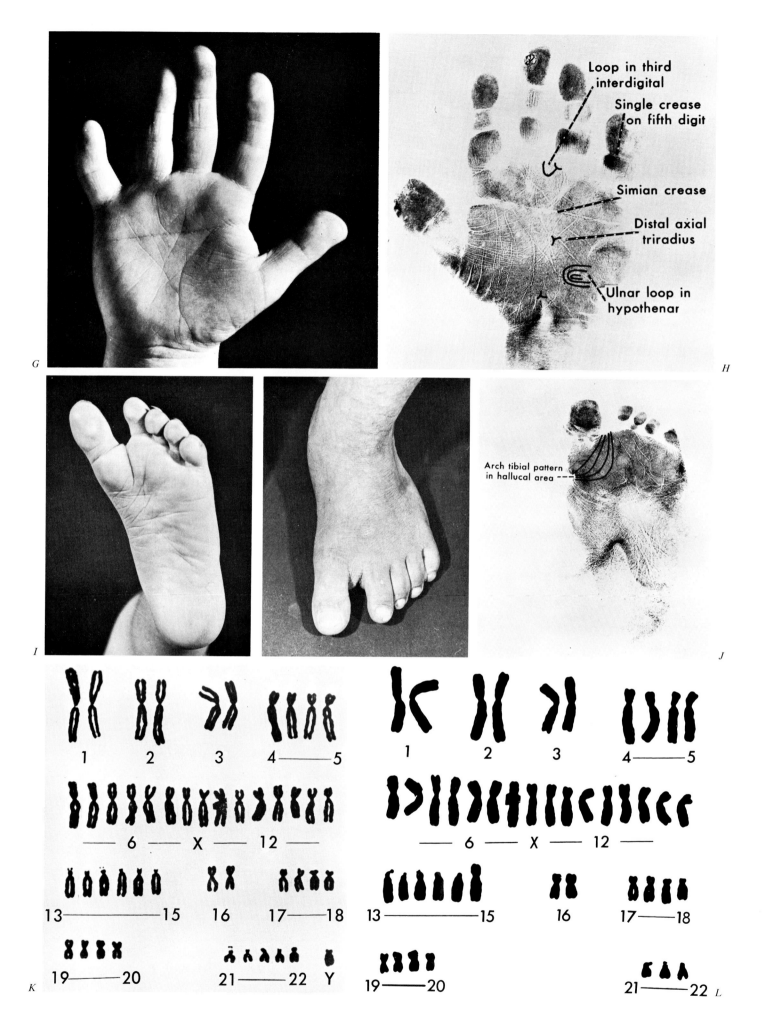

Plate IV-2. *G* and *H:* Hand and palm print showing some of the dermal ridge patterns in Down's syndrome. *I:* Shows the increased space between the first and second toes and the cleft on the ball of the foot between these toes. *J:* Sole print showing the most common dermal ridge pattern in Down's syndrome. *K:* Karyotype showing trisomy of 21–22 group. *L:* Karyotype of female carrier of translocation, showing a total of 45 chromosomes with one member of G (21–22) group translocated to a D (13–15) group chromosome. *(G, H,* and *J:* From J. R. Miller and J. Giroux, *J. Pediatr.,* **69:**302–12, 1966. *K* and *L:* Courtesy of Dr. L. Atkins, Boston, Mass.)

Group G Monosomy (45,XX,−G)

Absence of part or all of a small acrocentric chromosome, presumably 21 or 22, has been described in over ten patients. Three children [1–3] were thought to have complete absence of a G group chromosome. A fourth patient [4] had G monosomy plus mosaicism for a normal cell line. Other reported patients [5–13] have had partial deletions of a G group chromosome; their karyotypes showed either 45 chromosomes plus a G group fragment (45,XX,−G minute) or a ring G chromosome (46,XX,rG). It is appropriate to discuss patients with G monosomy and G deletion together because they have many phenotypic features in common. However, their abnormalities are nonspecific and clinical recognition is difficult.

It has been suggested [9,10] that there are two clinically distinct syndromes in which patients with either G monosomy or G deletion can be classified. The features proposed for syndrome I were hypertonia, antimongoloid slant, prominent nasal bridge, micrognathia, skeletal malformations, and growth retardation [3,5–7,12,13]; syndrome II included hypotonia, epicanthal folds, and syndactyly of toes [8–10,13]. However, all reported patients do not conform to this clinical differentiation. This lack of clear delineation may be related to uncertainty as to whether chromosome 21 or 22 is involved in a given case, the variation in the amount of deleted chromosomal material, or the presence of undetected mosaicism. Because of the limited amount of reported clinical and cytogenetic data, it seems appropriate at this time to consider the findings in these patients as one group.

Physical Features

FACE: Most patients have had epicanthic folds, a downward palpebral slant, and a small chin. The nose is prominent, and in some infants the tip has been misshapen [2–6] (*Figures A, B, C, D, and E*). One patient had cyclopia [11].

EYES: One patient had corneal opacities (*Figure E*) and a cataract in one eye [7]. Microphthalmia and Brushfield spots were each noted in separate patients [13].

EARS: The ears have been described as large, low-set, and misshapen [2,3] (*Figures B, C, D, and E*) and as having large external auditory canals [5,6].

GENITALIA: Three reported males had hypospadias and three had cryptorchidism [2,5–7].

LIMBS: Short and spadelike hands [1], a short index finger [4], short fifth fingers [10], dystrophic nails, clubfeet [4–6], rocker-bottom feet [7] (*Figure E*), and syndactyly between toes 2 and 3 [8–10] have been described.

Nervous System

All of the reported patients have been mentally retarded, usually to a severe degree. One had myoclonic seizures as a neonate and subsequently had spastic hemiparesis [1]. Another had severe muscular hypotonia as a newborn [2]. Muscular hypertonia [3] and spastic tetraplegia [4] were noted in two other patients.

Pathology

No anomalies have been consistently described, although porencephaly [4], pyloric stenosis [5,6,8], Meckel's diverticulum and common mesentery [5], and ventricular and atrial septal defects [2,13], pulmonary artery hypoplasia, and unilateral renal agenesis [13] have been reported. The child with cyclopia [11] had many brain anomalies, including a single cerebral ventricle and absence of the septum pellucidum and corpus callosum.

Laboratory Studies

One patient had a diminished serum IgA level [1] and another had decreased IgA and IgG [5]. The leukocyte alkaline phosphatase levels have been either normal [6,7,9] or increased [1,5]. Some patients have had thrombocytopenia and eosinophilia [5,6].

Treatment and Prognosis

Many of the reported patients died in the first year of life.

Genetics

Until these descriptions of 21 monosomy [1–3], complete absence of an autosome had been considered incompatible with survival. Because of the limitation of study methods, one can never rule out mosaicism in patients with apparent complete monosomy. Furthermore, an apparent monosomy may actually be a subtle chromosome rearrangement. Wyandt et al. [14] showed that a child with apparent monosomy 21 actually had a *de novo* 18/21 translocation that was evident only by autoradiography, measurements of chromosomes, and quinacrine staining.

References

1. Al-Aish, M. S., de la Cruz, F., Goldsmith, L. A., Volpe, J., Mella, G., and Robinson, J. C. Autosomal monosomy in man. Complete monosomy G (21–22) in a four-and-one-half-year-old mentally retarded girl. *N. Engl. J. Med.,* **227**:777–84, 1967.
2. Hall, B., Fredga, K., and Svenningsen, N. A case of monosomy G? *Hereditas,* **57**:356–64, 1967.
3. Thorburn, M. J., and Johnson, B. E. Apparent monosomy of a G autosome in a Jamaican infant. *J. Med. Genet.,* **3**:290–92, 1966.
4. Böhm, R., and Fuhrmann, W. Lebensfähigkeit bei Monosomie G. *Monatsschr. Kinderheilkd.,* **117**:184–87, 1969.
5. Lejeune, J., Berger, R., Réthoré, M. O., Archambault, L., Jérôme, H., Thieffry, S., Aicardi, J., Broyer, M., Lafourcade, J., Cruveiller, J., and Turpin, R. Monosomie partielle pour un petit acrocentrique. *C. R. Acad. Sci. (D) (Paris),* **259**:4187–90, 1964.
6. Reisman, L. E., Kasahara, S., Chung, C. Y., Darnell, A., and Hall, B. Anti-mongolism: studies in an infant with a partial monosomy of the 21 chromosome. *Lancet,* **1**:394–97, 1966.
7. Challacombe, D. N., and Taylor, A. Monosomy for a G autosome. *Arch. Dis. Child.,* **44**:113–19, 1969.
8. Reisman, L. E., Darnell, A., Murphy, J. W., Hall, B., and Kasahara, S. A child with partial deletion of a G-group autosome. *Am. J. Dis. Child.,* **114**:336–39, 1967.
9. Weleber, R. G., Hecht, F., and Giblett, E. R. Ring-G chromosome, a new G-deletion syndrome? *Am. J. Dis. Child.,* **115**:489–93, 1968.
10. Warren, R. J., and Rimoin, D. L. The G deletion syndromes. *J. Pediatr.,* **77**:658–63, 1970.
11. Cohen, M. M. Chromosomal mosaicism associated with a case of cyclopia. *J. Pediatr.,* **69**:793–98, 1966.
12. Nevin, N. C., MacLaverty, B., and Campbell, W. A. B. A child with a ring G chromosome (46,XX,Gr). *J. Med. Genet.,* **8**:231–34, 1971.
13. Kelch, R. P., Franklin, M., and Schnickel, R. D. Group G deletion syndromes. *J. Med. Genet.,* **8**:341–45, 1971.
14. Wyandt, H. E., Hecht, F., Lovrien, E. W., and Stewart, R. E. Study of a patient with apparent monosomy 21 due to translocation: 45,XX,21−,t(18q+). *Cytogenetics* (1972, in press).

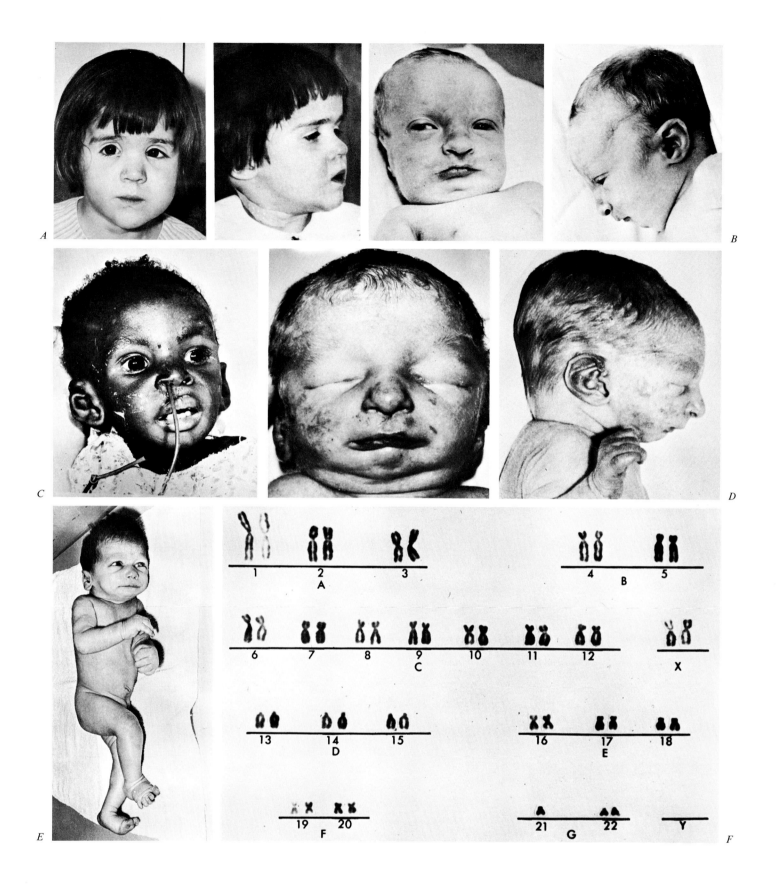

Plate IV-3. *A:* A 3½-year-old girl with wide-set, downward-slanting eyes, epicanthal folds, and spastic hemiplegia who had monosomy G. *B:* A male infant with narrow palpebral fissures, depressed tip of the nose, small chin, and monosomy G. *C:* A 1-year-old girl with hypertelorism, large malformed ears, and monosomy G. *D:* A male infant with a downward palpebral slant, depressed tip of the nose, and small chin who had mosaicism with two cell lines, 21 monosomy and 21 monosomy plus a centric fragment. *E:* A newborn male with bilateral corneal opacities, malformed ears, "rocker-bottom" feet, and mosaicism for two cell lines, 45,XY,G— and 46,XY,Gr. *F:* Karyotype showing absence of a number 21 chromosome. (*A:* From M. S. Al-Aish *et al., N. Engl. J. Med.,* **277:**777–84, 1967. *B:* From B. Hall *et al., Hereditas,* **57:**356–64, 1967. *C:* Courtesy of Dr. M. J. Thorburn, Kingston, Jamaica, W.I. *D:* From L. E. Reisman *et al., Lancet,* **1:**394–97, 1966. *E:* From D. N. Challacombe and A. Taylor, *Arch. Dis. Child.,* **44:**113–19, 1969. *F:* Courtesy of Dr. F. de la Cruz, Bethesda, Md.)

Chromosome 18 Trisomy (47,XX,+18)

In 1960 Edwards and his associates [1] reported a female infant with a peculiar facies, webbing of the neck, congenital heart disease, neonatal hepatitis, and many minor abnormalities in association with an extra E group chromosome. Since that time, more than 150 patients with this syndrome have been identified [2]. Studies have shown that the extra chromosome is number 18. Apparently this congenital anomaly syndrome, like the 4p−, 18p−, and 18q− syndromes, was never recognized as a specific clinical entity until the advent of chromosome analysis. The incidence of the 18 trisomy syndrome in newborns was estimated as 1 : 6800 in 1968 [2].

Physical Features

HEAD: Prominence of the occiput (*Figure D*) or an elongated skull is present in almost all patients. Microcephaly is uncommon.

FACE: The most common facial features are hypertelorism, epicanthic folds, narrow palpebral fissures, hypoplastic supraorbital ridges, ptosis, and a small chin [2,3] (*Figures A, H, and I*).

EYES: Corneal opacities, cataracts, and either an excess or a paucity of eyebrows and eyelashes have been described in a few patients [3]. Microphthalmos was noted in 7 of 26 infants in one study [2].

EARS: The ears are often small, low-set, and malformed (*Figures C and F*). Overfolding of the helix is common.

MOUTH: In a series of 27 patients, 3 had a cleft palate and 1 had a cleft lip [2].

NECK: Most patients have a short neck with redundant skin folds. Webbing of the neck is present in about one third of the patients [2].

CHEST: The sternum is usually short; x-rays show that it is poorly ossified.

ABDOMEN: Inguinal and umbilical hernias are common.

GENITALIA: The testes are usually undescended in males. The labia majora are often hypoplastic in females.

LIMBS: The hands have an unusual appearance, with ulnar deviation at the wrist and the second and fifth fingers curved medially (*Figures G, H, and J*). Most patients have flexion contractures of the fingers (*Figures A and B*). In about half of the patients the thumb is retroflexible and distally placed. The nails are usually hypoplastic. Syndactyly (*Figures H and K*) is common; polydactyly is rare. Partial or complete absence of the radius occasionally occurs. Most of the patients have short, dorsiflexed great toes (*Figures A, D, and E*) and a prominent calcaneus. The most common foot abnormality is the calcaneovalgus deformity (*Figure K*).

DERMATOGLYPHICS: The dermal ridges are often difficult to delineate. Almost all patients have a predominance of arches on the digits, and about half have a transverse palmar crease [2]. An increased frequency of radial loops on the thumb tips and a paucity of whorls on the fingertips have also been noted [4].

SKIN: Capillary hemangiomas have been present on several patients.

HEIGHT: The few surviving older patients have had severe linear growth failure [5].

WEIGHT: Many of these patients have a low birth weight for their gestational age. The mean birth weight of 153 patients was 2242 grams for an average gestational age of 42 weeks [2]. The infants usually have feeding difficulties, and both weight gain and linear growth are very slow.

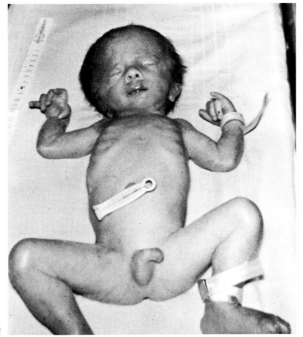

A

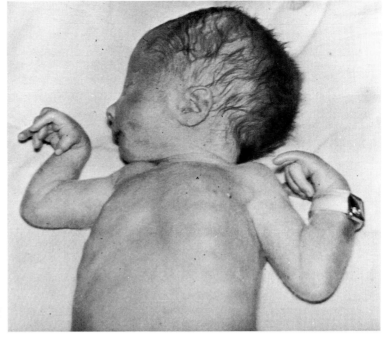

B

Plate IV-4. *A–C:* A newborn infant with hypoplastic supraorbital ridges, small chin, low-set ears, prominent occiput, flexion contractures of his right wrist and fingers 2 to 4, a dorsiflexed great toe, and small fingernails and toenails. *D:* A 4-month-old infant with a prominent occiput, small ventral hernia, "rocker-bottom" feet, and a medially curved fifth finger. *E* and *F:* An infant with extension of his legs, overlapping index finger, and malformed ear. (*D:* From I. A. Uchida *et al.*, *N. Engl. J. Med.,* **266:**1198–1201, 1962. *E* and *F:* Courtesy of Dr. D. Hoefnagel, Hanover, N.H.)

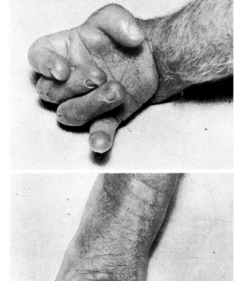

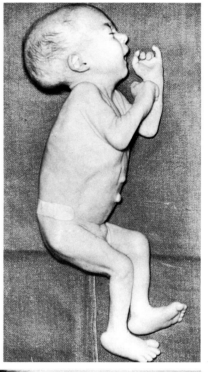

C

D

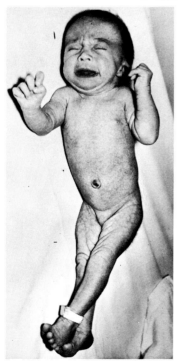

E

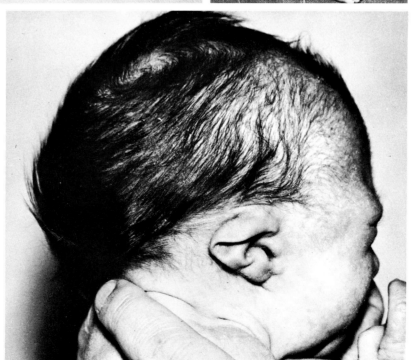

F

157

Nervous System

All patients have marked psychomotor retardation. Jitteriness and apnea are common neonatal problems. Either hypertonia or hypotonia of the muscles may be present. Seizures are common. Apparent deafness has also been noted in many patients [2].

Pathology

The brain weights are usually below average. Central nervous system abnormalities were noted in 15 out of 65 autopsies [6], but no anomaly is considered typical of 18 trisomy. The reported abnormalities include hydrocephalus, abnormal corpus callosum and cerebellum, absent occipital lobe and olfactory nerves, arhinencephaly, and meningomyelocele. Extensive cerebral heterotopias were found in periventricular areas of the brain in 13 of 16 infants in one study [7]. Asymmetric middle and inner ear anomalies were described in one patient [8].

Cardiac anomalies, especially atrial and ventricular septal defects and patent ductus arteriosus, are present in about half of the patients. Many different renal anomalies have been described. Diaphragmatic hernia, esophageal atresia, Meckel's diverticulum, malrotation of the colon, and a single umbilical artery are common findings [6,9]. Neonatal hepatitis was reported in 7 of 19 autopsies, including 2 patients with extrahepatic biliary atresia as well [10].

Treatment and Prognosis

In a survey of 153 patients, the mean survival was 71 days [2]. In a survey of 101 patients, one half survived for 2 months, one third for 3 months, and only one for 10 years [5].

Genetics

The identification of the extra chromosome as a number 18 has been done by autoradiography and quinacrine fluorescence staining [11]. A predominance of females has been noted in both liveborn infants and abortions. Of 143 patients, 113 (77 percent) were female [2]. Within this group of 143 there were several with an additional chromosomal abnormality; 4 females had XXX and 3 males XXY sex chromosome karyotypes. Advanced maternal age has been observed in 18 trisomy, as well as in the other autosomal trisomies.

Differential Diagnosis

1. Overlapping fingers, clinodactyly, malformed ears, and micrognathia are features of the patients with the pseudotrisomy 18 syndrome, but they have no chromosomal abnormalities. The disorder seems to be due to an autosomal recessive mutant gene (see page 336).
2. A small chin, overlapping fingers, syndactyly of the toes, and a calcaneovalgus deformity are features of patients with the Smith-Lemli-Opitz syndrome, but they also have ptosis, anteverted nostrils, a broad upper alveolar ridge, and hypospadias (see page 312).
3. Low birth weight, clinodactyly, and a small chin are features of patients with Silver-Russell syndrome, but they do not have multiple congenital malformations or severe mental deficiency (see page 310).
4. Neonatal hepatitis, congenital heart disease, deafness, and cataracts may also be found in infants with the rubella syndrome, but they do not have multiple minor and major anomalies (see page 118).
5. Cleft lip and palate and microphthalmos, which are found in a few patients with 18 trisomy, are typical phenotypic features of 13 trisomy (see page 164).

References

1. Edwards, J. H., Harnden, D. G., Cameron, A. H., Crosse, V. M., and Wolff, O. H. A new trisomic syndrome. *Lancet,* **1**:787–90, 1960.
2. Taylor, A. I. Autosomal trisomy syndromes: a detailed study of 27 cases of Edwards' syndrome and 27 cases of Patau's syndrome. *J. Med. Genet.,* **5**:227–52, 1968.
3. Ginsberg, J., Perrin, E. V., and Sueoka, W. T. Ocular manifestations of trisomy 18. *Am. J. Ophthalmol.,* **66**:59–67, 1968.
4. Ross, L. J. Dermatoglyphic observations in a patient with trisomy 18. *J. Pediatr.,* **72**:862–63, 1968.
5. Weber, W. W., Mamunes, P., Day, R., and Miller, P. Trisomy 17–18(E): studies in long-term survival with report of two autopsied cases. *Pediatrics,* **34**:533–41, 1964.
6. Passarge, E., True, C. W., Sueoka, W. T., Baumgartner, N. R., and Keer, K. R. Malformations of the central nervous system in trisomy 18 syndrome. *J. Pediatr.,* **69**:771–78, 1966.
7. Terplan, K. L., Lopez, E. C., and Robinson, H. B. Histologic structural anomalies in the brain in trisomy 18 syndrome. *Am. J. Dis. Child.,* **119**:228–35, 1970.
8. Kos, A. O., Schuknecht, H. F., and Singer, J. D. Temporal bone studies in 13–15 and 18 trisomy syndromes. *Arch. Otolaryngol.,* **83**:439–45, 1966.
9. Lewis, A. J. The pathology of 18 trisomy. *J. Pediatr.,* **65**:92–101, 1964.
10. Alpert, L. I., Strauss, L., and Hirschhorn, K. Neonatal hepatitis and biliary atresia associated with trisomy 17–18 syndrome. *N. Engl. J. Med.,* **280**:16–20, 1969.
11. Caspersson, T., Lomakka, G., and Zech, L. The 24 fluorescence patterns of the human metaphase chromosomes—distinguishing characters and variability. *Hereditas,* **67**:89–102, 1971.

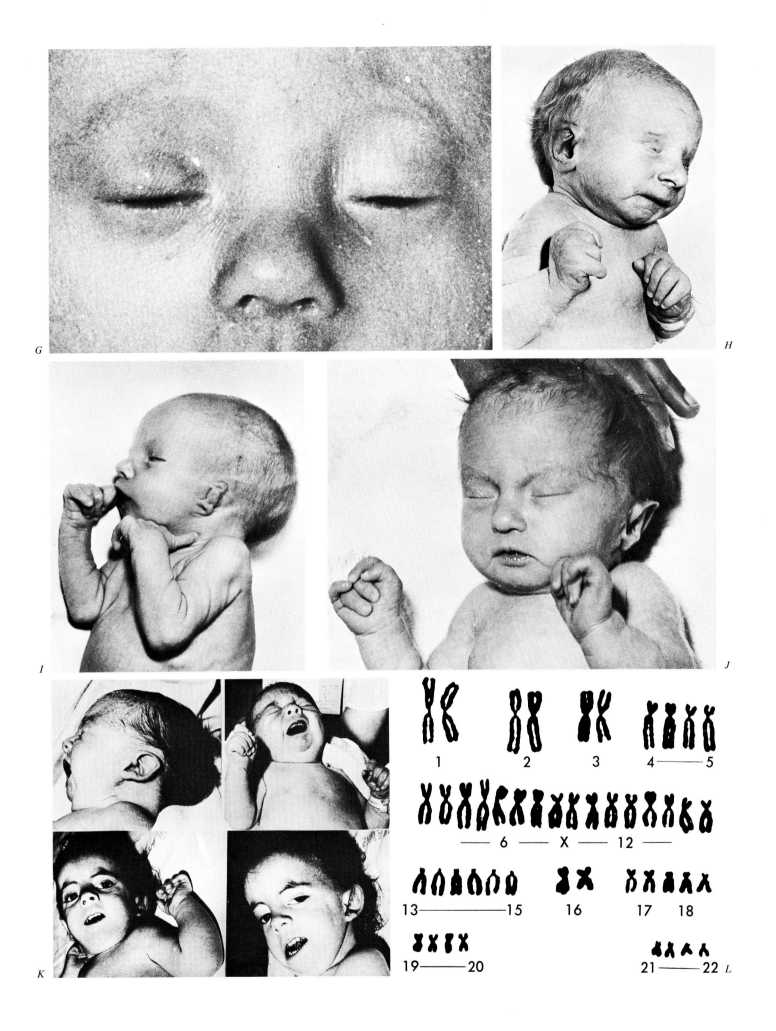

Plate IV-4. *G:* Close-up view showing hypertelorism, narrow palpebral fissures, and a lack of eyebrows, eyelashes, and supraorbital bony ridges. *H–J:* Three infants each showing a lack of eyebrows, eyelashes, and supraorbital ridges, small chin, overlapping of fingers 2 and 5, and small fingernails. Note the difference in the shapes of their ears. *K:* Shows the changes in the facial appearance of a child between 4 months and 4 years of age. *L:* Karyotype showing an extra number 18 chromosome. (*G–J:* Reprinted from A. I. Taylor, *J. Med. Genet.,* **5:**227, 1968, by permission of the author and editor. *K:* Courtesy of Dr. E. Passarge, Hamburg, Germany. *L:* Courtesy of Dr. L. Atkins, Boston, Mass.)

Chromosome 18, Deletion of Long Arm (46,XX,18q−)

In 1964 deGrouchy, Royer, Salmon, and Lamy [1] reported a deaf, microcephalic, and mentally retarded girl with a deletion of a portion of the long arm of a number 18 chromosome. Subsequent descriptions of more than 25 patients with the 18q− syndrome have shown that a fairly consistent phenotype is to be expected [2–6].

Physical Features

HEAD: Most patients are microcephalic.

FACE: The midportion of the face appears to be underdeveloped; the eyes are deeply set, the maxilla is flat, and the normal forehead and chin relatively prominent (*Figures A, B, and C*). The mouth has downward slanting corners and a "carp-shaped" appearance (*Figure E*). The tip of the nose has a broad, triangular appearance [2,3,6].

EYES: A tilted optic disc has been described in several patients [2].

EARS: The antihelix and antitragus are prominent, and the helix is poorly developed. The scaphoid fossa is deep, and the external auditory meatus is narrow or atretic [2,3] (*Figures B and D*).

CHEST: The nipples are often widely separated.

GENITALIA: In females the labia and clitoris are small. In males the penis and scrotum may be small and the testes undescended [2,4].

LIMBS: The fingers have a long, tapered appearance. The toes are irregularly aligned. A vertical talus is occasionally present. Dimples are often present on the elbows, shoulders, knees, and knuckles.

DERMATOGLYPHICS: A predominance of whorls on the digits is a frequent finding [2]. The triradius is displaced toward the radial margin of the palm [7].

WEIGHT: The birth weight is often below normal for the gestational age.

Nervous System

The reported patients have been severely retarded. Striking hypotonia during infancy has also been noted [2,3]. Five out of six patients in one series [3] had a hearing loss and four had nystagmus.

Pathology

Several patients have had congenital heart disease [3,5].

Laboratory Studies

Some, but not all, patients with the 18q− syndrome have low levels of the immunoglobulin IgA in the serum and saliva [6,8]. Tests of delayed hypersensitivity and other humoral antibodies have shown no abnormalities.

Genetics

Autoradiographic studies have shown that the deleted chromosome is a number 18 [3]. Most patients represent sporadic chromosomal abnormalities and their families are normal. In two families either the father [9] or the mother [10] was a balanced translocation carrier.

Differential Diagnosis

1. Microcephaly, maxillary hypoplasia, short stature, small external genitalia, and cryptorchidism are also features of the XXXXY syndrome (see page 190).
2. Underdevelopment of the middle portion of the face is also a feature of Apert's syndrome (see page 222) and Crouzon's disease (see page 230).

References

1. deGrouchy, J., Royer, P., Salmon, C., and Lamy, M. Délétion partielle des bras longs du chromosome 18. *Path. Biol.*, **12**:579–82, 1964.
2. deGrouchy, J.   The 18p−, 18q− and 18r syndromes. *Birth Defects: Original Article Series*, Vol. V, No. 5, May, 1969, pp. 74–87. Williams & Wilkins Co., Baltimore.
3. Wertelecki, W., and Gerald, P. S. Clinical and chromosomal studies of the 18q− syndrome. *J. Pediatr.*, **78**:44–52, 1971.
4. Insley, J.   Syndrome associated with a deficiency of part of the long arm of chromosome no. 18. *Arch. Dis. Child.*, **42**:140–46, 1967.
5. Kushnick, T., and Matsushita, G. Partial deletion of long arms of chromosome 18. *Pediatrics*, **42**:194–97, 1968.
6. Stewart, J., Go, S., Ellis, E., and Robinson, A. Absent IgA and deletions of chromosome 18. *J. Med. Genet.*, **7**:11–19, 1970.
7. Mavalwala, J., Wilson, M. G., and Parker, C. E. The dermatoglyphics of the 18q− syndrome. *Am. J. Phys. Anthropol.*, **32**:443–50, 1970.
8. Feingold, M., Schwartz, R. S., Atkins, L., Anderson, R., Bartsocas, C. S., Page, D. L., and Littlefield, J. W. IgA deficiency associated with partial deletion of chromosome 18. *Am. J. Dis. Child.*, **117**:129–36, 1969.
9. Day, E. J., Marshall, R., Macdonald, P. A. C., and Davidson, W. M. Deleted chromosome 18 with paternal mosaicism. *Lancet*, **2**:1307, 1967.
10. Nance, W. E., Higdon, S. H., Chown, B., and Engel, E. Partial E-18 long-arm deletion. *Lancet*, **1**:303, 1968.

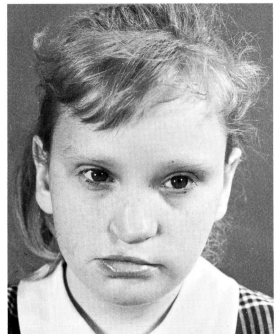

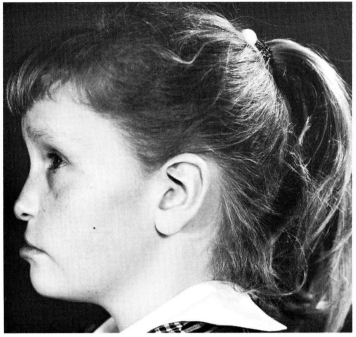

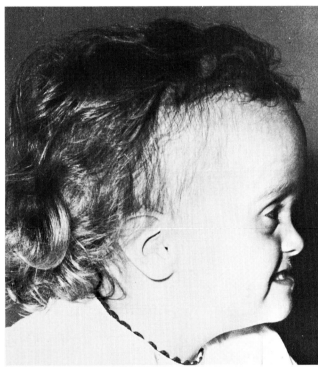

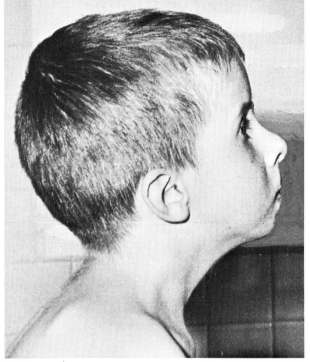

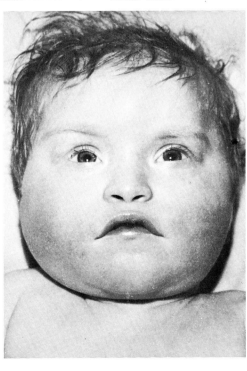

Plate IV-5. *A* and *B:* A 10-year-old girl with cleft lip and palate, upward palpebral slant, depressed middle portion of the face, narrow ear canals, and prominent anthelix. She also had a deficiency of serum IgA. *C:* A 4-year-old girl with marked prominence of the brow, maxillary hypoplasia, and stenotic ear canals, who also had an IgA deficiency. *D:* A 6-year-old boy with micrognathia, low-set ears, and small external auditory canals. *E:* Shows a 17-month-old boy with round face, upward eye slant, and carp-shaped mouth. *F:* Karyotype showing absence of part of the long arms of a number 18 chromosome (*arrow*). (*C:* Reprinted from J. M. Stewart *et al., J. Med. Genet.,* **7:**11, 1970, by permission of the authors and editor. *D:* From T. Kushnick and G. Matsushita, *Pediatrics,* **42:**194–97, 1968. *E:* Reprinted from J. Insley, *Arch. Dis. Child.,* **42:**140, 1967, by permission of the author and editor. *F:* Courtesy of Dr. L. Atkins, Boston, Mass.)

Chromosome 18, Deletion of Short Arm (46,XX,18p−)

In 1963 deGrouchy, Lamy, Thieffrey, Arthuis, and Salmon [1] reported a 6-year-old child with absence of part of the short arm of a number 18 chromosome in association with mental retardation, short stature, and several minor anomalies. More than 20 additional patients have subsequently been reported [2–4]. Although interpreted as an abnormal number 18, it has not been shown for most patients whether the abnormal chromosome was number 17 or 18. Possibly this explains why only a few phenotypic similarities have been observed in patients with this syndrome.

Physical Features

HEAD: The head is usually microcephalic and brachycephalic.

FACE: Hypertelorism, epicanthic folds, and ptosis are the most common facial features [2] (*Figures A and B*). The bridge of the nose is usually flat and the chin is often small. Patients with the cyclops malformation [5], cebocephaly [6], and hypotelorism with cleft lip [5] (*Figure E*) have also been reported.

EYES: Most patients have strabismus [2,3].

EARS: Large floppy ears [2] (*Figure C*), as well as small, low-set ears, have been described.

NECK: Webbing of the neck (*Figure D*) with a low posterior hairline has been described in several patients [2,3].

CHEST: A few patients have had a shieldlike chest.

LIMBS: Short, broad fingers, syndactyly, clinodactyly, cubitus valgus, congenital dislocation of the hips, talipes equinovarus, and pes planus have each been described in different patients [7].

HEIGHT: The height of the reported children and adults has been below normal [2,3].

WEIGHT: Failure to thrive is a common problem in infancy.

Nervous System

All of the reported patients have been retarded. In the first 12 reported patients the IQ range was 35 to 75 [7].

Pathology

Arhinencephaly has been present in the infants with the cyclops and cebocephaly malformations [5,6].

Laboratory Studies

One patient had hypothyroidism [6], one had diabetes mellitus [8], and one had renal tubular acidosis [7]. Absence of serum and salivary IgA has been reported in two patients [3,9].

Genetics

In two families the mother has had a deficiency of the short arm of chromosome 18 similar to that of the affected infant. One of these mothers was mentally retarded [6] and the other had normal intelligence [5].

Differential Diagnosis

Short stature, ptosis, webbing of the neck, and a shieldlike chest are also features of some patients with the XO syndrome (see page 180).

References

1. deGrouchy, J., Lamy, M., Thieffry, S., Arthuis, M., and Salmon, C. Dysmorphie complexe avec oligophrénie: délétion des bras courts d'un chromosome 17–18. *C. R. Acad. Sci. (D) (Paris)*, **256**:1028–29, 1963.
2. deGrouchy, J. The 18p−, 18q− and 18r syndromes. *Birth Defects: Original Article Series*, Vol. V, No. 5, May, 1969, pp. 74–87. Williams & Wilkins Co., Baltimore.
3. Reinwein, H., Struwe, F. E., Bettecken, F., and Wolf, U. Defizienz am Kurzen Arm eines Chromosoms Nr. 18 (46,XX,18p−). Ein einheitliches Missbildungssyndrom. *Monatsschr. Kinderheilkd.*, **116**:511–14, 1968.
4. Fischer, P., Golob, E., Friedrich, F., Kunze-Muhl, E., Doleschel, W., and Aichmair, H. Autosomal deletion syndrome. *J. Med. Genet.*, **7**:91–98, 1970.
5. McDermott, A., Insley, J., Barton, M. E., Rowe, P., Edwards, J. H., and Cameron, A. H. Arrhinencephaly associated with a deficiency involving chromosome 18. *J. Med. Genet.*, **5**:60–67, 1968.
6. Uchida, I. A., McRae, K. N., Wang, H. C., and Ray, M. Familial short arm deficiency of chromosome 18 concomitant with arhinencephaly and alopecia congenita. *Am. J. Hum. Genet.*, **17**:410–19, 1965.
7. Migeon, B. R. Short arm deletions in group E and chromosomal "deletion" syndromes. *J. Pediatr.*, **69**:432–38, 1966.
8. Van Dyke, H. E., Valdmanis, A., and Mann, J. D. Probable deletion of the short arm of chromosome 18. *Am. J. Hum. Genet.*, **16**:364–74, 1964.
9. Ruvalcaba, R. H. A., and Thuline, H. C. IgA absence associated with short arm deletion of chromosome No. 18. *J. Pediatr.*, **74**:964–66, 1969.

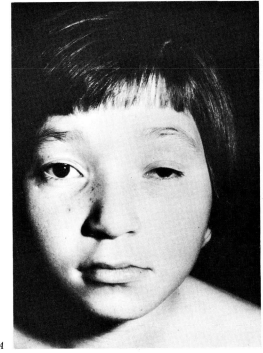

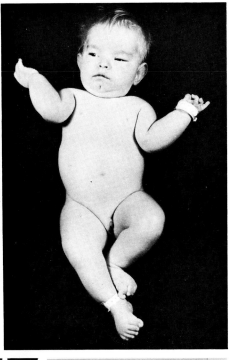

A

B

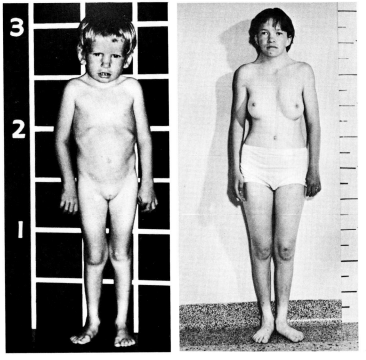

Plate IV-6. *A:* An 11-year-old girl with hypertelorism and ptosis of the left eye. *B:* A 3-month-old boy with a round face, hypertelorism, epicanthal folds, large ears, and edema of dorsum of hands and feet. *C:* A 5-year-old girl with a small chin and webbing of the neck. *D:* A 16-year-old girl with neck webbing and strabismus. *E:* A newborn male with arhinencephaly, hypotelorism, absence of the nose, and bilateral cleft lip and palate. *F:* Karyotype showing deletion of the short arms of a number 18 chromosome (*arrow*). (*A:* From S. Gilgenkrantz *et al., Ann. Genet.,* **11:**17–21, 1968. *B:* Courtesy of Dr. B. R. Migeon, Baltimore, Md. *C:* From R. L. Summitt, *G.P.,* **39:**96–113, 1967. *D:* From H. E. Van Dyke *et al., Am. J. Hum. Genet.,* **16:**364–74, 1964. *E:* Reprinted from A. McDermott, *J. Med. Genet.,* **5:**60, 1968, by permission of the author and editor. *F:* From J. deGrouchy *et al., Ann. Genet.,* **10:**221–23, 1967.)

C

D

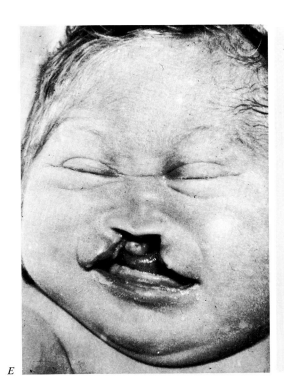

E

F

Chromosome 13 Trisomy
(D Trisomy; 47,XX, + 13)

Patau, Smith, Therman, Inhorn, and Wagner [1] described in 1960 the first patient with trisomy 13, an infant with a cerebral defect, anophthalmia, cleft lip and palate, simian creases, "trigger thumbs," polydactyly, capillary hemangiomas, and a heart defect. A survey of the medical literature showed that several similarly affected patients had been reported before chromosome analysis was available. The earliest, described by Bartolin in 1657, was an infant with no eyes, a broad nose, facial bone anomalies, and polydactyly [2]. By 1968 a total of 178 patients with 13 trisomy had been ascertained [3], and the incidence of the syndrome was estimated as 1:7600 newborns [4].

Physical Features

HEAD: Most patients are microcephalic. A keel-shaped forehead (trigonocephaly) due to premature closure of the metopic suture is often present (*Figures A, B, C, D and F*). Prominence of the occiput has been noted in a few patients [4].

FACE: The common facial anomalies are cleft lip, hypertelorism, shallow supraorbital ridges, and a small chin (*Figures A–D, F–K*). However, several infants have had a bulbous nose and no cleft lip or palate (*Figures C, G, and I*). A few patients have had the cyclops, cebocephaly, and ethmocephaly malformations [5].

EYES: The most common eye anomalies are microphthalmia, iris colobomas, and cataracts. Anophthalmia is occasionally present, but is usually unilateral (*Figure F*).

EARS: Most patients have small, low-set, and malformed ears (*Figures B, F–K*).

MOUTH: Over half of the patients have either a bilateral (*Figures F and H*) or a unilateral (*Figure A*) cleft lip in association with a cleft palate [4].

NECK: The neck is usually short. Extra skin folds are often present in infants, but webbing of the neck is rare.

ABDOMEN: Inguinal and umbilical hernias are common.

GENITALIA: Almost all males have undescended testes.

LIMBS: Polydactyly and flexion deformities of the fingers are present in most patients (*Figures A and B*). The nails are long and hyperconvex. Less common findings are a distally placed thumb, syndactyly, and hypoplastic nails. Six of the 27 patients in one study had a clubfoot deformity [4]. Fibular polydactyly may be present on one or both feet (*Figures A and B*). Broad thumbs and great toes have also been reported [6] (*Figure G*).

DERMATOGLYPHICS: The dermal ridges are often hypoplastic. Many patients have distally placed palmar axial triradii, an increased number of arches and radial loops on the digits, and transverse palmar creases. An arch fibular pattern is often found in the hallucal area of the foot.

SKIN: Most patients have capillary hemangiomas (*Figure A*). Skin defects are sometimes present on the scalp.

HEIGHT AND WEIGHT: In a survey of 74 patients [4] the average birth weight was 2609 g with an average gestational age of 39 weeks. Almost all infants have feeding difficulties and slow weight gain. The height and weight are always far below the average for their chronologic age.

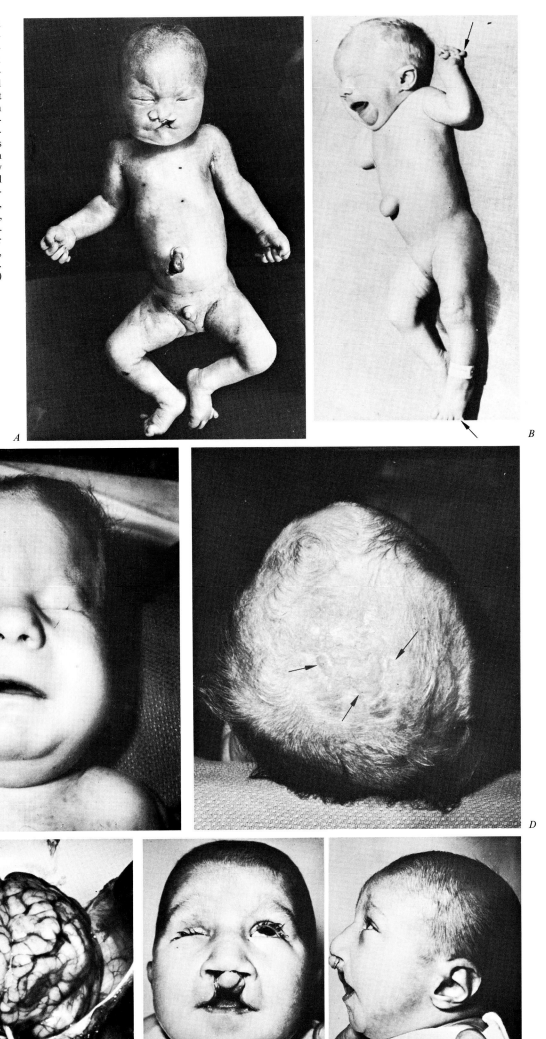

Plate IV-7. *A:* A newborn with trigonocephaly, cleft lip, hemangiomas, and postaxial polydactyly of both hands and feet. *B:* A 6-week-old infant with low-set ears, an umbilical hernia, and postaxial polydactyly of the left hand and foot (*arrow*). *C–E:* An infant with a keel-shaped forehead (trigonocephaly), microphthalmia, and scalp defects (*arrows*). The forebrain is shown with absence of both olfactory bulbs. *F:* A child with bilateral cleft lip and unilateral anophthalmia. (*A:* From P. Conen *et al., Am. J. Dis. Child.,* **111:**236–47, 1966. *B:* Courtesy of Dr. L. Atkins, Boston, Mass. *C–E:* Courtesy of Dr. G. R. Hogan, Boston, Mass. *F:* Courtesy of Dr. D. Hoefnagel, Hanover, N.H.)

Nervous System

All of the patients have severe mental retardation. During early infancy jitteriness and apnea are common. Eight of 16 infants in one study [4] were presumed to be deaf. Most patients have either muscular hypotonia or hypertonia. Minor motor seizures often occur.

Pathology

Arhinencephaly is a frequent cerebral malformation, but it is not always present. In general, there are usually abnormalities of fissures and gyri formation and areas of cortical dysgenesis [7]. The olfactory bulbs and tracts are often absent (*Figure E*). Extensive heterotopias are usually seen in the cerebellum. In some instances there is hypoplasia or aplasia of the vermis [8]. Either septal defects or patent ductus arteriosus is found in half of the patients. Various rotational anomalies are a less common finding. Few patients have a normal heart. Hydronephrosis and a polycystic renal cortex are the most common renal anomalies. A biseptate uterus was present in 5 of 12 females in one series [4]. Intraocular cartilage, extending from the retrolental region to the sclera, is a common finding [9]. Patients with no response to sound have had inner ear anomalies, primarily of the cochlea and saccule [10].

Laboratory Studies

Several hematologic abnormalities have been observed in newborns with 13 trisomy. Hemoglobins Gower 2 and Bart's, which are normally present only in the fetus, have been found in newborn infants. Also, a high level of fetal hemoglobin and low level of hemoglobin A_2 has been shown to persist throughout the first several months of life [11]. An increased number of projections on the nuclei of polymorphonuclear leukocytes has also been observed [12].

Treatment and Prognosis

In a review of 221 patients with 13 trisomy, it was found that approximately half lived to 1 month, one third to 3 months, and one twentieth to 3 years of age. The 30 patients with translocation 13 trisomy and the thirteen with 13 trisomy plus mosaicism for a normal cell line survived longer than the 178 with trisomy [3].

Genetics

The extra D chromosome has consistently been shown to be a number 13 both by autoradiography and quinacrine fluorescence staining [13]. The usual karyotype for 13 trisomy is a total of 47 chromosomes with an extra D group chromosome (*Figure L*). Translocation occurred in 14 percent, or 30 of 221 patients. In translocation there is usually a total of 46 chromosomes and the long arm of extra chromosome 13 is usually attached to another D chromosome, although translocation may also occur to another chromosome. The phenotypic features of patients with 13 trisomy and those with translocation 13 trisomy are the same. An increase in maternal age is associated with 13 trisomy, whereas translocation appears to occur independently of maternal age [3].

Differential Diagnosis

1. Microphthalmia, cleft lip and palate, polydactyly, clubfeet, and polycystic kidneys are features of infants with the Meckel syndrome, but they usually have an encephalocele and median cleft lip and autosomal recessive mode of inheritance (see page 292).
2. Arhinencephaly in association with a medial cleft lip, cyclopia, ethmocephaly, or cebocephaly may occur in patients who have normal chromosomes. In some families the arhinencephaly may be due to an autosomal recessive mutant gene (see pages 206 and 208).
3. Hypertelorism, cleft lip and palate, and capillary hemangiomas are features of patients with the 4p− syndrome (see page 174).
4. Males with X-linked anophthalmia may have mental retardation and microcephaly, but they usually have no other anomalies and, of course, have a normal karyotype (see page 242).

References

1. Patau, K., Smith, D. W., Therman, E., Inhorn, S. L., and Wagner, H. P. Multiple congenital anomaly caused by an extra autosome. *Lancet*, 1:790–93, 1960.
2. Warburg, M. Anophthalmos complicated by mental retardation and cleft palate. *Acta Ophthalmol. (Kbn.)*, 38:394–404, 1960.
3. Magenis, R. E., Hecht, F., and Milham, S., Jr. Trisomy 13 (D₁) syndrome: studies on parental age, sex ratio and survival. *J. Pediatr.*, 73:222–28, 1968.
4. Taylor, A. I. Autosomal trisomy syndromes: a detailed study of 27 cases of Edwards' syndrome and 27 cases of Patau's syndrome. *J. Med. Genet.*, 5:227–52, 1968.
5. Snodgrass, G. J. A. I., Butler, L. J., France, N. E., Crome, L., and Russell, A. The "D" (13–15) trisomy syndrome: an analysis of 7 examples. *Arch. Dis. Child.*, 41:250–61, 1966.
6. Wilson, M. G. Rubinstein-Taybi and D₁ trisomy syndromes. *J. Pediatr.*, 73:404–408, 1968.
7. Hogan, G. R. Personal communication, 1970.
8. Terplan, K. L., Sandberg, A. A., and Aceto, T., Jr. Structural anomalies in the cerebellum in association with trisomy. *J.A.M.A.*, 197:557–68, 1966.
9. Cogan, D. G., and Kuwabara, T. Ocular pathology of the 13–15 trisomy syndrome. *Arch. Ophthalmol. (Chicago)*, 72:246–53, 1964.
10. Maniglia, A. J., Wolff, D., and Herques, A. J. Congenital deafness in 13–15 trisomy syndrome. *Arch. Otolaryngol.*, 92:181–88, 1970.
11. Wilson, M. G., Schroeder, W., A., Graves, D. A., and Kach, V. D. Hemoglobin variations in D-trisomy syndrome. *N. Engl. J. Med.*, 277:953–58, 1967.
12. Huehns, E. R., Lutzner, M., and Hecht, F. Nuclear abnormalities of the neutrophils in D₁ (13–15) trisomy syndrome. *Lancet*, 1:589–90, 1964.
13. Miller, D. A., Allderdice, P. W., Miller, O. J., and Breg, W. R. Quinacrine fluorescence patterns of human D group chromosomes. *Nature (Lond.)*, 232:24–27, 1971.

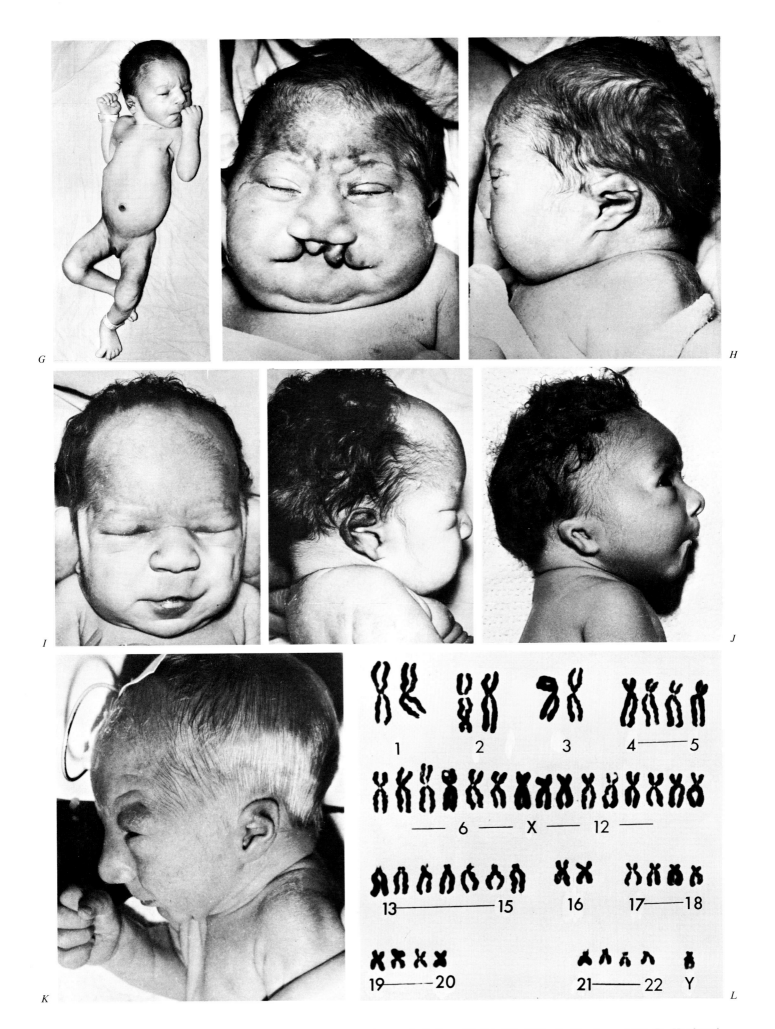

Plate IV-7. *G:* An infant with a prominent nose, malformed ear, and broad, medially deviated great toe. *H:* An infant with a capillary hemangioma of the forehead, upward palpebral slant, and malformed ear. *I:* An infant with a bulbous nose and malformed ear. *J* and *K:* Two infants with small chins and malformed ears. *L:* Karyotype showing extra D group (13–15) chromosome. (*G:* From M. G. Wilson, *J. Pediatr.,* **73:**404–408, 1968. *H:* Courtesy of Dr. D. Hoefnagel, Hanover, N.H. *I:* Courtesy of Dr. M. G. Wilson, Los Angeles, Calif. *J* and *K:* Reprinted from G. J. A. I. Snodgrass *et al., Arch. Dis. Child.,* **41:**253, 1966, by permission of the authors and editor. *L:* Courtesy of Dr. L. Atkins, Boston, Mass.)

Chromosome 13, Deletion of Long Arm (46,XX,13q−) and Ring D (46,XX,r13)

More than 30 patients with either the 13q− or the r13 syndromes have been reported [1–4,4a,4b]. There seems to be no phenotypic difference between the patients with 13q− and r13 karyotypes. Several authors [2–4] have noted that some, but not all, of these patients have similar physical features. In some cases this is a clinically recognizable syndrome.

Physical Features

HEADS: These patients are microcephalic. Many have prominence of the midportion of the brow, as in trigonocephaly due to premature closure of the metopic suture [4] (*Figures A and E*).

FACE: The most common facial features are hypertelorism, narrow palpebral fissures, a prominent bridge of the nose, epicanthic folds, ptosis, a small chin, and facial asymmetry (*Figures A, B, C, E, and F*).

EYES: In a review of 23 patients, 8 had microphthalmos, 6 had iris colobomas, 4 had a cataract, and 3 had retinoblastoma [4]. In another review [4b] it was noted that 7 of 12 patients with the 13q− syndrome had retinoblastoma, with the tumor in both eyes in 5. By contrast only 1 of 18 patients with r13 had retinoblastoma.

EARS: The ears are often large and rotated posteriorly (*Figures A, C, and F*).

MOUTH: Some patients have a protruding maxilla [4].

NECK: The neck is often short.

GENITALIA: The males usually have cryptorchidism and hypospadias; only a few females have had abnormal external genitalia [4].

RECTUM: Four out of 23 patients [4] had imperforate anus and perineal fistulas.

LIMBS: Absence or hypoplasia of the thumb is the most striking skeletal anomaly; 7 of 23 patients had this finding [1–4] (*Figures A, E, and F*). Six patients had short fifth fingers. Clubfoot and hip dislocation were noted in a few patients.

HEIGHT AND WEIGHT: The birth weight is usually low for the gestational age. During infancy and childhood these patients usually have severe growth retardation.

Nervous System

Almost all of these patients are severely retarded. One child had arthrogryposis of both legs [4a].

Pathology

Two patients had arhinencephaly [1,3] and one had a small occipital meningocele [4]. Seven of 23 had congenital heart disease [4].

Laboratory Studies

Ten out of 23 patients [4] had pelvic-girdle and lower spine anomalies on x-ray.

Genetics

The deleted chromosome has been shown by autoradiography to be a number 13 (*Figure D*) [4,4a].

Differential Diagnosis

1. Hypertelorism, iris colobomas, congenital heart disease, and imperforate anus are features of some patients with the syndrome of the extra small acrocentric chromosome (cat's eye syndrome) (see page 176).
2. Thumb anomalies, microphthalmos, and intestinal malformations are also features of patients with thalidomide embryopathy, but they often have malformed ears and phocomelia and rarely are severely retarded (see page 132).
3. Absent or hypoplastic thumbs and congenital heart disease are features of patients with Fanconi's anemia (see page 282) and the Holt-Oram syndrome [5].
4. Narrow palpebral fissures, epicanthus inversus, and ptosis comprise a hereditary malformation syndrome that is not associated with mental retardation, skeletal anomalies, or gross chromosome abnormality. This syndrome is due to an autosomal dominant mutant gene [6].
5. Bilateral retinoblastoma unassociated with congenital malformations is usually due to an autosomal dominant mutant gene, whereas only about 15 percent of the unilateral retinoblastomas are hereditary [7].

References

1. Bain, A. D., and Gauld, I. K. Multiple congenital abnormalities associated with ring chromosome. *Lancet,* **2:**304–305, 1963.
2. Sparkes, R. S., Carrel, R. E., and Wright, S. W. Absent thumbs with a ring D2 chromosome: a new deletion syndrome. *Am. J. Hum. Genet.,* **19:**644–59, 1967.
3. Juberg, R. C., Adams, M. S., Venema, W. J., and Hart, M. G. Multiple congenital anomalies associated with a ring-D chromosome. *J. Med. Genet.,* **6:**314–21, 1969.
4. Allderdice, P. W., Davis, J. G., Miller, O. J., Klinger, H. P., Warburton, D., Miller, D. A., Allen, F. H., Jr., Abrams, C. A. L., and McGilvray, E. The 13q− deletion syndrome. *Am. J. Hum. Genet.,* **21:**499–512, 1969.
4a. Grace, E., Drennan, J., Colver, D., and Gordon, R. R. The 13q− deletion syndrome. *J. Med. Genet.,* **8:**351–57, 1971.
4b. Taylor, A. I. Dq−, Dr and retinoblastoma. *Humangenetik,* **10:**209–17, 1970.
5. Holt, M., and Oram, S. Familial heart disease with skeletal malformations. *Br. Heart J.,* **22:**236–42, 1960.
6. Johnson, C. C. Surgical repair of the syndrome of epicanthus, blepharophimosis and ptosis. *Arch. Ophthalmol. (Chicago),* **71:**510–16, 1964.
7. Jensen, R. D., and Miller, R. W. Retinoblastoma: epidemiologic characteristics. *N. Engl. J. Med.,* **285:**307–11, 1971.

Plate IV-8. *A* and *B:* Show an 18-month-old boy with the 13q— syndrome and trigonocephaly, hypertelorism, narrow palpebral fissures with a downward slant, bilateral radioulnar synostosis, and absent right thumb. *C:* A 21-month-old boy with the 13 ring syndrome who has hypertelorism, narrow palpebral fissures, and facial asymmetry. *D:* The D group chromosomes from several metaphase plates along with the tritiated thymidine labeling patterns for both of these patients. The columns of abnormal number 13 chromosomes (both 13q— and 13r) are indicated by the *arrows. E* and *F:* A 1-month-old girl with the 13 ring syndrome with narrow palpebral fissures, a small chin, and posteriorly rotated ears. The x-rays of both hands show absence of the thumbs, the first metacarpals, and the middle phalanx of the fifth fingers and fusion of the fourth and fifth metacarpals. (*A:* Courtesy of Dr. P. W. Allderdice, New York, N.Y. *B–D:* From P. W. Allderdice *et al., Am. J. Hum. Genet.,* **21:**499–512, 1969; University of Chicago Press, publisher. *E* and *F:* Reprinted from R. C. Juberg, *J. Med. Genet.,* **6:**314, 1969, by permission of the author and editor.)

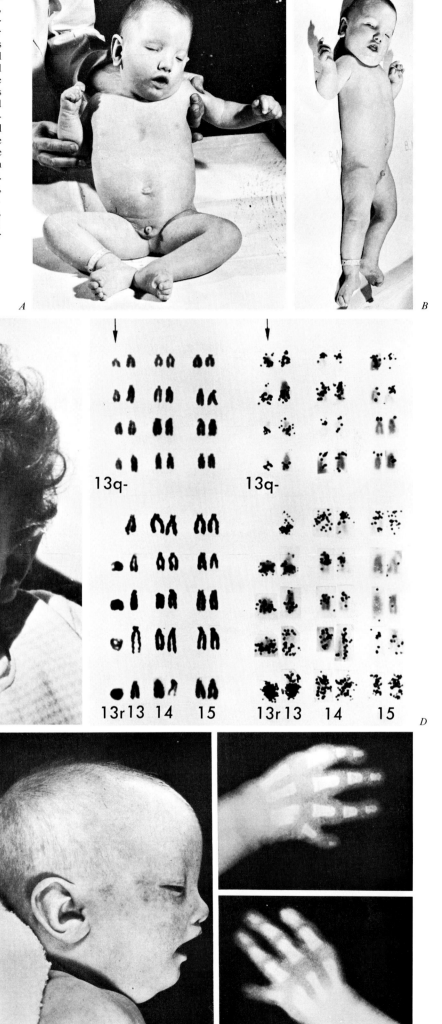

A

B

C

13q-   13q-

13r 13 14   15   13r 13 14   15

D

E

F

169

Chromosome 5, Deletion of Short Arm (Cri du Chat Syndrome; 46,XX,5p—)

In 1963 Lejeune and his associates [1] described several infants with a mewing or catlike cry, multiple deformities, and mental retardation in association with a deletion of a portion of the short arm of a group B (4–5) chromosome. Subsequently, other infants were reported who had a similar group B short arm deletion, but different anomalies and no catlike cry. Studies of chromosome morphology and DNA replication patterns showed that this second group of patients had a deletion of chromosome number 4 and that the cri du chat syndrome is associated with a deletion of number 5 [2]. While more than 70 patients with a group B deletion have been reported, only in a smaller number has it been shown by autoradiography that chromosome 5 is the deleted member. In the years before chromosome analysis was available, some patients with the 5p— syndrome were being ascertained and were apparently diagnosed as having congenital laryngeal stridor [3]. However, the association of the mental retardation, congenital anomalies, and abnormal cry was not established until the chromosome abnormality was identified. The incidence of the 5p— syndrome is not known, but it may be a relatively common cause of severe mental retardation. In one study [4], 7 of 744 patients with IQ's below 35 had this syndrome.

Physical Features

HEAD: Almost all patients are microcephalic.

FACE: The typical infant has a round face with hypertelorism, epicanthal folds, a downward eye slant, and a small chin (*Figures A, B, C, G, and H*). The nose is prominent and in profile it is considered beaklike [5]. These facial features are most distinctive in infants and may not be present in older patients. In a study [4] of 13 older patients the faces were thin and sometimes asymmetric. The base of the nose was broad (*Figures D, I, and J*). The philtrum was short. Some had micrognathia (*Figure F*) and others prognathia.

EYES: Strabismus is common. A few patients have had optic atrophy and iris colobomas [4].

EARS: The ears are usually low-set. Several patients have had preauricular skin tags and malformed ears (*Figures B and F*).

MOUTH: The palate is high. Malocclusion was present in most older patients in one study [4].

NECK: The neck is short.

VOICE: The high-pitched, wailing, catlike cry is present during the first weeks of life. The epiglottis is flaccid, and the larynx is very narrow. During inspiration the elongated epiglottis flops down over or into the larynx, causing the stridor. During phonation and crying, the voice is weakened because the cords fail to approximate posteriorly, and the high-pitched cry is emitted from the approximated anterior portion of the cords [3] (*Figure K*).

BACK: Seven of 13 adults in one study had scoliosis [4].

LIMBS: In the same study 11 of 13 had short metacarpals and metatarsals. Clinodactyly and various types of clubfoot deformity have been reported, but are uncommon.

DERMATOGLYPHICS: The common findings are an increased frequency of arches and whorls on the digits, thenar patterns on the palms, transverse palmar creases, and distally placed palmar triradii [6].

HAIR: Premature graying of hair was present in 5 of 12 older patients [4].

HEIGHT AND WEIGHT: Many infants are small for their gestational age at birth and remain retarded in height and weight throughout their lives.

GROWTH AND DEVELOPMENT: No abnormalities of sexual development have been noted in adults [4].

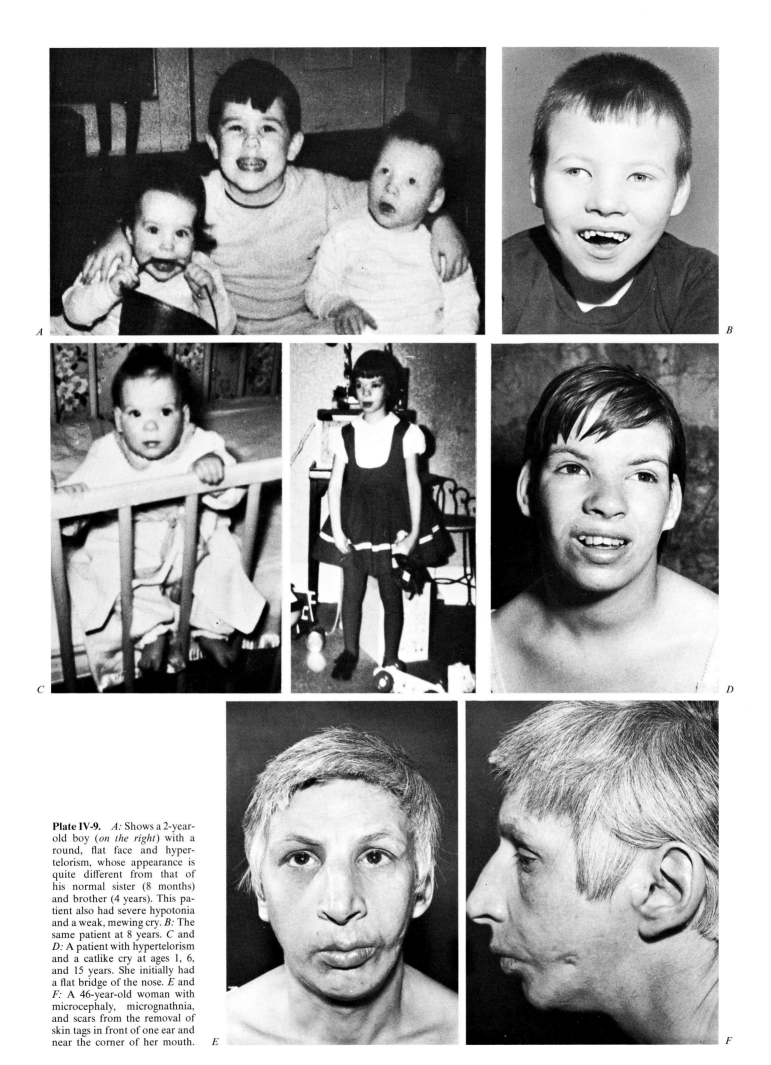

Plate IV-9. *A:* Shows a 2-year-old boy (*on the right*) with a round, flat face and hypertelorism, whose appearance is quite different from that of his normal sister (8 months) and brother (4 years). This patient also had severe hypotonia and a weak, mewing cry. *B:* The same patient at 8 years. *C* and *D:* A patient with hypertelorism and a catlike cry at ages 1, 6, and 15 years. She initially had a flat bridge of the nose. *E* and *F:* A 46-year-old woman with microcephaly, micrognathnia, and scars from the removal of skin tags in front of one ear and near the corner of her mouth.

Nervous System

All of the reported patients have been severely retarded. Most do not speak, and many have not learned to walk before the age of 10 years. In many the IQ is estimated to be less than 10. Both muscular hypertonia and hypotonia have been described in infants. Older patients often have a waddling gait and poor muscular development. Hyperactive deep tendon reflexes, extensor plantar responses, and muscular hypertonia have also been noted in older patients [12]. Seizures are uncommon [3,4,7].

Pathology

Few neuropathologic data are available. The brain of a severely retarded 19-year-old girl was mature, fully developed, and of uniformly small size. There was no evidence of loss of myelin, and the microscopic examination showed no abnormalities [7]. Another patient had a small brain with slight ventricular dilation [4], and a third had a small left cerebellar hemisphere [8]. Several patients have had cardiac anomalies.

Laboratory Studies

The few pneumoencephalograms reported have shown dilated ventricles. The frontal sinuses of adults are often large [4]. Abnormalities are often present on the electroencephalogram [7].

Genetics

Differentiation between chromosomes 4 and 5 is possible because in chromosome 5 DNA replication terminates earlier [2]. Further differentiation between chromosomes 4 and 5 is provided by quinacrine mustard fluorescence [13]. In general, a simple deletion of the short arm of one of the number 5 chromosomes is considered the primary abnormality; in some patients the deletion may be minute, involving as little as 4 percent of the short arm [9]. Recent studies using the new reverse Giemsa method [14] for staining chromosomes have shown that the 5p− syndrome may sometimes result from chromosome inversion and deletion, instead of a simple deletion [15].

It has been estimated that a familial unbalanced translocation accounts for about 13 percent of the cases of the cri du chat syndrome. Either parent may have the balanced translocation; they will, of course, be phenotypically normal. In one reported family [9] the mother was normal, but her karyotype showed mosaicism with both a normal cell line and a 5p− cell line. She had two children with the cri du chat syndrome.

Differential Diagnosis

1. A round face with epicanthic folds and hypertelorism may be seen in children with many other disorders, such as the XXXXY syndrome (see page 190) and Carpenter's syndrome (see page 232).
2. Hypertelorism and a prominent nose are features of patients with the telecanthus-hypospadias syndrome (see page 346) and the 4p− syndrome (see page 174).
3. A catlike cry has also been reported in a few patients with chromosome 18 trisomy (see page 156).

References

1. Lejeune, J., Lafourcade, J., Berger, R., Vialatte, J., Boeswillwald, M., Seringe, P., and Turpin, R. Trois cas de délétion partielle du bras court d'un chromosome 5. *C. R. Acad. Sci.* (D) (Paris), **257**:3098–3102, 1963.
2. Warburton, D., Miller, D. A., Miller, O. J., Breg, W. R., deCapoa, A., and Shaw, M. W. Distinction between chromosome 4 and chromosome 5 by replication pattern and length of long and short arms. *Am. J. Hum. Genet.,* **19**:399–415, 1967.
3. Ward, P. H., Engel, E., and Nace, W. E. The larynx in the cri du chat (cat cry) syndrome. *Trans. Am. Acad. Ophthalmol. Otolaryngol.,* **72**:90–102, 1968.
4. Breg, W. R., Steele, M. W., Miller, O. J., Warburton, D., deCapoa, A., and Allderdice, P. W. The cri du chat syndrome in adolescents and adults: clinical findings in 13 older patients with partial deletion of the short arm of chromosome No. 5 (5p−). *J. Pediatr.,* **77**:782–91, 1970.
5. Gordon, R. R., and Cooke, P. Facial appearance in cri du chat syndrome. *Dev. Med. Child Neurol.,* **10**:69–76, 1968.
6. Warburton, D., and Miller, O. J. Dermatoglyphic features of patients with a partial short arm deletion of a B-group chromosome. *Ann. Hum. Genet.,* **31**:189–207, 1967.
7. Solitare, G. B. The cri du chat syndrome: neuropathologic observations. *J. Ment. Defic. Res.,* **11**:267–77, 1967.
8. Lejeune, J., Lafourcade, J., deGrouchy, J., Berger, R., Gautier, M., Salmon, C., and Turpin, R. Délétion partielle du bras court du chromosome 5. Individualisation d'un nouvel état morbide. *Sem. Hop. Paris,* **40**:1069–79, 1964.
9. Warburton, D., Miller, D. A., Miller, O. J., Allderdice, P. W., and deCapoa, A. Detection of minute deletions in human karyotypes. *Cytogenetics,* **8**:97–108, 1969.
10. deCapoa, A., Warburton, D., Breg, W. R., Miller, D. A., and Miller, O. J. Translocation heterozygosis: a cause of five cases of the cri du chat syndrome and two cases with a duplication of chromosomes number 5 in three families. *Am. J. Hum. Genet.,* **19**:586–603, 1967.
11. Philip, J., Brandt, N. J., Friis-Hansen, B., Mikkelsen, M., and Tygstrup, I. A deleted B chromosome in a mosaic mother and her cri du chat progeny. *J. Med. Genet.,* **7**:33–36, 1970.
12. Platt, M., and Holmes, L. B. Hypertonia in older patients with the 5p− syndrome. *Lancet,* **2**:1429, 1971.
13. Caspersson, T., Lindsten, J., and Zech, L. Identification of the abnormal B group chromosome in the "cri du chat" syndrome by QM-fluorescence. *Exp. Cell Res.,* **61**:475–76, 1970.
14. Dutrillaux, B., and LeJeune, J. Sur une nouvelle technique d'analyse du caryotype humain. *C.R. Acad. Sci.* [D] (*Paris*), **272**:2638–40, 1971.
15. Hecht, F., Wyandt, H. E., and Erbe, R. W. Revolutionary cytogenetics. *N. Engl. J. Med.,* **285**:1482–84, 1971.

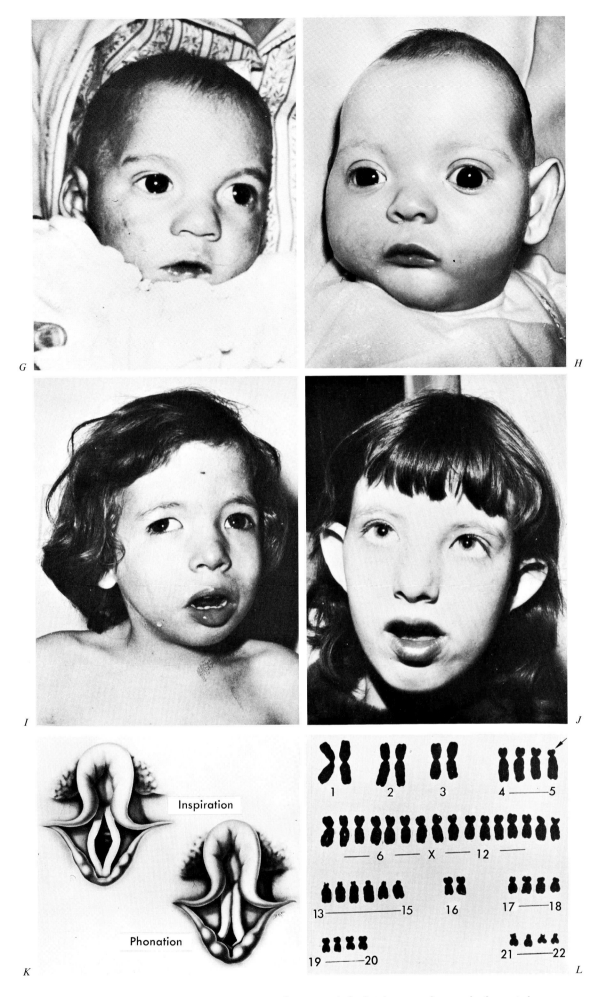

Plate IV-9. *G* and *H:* Two infants with a round face and hypertelorism. *I:* A 4½-year-old girl with epicanthal folds, hypertelorism, a downward palpebral slant, and divergent strabismus. *J:* A 12-year-old girl with hypertelorism and epicanthal folds. *K:* A drawing of the appearance of the larynx during inspiration and phonation. The epiglottis is long and limp, the larynx is narrow, and the glottic chink is diamond-shaped during inspiration. During phonation the cords approximate anteriorly, but leave an air space in the posterior commissure area. *L:* Karyotype showing the absence of part of the short arms of a number 5 chromosome (*arrow*). (*G* and *I–K:* From P. Ward *et al., Trans. Am. Acad. Ophthalmol. Otolaryngol.,* **72:**90–102, 1968. *H:* From R. R. Gordon and P. Cooke, *Dev. Med. Child Neurol.,* **10:**69–76, 1968. *L:* Courtesy of Dr. L. Atkins, Boston, Mass.)

Chromosome 4, Deletion of Short Arm (46,XX,4p−)

Deletion of the short arm of a B group (4–5) chromosome was initially thought to be associated with only one clinical syndrome, the cri du chat (cat-cry) syndrome. However, in 1965 Wolf, Reinwein, Porsch, Schroter, and Baitsch [1] described a child with a B group deletion who had severe facial anomalies and no catlike cry. Autoradiographic studies showed the abnormality in this patient to be in a number 4 chromosome. Since then more than 20 patients with the 4p− syndrome have been described [2–8]. It is likely that some of the patients previously reported to have B group deletions would have been shown to have the 4p− syndrome if autoradiography had been performed to identify the abnormal chromosome. Based on the reported cases, this seems to be a clinically recognizable disorder.

Physical Features

HEAD: Most of the reported patients have had microcephaly. Midline scalp defects were present in 5 of 12 patients in one review [5].

FACE: The face is characterized by a prominent glabella, a broad nasal bridge, a beaked or deformed nose, hypertelorism, epicanthic folds, a carp-shaped mouth, a small chin, and ptosis [4–7] (*Figures A-E*). Several patients have had facial asymmetry.

EYES: Prominent eyes, strabismus, and iris defects, such as coloboma, ectopic pupil, and coarse iris, have been present in many patients [5].

EARS: Almost all patients have had simple, low-set ears. The cartilage of the outer ear is often underdeveloped. Preauricular sinuses are common [3,7], and 6 of 9 patients in one review [5] had preauricular tags.

MOUTH: Seven of 13 reported infants had a cleft lip and/or palate [5,7] (*Figures A and B*).

VOICE: One of the reported patients had a catlike cry [4].

ABDOMEN: Inguinal hernias have been present in several males and females.

GENITALIA: All males have had hypospadias, and many have also had cryptorchidism [7].

LIMBS: Flexion deformities of the fingers, clinodactyly, and clubbed feet were each noted in a few patients [5–7].

DERMATOGLYPHICS: Most patients have transverse palmar creases, hypoplastic dermal ridges, and low dermal ridge counts [7,8].

SKIN: A capillary hemagioma (*Figures A and D*) on the forehead was noted in two patients [1,2].

HEIGHT AND WEIGHT: All of the patients have had a low birth weight for their gestational age and severe retardation of linear growth.

Nervous System

All of the reported patients have been severely retarded. Several patients have had hypotonia, seizures, and indifference to painful stimuli [5].

Pathology

Five of 12 patients in one review [5] had congenital heart disease, all probably atrial septal defects. A variety of other cardiac anomalies have also been reported [8]. Dilatation of the cerebral ventricles has been noted in 5 patients [5].

Laboratory Studies

A marked delay in the ossification of the carpals, tarsals, and pubic bones had been noted in several patients [7].

Treatment and Prognosis

Death often occurs in the first months of life with congestive heart failure and pulmonary infections frequent causes [8].

Genetics

Differentiation between chromosomes 4 and 5 can be made by autoradiography because DNA replication terminates later in chromosome number 4 [5]. Identification of number 4 can also be made using quinacrine mustard fluorescence [9]. No reported patient has represented a familial unbalanced translocation, in contrast to the frequency of this finding in families in which the 5p− syndrome has occurred [8].

Differential Diagnosis

1. A prominent nose, iris defects, cleft lip and palate, microcephaly, hemangiomas, growth failure, and severe mental retardation have been found in several patients with 13 trisomy (see page 164).
2. Hypertelorism, a prominent nose, and hypospadias are features of males with the telecanthus-hypospadias syndrome (see page 346) and the 5p− syndrome (see page 170).
3. Microcephaly, a prominent nose, and cleft lip are features of patients with the oral-facial-digital syndrome, but they also have multiple oral frenula, alopecia, and syndactyly (see page 300).

References

1. Wolf, U., Reinwein, H., Porsch, R., Schroter, R., and Baitsch, H. Defizienz an den kurzen Armen eines Chromosoms Nr. 4. *Humangenetik*, **1**:397–413, 1965.
2. Leão, J. C., Bargman, G. J., Neu, R. L., Kajii, T., and Gardner, L. I. New syndrome associated with partial deletion of short arms of chromosome no. 4. *J.A.M.A.*, **202**:434–37, 1967.
3. Pfeiffer, R. A. Neue Dokumentation zur Abgrenzung eines Syndroms der Deletion des kurzen Arms eines Chromosoms Nr. 4. *Z. Kinderheilkd.*, **102**:49–61, 1968.
4. Subrt, I., Blehova, B., and Sedlackova, E. Mewing cry in a child with the partial deletion of the short arm of chromosome 4. *Humangenetik*, **8**:242–48, 1969.
5. Arias, D., Passarge, E., Engle, M. A., and German, J. Human chromosomal deletion: two patients with the 4p− syndrome. *J. Pediatr.*, **76**:82–88, 1970.
6. Wilcock, A. R., Adams, F. G., Cooke, P., and Gordon, R. R. Deletion of short arm of no. 4 (4p−)—a detailed case report. *J. Med. Genet.*, **7**:171–76, 1970.
7. Miller, O. J., Breg, W. R., Warburton, D., Miller, D. A., deCapoa, A., Allderdice, P. W., Davis, J., Klinger, H. P., McGilvray, E., and Allen, F. H., Jr. Partial deletion of the short arm of chromosome no. 4 (4p−): clinical studies in five unrelated patients. *J. Pediatr.*, **77**:792–801, 1970.
8. Guthrie, R. D., Aase, J. M., Asper, A. C., and Smith, D. W. The 4p− syndrome. A clinically recognizable chromosomal deletion syndrome. *Am. J. Dis. Child.*, **122**:421–25, 1971.
9. Caspersson, T., Zech, L., and Johansson, C. Quinacrine mustard fluorescence of human chromosomes 4, 5 and X. *Exp. Cell. Res.*, **61**:474–75, 1970.

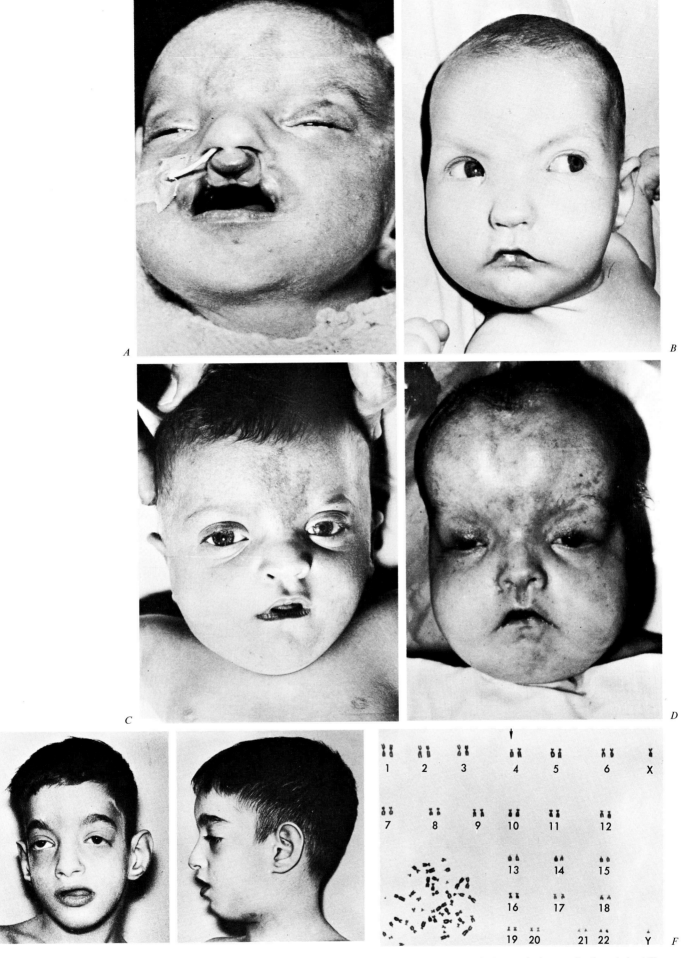

Plate IV-10. *A:* The first reported patient at 2 months of age. He had a bilateral cleft lip, hypertelorism, a downward palpebral slant, strabismus, a corneal opacity, and a capillary hemangioma on his forehead. *B:* An infant with round face, hypertelorism, and prominent glabella. *C:* A newborn infant with a large head, prominent forehead and supraorbital ridges, hypertelorism, an ectopic left pupil, and small chin. *D:* A 4-month-old infant with facial asymmetry, hemangioma of forehead, prominent glabella, and hypertelorism. *E:* An 8-year-old boy with microcephaly, ptosis, hypertelorism, and a broad, beaklike nose. *F:* Karyotype showing absence of part of the short arms of a number 4 chromosome (*arrow*). (*A:* From U. Wolf *et al., Humangenetik,* **1:**397–413, 1965. *B* and *F:* Courtesy of Dr. J. German, New York, N.Y. *C:* Reprinted from A. R. Wilcock *et al., J. Med. Genet.,* **7:**171, 1970, by permission of the authors and editor. *D:* From J. C. Leão *et al., J.A.M.A.,* **202:**434–37, 1967. *E:* Courtesy of Dr. W. R. Breg, Southbury, Conn.)

Syndrome of Extra Small Acrocentric Chromosome (Cat's Eye Syndrome; 47, XX, + ?G)

In 1965 Schachenmann and his associates [1] described three children with iris colobomas and either anal atresia or imperforate anus in association with an additional small acrocentric chromosome, smaller than the G group (21–22) chromosomes. At least six more affected patients have since been described [2–5], including three in one family [2]. The alternate designation of the "cat's eye" syndrome has been suggested because the associated iris coloboma is similar in appearance to the vertical pupil of a cat [2]. Most, if not all, patients have been ascertained because they had an imperforate anus.

Physical Features

FACE: The reported patients have had a few similar facial features, which include hypertelorism, a downward palpebral slant, strabismus, and a small chin [1,3–5] (*Figures A and D*).

EYES: Most of the reported patients have had unilateral or bilateral iris (*Figure D*) and choroid colobomas. A cataract in one eye and bilateral iris colobomas were present in one child's mother, who also had the same chromosomal abnormality [1]. Microphthalmia has been noted in two children [1,5] (*Figure E*).

EARS: Most patients have had preauricular fistulas and skin tags [1–5] (*Figure B*).

RECTUM: Either imperforate anus or anal atresia has been present in all of the reported children. Rectovaginal and rectovesicular fistulas have often been associated abnormalities.

LIMBS: One child had bilateral congenital dislocation of the hips [1].

Nervous System

Most, but not all, of the reported children have had retarded psychomotor development [1–5].

Laboratory Studies

Four children had urinary tract malformations [2–4], two had either rib or vertebral anomalies [4,5], and two had congenital heart disease [2].

Genetics

In the families in which several members have had the extra small acrocentric chromosome, some had no phenotypic abnormalities and others have had only one anomaly, an imperforate anus. Mosaicism for the extra chromosome was found in one child's maternal grandfather, but the child's mother showed no mosaicism [2]. The precise origin of the extra chromosome is still uncertain.

Differential Diagnosis

1. Iris colobomas and hypertelorism are features of patients with 13 trisomy, but they often have microphthalmia, cleft lip and palate, and many additional malformations (see page 164).
2. Preauricular sinuses and skin tags and hypertelorism are features of patients with the 5p− syndrome (see page 170).
3. Imperforate anus and vertebral anomalies are features of a new malformation syndrome described by Say and Gerald [6], but these patients also have polydactyly and no eye anomalies.

References

1. Schachenmann, G., Schmid, W., Fraccaro, M., Mannini, A., Tiepolo, L., Perona, G. P., and Sartori, E. Chromosomes in coloboma and anal atresia. *Lancet*, **2**:290, 1965.
2. Gerald, P. S., Davis, C., Say, B. M., and Wilkins, J. L. A novel chromosomal basis for imperforate anus (the "cat's eye" syndrome). *Pediatr. Res.*, **2**:297, 1968.
3. Nielsen, J., Tsuboi, T., Friedrich, U., Mikkelsen, M., Lund, B., and Steinicke, O. Additional small acrocentric chromosome: two cases. *J. Ment. Defic. Res.*, **13**:106–22, 1969.
4. Thomas, C., Cordier, J., Gilgenkrantz, S., Reny, A., and Raspiller, A. Un syndrome rare: atteinte colobomateuse du globe oculaire, atrésie anale, anomalies congénitales multiples et présence d'un chromosome surnuméraire. *Ann. Ocul. (Paris)*, **202**:1021–31, 1969.
5. Weber, F. M., Dooley, R. R., and Sparkes, R. S. Anal atresia, eye anomalies, and an additional small abnormal acrocentric chromosome (47,XX,mar+): report of a case. *J. Pediatr.*, **76**:594–97, 1970.
6. Say, B., Balci, S., Pirnar, T., and Hicsonmez, A. Imperforate anus/polydactyly/vertebral anomalies syndrome: a hereditary trait? *J. Pediatr.*, **79**:1033–34, 1971.

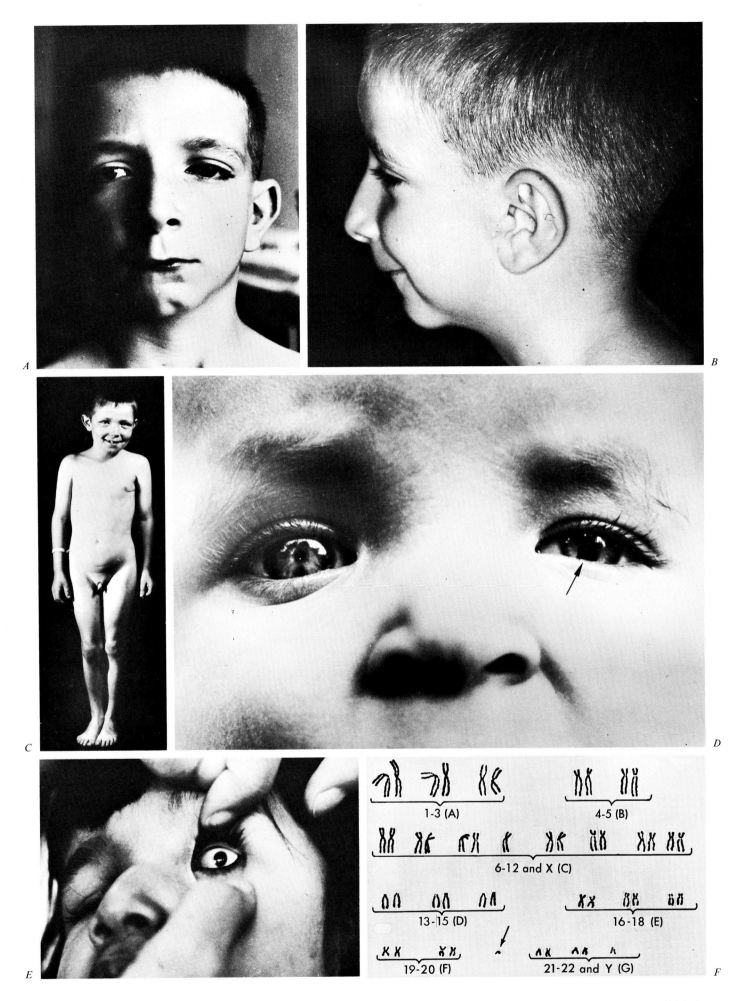

Plate IV-11. *A* and *B:* A 9-year-old boy with a downward eye slant, small chin, and scar from removal of a preauricular tag. He also had an imperforate anus and total anomalous pulmonary venous drainage; his IQ was 83. *C:* An 11-year-old boy with a chest scar from repair of tetralogy of Fallot. He also had an imperforate anus and slightly subnormal intelligence. *D:* A 6-month-old infant with bilateral iris colobomas (*arrow*), hypertelorism, a downward palpebral slant, and a preauricular fistula. *E:* Shows microphthalmia and small iris in another patient. *F:* Karyotype showing extra small acrocentric chromosome (*arrow*), smaller than any other chromosome. (*A–C* and *F:* Courtesy of Dr. P. S. Gerald, Boston, Mass. *D:* Courtesy of Dr. W. Schmid, Zurich, Switzerland. *E:* From F. M. Webber *et al., J. Pediatr.,* **76:**594–97, 1970.)

177

Sex Chromosome Syndromes
XO Syndrome (Turner's Syndrome, Gonadal Dysgenesis; 45,X)

In 1938 Turner [1] described seven young girls with sexual infantilism, webbing of the neck, deformity of the elbow, and short stature. Subsequently, a number of patients with these clinical features were shown to be chromatin negative and to have a 45,X karyotype. The frequency of the 45,X syndrome in newborns is 1:3300 [2]. This does not indicate the true incidence, however, for studies of early spontaneous abortuses have shown that about 3.5 percent have a 45,X karyotype and that 97 percent of the 45,X conceptions die in utero [3].

Physical Features

FACE: Many of these patients resemble each other; often the face is triangular and the chin is small (Figures *A, B, and C*). Some patients also have a flat nasal bridge, hypertelorism, epicanthal folds, and ptosis [4–6].

EYES: Strabismus and corneal opacities are occasionally present.

EARS: The ears are usually large and prominent.

MOUTH: The palate may be high and narrow.

NECK: The posterior hairline is low (*Figure D*). Neck webbing is present in about half of the patients [4,6].

CHEST: The chest is often broad with small, widely spaced nipples and a shieldlike appearance (*Figure C*). Pectus excavatum is sometimes present.

LIMBS: The common findings are pitting edema of the hands and feet (*Figures A and E*), clinodactyly of the fifth finger, a short fourth metacarpal, cubitus valgus, and nails that are hypoplastic in the newborn and small and hyperconvex in the older patient.

DERMATOGLYPHICS: The common findings are a distal axial triradius, increased incidence of hypothenar patterns, and high ridge counts [7].

SKIN: Scattered small brown moles and pigmented nevi are common in older children and adults, but few are seen in young infants.

HEIGHT: The average length at birth is below normal [5]. The adult height is usually less than 58 inches (148 cm), with an average of 55 inches (140 cm) [4–6].

GROWTH AND DEVELOPMENT: At the time of expected puberty, feminization and menarche do not occur.

Nervous System

The average IQ is only slightly below normal. In a series of 27 patients, 2 had mild mental deficiency [6]. Severe mental retardation is uncommon. Studies of a small number of patients have indicated that a deficiency in space-form perception and orientation is common [8]. The incidence of nerve deafness is much higher than in the normal population [4,6].

Pathology

In place of normal gonads these patients have ovarian streaks which are parallel to and below the fallopian tubes and are composed largely of collagenous tissue organized in whorls. No true follicles or secretory cells are present. In a few adults gonadoblastomas and dysgerminomas have developed in the streak gonads. Congenital heart disease and renal anomalies are found in one third of the patients. Coarctation of the aorta is the most common cardiac lesion. Rotational abnormalities, hydronephrosis, and horseshoe kidneys are the most frequent renal anomalies [6].

Laboratory Studies

Because of the failure of gonad development, there are elevated levels of gonadotropins after the age of expected puberty. Serum growth hormone levels are normal. An increased incidence of thyroiditis, achlorhydria, and diabetes mellitus has been observed in older patients. Most patients have serum antibodies to thyroid, gastric, or ovarian tissue [9]. In patients with lymphedema small, presumably hypoplastic, lymph vessels are usually demonstrated by lymphangiography.

Treatment and Prognosis

Estrogen therapy after the age of expected puberty is recommended to promote feminization and social acceptability. Except for recurrent otitis media, these patients generally enjoy good health. Individuals with mosaicism which includes the 46,XX cell line may be fertile.

Genetics

While most patients with Turner's syndrome have a 45,X karyotype, many patients have either 45,X/46,XX mosaicism [3] or 46 chromosomes including an abnormal X, such as an isochromosome X. Patients with 46,XX,Xp– and 46,XX,Xq– both may have features of Turner's syndrome [10].

Differential Diagnosis

1. Ptosis, hypertelorism, short stature, cubitus valgus, and clinodactyly are features of patients with Noonan's syndrome, but they have prognathism, pectus carinatum or excavatum, a higher incidence of mental retardation, normal secondary sexual characteristics, and normal chromosomes (see page 298).
2. Individuals with familial XY gonadal dysgenesis have a normal female phenotype, streak ovaries, and a 46,XY karyotype. This disorder is thought to be due to a mutant gene that is either X-linked or autosomal with expression only in chromosomal males [11].
3. Individuals with 46,XX gonadal dysgenesis have streak ovaries, but a normal female habitus. This syndrome is probably due to an autosomal recessive mutant gene [12].
4. Neck webbing, lymphedema, shield chest, and short stature are occasional features of the 46,XX,18q– syndrome (see page 160).
5. Excessive skin folds of the neck, epicanthic folds, a broad nasal bridge, strabismus, and clinodactyly are also features of patients with Down's syndrome (see page 150).

References

1. Turner, H. H. A syndrome of infantilism, congenital webbed neck and cubitus valgus. *Endocrinology,* **23**:566–74, 1938.
2. Court Brown, W. M. Sex chromosome anenploidy in man and its frequency with special reference to mental subnormality and criminal behavior. *Int. Rev. Exp. Pathol.,* **7**:31–97, 1969.
3. Hecht, F., and Macfarlane, J. P. Mosaicism in Turner's syndrome reflects the lethality of XO. *Lancet,* **2**:1197–98, 1969.
4. Lemli, L., and Smith, D. W. The XO syndrome: a study of the differentiated phenotype in 25 patients. *J. Pediatr.,* **63**:577–88, 1963.
5. Engel, E., and Forbes, A. P. Cytogenetic and clinical findings in 48 patients with congenitally defective or absent ovaries. *Medicine,* **44**:135–64, 1965.
6. Goldberg, M. B., Scully, A. L., Solomon, I. L., and Steinbach, H. L. Gonadal dysgenesis in phenotypic female subjects. A review of eighty-seven cases, with cytogenetic studies in fifty-three. *Am. J. Med.,* **45**:529–43, 1968.
7. Forbes, A. P. Fingerprints and palm prints (dermatoglyphics) and palmar-flexion creases in gonadal dysgenesis, pseudohypoparathyroidism and Klinefelter's syndrome. *N. Engl. J. Med.,* **270**:1268–77, 1964.
8. Money, J., Alexander, D., and Ehrhardt, A. Visual-constructional deficit in Turner's syndrome. *J. Pediatr.,* **69**:126–27, 1966.
9. Vallotton, M. B., and Forbes, A. P. Autoimmunity in gonadal dysgenesis and Klinefelter's syndrome. *Lancet,* **1**:648–51, 1967.
10. Hecht, F., Jones, D. L., Delay, M., and Klevit, H. Xq– Turner's syndrome: reconsideration of hypothesis that Xp– causes somatic features in Turner's syndrome. *J. Med. Genet.,* **7**:1–4, 1970.
11. Espiner, E. A., Veale, A. M. O., Sands, V. E., and Fitzgerald, P. H. Familial syndrome of streak gonads and normal male karyotype in five phenotypic females. *N. Engl. J. Med.,* **283**:6–11, 1970.
12. Simpson, J. L., and Christakos, A. C. Hereditary factors in obstetrics and gynecology. *Obstet. Gynecol. Survey,* **24**:580–601, 1969.

Plate IV-12. *A:* A newborn female
with severe pitting edema of the legs
and a small chin. *B:* An 8-year-old girl
with short stature (48 in., 123 cm) and
a webbed neck. *C–E:* A 13-year-old
girl with a webbed neck, ptosis, shield
chest, small and widely spaced nipples,
a low posterior hairline, and slight
puffiness of the dorsum of her fingers.
F: A karyotype with 45 chromosomes,
including only one X chromosome. (*A:*
Courtesy of Dr. C. R. Scott, Seattle,
Wash. *B:* Courtesy of Dr. J. D. Crawford, Boston, Mass. *F:* Courtesy of Dr.
L. Atkins, Boston, Mass.)

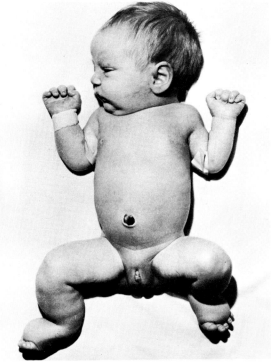

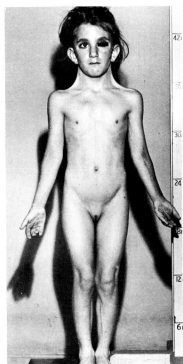

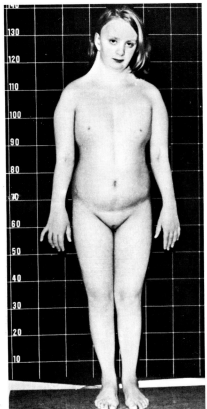

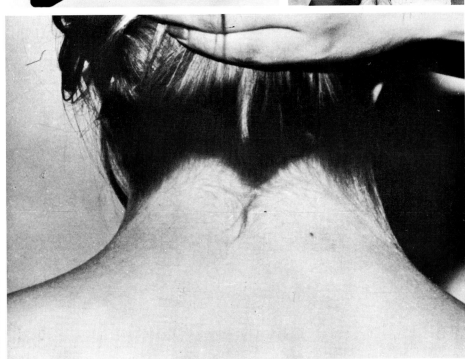

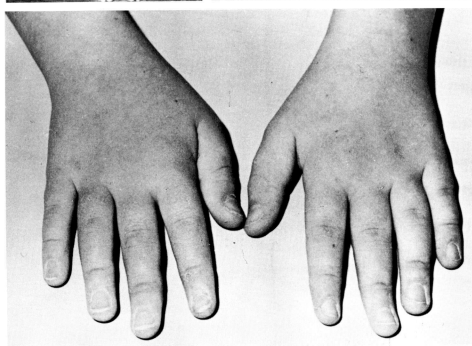

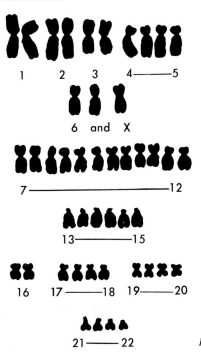

XXXX Syndrome (48,XXXX)

In 1961 Carr, Barr, and Plunkett [1] described two mentally retarded females with a 48,XXXX karyotype. Since then, more than ten additional affected females have been described [2–10]. As most of these patients were ascertained through the screening of mentally retarded individuals, the relationship of this syndrome to mental deficiency remains uncertain. The reported patients have had a variety of major and minor anomalies, but no specific phenotype. This discussion and the accompanying pictures are included to emphasize and illustrate this phenotypic variability.

Physical Features

FACE: Three females have been considered to have a peculiar facial appearance, two having hypertelorism [3,4] and two with an appearance suggestive of that seen in Down's syndrome [4,5].

LIMBS: Dislocated hips [2], short middle and distal phalanges [6], and clinodactyly of the fifth fingers [7] have each been reported in one patient. Two patients have had radioulnar synostosis [8].

DERMATOGLYPHICS: These patients have a reduced total finger ridge count [8].

GROWTH AND DEVELOPMENT: Some women have had normal menses, and others have had irregular menses [8,9].

Nervous System

The intelligence quotients of the reported patients have ranged from 30 [1] to 80 [3], with most having an IQ above 50.

Genetics

One affected female has had two children, one of whom was apparently a normal female and the other with Down's syndrome [10].

References

1. Carr, D. H., Barr, M. L., and Plunkett, E. R. An XXXX sex chromosome complex in two mentally defective females. *Can. Med. Assoc. J.,* **84:**131–37, 1961.
2. Davies, T. S. Buccal smear surveys for sex chromatin. *Br. Med. J.,* **1:**1541–42, 1963.
3. DiCagno, L., and Franceschini, P. Feeblemindedness and XXXX karyotype. *J. Ment. Defic. Res.,* **12:**226–36, 1968.
4. Lejeune, J., and Abonyi, D. Syndrome 48,XXXX chez une fille de quatorze ans. *Ann. Genet. (Paris),* **11:**117–19, 1968.
5. deGrouchy, J., Brissaud, H. E., Richardet, J. M., Repéssé, G., Sanger, R., Race, R. R., Salmon, C., and Salmon, D. Syndrome 48,XXXX chez une enfant de six ans: transmission anormale du groupe Xg. *Ann. Genet. (Paris),* **11:**120–24, 1968.
6. Berkeley, M. I. K., and Faed, M. J. W. A female with the 48,XXXX karyotype. *J. Med. Genet.,* **7:**83–85, 1970.
7. Duncan, B. P., Nicholl, J. O., and Downes, R. An XXXX sex chromosome complement in a female with mild mental retardation. *Can. Med. Assoc. J.,* **102:**969–70, 1970.
8. Telfer, M. A., Richardson, C. E., Helmken, J., and Smith, G. F. Divergent phenotypes among 48,XXXX and 47,XXX females. *Am. J. Hum. Genet.,* **22:**326–35, 1970.
9. Park, I.-J., Tyson, J. E., and Jones, H. W., Jr. A 48,XXXX female with mental retardation. Report of a case. *Obstet. Gynecol.,* **35:**248–52, 1970.
10. Bergemann, E. Die Häufigkeit des Abweichens vom normalen Geschlechtschromatin und eine Familienuntersuchung bei Triplo-X. *Helv. Med. Acta,* **29:**420–22, 1962.

Plate IV-13. *A* and *B:* An 11-year-old girl with bilateral congenital hip dislocation and a large port wine nevus. *C:* A 12-year-old girl with mild strabismus and an accessory nipple. *D:* An 8-year-old girl who had a patent ductus arteriosus and clinodactyly. *E:* A 3½-year-old girl with microcephaly and deformed ears. *F:* A 28-year-old woman with a short, wide neck. She also had extreme myopia, exotropia, nystagmus, underdeveloped breasts, and radioulnar synostosis. (*A* and *B:* Courtesy of Dr. T. S. Davies, Monmouthshire, England. *C:* From D. H. Carr *et al., Can. Med. Assoc. J.,* **84:**131–37, 1961. *D:* Courtesy of Dr. F. A. Baughman, Jr., Grand Rapids, Mich. *E* and *F:* From M. A. Telfer *et al., Am. J. Hum. Genet.,* **22:**326–35, 1970.)

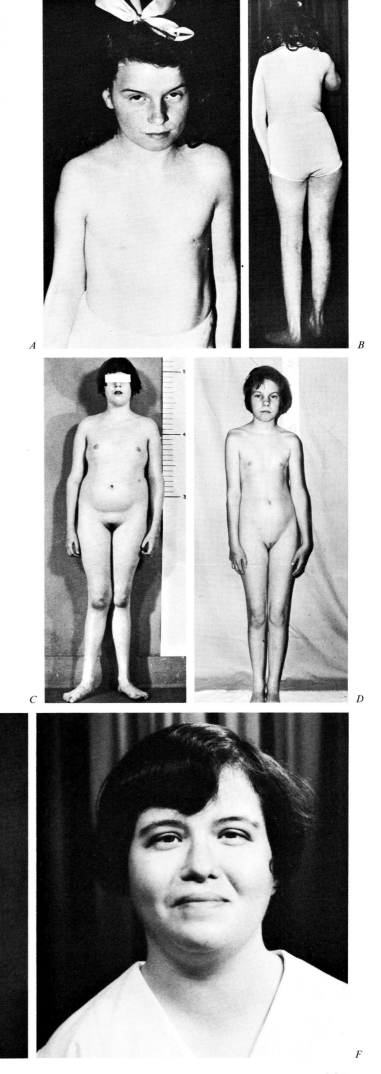

XXXXX Syndrome (49,XXXXX)

Only four females with the XXXXX syndrome have been described, the first in 1963 by Kesaree and Woolley [1]. Three were young children [1-3], and the fourth [4] was 16 years old, an age difference that limits the comparison of their phenotypic features.

Physical Features

HEAD: Three were microcephalic. One had a flattened occiput [4].

FACE: All had hypertelorism. Two children had an upward slant of the palpebral fissures (*Figures A, B, C, and D*) [1,2]. Two had epicanthal folds [2,3].

EARS: The ears were normal, but were low-set in one [2].

NECK: Two of the patients had a very short neck [2,3].

CHEST: The 16-year-old girl had infantile breasts (*Figure D*) [4].

GENITALIA: The older girl had scanty pubic hair and prepubescent external genitalia. Her uterus was considered small by palpation [4].

BACK: Moderate scoliosis of the dorsal spine was present in the older girl [4].

LIMBS: The hands of the two of the younger children were considered small [1,2]. Three had clinodactyly of the fifth fingers. One child had a unilateral talipes equinovarus deformity [2] (*Figure B*). Another had small feet with overlapping toes [1] (*Figure A*). The third child also had overlapping toes [3]. The older girl had flexed elbows and knees (*Figure D*).

DERMATOGLYPHICS: One patient [1] had bilateral and another [3] had unilateral transverse palmar creases. Ten digital arches were the only other dermatoglyphic finding noted [4], this in the 16-year-old.

Nervous System

All four were mentally retarded. One had periodic upward rolling of her eyes [2]. Another had incoordinated eye movements [4].

Pathology

Surgical ligation of a patent ductus arteriosus was performed in the first two children [1,2]. The third child was thought to have an endocardial cushion defect, which caused cardiac failure and death at $2^{5}/_{12}$ years [3].

Laboratory Studies

Buccal smears show multiple nuclear sex chromatin bodies up to 4 in number. Only the older girl has had extensive radiologic studies. These showed many malformations, the most prominent being a thick sternum, scoliosis of the lumbar spine, and subluxation of the elbow joints with radioulnar synostosis [4].

Genetics

Many cases of the XXXXY syndrome have been reported during the time when only these four patients with the XXXXX syndrome have been described. The reason for this apparent difference in the prevalence of these two syndromes with 49 chromosomes is not known.

References

1. Kesaree, N., and Woolley, P. V., Jr. A phenotypic female with 49 chromosomes, presumably XXXXX. A case report. *J. Pediatr.,* **63:**1099–1103, 1963.
2. Brody, J., Fitzgerald, M. C., and Spiers, A. S. D. A female child with five X chromosomes. *J. Pediatr.,* **70:**105–109, 1967.
3. Yamada, Y., and Neriishi, S. Penta X (49,XXXXX) chromosome constitution: a case report. *Jap. J. Hum. Genet.,* **16:**15–21, 1971.
4. Sergovich, F., Uilenberg, C., and Pozsonyi, J. The 49,XXXXX chromosome constitution: similarities to the 49,XXXXY condition. *J. Pediatr.,* **78:**285–90, 1971.

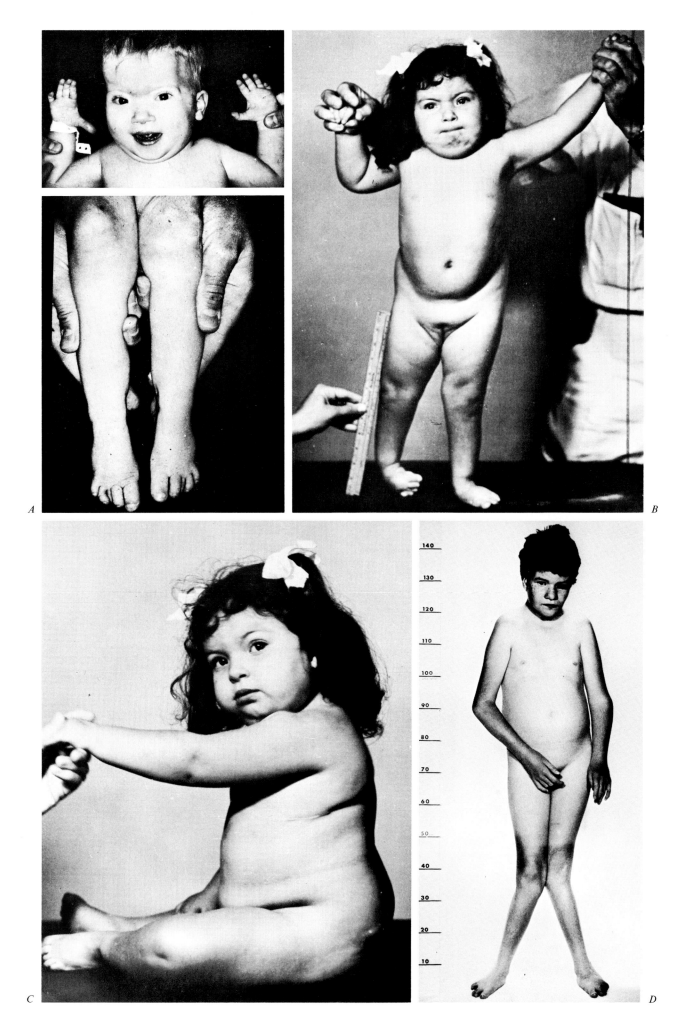

Plate IV-14. *A:* A 2-year-old girl with hypertelorism, an upward eye slant, small hands, clinodactyly of the fifth fingers, and overlapping toes. *B* and *C:* A 2-year-old girl with a short neck and equinovarus deformity of her right foot. *D:* A 16-year-old girl with a small chest, infantile breasts, and flexed elbows and knees. (*A:* From N. Kesaree and P. V. Woolley, Jr., *J. Pediatr.,* **63:**1099–1103, 1963. *B:* From J. Brody *et al., J. Pediatr.,* **70:**105–109, 1967. *C:* Courtesy of Dr. J. Brody, Gordonvale, Queensland, Australia. *D:* Courtesy of Dr. F. R. Sergovich, London, Ontario, Canada.)

XXY Syndrome (Klinefelter's Syndrome; 47,XXY)

In 1942 Klinefelter, Reifenstein, and Albright [1] described nine men with gynecomastia, small testes, aspermia, and increased excretion of follicle-stimulating hormone. This clinical syndrome, which is usually referred to as Klinefelter's syndrome, has since been shown to be associated with a single nuclear sex chromatin body and a 47,XXY karyotype. Confusion has arisen from the use of the term *Klinefelter's syndrome* to refer also to patients with the 48,XXXY, 49,XXXXY, and 48,XXYY karyotypes. Furthermore, phenotypic males with gynecomastia and hypogonadism and a 46,XY karyotype have sometimes been classified as chromatin-negative Klinefelter's syndrome. In this discussion the term *Klinefelter's syndrome* is used only to refer to the 47,XXY syndrome. The incidence is approximately 1:1400 livebirths [2].

Physical Features

BREASTS: Most adolescent and adult patients have bilateral or unilateral breast enlargement with glandular tissue responsible for most of the increase in size (*Figures A, B, and C*).

GENITALIA: In a study of 50 adults [3], the penis was normal in size in 90 percent of the patients and smaller than normal in the remainder. All had small testes, which were usually firm in consistency. The prostate was smaller than normal in 46 percent of the patients. In a study [3a] of 9 prepubertal boys, 8 had small testes.

LIMBS: The most common minor anomalies are clinodactyly and cubitus valgus. These were found in 11 and 4 patients, respectively, in a study of 24 individuals [4].

DERMATOGLYPHICS: A low ridge count in the digit patterns is the most striking difference from normal. In general, the dermal patterns of these individuals are more similar to normal females than to normal males [5].

HAIR: Most adults have diminished facial hair. The pubic hair followed a feminine distribution in 13 of 32 patients in one study [3]. Many patients have less than the normal amount of body hair. Frontal balding occurs in only a few patients.

HEIGHT: The adult height ranged from 64 to 80 inches (162 to 204 cm) in two studies, with averages of 70 [4] and 71¼ [3] inches (179 and 181 cm). The increased height is chiefly in the lower body segment.

WEIGHT: Obesity is common and often develops in patients who were of normal weight as adolescents. Nine of 30 patients in one series had a eunuchoid appearance [3] (*Figure B*).

Nervous System

While mental deficiency is uncommon in patients with Klinefelter's syndrome, surveys of mental institutions have shown that the frequency of the 47,XXY syndrome in such institutions is three times greater than in the normal population [2]. Many patients have a blustery manner and are very talkative, but what they say has little meaning. Most are unable to complete high school. A high incidence of divorce, unemployment, alcoholism, and various psychiatric disorders has also been reported [3,4].

Pathology

Testicular biopsies of adults show hypoplasia and hyalinization of the seminiferous tubules. The Leydig cells are clumped (*Figure D*) and in some patients hyperplastic. Little evidence of spermatogenesis can be found.

Laboratory Studies

The buccal smear shows a single sex chromatin body (*Figure E*). No spermatozoa could be found in the semen analysis of 17 adult patients [4]. No patients have been fertile. The urinary gonadotropins are elevated in the adults. The urinary 17-ketosteroids are usually normal. The plasma testosterone level before and after stimulation with chorionic gonadotropin is less than that of normal males [6]. A high incidence of diabetes mellitus, hyperlipemia, and hypercholesterolemia has been reported [3,4].

Treatment and Prognosis

While these patients have a normal life expectancy, most have very chaotic and unpredictable life patterns, which works against any therapeutic or rehabilitative efforts. Treatment of three adolescents with testosterone produced a more masculine appearance and more assertive and goal-directed behavior [7].

Genetics

It is postulated that nondisjunction is the source of the extra X chromosome in Klinefelter's syndrome. In some patients the extra X is of maternal origin, and in others it is of paternal origin [8]. Among individuals with Klinefelter's syndrome an increased incidence of twins concordant for 47,XXY has been noted [8a].

Differential Diagnosis

1. Hypogonadism and gynecomastia occur in patients with the 48,XXYY (see page 186), 48,XXXY (see page 188), and 49,XXXXY syndromes (see page 190), but they are differentiated by a higher incidence of skeletal anomalies and mental retardation than in the 47,XXY syndrome.
2. Several hereditary syndromes have been described in which hypogonadism is associated with either a primary gonadotropin deficiency or a primary testicular abnormality and a normal karyotype, but the testis pathology and body habitus may be similar to those of patients with Klinefelter's syndrome [9].
3. Phenotypic males with a 46,XX karyotype also have gynecomastia and small testes [10].

References

1. Klinefelter, H. F., Jr., Reifenstein, E. C., Jr., and Albright, F. Syndrome characterized by gynecomastia, aspermatogenesis without A-Leydigism, and increased excretion of follicle-stimulating hormone. *J. Clin. Endocrinol.,* **2**:615–27, 1942.
2. Ratcliffe, S. G., Stewart, A. L., Melville, M.M., and Jacobs, P. A. Chromosome studies on 3500 new-born male infants. *Lancet,* **1**:121–22, 1970.
3. Becker, K. L., Hoffman, D. L., Albert, A., Underdahl, L. O., and Mason, H. L. Klinefelter's syndrome. Clinical and laboratory findings in 50 patients. *Arch. Intern. Med.,* **118**:314–21, 1966.
3a. Laron, Z., and Hoehman, I. H. Small testes in prepubertal boys with Klinefelter's syndrome. *J. Clin. Endocrinol. Metab.,* **32**:671–72, 1971.
4. Zuppinger, K., Engel, E., Forbes, A. P., Mantooth, L., and Claffey, J. Klinefelter's syndrome, a clinical and cytogenetic study in twenty-four cases. *Acta Endocrinol. (Kbh),* **54**(Suppl. 113):5–48, 1967.
5. Cushman, C. J., and Soltan, H. C. Dermatoglyphics in Klinefelter's syndrome (47,XXY). *Hum. Hered.,* **19**:641–53, 1969.
6. Kliman, B., and Briefer, C. Cited by Federman, D. D. *Abnormal Genital Development.* W. B. Saunders Co., Philadelphia, 1967, pp. 31–32.
7. Myhre, S. A., Ruvalcaba, R. H. A., Johnson, H. R., Thuline, H. C., and Kelley, V. C. The effects of testosterone treatment in Klinefelter's syndrome. *J. Pediatr.,* **76**:267–76, 1970.
8. Frøland, A., Sanger, R., and Race, R. R. Xg blood groups of 78 patients with Klinefelter's syndrome and of some of their patients. *J. Med. Genet.,* **5**:161–64, 1968.
8a. Vague, J., Boyer, J., Nicolino, J., Mattei, A., Luciani, J., Arnaud, A., Pouch, J., and Valette, A. Maladie de Klinefelter chez deux jumeaux monozygotes. *Ann. Endocrinol. (Paris),* **29**:709–29, 1968.
9. Rimoin, D. L., Borgaonkar, D. S., Asper, S. P., Jr., and Blizzard, R. M. Chromatin-negative hypogonadism in phenotypic men. *Am. J. Med.,* **44**:225–33, 1968.
10. Sebaoun, M., Fournier, M., Gilbert-Dreyfus, and Netter, A. Les hommes de caryotype 46XX. A propos de deux nouvelles observations. *Ann. Endocrinol. (Paris),* **30**:741–58, 1969.

Plate IV-15. *A:* Shows a teen-age boy with gynecomastia. *B* and *C:* Two adults with gynecomastia who also had small testes. *D:* Testicular biopsy showing clumping of the Leydig cells and absence of spermatogonia. *E:* Buccal smear showing single sex chromatin body (*arrow*). *F:* An XXY karyotype with an extra chromosome in the 6-X-12 group. (*A:* Courtesy of Dr. J. D. Crawford, Boston, Mass. *B:* Courtesy of Dr. B. Kliman, Boston, Mass. *C* and *D:* From D. D. Federman, *Abnormal Sexual Development,* W. B. Saunders Co., Philadelphia, 1967. *E:* Courtesy of Dr. P. Taft, Boston, Mass. *F:* Courtesy of Dr. L. Atkins, Boston, Mass.)

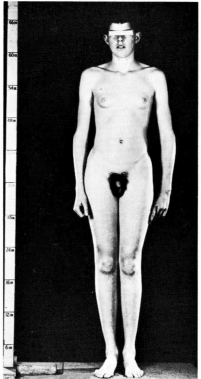
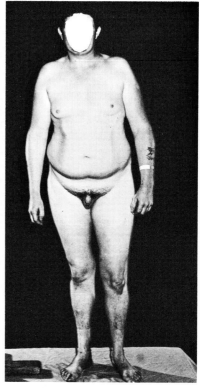

A

B

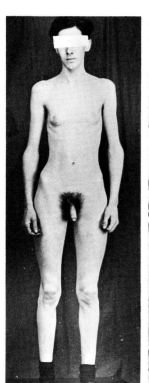

C

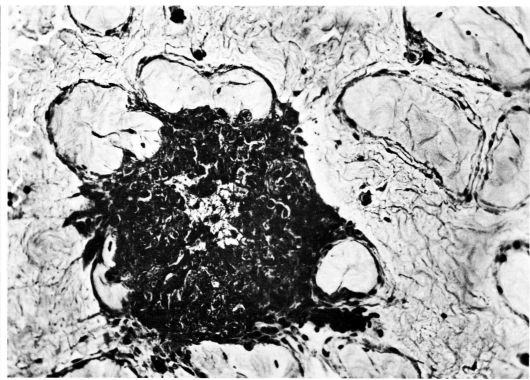

D

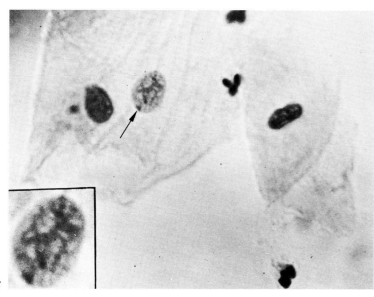

E

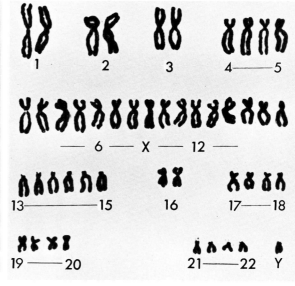

F

185

XXYY Syndrome (48,XXYY)

The first patient with the XXYY syndrome was reported in 1960 by Muldal and Ockey [1]. Since then over 50 individuals with this syndrome have been ascertained usually through the study of patients with either mental retardation and skeletal deformities or with genital anomalies [2–6, 6a]. Because of the bias of this method of ascertainment, the complete clinical spectrum of this disorder has not been established.

Physical Features

FACE: Prognathism has been noted in several patients.

NECK: Several patients have had webbing of the neck.

BREASTS: Many patients have either unilateral or bilateral gynecomastia [3] (*Figures A and B*).

GENITALIA: The phallus is normal in size in most individuals, but the testes are small.

DERMATOGLYPHICS: The most common findings are a predominance of arches and very small loops on the fingers, a low total ridge count, and a high incidence of hypothenar patterns [5].

SKIN: Several patients have had stasis dermatitis at an early age. Varicose veins, cutaneous angiomas, and acrocyanosis are also common [4,6].

HAIR: The amount of facial, axillary, and pubic hair is often less than normal.

HEIGHT: Many of the reported patients have been excessively tall (*Figures B and C*).

WEIGHT: Eunuchoid proportions with excessive abdominal and hip fat have been described in several adults [4,5] (*Figure C*).

Nervous System

All of the patients have been mildly to severely mentally retarded. In a review [6a] of 33 patients, 20 had IQ's below 70. A few patients have shown aggressive or bizarre behavior [2].

Pathology

In pubertal patients the testes have shown hyalinization of the tubules, an absence of germinal cells, and prominence of the Leydig cells [5] (*Figures D and E*). Testicular biopsies have been performed on two prepubertal patients, one showing no abnormalities and the other small seminiferous tubules with a diminished number of spermatogonia [3].

Laboratory Studies

An abnormal elevation of follicle-stimulating hormone and urinary gonadotropins is usually present after the age of expected puberty [6a]. The levels of urinary 17-ketosteroids are low to normal.

Genetics

It is thought that the 48,XXYY cell line is due to two successive nondisjunction events in the father, producing an XYY sperm, but a single nondisjunctive event in both parents has not been ruled out [4,6a].

Differential Diagnosis

1. Individuals with the XXY syndrome (Klinefelter's syndrome) also have hypogonadism and gynecomastia, but as a group these patients do not have as high an incidence of tall stature and mental retardation as is associated with the XXYY syndrome (see page 184).
2. Tall stature and abnormal behavior have been features of some patients with the 47,XYY karyotype [7].

References

1. Muldal, S., and Ockey, C. H. The "double male": a new chromosome constitution in Klinefelter's syndrome. *Lancet*, 2:492–93, 1960.
2. Garcia, H. O., Borgaonkar, D. S., and Richardson, F. XXYY syndrome in a prepubertal male. *Johns Hopkins Med. J.*, 121:31–37, 1967.
3. Ferrier, P. E., and Ferrier, S. A. XXYY Klinefelter's syndrome: case report and a study of the Y chromosomes' DNA replication pattern. *Ann. Genet.* (*Paris*), 11:145–51, 1968.
4. Waterman, D. F., London, J., Valdmanis, A., and Mann, J. D. The XXYY chromosome constitution. *Am. J. Dis. Child.*, 111:421–25, 1966.
5. Parker, C. E., Mavalwala, J., Melnyk, J., and Fish, C. H. The 48,XXYY syndrome. *Am. J. Med.*, 48:777–81, 1970.
6. Peterson, W. C., Gorlin, R. J., Peagler, F., and Bruhl, H. Cutaneous aspects of the XXYY genotype. *Arch. Dermatol.*, 94:695–98, 1966.
6a. Borgaonkar, D. S., Mules, E., and Char, F. Do the 48,XXYY males have a characteristic phenotype? *Clin. Genet.*, 1:272–93, 1970.
7. Court Brown, W. M. Males with an XYY sex chromosome complement. *J. Med. Genet.*, 5:341–59, 1968.

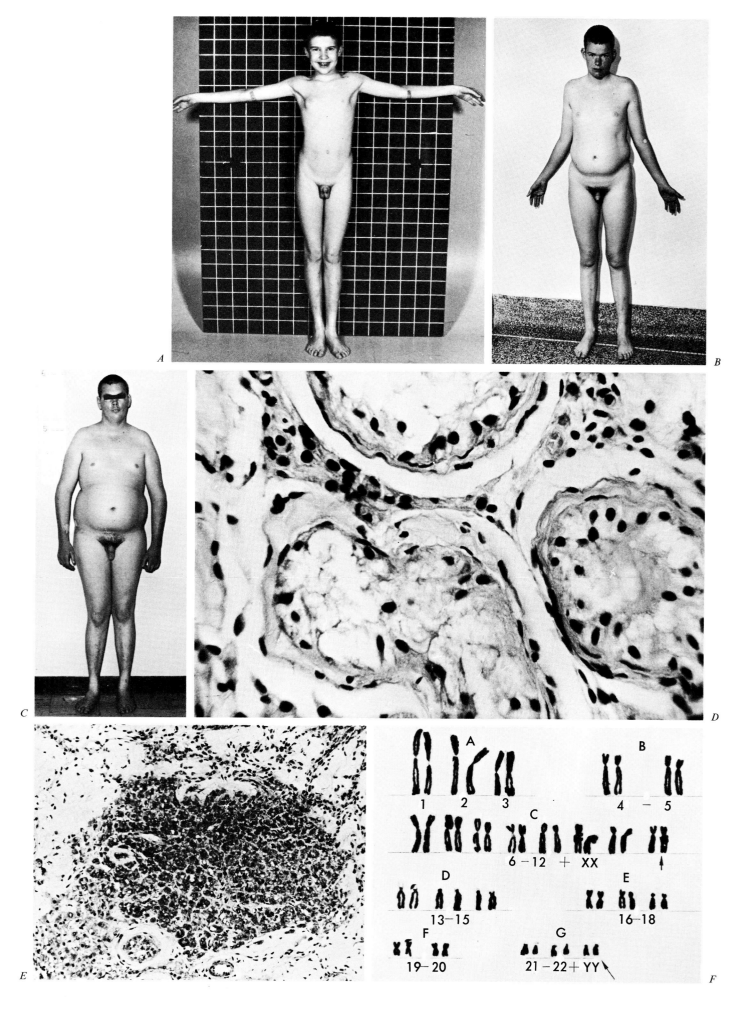

Plate IV-16. *A:* A 15-year-old boy with unilateral gynecomastia. *B:* A tall (71 in., 182 cm), obese 15-year-old boy who had gynecomastia and small, hard testes. *C:* A 19-year-old who was tall (72 in., 185.4 cm) and had a eunuchoid habitus. *D* and *E:* Testes biopsies from this boy show thick hyaline membranes of the spermatic tubules and clumps of Leydig cells. *F:* A karyotype showing 48 chromosome with an extra X and Y (*arrow*) chromosome. (*A:* From P. E. Ferrier and S. A. Ferrier, *Ann. Genet.*, **11:**145–51, 1968. *B:* From D. F. Waterman *et al., Am. J. Dis. Child.*, **111:**421–25, 1966. *C–F:* From C. E. Parker *et al., Am. J. Med.*, **48:**777–81, 1970.)

XXXY Syndrome (48,XXXY)

In 1959 Barr, Shaver, Carr, and Plunkett [1] reported three males with mental retardation, hypogonadism, and a 48,XXXY karyotype (*Figures A and B*). Since that time more than 25 more patients have been reported [2–9]. As most of the reported patients were ascertained through screening of mentally retarded patients, both the spectrum of the associated physical features and the relationship of this syndrome to mental retardation remain unknown. While the incidence of the XXXY syndrome is not known, only one patient was discovered in nuclear chromatin studies of 23,000 newborn males [8].

Physical Features

FACE: Several patients had a flat bridge of the nose, epicanthal folds, and mild prognathism [5,6] (*Figure C*).

BREASTS: Five of 12 patients 14 or more years old in one review had gynecomastia [5].

GENITALIA: The phallus was normal in size, but the testes were small in most patients. In the adults the prostate was smaller than normal [1–7].

LIMBS: Three patients had bilateral radioulnar synostosis [2,6,7] (*Figure D*). Seven of nineteen had clinodactyly of the fifth fingers [5–7].

SKIN: The facial and body hair was less than normal in some of the patients.

HEIGHT: The height of the reported adults was between 64 and 73 inches (164 and 188 cm) [5].

Nervous System

The reported patients have had intelligence quotients ranging from 20 to 76 [1–7], with most between 40 and 60. Muscular hypotonia is often present, especially in infants [5].

Pathology

The testis biopsies in seven patients [1–4] showed similar abnormalities: small or atrophic seminiferous tubules, large islands of Leydig cells, and an absence of germinal cells. The histologic structure in one patient's biopsy was considered nearly normal [1].

Laboratory Studies

The urinary gonadotropins were elevated in all of the adults who had small testes and abnormal testicular histology. The buccal smear shows some cells have none, some one, and others two nuclear sex chromatin bodies (*Figure E*).

Genetics

Xg[a] blood group antigen studies in one family [5] showed that all of the affected boy's X chromosomes came from his mother. Two sets of twins concordant for the 48,XXXY karyotype have been reported [9,10].

Differential Diagnosis

Hypogenitalism, gynecomastia, prognathism, and skeletal anomalies are also features of males with the 49,XXXXY syndrome (see page 190).

References

1. Barr, M. L., Shaver, E. L., Carr, D. H., and Plunkett, E. R. An unusual sex chromatin pattern in three mentally deficient subjects. *J. Ment. Defic. Res.,* 3:78–87, 1959.
2. Ferguson-Smith, M. A., Johnston, A. W., and Handmaker, S. D. Primary amentia and micro-orchidism associated with an XXXY sex-chromosome constitution. *Lancet,* 2:184–87, 1960.
3. Carr, D. H., Barr, M. L., Plunkett, E. R., Grumbach, M. M., and Morishima, A. and Chu, E. H. Y. An XXXY sex chromosome complex in Klinefelter subjects with duplicated sex chromatin. *J. Clin. Endocrinol.,* 21:491–505, 1961.
4. Takayasu, H., Kinoshita, K., Tsuboi, T., and Kurihara, T. Twins with Klinefelter's syndrome. *Lancet,* 2:1424, 1967.
5. Zollinger, H. Das XXXY- Syndrom. Zwei neue Beobachtungen im Kleinkindesalter und eine Literaturubersicht. *Helv. Paediatr. Acta,* 24:589–99, 1969.
6. Greenstein, R. M., Harris, D. J., Luzzatti, L., and Cann, H. M. Cytogenetic analysis of a boy with the XXXY syndrome: origin of the X-chromosomes. *Pediatrics,* 45:677–86, 1970.
7. McGann, B. R., Alexander, M., and Fox, F. A. XXXY chromosomal abnormality in a child. *Calif. Med.,* 112:30–32, 1970.
8. Taylor, A. I., and Moores, E. C. A sex chromatin survey of newborn children in two London hospitals. *J. Med. Genet.,* 4:258–59, 1967.
9. Simpson, J. L., Morillo-Cucci, G., Horwith, M. I., Stiefel, F., and Feldman, F. Monozygotic twins with 48,XXXY Klinefelter's syndrome. (Abstract.) IVth International Congress of Human Genetics, Paris, 1971.
10. Takayasu, H., Kinoskita, K., Tsuboi, T., and Kurihara, T. Twins with Klinefelter's syndrome. *Lancet,* 2:1424, 1967.

Plate IV-17. *A* and *B:* Two of the first three reported patients, who were ages 15 and 31 years and had a normal facial appearance and habitus. *C:* A 3¾-year-old Oriental boy with a flattened bridge of the nose, epicanthal folds, and mild prognathia. *D:* Shows the proximal radioulnar synostosis in this boy. *E:* The buccal epithelial cell in center shows the two nuclear chromatin bodies (*arrows*). *F:* Karyotype showing three X chromosomes. (*A* and *B:* From M. L. Barr *et al., J. Ment. Defic. Res.,* **3:**78–87, 1959. *C, D,* and *F:* From R. M. Greenstein *et al., Pediatrics,* **45:**677–86, 1970. *E:* Courtesy of Dr. R. M. Greenstein, Hartford, Conn.)

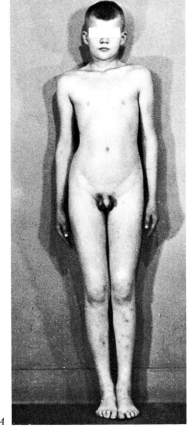
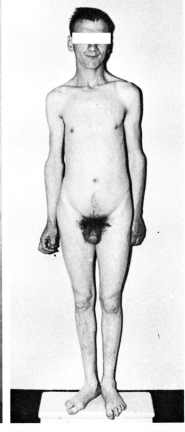

A

B

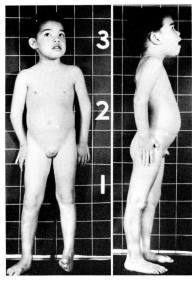
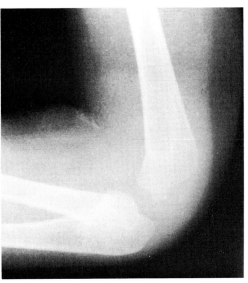
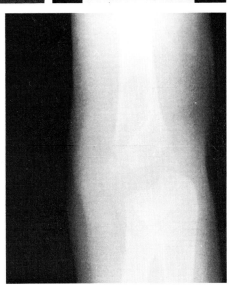

C

D

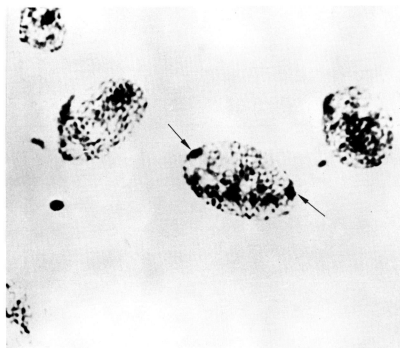

E

F

189

XXXXY Syndrome (49,XXXXY)

In 1960 Fraccaro, Kaijser, and Lindsten [1] reported the first patient with the XXXXY syndrome, a 7-year-old boy who was mentally retarded and had ambiguous external genitalia. Subsequently, over 60 additional patients with this syndrome have been described [2–6]. Since most of these patients were found through the study of either mentally retarded or deformed individuals, the full clinical spectrum of this syndrome has not been established. The incidence of the 49,XXXXY syndrome is not known.

Physical Features

HEAD: Several different head sizes and shapes have been described: microcephaly [2], dolichocephaly, and brachycephaly [3].

FACE: The eyes are widely spaced and the nose is broad and flat (*Figures B, C, and D*). A slight upward eye slant, epicanthic folds, and strabismus are often present. In profile, prognathism is evident in many patients [4] (*Figure B*).

EARS: In some reported patients the ears have been large and malformed and in others small, simple and low-set.

MOUTH: In those who have prognathism, the mandibular teeth protrude beyond the maxillary teeth. A few patients have had a bifid uvula and cleft palate.

NECK: Some patients have had a short, broad neck with a mild degree of webbing [4].

BACK: Kyphosis, increased lordosis, and scoliosis are common (*Figures B and D*).

GENITALIA: In postpubertal patients the penis is small and the scrotum is poorly rugated. One or both of the testes are often undescended.

LIMBS: In one review [4] 25 of 28 patients had both limitation of movement of the elbow and clinodactyly. Many patients also have coxa valga, genu valgum, and pes planus (*Figures C and D*). Several have had malformed toes, especially hallux valgus (*Figure A*).

HEIGHT: The height of adults is usually below average.

WEIGHT: The birth weight may be normal or low for the gestational age. Feeding problems and a slow weight gain are common in infancy.

Nervous System

Most, but not all, of the reported patients have been mentally retarded with intelligence quotients of less than 60 [3,4,6]. During infancy muscular hypotonia and hyperextensibility of the joints are common [6a]. One infant had normal intellect development at 15 months of age and later was mentally retarded [5]. In older children the deep tendon reflexes may be hyperactive. Several patients have had either seizures or abnormal electroencephalograms.

Pathology

Abnormalities of the testes have been found in almost all patients. Usually the germ cell maturation has been incomplete. Many prepubescent patients have had a lack of spermatogonia; some patients have had seminiferous tubule atrophy and others an absence of Leydig cells. The adult patients have had more advanced tubular atrophy, fibrosis, no Leydig clumps, and a lack of spermatogonia [2,4].

Laboratory Studies

Skull x-rays have revealed sclerotic cranial sutures, a widened interorbital distance, a thick cranial vault, and prognathism in many patients. In a series of 19 patients, radioulnar synostosis was present in 8 and a proximal radioulnar dislocation in 7. The intercondylar fossa was shallow in 11 of 12 patients. Most patients also had vertebral anomalies and scoliosis, and a retarded bone age [4].

At the age of expected puberty these patients have an abnormal rise in urinary gonadotropins. The buccal smear shows up to three nuclear chromatin bodies, which reflect the three late-replicating, extra X chromosomes [6] (*Figure E*).

Genetics

The three extra X chromosomes are thought to be the result of two sequential nondisjunctional events in either meiosis or mitosis or in both. Xg^a blood group antigen studies in two families showed that the two affected males with the 49,XXXXY karyotype received all four X chromosomes from their mothers [7].

Differential Diagnosis

1. The flat nasal bridge, epicanthic folds, strabismus, upward palpebral slant, short neck, clinodactyly, muscular hypotonia, and hyperextensible joints are also features of Down's syndrome, but these patients usually do not have prognathism or scoliosis (see page 150).
2. Patients with Klinefelter's (47,XXY) syndrome are differentiated by the lack of both skeletal anomalies and severe mental retardation and by often having a normal-size penis and gynecomastia (see page 184).
3. Hypogenitalism, gynecomastia, hypotonia in infancy, and clinodactyly are also features of the XXXY syndrome (see page 188).
4. Prognathism and kyphoscoliosis are features of patients with the syndrome of acromegaloid features, hypertelorism, and pectus carinatum, but these patients also have coarse facial features and large hands (see page 316).

References

1. Fraccaro, M., Kaijser, K., and Lindsten, J. A child with 49 chromosomes. *Lancet*, **2**:899–902, 1960.
2. Barr, M. L., Carr, D. H., Pozsonyi, J., Wilson, R. A., Dunn, H. G., Jacobson, T. S., and Miller, J. R. The XXXXY sex chromosome abnormality. *Can. Med. Assoc. J.*, **87**:891–901, 1962.
3. Scherz, R. G., and Roeckel, I. E. The XXXXY syndrome. A report of a case and review of the literature. *J. Pediatr.*, **63**:1093–98, 1963.
4. Zaleski, W. A., Houston, C. S., Pozsonyi, J., and Ying, K. L. The XXXXY chromosome anomaly: report of three new cases and review of 30 cases from the literature. *Can. Med. Assoc. J.*, **94**:1143–54, 1966.
5. Shapiro, L. R., Brill, C. B., Hsu, L. Y. F., Calvin, M. E., and Hirschhorn, K. Deceleration of intellectual development in a XXXXY child. *Am. J. Dis. Child.*, **122**:163–64, 1971.
6. Rowley, J., Muldal, S., Gilbert, C. W., Lajtha, L. G., Lindsten, J., Fraccaro, M., and Kaijser, K. Synthesis of deoxyribonucleic acid on X-chromosomes of an XXXXY male. *Nature*, **197**:251–52, 1963.
6a. Hayek, A., Riccardi, V., Atkins, L., and Hendren, H. 49,XXXXY chromosomal anomaly in a neonate. *J. Med. Genet.*, **8**:220–21, 1971.
7. Lewis, F. J. W., Frøland, A., Sanger, R., and Race, R. R. Source of the X chromosomes in two XXXY males. *Lancet*, **2**:589, 1964.

Plate IV-18. *A:* A 2-week-old infant with striking muscular hypotonia and a short neck with excessive skin folds. *B:* A 14-year-old boy with marked lumbar lordosis, prognathism, and a flat nasal bridge. *C:* A 15½-year-old boy with webbing of the neck, flexed elbows (due to a dislocated right ulna and left radius), small genitalia, and hallux valgus. He also had congenital dislocation of both hips. *D:* A 13-year-old boy with severe vertebral deformities, bilateral dislocation of the radius, genu valgum, clinodactyly, clubfoot deformity, and small testes. *E:* A buccal epithelial cell in which three sex chromatin bodies are visible (*arrows*) along the edge of the nucleus. *F:* A 49,XXXXY karyotype with the four X chromosomes shown with pair 6. Three of the X's were identified as late-labeling by autoradiography. (*A:* From A. Hayek *et al.*, *J. Med. Genet.*, **8:**220–21, 1971, by permission of the author and editor. *B:* Courtesy of Dr. J. Galindo, Glens Falls, N.Y. *C:* From D. D. Federman, *Abnormal Sexual Development*, W. B. Saunders Co., Philadelphia, 1967. *D:* From J. Jancar, *Int. Copenhagen Congress on M.R.* [J. Øster, ed.], Vol. 1, pp. 179–95, 1964. *E* and *F:* Courtesy of Dr. L. Atkins, Boston, Mass.)

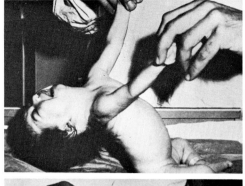
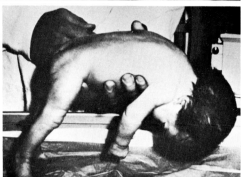
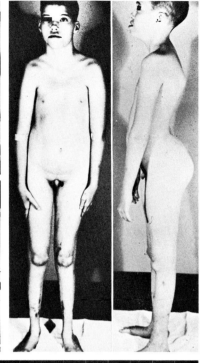
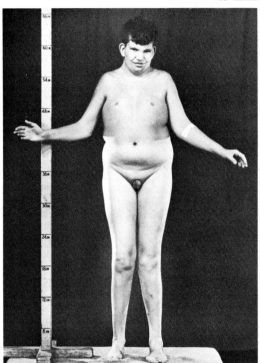
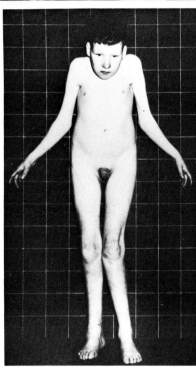
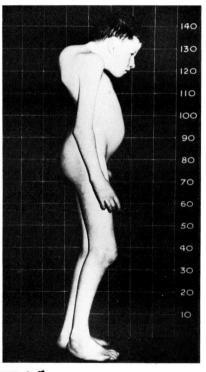
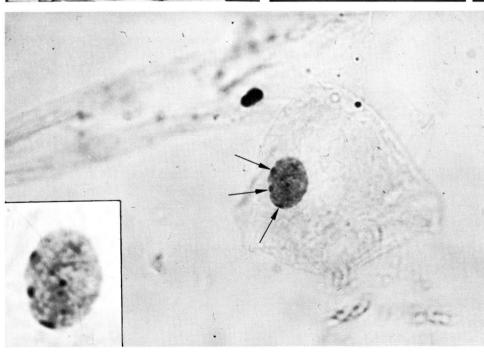

Chapter V
Central Nervous System Malformations

Introduction

This chapter is concerned with central nervous system malformations that can be diagnosed by their associated physical features. The disorders discussed are quite heterogenous and relate to many different parts of the nervous system. To put these malformations in proper perspective one should know the incidence of all malformations in both individuals with normal intelligence and those with mental retardation. These data are not available. Two limited types of data are (1) the prevalence of nervous system malformations in newborn infants and (2) the neuropathologic diagnoses from the autopsies of patients in institutions for the mentally retarded.

Studies of liveborn and stillborn infants have shown that nervous system malformations are the most common major malformations. In a study of 8684 births by Nelson and Forfar [1], 133 major malformations were found in 8512 liveborns and 54 major malformations in 172 stillborns. The prevalence of all nervous system malformations in relation to other major malformations and the prevalence of the most common types of nervous system malformations were as follows:

	Number Liveborn	Prevalence per 1000 Livebirths	Number Stillbirths	Prevalence per 1000 Stillbirths	Total Number Births	Prevalence per 1000 Total Births
A. Central Nervous System Anomalies 39%*						
1. Anencephaly	4	0.5	27	157	31	3.6
2. Spina bifida (including meningomyelocele)	16	1.9	12	70	28	3.2
3. Hydrocephaly	5	0.6			5	0.6
4. Encephalocele	5	0.6	1	6	6	0.7
5. Microcephaly	2	0.2			2	0.2
Total	32	3.8	40	233	72	8.4
B. Cardiovascular 21%*	39	4.5	1	6	40	4.5
C. Alimentary 16%	24	2.8	5	29	29	3.4
D. Skeletal 6%	10	1.2	2	12	12	1.4
E. Renal 4%	6	0.7	1	6	7	0.8
F. Respiratory 2%	3	0.3	1	6	4	0.4
G. Other 6%	9	0.9	3	18	12	1.2
H. Chromosomal abnormalities 6%	10	1.2	1	6	11	1.3

*Percentage of all congenital anomalies.

These data indicate that many of the disorders discussed in this chapter could be considered common structural malformations, with the incidence ranging from 0.2 per 1000 to 1.9 per 1000 livebirths. However, there are obvious limitations in data obtained from examining newborns. First, one of the most common anomalies, anencephaly, is incompatible with survival. Second, some types of malformations, such as microcephaly and hydrocephalus, are often not evident at birth.

The neuropathologic diagnoses made in autopsied patients from institutions for the retarded provide another perspective. It should be remembered that such patients are highly selected; not only have they survived long enough to be admitted to an institution, but in general a low IQ (often less than 70) is required for admission. The data from three studies are tabulated as follows:

	Freytag and Lindenberg [2]	Benda [3]	Malamud [4]
Total deaths	712		
Total autopsies	359		
Autopsies with pathologic conditions	297	258	512
Malformations	93	36	107
Arnold-Chiari anomalies	18		
Microgyria, pachygyria, and agyria	18		
Microcephaly	9		
Agenesis of corpus callosum	8		
Porencephaly	7		
Ectopic gray matter	6		
Abnormal convolutional pattern	6		
Arhinencephaly	4		
Malformation of brainstem	4		
Meningoencephalocele	3		
Hydranencephaly	2		
Macrocephaly	1		
Other anomalies	7		
Oligoencephaly*		40	175
Mongolism	31	55	97
Other diagnoses	173	127	133

*This term refers to patients whose brains showed no specific lesions that could be otherwise classified. In many instances these brains showed asymmetry, anomalous cells, and disorders of differentiation. They showed insufficient structural development of the nervous system which was the basis for considering these brains as different from true microcephaly [3].

Many of these malformations can be diagnosed by physical examination. The challenge for the clinician is to see if more cerebral malformations can be clinically recognized. The best recent example of progress in this area is the recognition of craniofacial anomalies associated with lissencephaly (see page 198). Another possibility is the association of a specific facial appearance in individuals with agenesis of the corpus callosum [5,6].

The practical value of the early detection of the malformations in this chapter is related to both the child and his family. Often the child's survival and intelligence are affected by the early recognition of lesions that can be surgically repaired. Also, the family benefits from knowing the affected child's prognosis and the risk of recurrence of the same disorder in subsequent children.

References

1. Nelson, M. M., and Forfar, J. O. Congenital abnormalities at birth: their association in the same patient. *Dev. Med. Child. Neurol.*, 11:3–16, 1969.
2. Freytag, E., and Lindenberg, R. Neuropathologic findings in patients of a hospital for the mentally deficient. A survey of 359 cases. *Johns Hopkins Med. J.*, 121:379–92, 1967.
3. Benda, C. E. Structural cerebral histopathology of mental deficiencies. In *Proceedings of First International Congress of Neuropathology* (Rome), Vol. 2, 1952, pp. 7–50.
4. Malamud, N. *Proceedings of First International Congress of Neuropathology* (Rome), 1952, Vol. 2, pp. 261–74.
5. Andermann, E., Andermann, F., and Melancon, D. Three familial midline malformation syndromes of the central nervous system. (Abstract.) IVth International Congress of Human Genetics, Paris, 1971, p. 15.
6. Passarge, E., and Colmant, H. G. A familial disorder of dolicocephaly, agenesis of the corpus callosum, hydrocephaly, and diffuse myelin defects with sclerosis of the telencephalon and cerebellum. (Abstract.) IVth International Congress of Human Genetics, Paris, 1971, p. 139.

Microcephaly Syndromes

A child is considered microcephalic if its head circumference is more than two standard deviations below the mean for children of its age and sex [1]. In general, the children with the smallest heads are the most severely retarded. However, it must also be stressed that every microcephalic individual is not mentally retarded [2]. The causes of microcephaly include a variety of environmental factors, acquired conditions, and hereditary disorders:

1. Maternal factors
   a. Intrauterine infections (e.g., rubella, cytomegalovirus) (see Chapter III)
   b. Hyperphenylalaninemia [3] (see page 46)
   c. Radiation [4]
2. Perinatal factors
   a. Perinatal anoxia
   b. Meningitis
3. Head trauma with multiple skull fractures and subdural hematomas (see page 140)
4. Chromosomal abnormalities (e.g., trisomy 13, 5p— syndrome) (See Chapter IV)
5. Hereditary multiple congenital anomaly syndromes (e.g., Seckel's bird-headed dwarfism, Fanconi's anemia) (see Chapter VI)
6. Microcephaly syndromes
   a. Alpers' disease (see page 74)
   b. Chorioretinopathy with hereditary microcephaly [5]
   c. Tapetoretinal degeneration with microcephaly [6]
   d. Congenital microcephaly with hiatus hernia and nephrotic syndrome [7]
   e. Cutis verticis gyrata [8] (*Figures A, B, C, and D*)
   f. Polymicrogyria [9]
   g. Lissencephaly syndrome (see page 198)
   h. Autosomal recessive microcephaly [10–12]
   i. X-linked microcephaly [13]
   j. "Pure" microcephaly (see below)

"Pure" or "True" Microcephaly (Microcephaly Vera)

"Pure" or *"true" microcephaly* is the term used to refer to patients whose microcephaly is unexplained and who have no associated congenital anomalies. Presumably patients with autosomal recessive [10–12] and X-linked [13] microcephaly are often placed in this group, for they have a similar appearance. The most striking feature is the contrast between the small size of the cranium and the normal size of the face. The forehead is low and narrow and recedes sharply; the occiput is flat and the vertex is somewhat pointed (*Figures A, B, C, E, and F*). Microcephaly may be evident at birth (*Figure E*) or not until the child is several months old. Many of these patients are below normal in height. Spasticity of all limbs, but especially the legs, is common. True microcephalics are usually retarded, often severely so. Skull x-rays show a small cranium, normal sutures, and no evidence of increased intracranial pressure (*Figure D*).

References

1. Pryor, H. B., and Thelander, H. Abnormally small head size and intellect in children. *J. Pediatr.,* **73**:593–98, 1968.
2. Martin, H. P. Microcephaly and mental retardation. *Am. J. Dis. Child.,* **119**:128–31, 1970.
3. Frankenburg, W. K., Duncan, B. R., Coffelt, R. W., Koch, R., Coldwell, J. G., and Son, C. D. Maternal phenylketonuria: implications for growth and development. *J. Pediatr.,* **73**:560–70, 1968.
4. Wood, J. W., Johnson, K. G., and Omori, Y. *In utero* exposure to the Hiroshima atomic bomb. An evaluation of head size and mental retardation: Twenty years later. *Pediatrics,* **39**:385–92, 1967.
5. McKusick, V. A., Stauffer, M., Knox, D. L., and Clark, D. B. Chorioretinopathy with hereditary microcephaly. *Arch. Ophthalmol.,* **75**:597–600, 1966.
6. Schmidt, B., Jaeger, W., and Newbauer, H. Ein Mikrozephalie-Syndrom mit atypischer tapetoretinaler Degeneration bei 3 Geschwistern. *Klin. Monatsbl. Augenheilkd.,* **150**:188–96, 1967.
7. Galloway, W. H., and Mowat, A. P. Congenital microcephaly with hiatus hernia and nephrotic syndrome in two sibs. *J. Med. Genet.,* **5**:319–21, 1968.
8. MacGillivray, R. C. Cutis verticis gyrata and mental retardation. *Scott. Med. J.,* **12**:450–54, 1967.
9. Crome, L. Microgyria. *J. Pathol.,* **64**:479–95, 1952.
10. Kloepfer, H. W., Platou, R. V., and Hansche, W. J. Manifestations of a recessive gene for microcephaly in a population isolate. *J. Genet. Hum.,* **13**:52–59, 1964.
11. van den Bosch, J. Microcephaly in the Netherlands: a clinical and genetical study. *Ann. Hum. Genet.,* **23**:91–116, 1959.
12. Böök, J. A., Schut, J. W., and Reed, S. C. A clinical and genetical study of microcephaly. *Am. J. Ment. Defic.,* **57**:637–60, 1953.
13. Paine, R. S. Evaluation of familial biochemically determined mental retardation in children, with special reference to aminoaciduria. *N. Engl. J. Med.,* **262**:658–65, 1960.

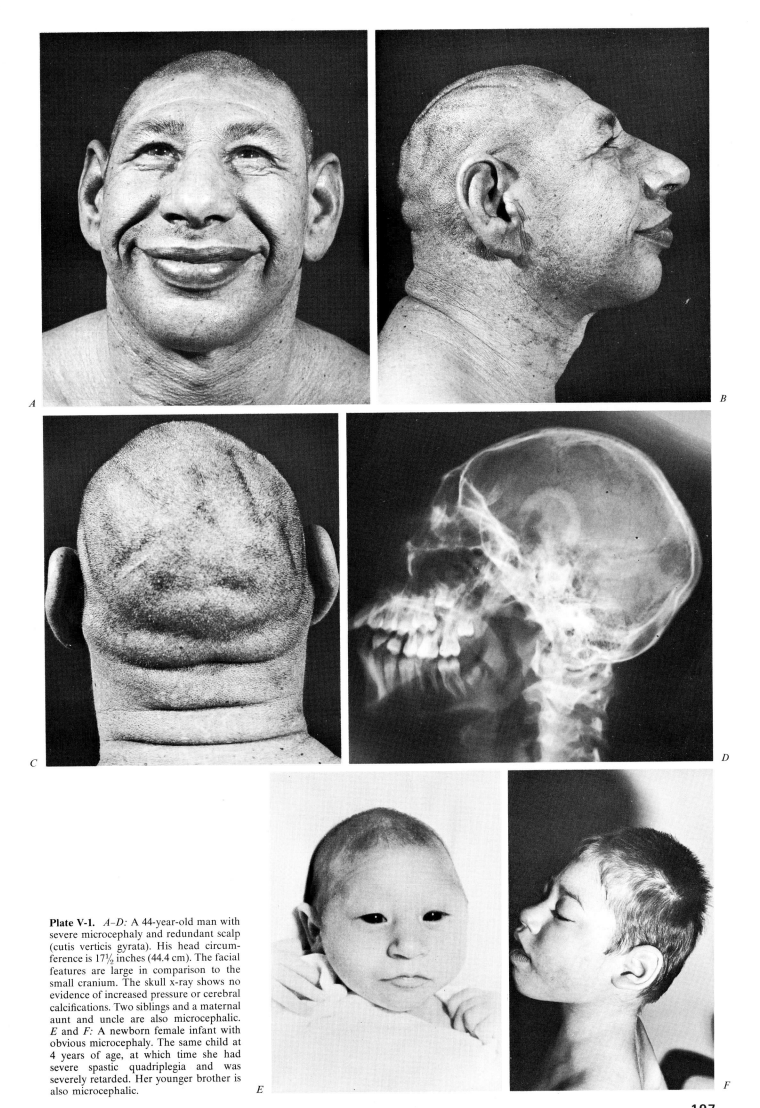

Plate V-1. *A–D:* A 44-year-old man with severe microcephaly and redundant scalp (cutis verticis gyrata). His head circumference is 17½ inches (44.4 cm). The facial features are large in comparison to the small cranium. The skull x-ray shows no evidence of increased pressure or cerebral calcifications. Two siblings and a maternal aunt and uncle are also microcephalic. *E* and *F:* A newborn female infant with obvious microcephaly. The same child at 4 years of age, at which time she had severe spastic quadriplegia and was severely retarded. Her younger brother is also microcephalic.

197

Lissencephaly Syndrome

The term *lissencephaly* means "smooth brain." It refers to a severe form of cerebral maldevelopment in which the gyri are wide and the sulci shallow, or both are entirely absent. Until recently this diagnosis could be made only at autopsy. However, seven infants with lissencephaly have been described [1–4] who had similar facial anomalies, which suggests that this syndrome may now be recognized clinically. Whether the clinically recognizable patients are a specific subgroup of the patients with lissencephaly will only be known when careful clinical-neuropathologic examinations have been performed on a large number of children with lissencephaly.

Physical Features

HEAD: All of the patients were microcephalic. Several had a hollowing or groove in the anterior temporal area.

FACE: The child described by Josephy [1] in 1944 had a slanting forehead and the facial features were "ferretlike." The other six patients [2–4] have been described in more detail and seem to have similar features: a high forehead, slight anteversion of the nostrils, slight upward palpebral slant, widely spaced eyes, and micrognathia (*Figures A, B, C, D, and E*).

EYES: Two patients had circumlimbal corneal clouding [4].

EARS: The ears were considered low-set in two patients [2]; in four patients they were posteriorly rotated and had incomplete or abnormal development of the helix [3,4].

ABDOMEN: Three patients had an enlarged liver and spleen [3,4]. The males have had undescended testes associated with inguinal hernias.

LIMBS: Two patients had unilateral polydactyly [2,4].

Nervous System

At birth these patients were quite hypotonic and had a weak cry, difficulty with feeding, and little spontaneous movement. They were often apneic and had feeble respirations. Gradually they developed opisthotonic posturing and, in some cases, hyperactive deep tendon reflexes. In general, these patients showed no psychomotor development and their posture became decerebrate. They had little response to any visual stimuli, light, or sound. Seizures, which were often difficult to control, occurred within the first weeks of life.

Pathology

The brains were smooth and had few, if any, visible sulci or gyri (*Figure F*). The ventricles were large and the white matter was hypoplastic. In general, the cortex was wide and the normal cortical laminations were absent. There were heterotopias of neurons in both the medulla and cerebellum [1–4]. Cardiac anomalies of several different types were de-scribed in four out of six patients in whom the complete postmortem findings were recorded [2–4]. Two siblings had agenesis of one kidney; one child also had duodenal atresia [2].

Laboratory Studies

Pneumoencephalograms showed dilated ventricles. A variety of electroencephalographic changes, especially generalized hypsarrhythmia, were described.

Treatment and Prognosis

All seven patients died within the first year of life. Their clinical course was characterized by a poor suck, regurgitation, aspiration, and severe failure to thrive.

Genetics

Autosomal recessive inheritance is suggested by the fact that there were two affected siblings in each of two unrelated families [2,4] in a total of seven cases.

Differential Diagnosis

1. Lissencephaly, severe hypotonia, microcephaly, a prominent forehead, hepatomegaly, cryptorchidism and death in infancy are features of patients with the cerebrohepatorenal syndrome, but they also have flexion contractures, renal cortical cysts, and ocular anomalies (see page 270).
2. Anteverted nostrils, a wide medial canthus, polydactyly, and cryptorchidism are features of patients with the Smith-Lemli-Optiz syndrome, but they have a broad maxillary alveolar ridge, ptosis, hypospadias in males, and less severe neurologic deficits (see page 312).
3. Two brothers have been described with lissencephaly, mental retardation, and hypertelorism who also had progressive spastic paraplegia and died at the ages of 9 and 19 years. Their mother had hypertelorism and mild seizures [5].

References

1. Josephy, H. Congenital agyria and defect of the corpus callosum. *J. Neuropathol. Exp. Neurol.,* **3**:63–68, 1944.
2. Miller, J. Q. Lissencephaly in two siblings. *Neurology (Minneap.),* **13**:841–50, 1963.
3. Daube, J. R., and Chou, S. M. Lissencephaly: two cases. *Neurology (Minneap.),* **16**:179–91, 1966.
4. Dieker, H., Edwards, R. H., ZuRhein, G., Chou, S. M., Hartman, H. A., and Opitz, J. M. The lissencephaly syndrome. *Birth Defects: Original Article Series,* Vol. V, No. 2., Feb., 1969, pp. 53–64. Williams & Wilkins Co., Baltimore.
5. Reznik, M., and Alberca-Serrano, R. Forme familiale d'hypertélorisme avec lissencéphalie se présentant cliniquement sous forme d'une arriération mentale avec epilepsie et paraplégie spasmodique. *J. Neurol. Sci.,* **1**:40–58, 1964.

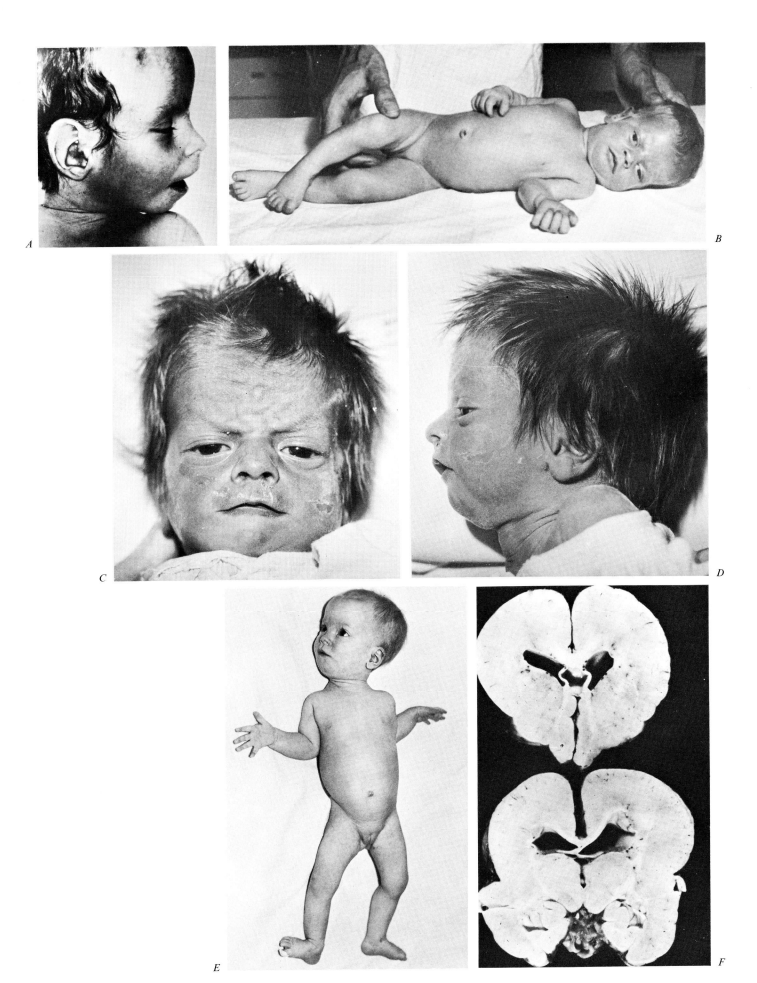

Plate V-2. *A:* One of two affected siblings, both of whom had a flat nasal bridge, a "hollowed-out" temporal area, and a small chin. *B:* A 4-month-old infant, a first cousin of the patient shown in *C* and *D*, with a prominent forehead, microcephaly, and hypotonia. *C* and *D:* A 2-week-old infant with a prominent forehead, marked wrinkling of the skin, a downward palpebral slant, a small chin, and microcephaly. *E* and *F:* A 7-month-old infant with a prominent forehead and occiput, temporal grooving, a small chin, persistent turning of the head to the right, and hypotonia. Cross sections of her brain at two levels show smoothness of the cortex, absence of sulci, and large ventricles. (*A:* From J. Q. Miller, *Neurology* [*Minneap.*], **13:**841–50, 1963. *B–E:* From H. Dieker *et al., Birth Defects: Original Article Series,* Vol. V, No. 2, Feb., 1969, pp. 53–64. Williams & Wilkins Co., Baltimore. *F:* From J. R. Daube and S. M. Chou, *Neurology* [*Minneap.*], **16:**179–91, 1966.)

Macrocephaly Syndromes
Stenosis of the Aqueduct of Sylvius

Obstruction of the aqueduct of Sylvius may result from a variety of pathologic conditions: congenital narrowing of the aqueduct, a membrane across the aqueduct, ependymitis, periaqueductal gliosis, pressure from an adjacent tumor, or herniation of the cerebellum and fourth ventricle (as in the Arnold-Chiari malformation) [1]. Among infants with hydrocephalus, aqueductal narrowing or stenosis is common; in a study of 44 hydrocephalic infants Elvidge [2] found aqueductal stenosis in 30 percent. Most patients with aqueductal stenosis have no similarly affected family members, but there are at least two types of hereditary aqueductal stenosis, which will be briefly described.

X-Linked Aqueductal Stenosis

In 1949 Bickers and Adams [3] reported a family in which seven male infants in two generations had had massive head enlargement at birth. Subsequently, more than 30 additional patients have been reported [4–8]. The head enlargement is generalized and is often present at birth (*Figure A*). Often the head is so large that ventriculotomy is necessary before vaginal delivery can be completed. A few patients have had less severe hydrocephalus at birth and have lived for several years, but have been mentally retarded [4] (*Figure B*). Autopsy studies [3–5,7,8] have shown that the most severe aqueductal narrowing is at the level of the trochlear nerve. It was initially presumed that only aqueductal narrowing would be present, but forking has also been observed in two families, including the first reported family [7–9]. X-linked aqueductal stenosis appears to be a relatively localized malformation, and there are usually no extracranial anomalies. Abnormally flexed thumbs have been reported, but they appear to be the result of the hydrocephalus. A few patients have been treated with ventriculoatrial shunts [6]. However, the patients with marked hydrocephalus at birth would have a poor prognosis for adequate psychomotor development even if the surgery were successful. In five families [3–8] with 37 affected males this deformity was transmitted as an X-linked recessive mutant gene.

Familial Aqueductal Stenosis and Basilar Impression

In 1968 Sajid and Copple [10] reported two brothers in whom the symptoms of hydrocephalus developed insidiously when they were young adults. The first had mildly delayed developmental milestones and an IQ of 84 at 15 years of age. At 18 he began to have difficulty in walking and subsequently developed optic atrophy, spastic diplegia, dysarthria, and athetoid posturing. At 39 he had a large, brachycephalic skull (circumference, 56 cm) (*Figure C*). Skull x-rays showed basilar impression and evidence of chronically increased intracranial pressure (*Figure D*). Pneumoencephalography and ventriculography (*Figure E*) showed complete aqueductal obstruction. The second patient was studied because he also had a brachycephalic appearance (*Figure F*). At 27 years he had a mildly spastic gait, hyperactive deep tendon reflexes in the legs, and a large head (circumference, 56.8 cm). The visual fields were mildly constricted in the periphery. X-ray studies showed findings almost identical with those of his brother: basilar impression, aqueductal stenosis, and obstructive hydrocephalus. Both patients benefited from the insertion of ventriculoatrial shunts.

References

1. Drachman, D. A., and Richardson, E. P., Jr. Aqueductal narrowing, congenital and acquired. *Arch. Neurol.* (*Chicago*), **5**:552–59, 1961.
2. Elvidge, A. R. Treatment of obstructive lesions of the aqueduct of Sylvius and the fourth ventricle by interventriculostomy. *J. Neurosurg.*, **24**:11–23, 1966.
3. Bickers, D. S., and Adams, R. D. Hereditary stenosis of the aqueduct of Sylvius as a cause of congenital hydrocephalus. *Brain*, **72**:246–62, 1949.
4. Edwards, J. H., Norman, R. M., and Roberts, J. M. Sex-linked hydrocephalus: report of a family with 15 affected members. *Arch. Dis. Child.*, **36**:481–85, 1961.
5. Warren, M., Lu, A. T., and Ziering, W. H. Sex-linked hydrocephalus with aqueductal stenosis. *J. Pediatr.*, **63**:1104–10, 1963.
6. Shannon, M. W., and Nadler, H. L. X-linked hydrocephalus. *J. Med. Genet.*, **5**:326–28, 1968.
7. Opitz, J. M., ZuRhein, G. M., Bilbo, R. E., and Eggman, L. D. Hydrocephalus due to a recessive X-linked gene. (Abstract.) Society for Pediatric Research, Atlantic City, 1963.
8. Holmes, L. B., and Nash, A. Hereditary aqueductal stenosis: a comparison of pathology in two generations. (Abstract.) American Society of Human Genetics, Toronto, 1967.
9. Opitz, J. M. Personal communication, 1969.
10. Sajid, M. H., and Copple, P. J. Familial aqueductal stenosis and basilar impression. *Neurology* (*Minneap.*), **18**:260–62, 1968.

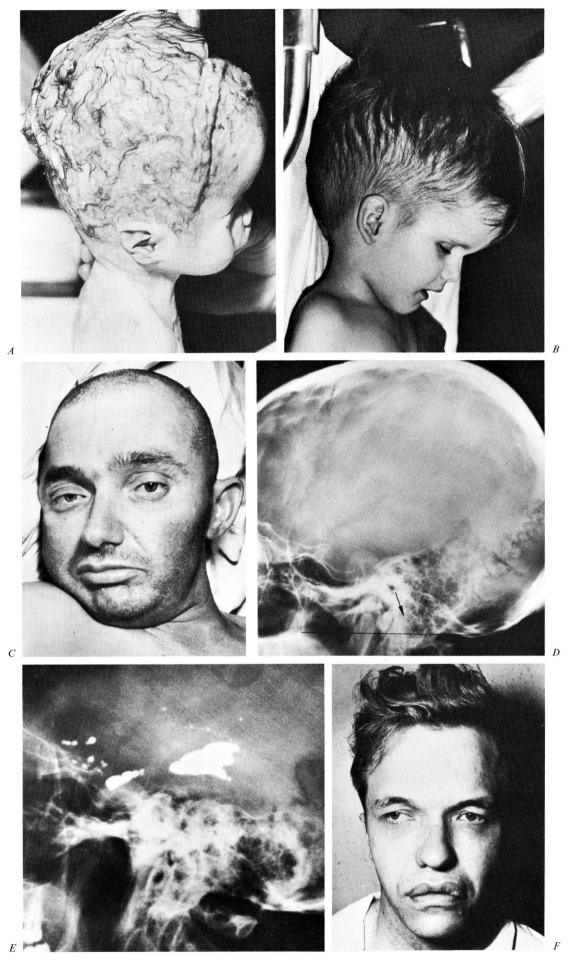

A

B

C

D

E

F

Plate V-3. *A:* A postmortem photograph of a child in the first reported family, showing generalized head enlargement (circumference 53 cm) which necessitated ventriculotomy and the removal of 1500 ml of ventricular fluid before vaginal delivery could be completed. *B:* Another male with hydrocephalus due to X-linked aqueductal stenosis. *C:* Shows an obtunded 39-year-old man with the second syndrome of aqueductal stenosis and basilar impression; he had signs of progressive increased intracranial pressure and a head circumference of 56 cm. *D.* Shows in this man the projection of the odontoid process (*arrow*) 11 mm above McGregor's line, demineralization of posterior clinoid processes, and prominent convolutional markings. *E:* The ventriculogram in this man, showing complete aqueductal obstruction. *F:* The 27-year-old brother of the man shown above. He also had obstructive hydrocephalus, aqueductal stenosis, and basilar impression, but was not mentally retarded. (*B:* Courtesy of Dr. J. M. Opitz, Madison, Wisc. *C* and *F:* Courtesy of Dr. P. J. Copple, Portland, Ore. *D* and *E:* From M. H. Sajid and P. J. Copple, *Neurology* [*Minneap.*], **18:**260–62, 1968.)

Dandy-Walker Syndrome

Hydrocephalus due to cystic enlargement of the fourth ventricle is called the Dandy-Walker syndrome because of the contributions of these two men in describing this malformation [1-3]. The enlargement is usually associated with atresia of the foramina of Luschka and Magendie in the roof of the fourth ventricle and distortion of the midline portion of the cerebellum. While the cause is not known, two theories of the origin of this anomaly are that there is failure of development of these foramina [4] and that there is a meningocelelike sac in place of the posterior medullary velum with cleft formation of the cerebellum [5]. The incidence of the Dandy-Walker syndrome is not known.

Physical Features

HEAD: Some newborns have head enlargement at birth [5]. Others have a normal head size at birth, but rapid enlargement in the first weeks of life [6]. The most characteristic feature is prominence of the occiput. Increased transillumination may be demonstrated over the occiput. Some patients later develop prominence of the brow and a dolichocephalic head shape with a long anteroposterior diameter [5] (*Figure A*).

Nervous System

These infants are often first evaluated because of head enlargement, slow psychomotor development, and sometimes seizures. If the hydrocephalus is extensive, a "cracked-pot" sound may be elicited by tapping the occiput. They may also have increased muscle tone and deep tendon reflexes in the legs [4-7]. Signs of cerebellar dysfunction are usually not present.

Pathology

The dilated fourth ventricle expands posteriorly, laterally, and sometimes downward into the cervical spinal canal (*Figure B*). The cisterna magna is undeveloped. The midline structures of the cerebellum are deficient, and the cerebellar hemispheres are displaced laterally (*Figure C*). The pons, medulla, and upper cervical cord are flat, broad, and displaced anteriorly. The entire tentorium, including its site of attachment to the cranial vault, is displaced upward, carrying with it the transverse sinuses and the torcular. There is symmetric internal hydrocephalus involving the aqueduct of Sylvius and the third and lateral ventricles [5].

Laboratory Studies

X-rays show that the cranial vault is enlarged, the sutures are separated, and there is bulging in the occipital area. The lambdoid suture, which is usually the least separated in other types of hydrocephalus, is widely separated. The tentorial insertion, as outlined by the imprint of the transverse sinuses on the cranial vault, has an oblique slant [4,7] (*Figure D*). On pneumoencephalography the air fills the dilated fourth ventricle and may extend downward in the cervical canal (*Figure E*).

Treatment and Prognosis

Infants with early and successful excision of the fourth ventricle cyst may have normal psychomotor development. Most patients require an additional shunting procedure to control the hydrocephalus.

Genetics

There is no definite evidence that this malformation is inherited. However, one family has been reported [5] in which three siblings had the Dandy-Walker syndrome.

Differential Diagnosis

1. Extraaxial cysts originating from the pia-arachnoid in the posterior fossa can cause both increased transillumination of the posterior fossa and hydrocephalus. The differentiation of these cysts can be made by careful clinical and radiologic studies [8].
2. Patients with hydrocephalus due to hydranencephaly (see page 204), aqueductal stenosis (see page 200), or meningomyelocele with Arnold-Chiari malformation (see page 212) may also have head enlargement at birth. However, they do not have the same striking enlargement of the occipital area as patients with the Dandy-Walker syndrome.
3. Two infants with dysmorphogenesis of joints, brain, and palate also had a Dandy-Walker malformation (see page 278).
4. Three male siblings with a syndrome of aqueductal stenosis and polycystic kidneys have been reported with one child having hydrocephalus at birth and a Dandy-Walker malformation [6].

References

1. Dandy, W. E. The diagnosis and treatment of hydrocephalus due to occlusions of the foramina of Magendie and Luschka. *Surg. Gynecol. Obstet.,* **32:**112–24, 1921.
2. Taggart, J. K., and Walker, A. E. Congenital atresia of the foramens of Luschka and Magendie. *Arch. Neurol. Psychiatr.,* **48:**583–612, 1942.
3. Walker, A. E. A case of congenital atresia of the foramina of Luschka and Magendie: surgical cure. *J. Neuropathol. Exp. Neurol.,* **3:**368–73, 1944.
4. Gibson, J. B. Congenital hydrocephalus due to atresia of the foramen of Magendie. *J. Neuropathol. Exp. Neurol.,* **14:**244–62, 1955.
5. Benda, C. E. The Dandy-Walker syndrome or the so-called atresia of the foramen Magendie. *J. Neuropathol. Exp. Neurol.,* **13:**14–29, 1954.
6. D'Agostino, A. N., Kernohan, J. W., and Brown, J. R. The Dandy-Walker syndrome. *J. Neuropathol. Exp. Neurol.,* **22:**450–70, 1963.
7. Matson, D. D. Prenatal obstruction of the fourth ventricle. *Am. J. Roentgenol.,* **76:**499–506, 1956.
8. Haller, J. S., Wolpert, S. M., Rabe, E. F., and Hills, J. R. Cystic lesions of the posterior fossa in infants: a comparison of the clinical, radiological, and pathological findings in Dandy-Walker syndrome and extra-axial cysts. *Neurology (Minneap.),* **21:**494–506, 1971.

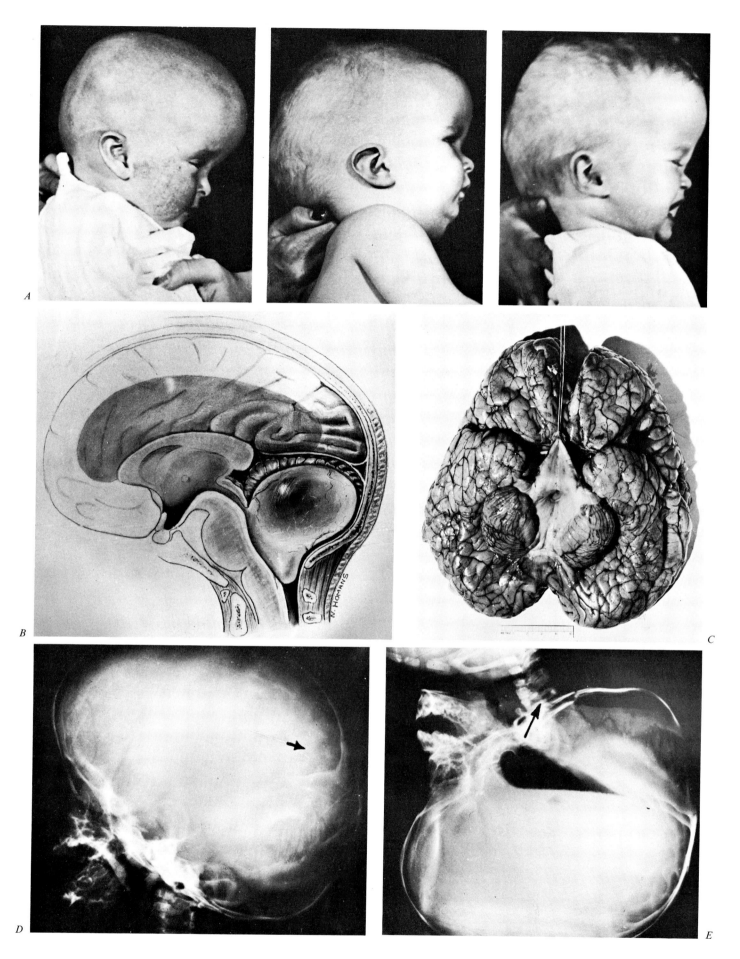

Plate V-4. *A:* Affected infants, aged 5, 5, and 1½ months, who have prominence of the frontal and occipital areas in varying degrees. *B:* Sagittal diagram showing the large fourth ventricle cyst and the elevation of the tentorium. *C:* View of the base of a brain showing the division of the cerebellum by the large fourth ventricle cyst, the top of which is retracted upward. *D:* Shows the high insertion of the tentorium (*arrow*) and the thin cranium; wide separation of the lambdoid sutures is barely visible. *E:* Pneumoencephalogram with the patient upside down, which shows the large air-filled cyst and the protrusion of this cyst down into the cervical vertebral canal (*arrow*) of this 8-week-old infant. (*A, C–E:* From D. D. Matson, *Am. J. Roentgenol.,* **76:**499–506, 1956. *B:* From F. D. Ingraham and D. D. Matson, *Neurosurgery of Infancy and Childhood,* 1954. Courtesy of Charles C Thomas, Publisher, Springfield, Ill.)

Hydranencephaly (Hydrencephaly)

The term *hydranencephaly* designates a severe cerebral defect in which the cerebral hemispheres are almost totally replaced by membranous sacs, but the meninges and cranium are intact. The term *hydrencephaly* has been suggested to distinguish this condition from anencephaly with fluid accumulation [1]. The incidence of hydranencephaly is not known; more than 60 cases had been reported by 1961 [2].

Physical Features

HEAD: At birth the infant may look normal, but a generalized head enlargement usually becomes evident in the first weeks of life (*Figure A*). The sutures become widely separated and a "cracked-pot" sound can be easily elicited. Increased transillumination of the skull is present over the area of the cerebral defect [3] (*Figures B and D*). However, increased transillumination may not be present in the first weeks of life, presumably because of the composition of the fluid, in particular protein and blood, within the membrane [4].

EYES: The optic discs are usually pale [2].

Nervous System

The affected newborn may show all of the normal neonatal reflexes and responses for several weeks. Thereafter, his lack of psychomotor development becomes apparent. Difficulty with swallowing, frequent screaming, incoordinated eye movements, deviations of conjugate gaze, strabismus, nystagmus, seizures, and hypothermia are other common signs of neurologic deterioration. The muscle tone may be normal initially, but the deep tendon reflexes soon become hyperactive. In a study [2] of three infants it was found that while they did not appear to see, the optical blinking reflex was preserved. This suggests that the pathways for this reflex were subcortical in these infants. Studies [4] on another 10-week-old infant showed behavioral responses to both auditory and visual stimuli.

Pathology

The cerebral hemispheres are entirely or almost entirely absent (*Figure C*), and a large thin-walled sac of fluid surrounded by a membrane of leptomeninges and a layer of glial tissue is present [1,4] (*Figure F*).

Laboratory Studies

The electroencephalogram usually shows complete absence of activity in all leads. One infant, who showed no response to visual stimuli on conventionally recorded electroencephalograms, was found by electronic averaging to have small-amplitude stereotyped responses [4]. In pneumoencephalography the cranium fills with air out to the periphery of the cavity, and the contour of the ventricles is not shown. Angiography usually shows attenuation of the cerebral vessels, particularly the branches of the internal carotid arteries, and normal external carotid circulation.

Treatment and Prognosis

Most affected infants are either stillborn or die in early infancy. One infant who survived to $4\frac{1}{2}$ years of age showed no psychomotor development [1]. A striking exception to the poor prognosis of these patients is one infant in whom no cerebral cortex could be demonstrated, but whose psychomotor development was normal at 21 months [5] (*Figure D*). At 5 years he had an IQ of 74 and was attending school [6].

Genetics

No similarly affected family members have been reported.

Differential Diagnosis

1. Increased transillumination over the cerebrum is also a feature of infants with porencephaly, but their cerebral defects are usually smaller and associated hydrocephalus is uncommon. The distinction can be made with certainty only at autopsy [7].
2. Infants with X-linked aqueductal stenosis will have severe generalized head enlargement at birth or in the first months of life with spreading of the sutures and marked transillumination, but show less transillumination and a more normal electroencephalogram (see page 200).
3. Infants with the Dandy-Walker syndrome gradually develop hydrocephalus, but usually the occiput is prominent and is the only area of increased transillumination (see page 202).

References

1. Crome, L., and Sylvester, P. E. Hydranencephaly (hydrencephaly). *Arch. Dis. Child.,* **33**:235–45, 1958.
2. Hill, K., Cogan, D. G., and Dodge, P. R. Ocular signs associated with hydranencephaly. *Am. J. Ophthalmol.,* **51**:267–75, 1961.
3. Hamby, W. B., Krauss, R. F., and Beswick, W. F. Hydranencephaly: clinical diagnosis. Presentation of seven cases. *Pediatrics,* **6**:371–83, 1950.
4. Barnet, A., Bazelon, M., and Zappella, M. Visual and auditory function in an hydranencephalic infant. *Brain Res.,* **2**:351–60, 1966.
5. Lorber, J. Hydranencephaly with normal development. *Dev. Med. Child Neurol.,* **7**:628–33, 1965.
6. Lorber, J. Personal communication, 1969.
7. Yakovlev, P. I., and Wadsworth, R. C. Schizencephalies. A study of the congenital clefts in the cerebral mantle. II. Clefts with hydrocephalus and lips separated. *J. Neuropathol. Exp. Neurol.,* **5**:169–205, 1946.

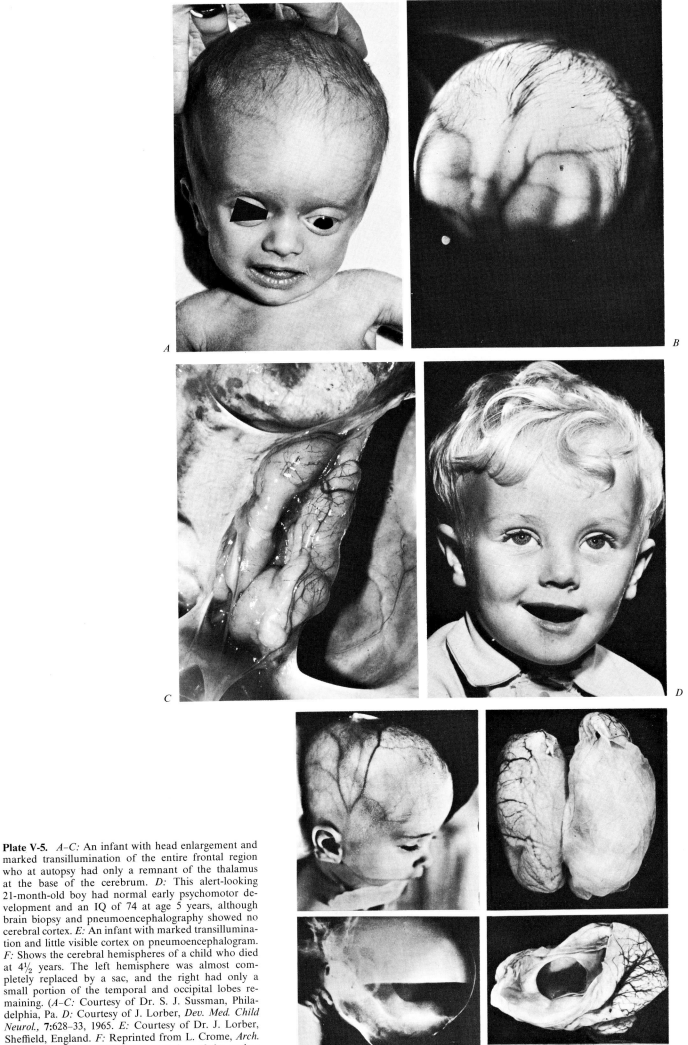

Plate V-5. *A–C:* An infant with head enlargement and marked transillumination of the entire frontal region who at autopsy had only a remnant of the thalamus at the base of the cerebrum. *D:* This alert-looking 21-month-old boy had normal early psychomotor development and an IQ of 74 at age 5 years, although brain biopsy and pneumoencephalography showed no cerebral cortex. *E:* An infant with marked transillumination and little visible cortex on pneumoencephalogram. *F:* Shows the cerebral hemispheres of a child who died at 4½ years. The left hemisphere was almost completely replaced by a sac, and the right had only a small portion of the temporal and occipital lobes remaining. (*A–C:* Courtesy of Dr. S. J. Sussman, Philadelphia, Pa. *D:* Courtesy of J. Lorber, *Dev. Med. Child Neurol.,* **7:**628–33, 1965. *E:* Courtesy of Dr. J. Lorber, Sheffield, England. *F:* Reprinted from L. Crome, *Arch. Dis. Child.,* **33:**235, 1958, by permission of the author and editor.)

Holotelencephaly (Arhinencephaly)

The term *holotelencephaly* refers to the group of anomalies in which there is only one cerebral ventricle, no sagittal cleavage into two cerebral hemispheres, defective evagination of olfactory and optic structures, and abnormalities of the corpus callosum, hippocampus, and basal ganglia (*Figure B*). This group of anomalies has also been designated as arhinencephaly. There are at least four types of facial anomalies associated with holotelencephaly: cyclopia, ethmocephaly, cebocephaly, and cleft lip with hypotelorism.

Cyclopia, Ethmocephaly, and Cebocephaly

These three rare facial deformities are discussed together because they constitute a morphologic spectrum. Also, they are all incompatible with prolonged survival. The incidence of these malformations is not known. As the reported patients have often had chromosomal abnormalities, the associated visceral and skeletal anomalies will not be enumerated.

Physical Features

FACE: The cyclops deformity consists of a single orbital fossa and a single diamond-shaped palpebral fissure (*Figures A and C*). The orbit may contain no globe tissue, a rudimentary eye, a single eye, or two small but fairly complete eyeballs that are closely adjacent. The eyelids are rudimentary or absent. There is no nose, but instead a proboscis above the eye. The proboscis is a tubular appendage with a single cavity that ends blindly at the surface of the skull and has no communication with the nasopharynx [1].

The term *ethmocephaly* designates severe orbital hypotelorism with two separate orbits, a proboscis above the eyes, and no normal nose (*Figures D and E*).

Individuals with cebocephaly have orbital hypotelorism and a proboscislike structure at the usual site of the nose (*Figure F*). This structure has no bony elements. Its single opening is lined with mucous epithelium and ends blindly [2].

MOUTH: In two patients with cyclopia there was a double cleft which started in the alveolar ridge and included both the hard and soft palate [1,3]. One patient had fusion of the tongue to the lower jaw by a thick frenulum [1]. Cleft palate is also present in some infants with cebocephaly.

Pathology

In addition to holotelencephaly, absence of the pituitary gland and olfactory bulbs and adrenal and thyroid hypoplasia have been observed in patients with cyclopia and cebocephaly [1-4].

Laboratory Studies

The cranium is small and the anterior and posterior fossae are also small. The anterior fossa is undivided and has only one opening through which the optic nerve passes. Absence of several bones has been noted, especially the crista galli, ethmoid, nasal, and premaxillary bones.

Treatment and Prognosis

In a report [2] of three patients with cebocephaly the two who died in the first five days of life had small adrenals and no pituitary. The infant who lived 14 weeks had a normal-sized pituitary and adrenals.

Genetics

Cyclopia has been described in association with chromosome 13 trisomy [5], 18p− syndrome [6], and monosomy G/normal mosaicism [7]. Ethmocephaly has been associated with 13 trisomy [7a]. Cebocephaly has been reported in association with 13 trisomy [8] and the 18p− syndrome [8a]. In one family four females bore offspring with cyclopia; a familial unbalanced translocation was suggested as the cause [9]. In one reported family there was one child with cyclopia (*Figure A*) and another with cebocephaly [10,11]. In another family [12] one child had cyclopia and the other ethmocephaly. Two brothers with cebocephaly were reported, one of whom was shown to have a normal karyotype [4]. In the last three families these malformations may have been due to autosomal recessive mutant genes.

References

1. Sedano, H. O., and Gorlin, R. J. The oral manifestations of cyclopia. *Oral Surg.*, **16**:823–38, 1963.
2. Haworth, J. C., Medovy, H., and Lewis, A. J. Cebocephaly with endocrine dysgenesis. *J. Pediatr.*, **59**:726–33, 1961.
3. Cohen, M. M., Jr., and Gorlin, R. J. Genetic considerations in a sibship of cyclopia and clefts. *Birth Defects: Original Article Series*, Vol. V, No. 2, February, 1969, pp. 113–17. Williams & Wilkins Co., Baltimore.
4. James, E., and Van Leeuwen, G. Familial cebocephaly. Case description and survey of the anomaly. *Clin. Pediatr. (Phila.)*, **9**:491–93, 1970.
5. Toews, H. A., and Jones, H. W., Jr. Cyclopia in association with D trisomy and gonadal agenesis. *Am. J. Obstet. Gynecol.*, **102**:53–56, 1968.
6. Nitowsky, H. M., Sindhvananda, N., Konigsberg, U. R., and Weinberg, T. Partial 18 monosomy in the cyclops malformation. *Pediatrics*, **37**:260–69, 1966.
7. Cohen, M. M. Chromosomal mosaicism associated with a case of cyclopia. *J. Pediatr.*, **69**:793–98, 1966.
7a. Diebold, J., Boué, J. G., Fayot-Petitmaire, M., Reymes, M., and Bègué, R. Trisomie 13–15: étude anatomo-pathologique d'une forme rare avec ethmocéphalie. *Arch. Anat. Pathol. (Paris)*, **15**:277–87, 1967.
8. Conen, P. E., Erkman, B., and Metaxotou, C. The "D" syndrome. *Am. J. Dis. Child.*, **111**:236–47, 1966.
8a. Gorlin, R. J., Yunis, J., and Anderson, V. E. Short arm deletion of chromosome 18 in cebocephaly. *Am. J. Dis. Child.*, **115**:473–76, 1968.
9. Pfitzer, P., and Müntefering, H. Chromosomentranslokation bei familiär gehäufter Cyclopie. *Virchows Arch. (Zellpath.)*, **1**:323–41, 1968.
10. Welter, E. S. Consecutive hydrocephalics. *Illinois Med. J.*, **133**:177–79, 1968.
11. Welter, E. S. Personal communication, 1968.
12. Ellis, R. On a rare form of twin monstrosity. *Trans. Obstet. Soc. London*, **7**:160–64, 1866.

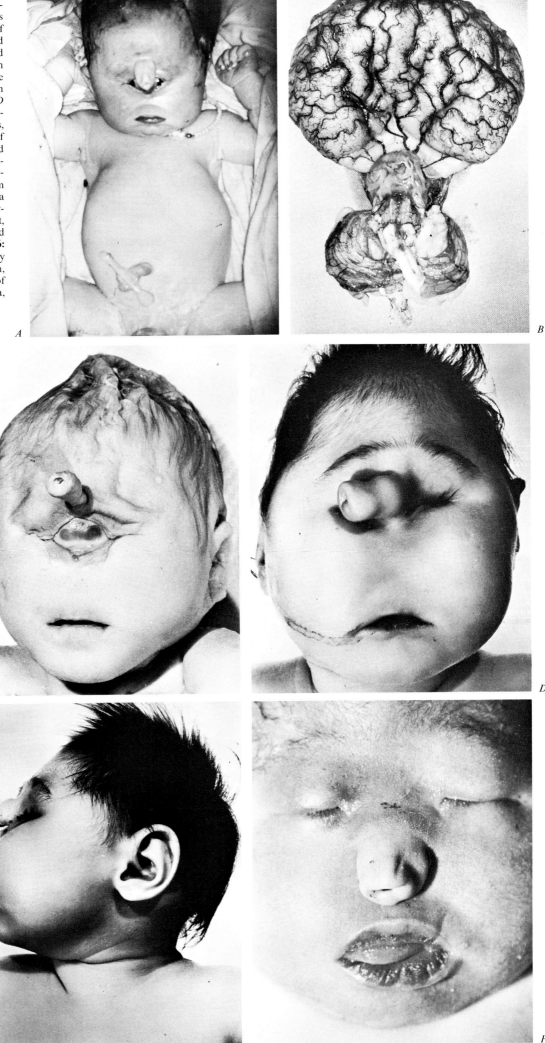

Plate V-6. *A* and *B:* This infant with cyclopia has two separate but fused eyeballs. His brain shows the absence of cleavage of the hemispheres and olfactory bulbs. His sister had cebocephaly. *C:* Shows fusion of the eyes and absence of the eyebrows, eyelids, and philtrum in an infant with cyclopia. *D* and *E:* An infant with ethmocephaly who has a proboscis, severe hypotelorism, absence of the nose and the philtrum, and eyebrows that meet in the midline. *F:* An infant with cebocephaly who has hypotelorism and a proboscislike nose with a single nostril. (*A* and *B:* Courtesy of Dr. E. S. Welter, Joliet, Ill. *C:* From H. Sedano and R. J. Gorlin, *Oral Surg.,* **16:** 823–38, 1963. *D* and *E:* Courtesy of Dr. P. Fleury, Amsterdam, Netherlands. *F:* Courtesy of Dr. S. Sussman, Philadelphia, Pa.)

Holotelencephaly with Cleft Lip and Hypotelorism

Since the advent of chromosome analysis, it has been customary to assume that the infant with holotelencephaly and cleft lip is likely to have chromosome 13 trisomy. However, several infants have been described who had these anomalies, but a normal chromosome karyotype [1-6]. Among infants with craniofacial anomalies associated with holotelencephaly, those with cleft lip and hypotelorism are the least severely malformed and the most likely to survive, albeit usually only for a few weeks or months.

Physical Features

HEAD: These patients are always microcephalic and sometimes have trigonocephaly (*Figure A*).

FACE: The cleft lip, absence of the nasal bridge, orbital hypotelorism, and an upward palpebral slant are the most striking facial features (*Figures A, C, D, E, and F*). Three types of cleft lip have been described: first, a triangular midline defect with the apex toward the columella (*Figures D and E*); second, a rectangular defect with the entire prolabium and premaxilla absent (*Figures A, C, E, and F*); third, bilateral lateral cleft lip with a median process representing the philtrum-premaxillary anlage. The nasal septum may be small or absent entirely. A cleft palate is often, but not always, present.

Nervous System

These patients are usually limp and apneic at birth. Those who survive may have extreme temperature fluctuations, nystagmus, disconjugate eye movements, no response to light or sound, hypertonic muscles and deep tendon reflexes, a poor suck, seizures, and little evidence of psychomotor development. Transillumination of the head shows an increased transmission of light, especially over the occiput [3,5,6].

Pathology

In addition to holotelencephaly (*Figure B*), these patients may have absence of the olfactory bulbs and tracts, cribriform plate, crista galli, septum pellucidum, and pituitary gland, and hypoplasia of the adrenal glands [1-6]. There have been few extracranial malformations.

Laboratory Studies

The cranium is small and the orbits are close together. The sella turcica is normal. Pneumoencephalography demonstrates the single cerebral ventricle [1,5,6].

Studies of pituitary function in one infant showed a diminished adrenocorticotropic hormone reserve and vasopressin-resistant diabetes insipidus. There was no evidence of defective release of either the thyroid-stimulating or growth hormones [5].

Treatment and Prognosis

Some infants have survived only a few hours, and others have survived several months.

Genetics

In three families [2,5,6] there were two or more affected siblings, which suggests that this disorder may be due to an autosomal recessive mutant gene.

Differential Diagnosis

1. Holotelencephaly, hypotelorism, and cleft lip have been associated with 13 trisomy (see page 164) and 18p— syndrome (see page 162). In both disorders there is a high incidence of additional congenital anomalies.
2. Hypotelorism and cleft lip and palate are features of patients with the Meckel syndrome, but they also have encephaloceles, polycystic kidneys, and polydactyly (see page 292).

References

1. Landau, J. W., Barry, J. M., and Koch, R. Arhinencephaly. *J. Pediatr.,* **62:**895–900, 1963.
2. DeMyer, W., Zeman, W., and Palmer, C. G. Familial alobar holoprosencephaly (arhinencephaly) with median cleft lip and palate. Report of a patient with 46 chromosomes. *Neurology (Minneap.),* **13:**913–18, 1963.
3. DeMyer, W., Zeman, W., and Palmer, C. G. The face predicts the brain: diagnostic significance of median facial anomalies for holoprosencephaly (arhinencephaly). *Pediatrics,* **34:**256–63, 1964.
4. Bishop, K., Connolly, J. M., Carter, C. H., and Carpenter, D. G. Holoprosencephaly. A case report with no extracranial abnormalities and normal chromosome count and karyotype. *J. Pediatr.,* **65:**406–14, 1964.
5. Hintz, R. L., Menking, M., and Sotos, J. F. Familial holoprosencephaly with endocrine dysgenesis. *J. Pediatr.,* **72:**81–87, 1968.
6. Khan, M., Rozdilsky, B., and Gerrard, J. W. Familial holoprosencephaly. *Dev. Med. Child Neurol.,* **12:**71–76, 1970.

Plate V-7. *A* and *B:* A newborn infant with a wide cleft lip and palate, absence of the nose and philtrum, and trigonocephaly with a palpable metopic suture. The brain was small; the gyri were wide and decreased in number. The view of the base of the brain shows fusion of the hemispheres and lateral ventricles and absence of the olfactory bulbs and tracts. *C* and *D:* Two affected siblings, the first of whom had hypoplasia of the adrenals and absence of the pituitary, and the second had multiple pituitary hormone deficiencies. *E:* Two infants with different lip defects, one a rectangular defect due to a bilateral lateral cleft lip (*left*) and the other a midline cleft shaped like an inverted V. The infant on the left had a similarly affected sister. *F:* An infant with severe hypotelorism, an upward palpebral slant, absence of the nose and premaxilla, and a wide midline cleft lip and palate. (*A* and *B:* From J. W. Landau *et al., J. Pediatr.,* **62:**895–900, 1963. *C* and *D:* From R. L. Hintz *et al., J. Pediatr.,* **72:**81–87, 1968. *E:* From W. DeMyer and W. Zeman, *Confin. Neurol.* **23:**1–36, 1963; courtesy of S. Karger, Basel/New York. *F:* Courtesy of Dr. W. A. Zaleski, Saskatoon, Saskatchewan, Canada.)

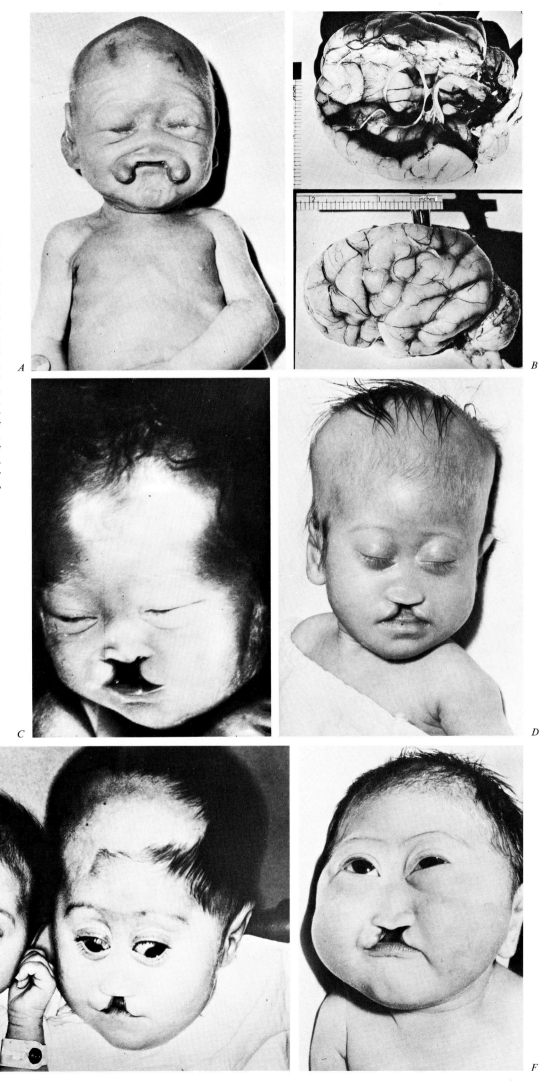

Other Central Nervous System Malformations
Cranium Bifidum with Encephalocele

Fusion defects of the skull may be of any size and in any location, but they are usually in the midline [1–3]. These midline defects are often referred to as cranium bifidum. If the defect is small, the dura will not herniate through and the brain is not involved. An example of this is cranium bifidum occultum frontalis [4]. However, the defect is usually large enough to be accompanied by protrusion of meninges. If this protrusion contains only spinal fluid it is called a meningocele. If it contains neural tissue, it is called an encephalocele or meningoencephalocele. Both meningoceles and encephaloceles may be located anywhere along the sagittal suture line, but the most common site is the occiput (*Figures B, C, D, E, and F*). Meningoceles (*Figure A*) have a good prognosis. Usually they can be successfully excised and the patients have normal intelligence [5,6]. A few have associated cerebral abnormalities and develop hydrocephalus.

Occipital encephalocele is much more common than occipital meningocele [6–8]. The skull defect is either located entirely within the squamous part of the cranium or the occipital arch is absent and the defect is confluent with the foramen magnum. The size of the swelling is no indication as to the extent of herniation of cerebral tissue. However, a poor prognosis is likely if the cranium is microcephalic or if hydrocephalus develops. Adding to the poor prognosis is a higher surgical risk in patients with encephaloceles than in those with meningoceles. In one series [7] of 45 patients, 20 survived, but only 4 had normal intelligence. In a series [6] of 23 patients, 15 survived and 8 had intelligence quotients estimated as greater than 70. In a series [8] of 40 patients whose occipital encephaloceles were excised, 25 were living after an average of 9 years after surgery. Fourteen had normal intelligence. Many patients have skeletal malformations, such as the Klippel-Feil syndrome, and brain anomalies, such as the Arnold-Chiari malformation. Hydrocephalus often develops and is usually treated with a ventriculoatrial shunt. Additional problems of patients who survive surgery for an occipital encephalocele are partial or complete blindness (usually of central cortical origin) and spasticity [7].

Genetics

A preponderance of females has been noted in several studies [5,7,8]. Cranium bifidum with meningocele and encephalocele are etiologically related to meningomyelocele and anencephaly [7]. Polygenic inheritance is likely. After the birth of one affected child, the parents' risk of having a subsequent child with one of these neural tube defects is about 5 percent.

Differential Diagnosis

1. Occipital encephaloceles are features of infants with the Meckel syndrome, but they also have microphthalmia, cleft lip and palate, polycystic kidneys, polydactyly, and clubfeet (see page 292).
2. Anterior encephaloceles were features of two infants with craniotelencephalic dysplasia, but they also had craniosynostosis and a protrusion of the frontal portion of the cranium (see page 236).

References

1. Ingraham, F. D., and Hamlin, H. Spina bifida and cranium bifidum. II. Surgical treatment. *N. Engl. J. Med.,* **228**:631–41, 1943.
2. Hoffman, E. P. The problems of spina bifida and cranium bifidum. *Clin. Pediatr. (Phila.),* **4**:709–16, 1965.
3. Epstein, J. A., and Epstein, B. S. Deformities of the skull surfaces in infancy and childhood. *J. Pediatr.,* **70**:636–47, 1967.
4. Terrafranca, R. J., and Zellis, A. Congenital hereditary cranium bifidum occultum frontalis. *Radiology,* **61**:60–66, 1953.
5. Barrow, N., and Simpson, D. A. Cranium bifidum. Investigation, prognosis and management. *Aust. Paediatr. J.,* **2**:20–26, 1966.
6. Guthkelch, A. N. Occipital cranium bifidum. *Arch. Dis. Child.,* **45**:104–109, 1970.
7. Lorber, J. The prognosis of occipital encephalocele. *Dev. Med. Child Neurol.,* Suppl. No. 13, pp. 75–87, 1967.
8. Mealey, J., Jr., Dzenitis, A. J., and Hockey, A. A. The prognosis of encephaloceles. *J. Neurosurg.,* **32**:209–18, 1970.

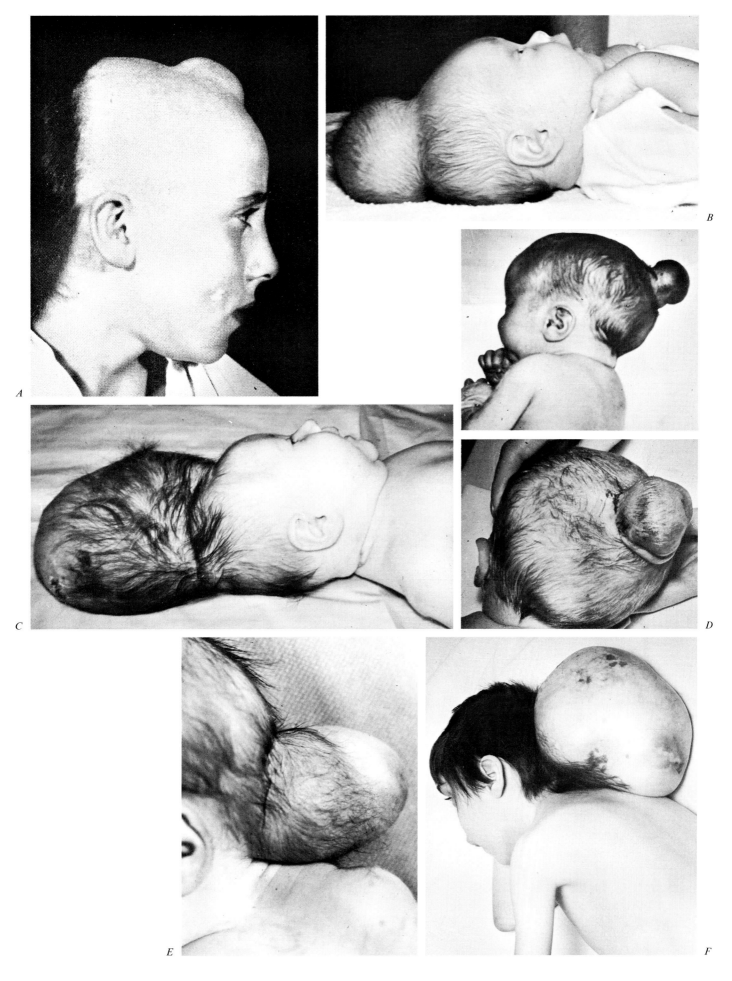

Plate V-8. *A:* A patient with a meningocele protruding through a midline frontal cranial defect. *B:* A severely retarded infant with a 4-cm midline midparietal defect and a meningocele which was subsequently closed. A ventriculogram showed large ventricles, absence of the septum pellucidum, and possible agenesis of the corpus callosum. *C:* An infant with a large encephalocele who at age 4 years had no appreciable psychomotor development. *D:* An infant with a small posterior encephalocele who subsequently developed hydrocephalus.

Absence of the corpus callosum was evident on the pneumoencephalogram. *E:* An infant with an occipital meningoencephalocele who also had stenosis of the aqueduct of Sylvius. *F:* A 13-year-old child with a large occipital meningoencephalocele. (*A:* From F. D. Ingraham and H. Hamlin, *N. Engl. J. Med.,* **228:**631–41, 1943. *B* and *C:* Courtesy of Dr. G. R. Hogan, Boston, Mass. *E:* Courtesy of Dr. N. P. Rosman, Boston, Mass.)

211

Meningomyelocele

A meningomyelocele is a herniation of the meninges and a portion of the spinal cord or nerve roots through a posterior defect in the vertebrae (*Figures A, B, and D*). The incidence of meningomyelocle varies according to socioeconomic and ethnic factors, and the range is between 1 and 9 per 1000 livebirths [1,2].

Physical Features

HEAD: These patients often have head enlargement due to hydrocephalus. The head enlargement, whether it is present at birth or develops later, is generalized and is characterized by prominence of the brow and occiput (*Figures C and D*).

BACK: There is considerable variation in the appearance and location of meningomyeloceles. Usually there is a central reddish plaque with a surrounding zone of thin translucent membrane, which in turn is encircled by a zone of thin pink or red skin (*Figure B*). The central red plaque consists of neural tissue, the expanded and everted spinal cord. The thin translucent membrane around the plaque is the arachnoid membrane, as the dura and skin persist up only a portion of the sac wall (*Figure A*). This arachnoid membrane varies in thickness and width and is often easily ruptured. Blood vessels ascend with the spinal cord or cauda equina to the fundus of the sac and give rise to the serous discharge on the free surface of the sac. Meningomyeloceles are most commonly located in the thoracolumbar region (*Figures B and D*). Less common locations are the upper thoracic areas, the sacral region, and the anterior lumbar area [3].

LIMBS: Many children have congenital dislocation of the hips and clubfoot deformities (*Figure C*) which are attributed to inadequate lower limb muscles in utero.

Nervous System

If these children do not develop hydrocephalus, they usually have normal intelligence. Those with hydrocephalus may have mild to severe mental retardation. A common finding in children with hydrocephalus is "cocktail party" or "chatterbox" conversation, terms used to indicate that the children are aggressive and fluent in social encounters, but upon questioning cannot respond in a consistent or meaningful manner [4].

Pathology

In patients with hydrocephalus, the greatest ventricular distention is near the vertex. Stretching and diminution in the depth of the sulci are also prominent in the frontal and parietal regions [5]. The hydrocephalus may be due to obstruction at any of several sites, such as the foramen of Monro, the aqueduct of Sylvius, foramina of Luschka and Magendie, and the foramen magnum. Extraventricular obstruction at the level of the foramen magnum may be caused by arachnoid adhesions from hemorrhage or infection or impaction of the cerebellum. The narrowing of the aqueduct of Sylvius often appears to be postinflammatory in nature, although congenital narrowing and forking are found in some children. Blockage of the fourth ventricle foramina may be a congenital failure to open or secondary to arachnoiditis, but often the fourth ventricle is obstructed because of herniation into the upper cervical spinal canal. This herniation of the hindbrain, referred to as a type II Chiari anomaly or Arnold-Chiari malformation, is often present in individuals with a meningomyelocele. In this malformation there is displacement of the inferior vermis of the cerebellum into the cervical canal accompanied by caudal displacement of the lower pons, the medulla, and the elongated fourth ventricle (*Figures E and F*).

Laboratory Studies

Vertebral anomalies are frequently present, such as fused vertebrae, hemivertebrae, diastematomyelia, scoliosis, and basilar impression of the first cervical vertebra.

Treatment and Prognosis

The age of the child, the presence of hydrocephalus and its severity, the degree of muscle paralysis in the legs, the presence of other major malformations, and the anatomic location of the meningomyelocele determine the therapeutic approach [6a]. An increase in survival and a decrease in the incidence of complete paralysis of the lower limbs has been reported following closure of the defect in the first 24 hours of life [3]. Treatment of the hydrocephalus may require a decompression procedure or the insertion of a bypass ventriculoatrial valve. Extraventricular obstruction associated with the Arnold-Chiari malformation is often best treated by suboccipital craniectomy and upper cervical laminectomy with wide decompression of the dura over the cerebellum and upper cervical spinal cord. Other aspects of medical care include careful observation for infection, especially in the nervous system and urinary tract, urologic investigation to detect obstruction, and orthopedic management for clubfoot and congenital hip dislocation.

Genetics

Meningomyelocele is usually considered to have a multifactorial or polygenic mode of inheritance [2]. However, the data are not completely compatible with this theory as monozygous twins have only a 5 percent concordance for this malformation, and the recurrence rate among maternal relatives is higher than that among paternal relatives [2a]. After the birth of one affected child, the risk of a subsequent sibling being affected is about 5 percent, which is seven times the incidence in the general population [2]. If there have been two affected children, the risk of having another affected child is 10 percent [6]; these data were obtained in England and none are available for other populations. This increased risk applies for all types of neural tube defects, such as meningomyelocele, meningocele, and anencephaly. Some national and ethnic groups have been shown to have an increased risk of this malformation and others a decreased risk [1].

Differential Diagnosis

Meningomyelocele also occurs as part of other syndromes, such as 18 trisomy (see page 156), the aminopterin embryopathy (see page 134), and the syndrome of cloacal exstrophy [7]. Each of these syndromes is readily distinguished by the associated malformations.

References

1. Naggan, L., and MacMahon, B. Ethnic differences in the prevalence of anencephaly and spina bifida in Boston, Massachusetts. *N. Engl. J. Med.*, **277**:1119–23, 1967.
2. Carter, C. O., David, P. A., and Laurence, K. M. A family study of major central nervous system malformations in South Wales. *J. Med. Genet.*, **5**:81–92, 1968.
2a. Nance, W. E. Anencephaly and spina bifida: an etiologic hypothesis. *Birth Defects: Original Article Series*, Vol. VII, No. 1, February, 1971, pp. 97–102. Williams & Wilkins Co., Baltimore.
3. Zachary, R. B., and Sharrard, W. J. W. Spinal dysraphism. *Postgrad. Med. J.* Suppl. Vol. 43, pp. 731–54, 1967.
4. Fleming, C. P. The verbal behavior of hydrocephalic children. *Dev. Med. Child Neurol.* Suppl. No. 15, pp. 74–82, 1968.
5. Emery, J. L., and Svitok, I. Intra-hemispherical distances in congenital hydrocephalus associated with meningomyelocele. *Dev. Med. Child Neurol.* Suppl. No. 15, pp. 21–29, 1968.
6. Carter, C. O., and Roberts, J. A. F. The risk of recurrence after two children with central-nervous-system malformations. *Lancet*, **1**:306–308, 1967.
6a. Lorber, J. Results of treatment of myelomeningocele. An analysis of 524 unselected cases, with special reference to possible selection for treatment. *Dev. Med. Child Neurol.*, **13**:279–303, 1971.
7. Spencer, R., and Geer, J. C. Ileocecal exstrophy with bifid intra-abdominal urinary bladder: incomplete exstrophy of the cloaca. *J. Pediatr. Surg.*, **2**:69–74, 1967.

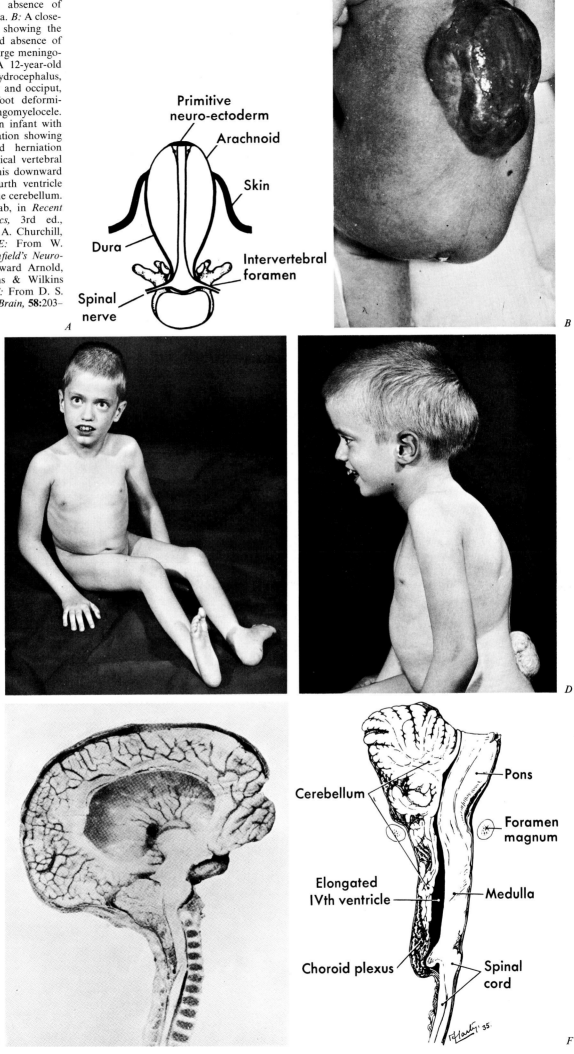

Plate V-9. *A:* Diagram of a meningo-myelocele showing the absence of coverage by skin and dura. *B:* A close-up view in a newborn showing the serous fluid exudate and absence of skin in the center of a large meningo-myelocele. *C* and *D:* A 12-year-old boy with arrested hydrocephalus, prominence of the brow and occiput, flaccid legs with clubfoot deformities, and a lumbar meningomyelocele. *E:* Sagittal section of an infant with Arnold-Chiari malformation showing bilateral ventricles and herniation of cerebellum into cervical vertebral canal. *F:* Diagram of this downward displacement of the fourth ventricle and inferior vermis of the cerebellum. (*A:* From G. H. Macnab, in *Recent Advances in Paediatrics,* 3rd ed., D. Gairdner [ed.], J. & A. Churchill, Ltd., London, 1965. *E:* From W. Blackwood *et al., Greenfield's Neuropathology,* 2nd ed., Edward Arnold, Ltd., London; Williams & Wilkins Co., Baltimore, 1963. *F:* From D. S. Russell and C. Donald, *Brain,* **58:**203–15, 1935.)

Primitive neuro-ectoderm

Arachnoid

Skin

Dura

Intervertebral foramen

Spinal nerve

A

B

C

D

Cerebellum

Pons

Foramen magnum

Elongated IVth ventricle

Medulla

Choroid plexus

Spinal cord

E

F

213

Chapter VI
Syndromes of Multiple Deformities

Syndrome of Elastic Tissue Deficiency, Corneal Dystrophy, Grimacing, and Mental Retardation

Syndrome of Dyschondroplasia, Facial Anomalies, and Polysyndactyly

Syndrome of Elbow Contractures, Corneal Opacities, Pointed Nose, and Mental Retardation

Syndrome of Facial Dysmorphism, Right-Sided Aortic Arch and Mental Deficiency

Syndrome of Malformed, Low-Set Ears and Conductive Hearing Loss

Syndrome of Marked Acceleration of Skeletal Maturation and Facial Anomalies

Syndrome of Microcephaly, Peculiar Appearance, Spasticity, and Choreoathetosis

Syndrome of Cryptorchidism, Chest Deformities, Contractures, and Arachnodactyly

Syndrome of Microcephaly, Snub Nose, Livedo Reticularis, and Low-Birth-Weight Dwarfism

Syndrome of Micromelia and Coarse Facial Features

Syndrome of Micrognathia, Malformed Ears, Clubfoot, and Flexion Deformities (Pseudotrisomy 18)

Syndrome of Oral, Cranial, and Digital Anomalies

Syndrome of Phocomelia, Flexion Deformities, and Facial Anomalies

Syndrome of Retinal Blindness, Polycystic Kidneys, and Brain Malformations

Syndrome of Tetraphocomelia, Cleft Lip and Palate, and Genital Hypertrophy (Roberts Syndrome)

Telecanthus-Hypospadias Syndrome

Treacher Collins Syndrome (Mandibulofacial Dysostosis, Franceschetti-Zwahlen-Klein Syndrome)

Trichorrhexis Nodosa with Mental Retardation

Introduction

Although this chapter on multiple deformity syndromes is the largest in the book, it does not include all disorders associated with deformities. Many are included in the other chapters. Some types of deformities discussed here relate primarily to one particular organ system, such as the eye or skeleton, and some are purely secondary, such as those associated with the neurologic syndromes.

The largest portion of this chapter is concerned with syndromes with major congenital anomalies. In part, this is a reflection of recent interest in the delineation of new syndromes. The frequency of these syndromes was suggested by the study [1] of 4412 newborns among whom 32 were found to have multiple anomalies. Nine of these were due to chromosomal abnormalities. Of the remaining 23 a clinical diagnosis could only be given to 3. As infants and children with multiple deformities are being studied more thoroughly, attention has been drawn to the value of the patients' minor anomalies in establishing the correct diagnoses [1,2]. By definition, minor anomalies have no serious surgical or cosmetic importance. They include physical features such as epicanthal folds, an upward slant of the palpebral fissures, indentations on the earlobes, a posterior rotation of the ears, and clinodactyly of the fifth finger. The interest in minor anomalies has pointed up the need for more data on normal variations and the incidence of the different minor anomalies in the general population. Unfortunately the definitions of what is abnormal vary and the incidence of single minor anomalies in normal infants has varied from 13 percent [1] to 2 percent [3] in different studies. Data are available on only some of the specific anomalies, such as epicanthal folds [4], the external ear [5], and the distance between the eyes [6,7].

Most of the syndromes with multiple congenital anomalies are due to single abnormal genes acting in either a recessive or dominant fashion. How a single gene can cause widely separated and seemingly unrelated malformations in different organ systems is not known. Such a gene is considered as having a pleiotropic effect. Experience with these diseases due to genes with a pleiotropic effect has shown that there are several important principles essential for their clinical recognition [2,2a]. First, no single minor anomaly is pathognomonic of any syndrome; all minor anomalies can occur in normal individuals. Second, the same major or minor anomaly can occur in several different syndromes. Third, a syndrome can occur without every associated malformation being present. Fourth, patients with the same syndrome often do not have the same number of anomalies or equally severe deformities.

It is certain that many more multiple deformity syndromes will be recognized among mentally retarded individuals. That this group has a high incidence of minor anomalies was established by Smith and Bostian [8]. In a study of 50 children with idiopathic mental retardation they found that 42 percent had three or more associated anomalies. Their study is augmented by others [9,10] which have shown that few mentally retarded individuals with multiple anomalies have chromosomal abnormalities.

References

1. Marden, P. M., Smith, D. W., and McDonald, M. J. Congenital anomalies in the newborn infant, including minor variations. A study of 4412 babies by surface examination for anomalies and buccal smear for sex chromatin. *J. Pediatr.*, **64**:357–71, 1964.

2. Opitz, J. M., Herrmann, J., and Dieker, H. The study of malformation syndromes in man. *Birth Defects: Original Article Series*, Vol. V, No. 2, February, 1969, pp. 1–10. Williams & Wilkins Co., Baltimore.

2a. Pinsky, L., and Fraser, F. C. Atypical malformation syndromes. *J. Pediatr.*, **80**:141–44, 1972.

3. Nelson, M. M., and Forfar, J. O. Congenital abnormalities at birth: their association in the same patient. *Dev. Med. Child Neurol.*, **11**:3–16, 1969.

4. Johnson, C. C. Epicanthus. *Am. J. Ophthalmol.*, **66**:939–46, 1968.

5. Lange, G. Familien-Untersuchungen uber die Erblichkeit metrischer und morphologischer Markmale des ausseren Ohres. *Z. Morphol. Anthropol.*, **57**:111–67, 1966.

6. Gerald, B. E., and Silverman, F. N. Normal and abnormal interorbital distances with specific reference to mongolism. *Am. J. Roentgenol.*, **95**:154–61, 1965.

7. Laestadius, N. D., Aase, J. M., and Smith, D. W. Normal inner canthal and outer orbital dimensions. *J. Pediatr.*, **74**:465–71, 1969.

8. Smith, D. W., and Bostian, K. E. Congenital anomalies associated with idiopathic mental retardation. Frequency in contrast to frequency in controls, in children with cleft lip and palate, and in those with ventricular septal defect. *J. Pediatr.*, **65**:189–96, 1964.

9. Summitt, R. L. Cytogenetics in mentally retarded defective children with anomalies: a controlled study. *J. Pediatr.*, **74**:58–66, 1969.

10. Daly, R. F. Chromosome aberrations in 50 patients with idiopathic mental retardation and in 50 control subjects. *J. Pediatr.*, **77**:444–53, 1970.

Craniosynostosis Syndromes

Premature fusion of the membranous cranial bones (craniosynostosis), causing a skull deformity, may occur as an isolated congenital anomaly or as part of a syndrome of multiple congenital anomalies. The most common type of craniosynostosis is closure of a single suture with no additional malformations. The sagittal suture is the most frequently involved, and the coronal and metopic sutures are the next most common [1–4] (*Figure A*).

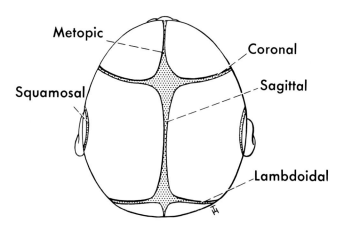

A. Normal Cranial Sutures in Infancy

The skull is deformed by craniosynostosis because normal skull growth in the direction perpendicular to the fused suture is inhibited and compensatory skull growth occurs parallel to the suture. The suture abnormality is therefore predictable from the clinical findings. For example, premature fusion of the sagittal suture produces an anteroposterior elongation of the skull, which is called scaphocephaly (*Figure B*). Fusion of one coronal suture results in flattening of the forehead on the same side and prominence of the frontal region of the opposite side. Fusion of both coronal sutures produces a flat forehead on both sides and absence of the brow ridges (*Figure C*). Fusion of the metopic suture results in a keel-shaped forehead due to the pinched-in appearance of the frontal bones, called trigonocephaly (*Figure D*). When more than one suture is fused prematurely, the skull is flattened over the closed sutures and expands in the direction of the open sutures. This means that patients with premature closure of both

the coronal and lambdoid sutures have upward growth of the cranium and a towerlike skull shape.

Patients with premature closure of only one suture almost always have normal intelligence [1,3]. In contrast, children with several sutures prematurely fused are more likely to be mentally retarded. This is thought to be because of increased intracranial pressure and impairment of normal brain growth, although it has not been well documented.

Early corrective surgery is recommended to obtain the greatest improvement in the child's appearance, as well as to possibly prevent brain damage that might otherwise occur in patients with several fused sutures [1,4]. The most common surgical technique consists of removal of a strip of bone from the site of the involved suture and the extension of the incision across the normal sutures. The pericranium is excised widely, and polyethylene film strips are placed around the bone edge throughout the entire length of the craniotomy. This postpones the time when the new bone, which is formed from the dura, will adhere to the old bone edges wrapped in film. The best results are achieved if surgery is performed in the first months of life. Although older children may not show as much cosmetic improvement as infants, surgery is indicated if there is evidence of elevated intracranial pressure.

Several syndromes in which craniosynostosis is often associated with mental retardation will be discussed in detail:

1. Premature closure of several sutures
2. Apert's syndrome (acrocephalosyndactyly, types I and II)
3. Chotzen's syndrome (acrocephalosyndactyly, type III)
4. Pfeiffer's syndrome (acrocephalosyndactyly, type VI)
5. Crouzon's disease (craniofacial dysostosis)
6. Carpenter's syndrome (acrocephalopolysyndactyly)
7. Cloverleaf skull (Kleeblattschädel syndrome)
8. Craniotelencephalic dysplasia
9. Syndrome of acrocephalosyndactyly, absent digits, and cranial defects
10. Syndrome of acrocephaly, cleft lip and palate, radial aplasia, and absent digits

References

1. Shillito, J., Jr., and Matson, D. D. Craniosynostosis: a review of 519 surgical patients. *Pediatrics*, **41**:829–53, 1968.
2. Anderson, F. M., and Geiger, L. Craniosynostosis. A survey of 204 cases. *J. Neurosurg.*, **22**:229–40, 1965.
3. Hemple, D. J., Harris, L. E., Svien, H. J., and Holman, C. B. Craniosynostosis involving the sagittal suture only: guilt by association? *J. Pediatr.*, **58**:342–55, 1961.
4. Anderson, H., and Gomes, S. P. Craniosynostosis. Review of the literature and indications for surgery. *Acta Paediatr. Scand.*, **57**:47–54, 1968.

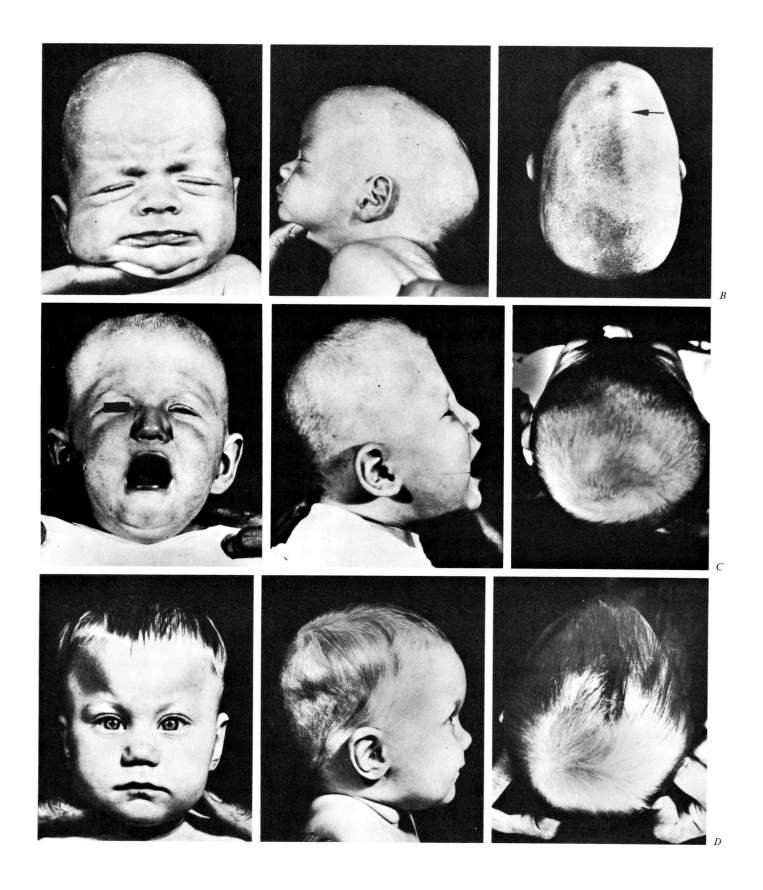

Plate VI-1. *A:* Diagram of the location of the cranial sutures. *B:* A 6-week-old boy with a long, narrow head and a prominent forehead due to sagittal synostosis. A ridge is visible (*arrow*) in the sagittal region posteriorly, where the greatest narrowing is also evident. In the picture of the top of his head, the child's face is pointing upward. *C:* A 5-month-old boy with flattening of the forehead due to bilateral coronal synostosis. *D:* An 8-month-old boy with a prominent ridge in the midforehead due to metopic synostosis. The frontal bones appear pinched on each side of the ridge. All of the children shown on this page have normal intelligence. (*A–D:* From J. Shillito, Jr., and D. D. Matson, *Pediatrics,* **41:**829–53, 1968.)

Premature Closure of Several Sutures

Children with premature closure of several cranial sutures may have a normal appearance or may be strikingly deformed at birth. The many different skull shapes reflect the variation in the time, extent, and sequence of suture closures. The incidence of patients with multiple suture closures is not known, but 47 patients were included in two studies [1,2] of 723 patients with all types of craniosynostosis.

Physical Features

HEAD: In a child with a normal head contour at birth the only abnormalities may be small or absent fontanels and thickening of the bone over the areas of premature suture closure. If all sutures are involved, the head remains small, the forehead is high and narrow, and the skull points toward the vertex (*Figures A and B*). In striking contrast to the infant with a normal head shape is the one with closure of several sutures in whom skull growth continued before birth in the direction of the anterior fontanel. Such a child may have a marked skull deformity at birth with a protrusion in the area of the anterior fontanel (*Figure E*).

Nervous System

Untreated patients often develop symptoms of elevated intracranial pressure. Subnormal intelligence is common.

Laboratory Studies

Skull x-rays show no visible sutures, and prominent convolutional impressions in the areas of premature fusion. In the child with a normal head shape at birth who is not treated, the anterior fossa is usually short and the skull comes to a peak at the vertex. Often the base angle is widened and the pituitary fossa is deformed [3] (*Figures C and D*).

Treatment and Prognosis

Early corrective surgery is recommended. Even with early surgery, some patients have subnormal intelligence. Others treated early, even those with severe skull deformities at birth, may have a normal appearance and normal intelligence [1] (*Figures E and F*).

Genetics

In some families there have been affected members in several generations, which suggests dominant inheritance [1,2].

Differential Diagnosis

Patients with "true" or "pure" microcephaly have a small head, but the forehead is usually short and slopes back. These patients do not have either clinical or x-ray evidence of increased intracranial pressure (see page 196).

References

1. Shillito, J., Jr., and Matson, D. D. Craniosynostosis: a review of 519 surgical patients. *Pediatrics,* **41:**829–53, 1968.
2. Anderson, F. M., and Geiger, L. Craniosynostosis. A survey of 204 cases. *J. Neurosurg.,* **22:**229–40, 1965.
3. Schurr, P. H. Craniosynostosis. *Dev. Med. Child Neurol.,* **10:**789–92, 1968.

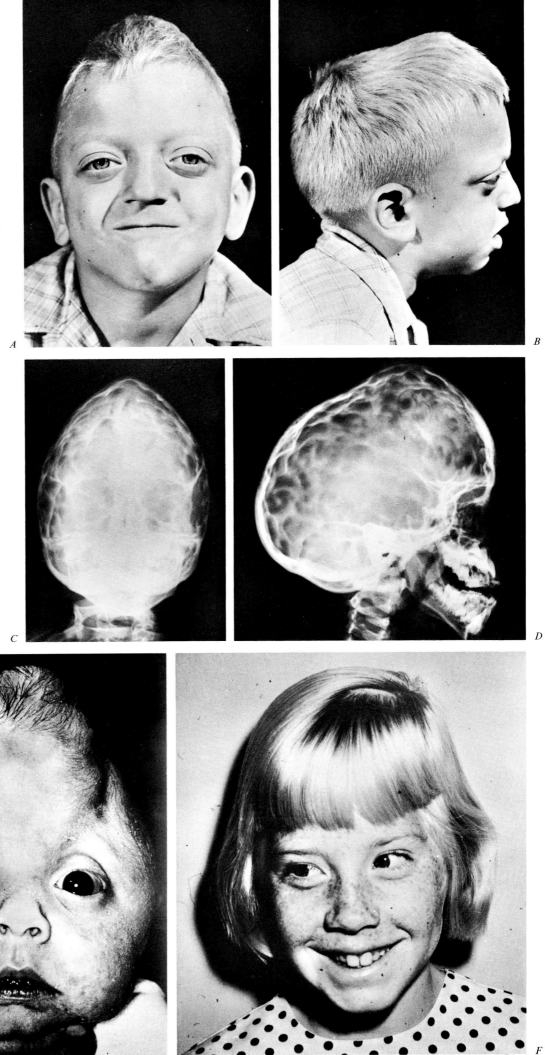

Plate VI-2. *A–D:* A moderately retarded 7-year-old boy with premature fusion of all sutures. His cranial vault is high and elongated, and peaks at the bregma. The skull x-rays show deep convolutional impressions, a short anterior fossa, and an enlarged sella. *E* and *F:* A newborn infant with protrusion of the cerebrum in the area of the anterior fossa, due to premature fusion of several sutures. Following multiple craniectomies in infancy, this child had an attractive appearance and normal intelligence. (*A, C,* and *D:* From F. M. Anderson and L. Geiger, *J. Neurosurg.,* **22:** 229–40, 1965. *B:* Courtesy of Dr. F. M. Anderson, Los Angeles, Calif. *E* and *F:* From J. Shillito, Jr., and D. D. Matson, *Pediatrics,* **41:**829–53, 1968.)

Apert's Syndrome
(Acrocephalosyndactyly, Types I and II)

In 1906 Apert [1] described one patient and reviewed eight previously reported patients with a tall skull, flat occiput, and syndactyly of the hands and feet. He proposed the term *acrocephalosyndactyly* to describe these patients. Subsequently many different disorders with both acrocephaly and syndactyly have been described, leading to confusion with terms such as *typical* and *atypical Apert's syndrome* [2]. Apert's syndrome has been classified as having two types, based on the extent of the syndactyly of the hands [3]. It seems likely that these two types are only phenotypic variations of the same disorder. Apert's syndrome is the most common craniosynostosis syndrome associated with mental retardation.

Physical Features

HEAD: The forehead is high and wide and the occiput is flat. The apex of the skull is at or near the bregma. The skull usually has a towerlike appearance because growth is predominantly directed upward (*Figures A, B, D, E, G, and H*).

FACE: The eyes are protuberant and widely placed. The palpebral fissures have a downward slant. The maxilla and the nasal bridge appear flat and underdeveloped, which gives the normal tip of the nose a beaklike appearance (*Figures E and H*). The chin is normal but is prominent because of the poorly developed maxilla. Facial asymmetry is also frequent (*Figure I*).

MOUTH: The palate is high and narrow. A posterior cleft palate and bifid uvula are common. The teeth are crowded and irregularly aligned.

LIMBS: The syndactyly involves all four limbs and is symmetric [4]. It may involve fusion of the skin alone or fusion of both skin and bone (*Figure J*). In the hands and feet all five digits may be involved, resulting in "mitten hands" (*Figure A*) and "sock feet" (*Figure C*), which are features of type I acrocephalosyndactyly [3]. The nails of the second to fifth fingers are often fused (*Figure J*). Syndactyly of digits 2, 3, and 4 with partial involvement of either or both the first and fifth digits (*Figure F*) is called type II acrocephalosyndactyly [3]. Children usually have some mobility of the interphalangeal joints, but this is not present in adults. When there is no syndactyly of the thumb and great toe, these digits are deviated, shortened, and enlarged (*Figure F*). Shortening of the arm and forearm with limitation of elbow motion and shoulder abduction are frequently present. A few patients have had radioulnar synostosis or absence of the radius, but these are infrequent findings.

SKIN: Forearm acne is common in postpubertal individuals [5].

Nervous System

The patients are usually moderately to severely retarded. Some have signs and symptoms of increased intracranial pressure. In one study [6] of six patients, all had dilated ventricles; one also had aqueductal stenosis. Four of the six had a normal cerebrospinal fluid pressure.

Pathology

One large series [2] included twelve patients on whom autopsies had been performed. Six had a variety of visceral malformations, including two with multiple cardiac anomalies, but no cerebral malformations; six had no additional anomalies. Another autopsied patient had absence of the posterior corpus callosum [6].

Plate VI-3. *A–C:* An infant with proptosis, a downward eye slant, maxillary hypoplasia, a beaklike nose, and bilateral coronal synostosis who is an example of acrocephalosyndactyly type I, because all five digits of the fingers and toes are fused together. The scar is from a recent craniectomy. *D–F:* A newborn with similar facial features, but classified as having acrocephalosyndactyly type II because the first digits are separate and the fifth digits are only partially fused to the fourth. At five $^{4}/_{12}$ years he had dull, normal to average intelligence.

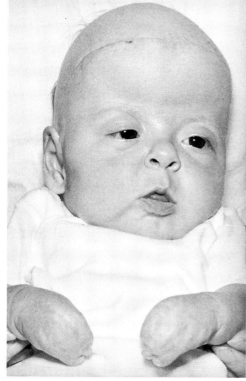

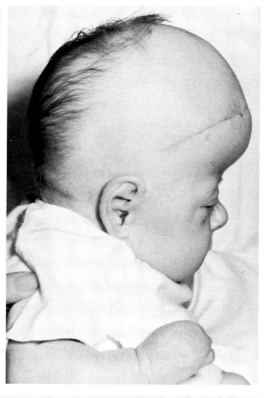

A

B

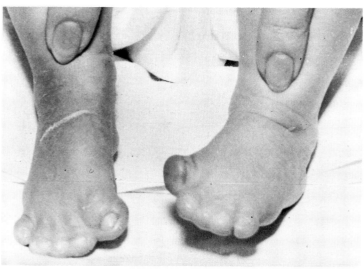

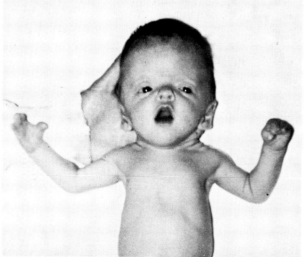

C

D

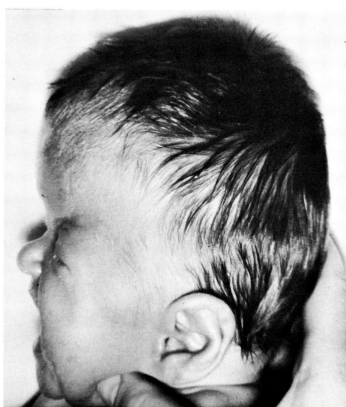

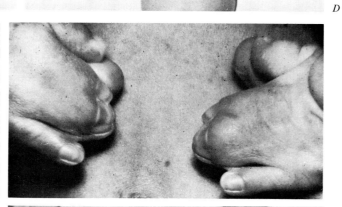

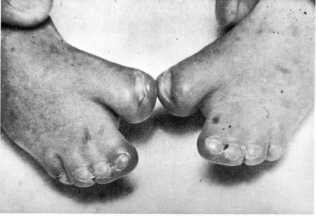

E

F

Laboratory Studies

The coronal and lambdoid are the cranial sutures that are most often prematurely fused. Early closure of facial sutures, such as zygomaticomaxillary and zygomaticotemporal, and other cranial sutures such as the sphenoparietal, squamosal, and sagittal is often present [7]. The closure may not be symmetric and the suture may not be fused throughout its entire length. As a result of the early closure of these sutures, there is usually shortening of the anteroposterior dimension and vertical lengthening of the calvarium (*Figure L*) and shallow and oblique orbital fossae. Progressive fusion between phalanges, carpals, metacarpals, metatarsals, and vertebrae has been described in several patients [4,8]. Trapezoid deformity and enlargement of the distal phalanx of the thumbs and great toes and enlargement of the first metacarpals and metatarsals are common (*Figure J*).

Treatment and Prognosis

It is recommended that the craniosynostosis be corrected in early infancy. It is not known whether this improves the intelligence of these patients. Repair of the syndactyly of the hands is often performed in the first few years to improve both the child's dexterity and appearance. A program of two surgical procedures to produce a three-fingered hand has been recommended for children less than 2 years old [4].

Genetics

Autosomal dominant. Because of the facial disfigurement and the associated mental retardation, the reproductive rate is low. As a result of this, most patients are thought to represent spontaneous mutations and only three examples of hereditary transmission have been reported [2,4,9]. In an analysis of 37 patients an elevated parental age was found [2].

Differential Diagnosis

1. Acrocephaly, maxillary hypoplasia, proptosis, a downward palpebral slant, and a beaklike nose are also features of patients with Crouzon's disease, but they have no limb anomalies (see page 230).
2. Four other types of acrocephalosyndactyly have been identified and are presumed to represent different gene mutations [3]: type III, Chotzen's syndrome, with mild acrocephaly and mild syndactyly of fingers and toes (see page 226); type IV, Mohr type, with acrocephaly and syndactyly of toes 4–5; type V, Waardenburg type, with plagiocephaly, buphthalmos, bifid terminal phalanges of digits 2 and 3, elbow and knee contractures, and cardiac malformations; type VI, Pfeiffer type, with acrocephaly and broad, short thumbs and big toes (see page 228).
3. Craniosynostosis and syndactyly are features of patients with Carpenter's syndrome, but they also have preaxial and postaxial polydactyly, less syndactyly of the hands, and a different facial appearance. This syndrome is inherited as an autosomal recessive trait (see page 232).
4. Acrocephaly and minimal syndactyly were features of the father and daughter described by Noack [10], but they also had normal intelligence and enlarged thumbs, and duplication of the great toe was evident by x-ray.
5. Syndactyly of the hands and feet and acrocephaly were features of two brothers described by Summitt, but they had normal intelligence and were obese [11].

References

1. Apert, E. De l'acrocéphalosyndactylie. *Bull. Soc. Med. Hop. Paris,* **23:**1310–30, 1906.
2. Blank, C. E. Apert's syndrome (a type of acrocephalosyndactyly)—observations on a British series of thirty-nine cases. *Ann. Hum. Genet.,* **24:**151–64, 1960.
3. McKusick, V. A. *Mendelian Inheritance in Man,* 2nd ed. Johns Hopkins Press, Baltimore, 1968, pp. 5–7.
4. Hoover, G. H., Flatt, A. E., and Weiss, M. W. The hand and Apert's syndrome. *J. Bone Joint Surg.,* **52:**878–95, 1970.
5. Cohen, M. M., Jr. Personal communication, 1970.
6. Hogan, G. R., and Bauman, M. L. Hydrocephalus in Apert's syndrome. *J. Pediatr.,* **79:**782–87, 1971.
7. Herrmann, J., Pallister, P. D., and Opitz, J. M. Craniosynostosis and craniosynostosis syndromes. *Rocky Mt. Med. J.,* **66:**45–56, 1969.
8. Schauerte, E. W., and St-Aubin, P. M. Progressive synosteosis in Apert's syndrome (acrocephalosyndactyly). *Am. J. Roentgenol.,* **97:**67–73, 1966.
9. Weech, A. A. Combined acrocephaly and syndactylism occurring in mother and daughter. A case report. *Bull. Hopkins Hosp.,* **40:**73–76, 1927.
10. Noack, M. Ein Beitrag zum Krankheitsbild der Akrozephalosyndaktylie (Apert). *Arch. Kinderheilkd.,* **160:**168–71, 1959.
11. Summitt, R. L. Recessive acrocephalosyndactyly with normal intelligence. *Birth Defects: Original Article Series,* Vol. V, No. 3, March, 1969, pp. 35–38, Williams & Wilkins Co., Baltimore.

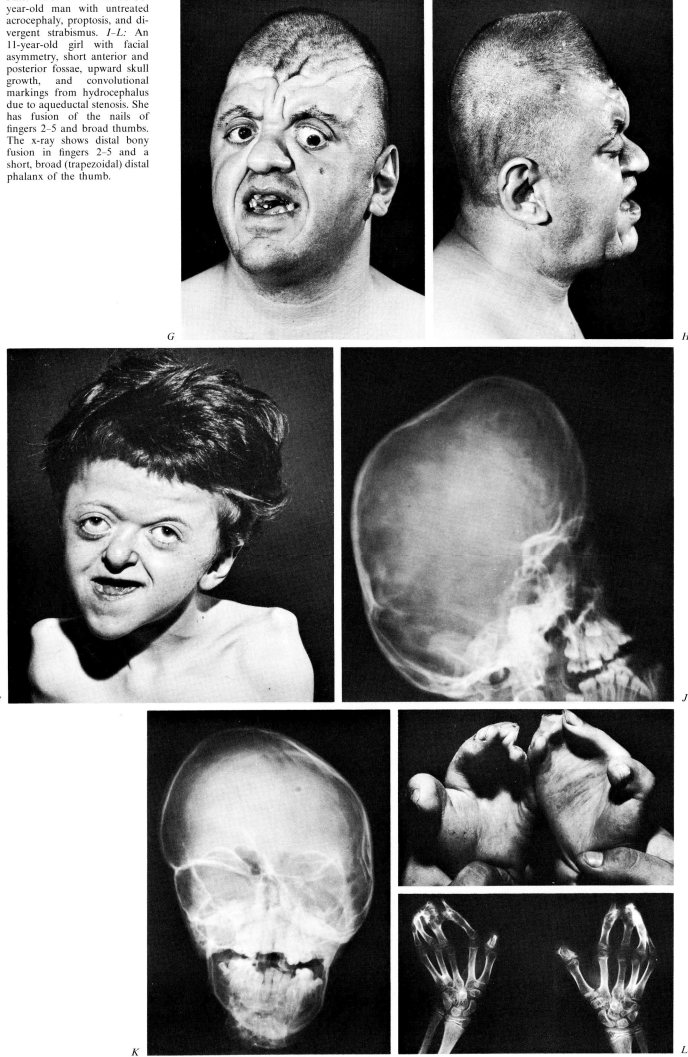

Plate VI-3. *G* and *H:* A 36-year-old man with untreated acrocephaly, proptosis, and divergent strabismus. *I–L:* An 11-year-old girl with facial asymmetry, short anterior and posterior fossae, upward skull growth, and convolutional markings from hydrocephalus due to aqueductal stenosis. She has fusion of the nails of fingers 2–5 and broad thumbs. The x-ray shows distal bony fusion in fingers 2–5 and a short, broad (trapezoidal) distal phalanx of the thumb.

G

H

I

J

K

L

225

Chotzen's Syndrome
(Acrocephalosyndactyly, Type III)

In 1932 Chotzen [1] described a father and two sons who had flat, high brows, hypertelorism, ptosis, prognathism, and syndactyly. A second family with ten affected members in three generations was reported in 1970 [2].

Physical Features

HEAD: The forehead and occiput are flat and the vertical diameter is increased (*Figures A, D, E, and F*).

FACE: The forehead is wide and flat. The eyes are widely spaced. The nose is prominent and the nasal septum is often deviated. Ptosis and prognathism are also common (*Figures A, B, E, and F*).

EARS: In one of the families [2] several individuals had small, low-set ears that were rotated posteriorly.

MOUTH: Severe early caries were noted in both families.

GENITALIA: Cryptorchidism is common.

LIMBS: The syndactyly involves only soft tissue and in the hands affects only the proximal portion of the fingers. In the family reported by Chotzen [1] the syndactyly involved the second and third fingers and the fourth and fifth toes. One child also had webbing between the second, third, and fourth toes of one foot. In the second family [2] the syndactyly involved primarily the second and third fingers (*Figure C*) and toes. Mild syndactyly also occurred between the third and fourth fingers, and one individual had syndactyly of the fourth and fifth toes (*Figure D*). One person had radioulnar synostosis.

HEIGHT: Short stature is common.

Nervous System

In Chotzen's report [1] both the father and his two sons were considered to have subnormal intelligence. In the second reported family [2] several members had measured IQ's between 50 and 60; the intelligence of the members without acrocephalosyndactyly was also considered low.

Laboratory Studies

In the second family [2] three members were shown to have coronal synostosis. One retarded girl with premature coronal suture closure also was shown by pneumoencephalography to have dilated lateral ventricles; another child with coronal synostosis had no evidence of hydrocephalus.

Treatment and Prognosis

Craniectomy in infants for the early closure of the coronal sutures will improve their appearance. The syndactyly is mild enough to not require surgery, except for cosmetic reasons.

Genetics

Autosomal dominant.

Differential Diagnosis

1. Acrocephaly and syndactyly are features of patients with Apert's syndrome, but they usually have extensive syndactyly of most digits and also have proptosis, maxillary hypoplasia, and a beaklike nose (see page 222).
2. Craniosynostosis, hypertelorism, deformed ears, and syndactyly are features of patients with Carpenter's syndrome, but they also have polysyndactyly of their feet, and the syndactyly of their hands when present involves digits 3 and 4 (see page 232).
3. Acrocephaly with a broad, flat forehead and prognathism are features of patients with Crouzon's disease, but they have proptosis, divergent strabismus, a beaked nose, and maxillary hypoplasia and do not have syndactyly (see page 230).

References

1. Chotzen, F.   Eine eigenartige familiäre Entwicklungsstörung. (Akrocephalosyndaktylie, Dysostosis craniofacialis and Hypertelorismus). *Monatsschr. Kinderheilkd.*, **55**:97–122, 1932.
2. Bartsocas, C. S., Weber, A. L., and Crawford, J. D.   Acrocephalosyndactyly type III: Chotzen's syndrome. *J. Pediatr.*, **77**:267–72, 1970.

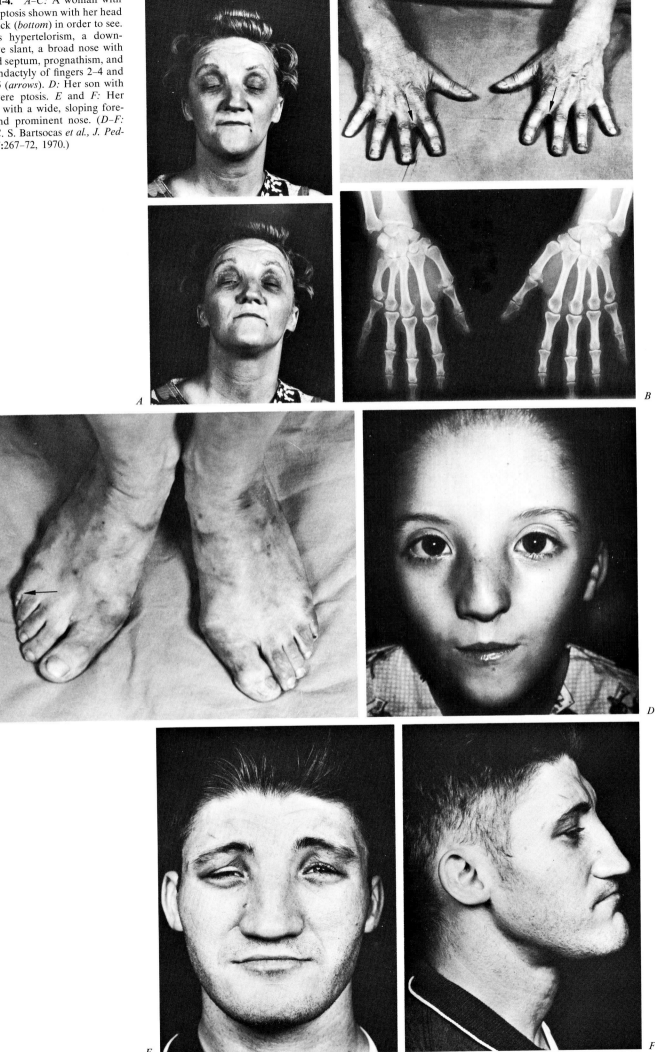

Plate VI-4. *A–C:* A woman with marked ptosis shown with her head tilted back (*bottom*) in order to see. She has hypertelorism, a downward eye slant, a broad nose with deviated septum, prognathism, and mild syndactyly of fingers 2–4 and toes 4–5 (*arrows*). *D:* Her son with less severe ptosis. *E* and *F:* Her brother with a wide, sloping forehead and prominent nose. (*D–F:* From C. S. Bartsocas *et al., J. Pediatr.,* **77:**267–72, 1970.)

Pfeiffer's Syndrome
(Acrocephalosyndactyly, Type VI)

In 1964 Pfeiffer [1] described eight members of one family with craniosynostosis, facial deformities, large thumbs and great toes, and syndactyly. Another patient was described in 1969 [2]. A third family with an affected father and two children has been studied, but not reported [3]. A fourth family was reported in 1971 [4]. While there is no definite association with subnormal intelligence, this disorder is included because of its importance as a separate form of acrocephalosyndactyly.

Physical Features

HEAD: These patients have a towerlike skull with increased upward growth, a prominent forehead, and flat occiput (*Figures A, C, and E*).

FACE: The eyes protrude and are widely spaced. The nose is flat and chin is prominent (*Figures A, C, and E*).

EYES: Many patients have divergent strabismus.

EARS: The ears are low-set.

MOUTH: The teeth are irregularly aligned and the palate is gothic. A few patients have had either a submucous cleft palate or bifid uvula [1].

LIMBS: The thumb and great toe are short, wide, and deviate medially. The syndactyly of the hands, when present, involves fingers 2-4, but does not always extend to the end of the digits [1] (*Figures B and F*). The syndactyly of the toes may involve only toes 1-2 [2] or may involve part or all of toes 1-4 (*Figures B, D, and F*). One child [2] had partially flexed elbows and a mild calcaneovarus deformity of the feet.

Nervous System

No neurologic abnormalities have been described in the published reports [1,2,4]. The father in the third family [3] has subnormal intelligence.

Laboratory Studies

X-rays show abnormally shaped phalanges in the thumbs and great toes, large first metatarsals, absence of the middle phalanges of the toes, ankylosed distal interphalangeal joints in the fingers, hypoplastic maxilla, a short anterior fossa of the skull, and a steep base of the skull [1]. One child had synostosis of the coronal sutures and radiohumeral and radioulnar synostosis [2]. Another had premature closure of the sagittal and coronal sutures, increased digital markings on the skull x-ray, shortening of the middle phalanges of the toes, and trapezoid-shaped proximal phalanges of the great toes [4].

Genetics

Autosomal dominant.

Differential Diagnosis

1. A towerlike skull, protruding eyes, large and deviated thumbs, and syndactyly are features of patients with Apert's syndrome, but they have more extensive syndactyly (see page 222).
2. A tower skull, hypertelorism, protruding eyes, and divergent strabismus are features of patients with Crouzon's disease, but they have normal hands and feet (see page 230).
3. Large, deviated thumbs and great toes are features of patients with the Rubinstein-Taybi syndrome, but they do not have protruding eyes or syndactyly and do have microcephaly, a prominent nose, and a downward palpebral slant (see page 306).
4. Broad thumbs and great toes and syndactyly are features of patients with the frontodigital syndrome, but they also have a prominent brow, preaxial polydactyly, and normal intelligence [4].

References

1. Pfeiffer, R. A. Dominant erbliche Akrocephalosyndactylie. Z. *Kinderheilkd.,* **90:**301–20, 1964.
2. Asnes, R. S., and Morehead, C. D. Pfeiffer syndrome. *Birth Defects: Original Article Series,* Vol. V, No. 3, March, 1969, pp. 198–203. Williams & Wilkins Co., Baltimore.
3. Pfeiffer, R. A. Personal communication, 1970.
4. Martsolf, J. T., Cracco, J. B., Carpenter, G. G., and O'Hara, A. E. Pfeiffer syndrome. An unusual type of acrocephalosyndactyly with broad thumbs and great toes. *Am. J. Dis. Child.,* **121:**257–62, 1971.
5. Marshall, R. E., and Smith, D. W. Frontodigital syndrome: a dominantly inherited disorder with normal intelligence. *J. Pediatr.,* **77:**129–33, 1971.

Plate VI-5. *A* and *B:* The propositus of the first reported family showing hypertelorism, a flat nasal bridge, repaired syndactyly of fingers 2–4, and syndactyly of toes 2–3. *C–F:* A son and father each with a high forehead, flat occiput, prominent chin, and large, short deviated thumbs and great toes. The son had syndactyly of toes 2–3 and the father of fingers 3–4 and toes 1–4. (*A:* From R. A. Pfeiffer, *Z. Kinderheilkd.,* **90:** 301–20, 1964. *B:* Courtesy of Dr. R. A. Pfeiffer, Münster, Germany, *C–F:* Courtesy of Dr. K. D. Ebel, Cologne, Germany.)

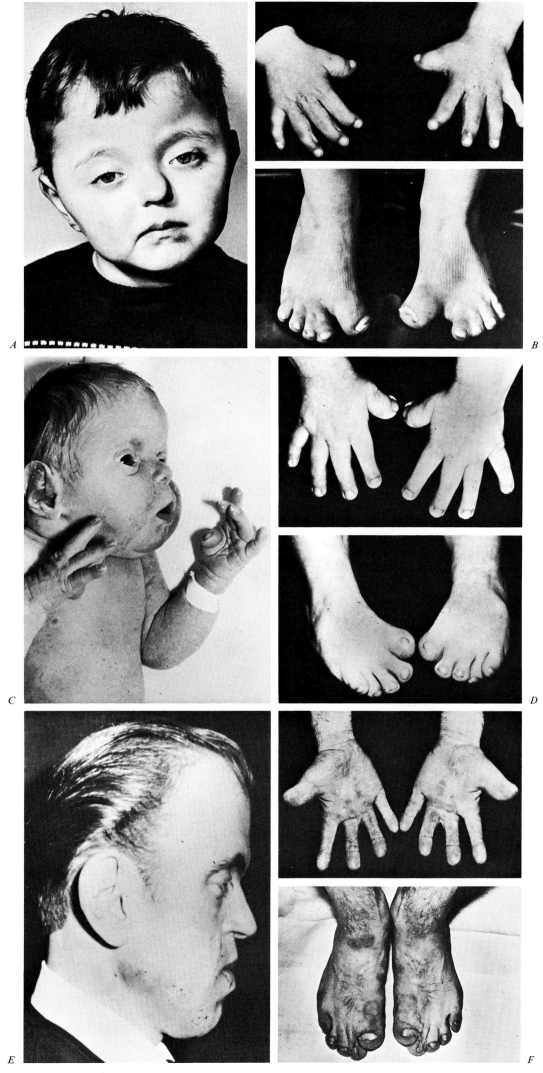

A

B

C

D

E

F

Crouzon's Disease
(Craniofacial Dysostosis)

In 1912 Crouzon [1] reported a mother and her son who had a widened skull with a protrusion in the region of the anterior fontanel, exophthalmos, a beaked nose, and hypoplasia of the maxilla. More than 100 additional patients had been reported by 1966 [2].

Physical Features

HEAD: Many different shapes have been described. One of the most common consists of a flat, wide forehead, an increased transverse skull diameter, and a decreased anteroposterior diameter, which occurs in patients with coronal and lambdoid synostosis (*Figures A and B*). A patient with marked upward skull growth in the area of the anterior fontanel (*Figure C*) has also been described [3]. Patients with premature closure of several sutures may be microcephalic, with the skull coming to a point at the vertex [4].

FACE: The eyes are proptosed and widely spaced. The palpebral slant is downward. The maxilla and zygomatic arches are underdeveloped. The nasal bridge is flat, and the tip of the nose, while normal, appears beaklike in the facial profile due to the mid-face hypoplasia. The chin is normal, but often appears to be prominent (*Figure B*).

EYES: Because of the exophthalmos these patients may not be able to converge or to fix on an object with both eyes. Strabismus is common [4].

EARS: Some patients have had malformed auditory canals and middle ear ossicles in association with a hearing loss [5].

MOUTH: The palate is high and narrow. The upper teeth are crowded and irregularly aligned.

Nervous System

These patients often have mild to moderate mental retardation. Some patients have had increased intracranial pressure due to the premature closure of several sutures and have developed optic atrophy and blindness.

Laboratory Studies

The skull x-rays show prominent convolutional markings in the areas of the prematurely fused sutures (*Figures A, B, and D*). The orbits are small and the maxilla is small and appears underdeveloped.

Treatment and Prognosis

Correction of severe skull deformity due to craniosynostosis is recommended in early infancy. It is not known whether early craniectomy improves the intelligence of these patients. Some adults, who had had no cranial surgery, had average or above average intelligence in association with increased intracranial pressure [6]. Cor pulmonale from upper airway obstruction has been reported [9].

Genetics

Autosomal dominant.

Differential Diagnosis

1. Acrocephaly (tower skull), proptosis, a downward palpebral slant, underdeveloped maxilla, and relative prognathism are also features of patients with Apert's syndrome, who can be distinguished only by the associated syndactyly (see page 222).

2. Acrocephaly, hypertelorism, and prognathism are features of patients with the Chotzen syndrome, but they also have ptosis, a broad nose, and syndactyly, and do not have protruding eyes (see page 226).

3. Craniosynostosis, hypertelorism, and a downward palpebral slant are features of individuals with the "pseudo-Crouzon's syndrome," but they do not have a beaklike nose, prognathism, or divergent strabismus [7].

4. A flat nasal bridge, hypertelorism, flat forehead, and prognathism are features of patients with the XXXXY syndrome, but they do not have proptosis or craniosynostosis and often have vertebral anomalies and hypogonadism (see page 190).

5. A flat nasal bridge and maxillary hypoplasia are features of patients with Larsen's syndrome [8], but they do not have either craniosynostosis, proptosis, or mental retardation, and do have multiple, recurrent joint dislocations.

References

1. Crouzon, O. Dysostose cranio-faciale héréditaire. *Bull. Soc. Med. Hop. Paris,* **33**:545–55, 1912.
2. Vulliamy, D. G., and Normandale, P. A. Cranio-facial dysostosis in a Dorset family. *Arch. Dis. Child.,* **41**:375–82, 1966.
3. Shiller, J. G. Craniofacial dysostosis of Crouzon: A case report and pedigree with emphasis on heredity. *Pediatrics,* **23**:107–12, 1959.
4. Flippen, J. H., Jr. Cranio-facial dysostosis of Crouzon. *Pediatrics,* **5**:90–96, 1950.
5. Boedts, D. La surdite dans la dysostose craniofaciale ou maladie de Crouzon. *Acta Otorhinolaryngol. Belg.,* **21**:143–55, 1967.
6. Cross, H. E., and Opitz, J. M. Craniosynostosis in the Amish. *J. Pediatr.,* **75**:1037–44, 1969.
7. Kernohan, D. C., Nevin, N. C., and Dodge, J. A. Familial craniosynostosis with oral anomalies. *Dev. Med. Child Neurol.,* **12**:315–20, 1970.
8. Latta, R. J., Graham, C. B., Aase, J., Scham, S. M., and Smith, D. W. Larsen's syndrome: a skeletal dysplasia with multiple joint dislocations and unusual facies. *J. Pediatr.,* **78**:291–98, 1971.
9. Don, N., and Siggers, D. C. Cor pulmonale in Crouzon's disease. *Arch. Dis. Child.,* **46**:394–96, 1971.

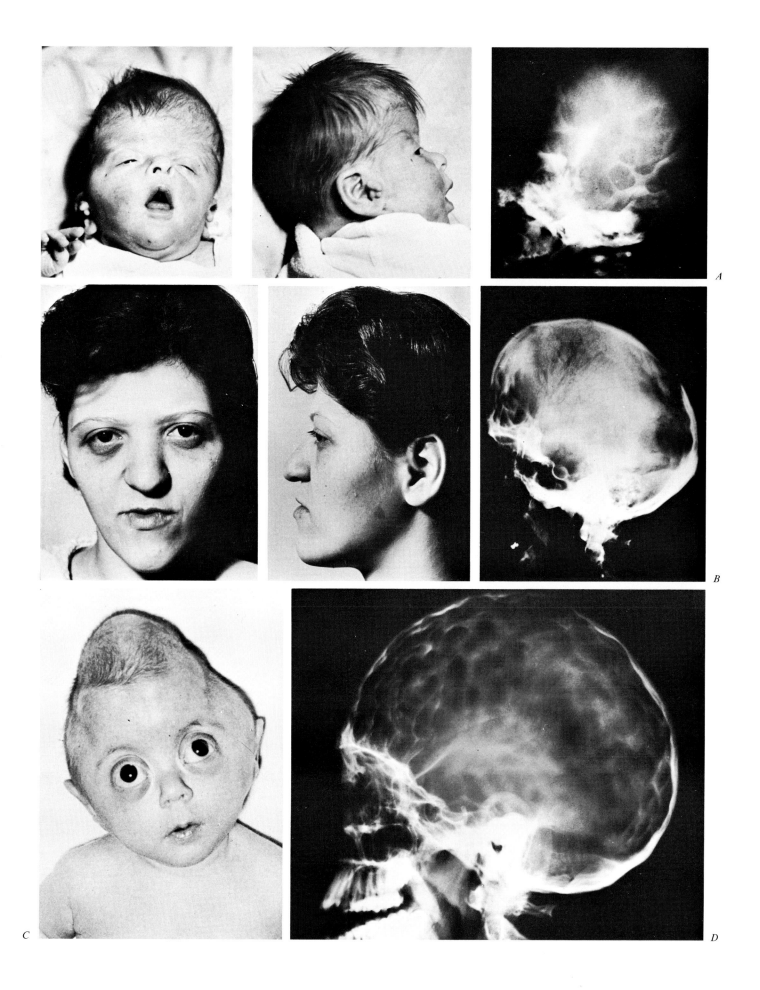

Plate VI-6. *A:* A newborn infant with a high forehead, downward slanting palpebral fissures, a beaklike nose, bilateral preauricular skin tags, and coronal and lambdoid synostosis. The lateral skull x-ray shows prominent convolutional markings in the anterior and posterior fossae. *B:* The mother of this infant. She had a wide, flat forehead, bilateral coronal synostosis, and prominent convolutional markings in the shortened anterior fossa. *C:* A 2-month-old infant with proptosis and protrusion of the skull and brain in the area of the anterior fontanel and the squamosal suture. Many family members in four generations had proptosis and hypertelorism. *D:* The skull x-ray of a patient with Crouzon's disease who had premature fusion of all sutures and prominent convolutional markings throughout the cranium. (*C:* From J. G. Shiller, *Pediatrics,* **23:**107–12, 1959. *D:* Courtesy of Dr. D. Hoefnagel, Hanover, N.H.)

231

Carpenter's Syndrome (Acrocephalopolysyndactyly)

In 1901 Carpenter [1] reported two sisters with acrocephaly, syndactyly between the third and fourth fingers, and polysyndactyly of the feet. Since that time several children with similar anomalies have been described under a variety of names. In 1966 Temtamy [2] reported one patient and reviewed 12 previously described patients, including several who had been originally reported as examples of the Laurence-Moon syndrome. This experience has shown that craniofacial anomalies, obesity, and a variety of skeletal deformities are also features of this syndrome.

Physical Features

HEAD: Patients with premature fusion of all sutures have a small head [2]. Those with premature closure of only the coronal and the lambdoid sutures have a wide, flat brow and occiput and increased vertical diameter of the skull.

FACE: The facial profile is flat (*Figure B*). The bridge of the nose is flat and the medial canthi are laterally displaced. The palpebral fissures have a slight downward slant (*Figures A and D*). Epicanthal folds and micrognathia are usually present.

EYES: Microcornea and corneal opacities have been described in some patients [2].

EARS: The ears are usually low-set and malformed (*Figure E*).

GENITALIA: The reported males have had hypogenitalism.

LIMBS: Partial syndactyly of the third and fourth fingers (*Figure C*) is the most common hand anomaly. Postaxial polydactyly has also been noted (*Figure F*). All patients have polysyndactyly of the toes with medial deviation and duplication of either the first or second toe (*Figures C and F*). Several patients have had genu valgum.

WEIGHT: These patients are usually obese.

Nervous System

Most of the reported patients have had subnormal intelligence [2].

Pathology

Postmortem findings are available on one of the patients reported by Carpenter [3] and two of three brothers who were originally reported as having the Laurence-Moon syndrome [4], but were considered by Temtamy [2] as examples of Carpenter's syndrome. The infant studied by Carpenter [3] had a cardiac anomaly. In the second report [4] one infant had a tetralogy of Fallot, unilateral hydroureter, a small phallus, and normal testes. The other infant had a single ventricle, transposition of the great vessels, biliary atresia, and hypergyria of the cerebral cortex.

Laboratory Studies

X-rays demonstrate the craniosynostosis, duplication of the first or second toe, triangular-shaped middle phalanges in those digits that are medially deviated, flaring of the iliac wings, flattening of the acetabulum, and coxa valga. Chromosome, amino acid, and mucopolysaccharide studies have been normal.

Treatment and Prognosis

Early correction of the craniosynostosis and polysyndactyly is recommended. Because the width of the foot prevents the wearing of normal shoes, one toe must be removed, usually one of the duplicated great toes. Cardiac anomalies were the cause of death in infancy of 3 out of 13 patients [2,3].

Genetics

Autosomal recessive.

Differential Diagnosis

1. Obesity, mental retardation, hypogenitalism, and polydactyly are features of patients with the Laurence-Moon syndrome, but they are distinguished by also having retinal degeneration and not having either craniofacial anomalies or syndactyly (see page 288).

2. Acrocephaly and syndactyly are features of patients with Apert's syndrome, but they are distinguished by having hypoplasia of the maxilla, proptosis, more extensive syndactyly of the hands, and the absence of polydactyly (see page 222).

3. Acrocephalosyndactyly, obesity, and genu valgum are features of the two brothers reported by Summit [5], but they had normal intelligence and did not have polydactyly.

4. Acrocephaly and polysyndactyly are features of the family with Noack's syndrome [6], but the syndactyly is minimal, the polydactyly is only visible in x-rays of the great toes, and the patients have normal intelligence.

5. Duplication of the great toe (and sometimes syndactyly of the fingers) and wide medial canthi are features of patients with the Mohr syndrome [7], but they have tongue and lip clefts, maxillary hypoplasia, and a conductive hearing loss.

References

1. Carpenter, G. Two sisters showing malformations of the skull and other congenital abnormalities. *Rep. Soc. Study Dis. Child. London,* **1**:110–18, 1901.
2. Temtamy, S. A. Carpenter's syndrome: acrocephalopolysyndactyly. An autosomal recessive syndrome. *J. Pediatr.,* **69**:111–20, 1966.
3. Carpenter, G. Case of acrocephaly with other congenital malformations—autopsy. *Proc. R. Soc. Med.,* **II** (part 1):199–201, 1909.
4. McLoughlin, T. G., and Shanklin, D. R. Pathology of Laurence-Moon-Bardet-Biedl syndrome. *J. Pathol.,* **93**:65–79, 1967.
5. Summitt, R. L. Recessive acrocephalosyndactyly with normal intelligence. *Birth Defects: Original Article Series,* Vol. V, No. 3, March, 1969, pp. 35–38. Williams & Wilkins Co., Baltimore.
6. Noack, M. Ein Beitrag zum Krankheitsbild der Akrozephalosyndaktylie (Apert). *Arch. Kinderheilkd.,* **160**:168–71, 1959.
7. Rimoin, D. L., and Edgerton, M. T. Genetic and clinical heterogeneity in the oral-facial-digital syndromes. *J. Pediatr.,* **71**:94–102, 1967.

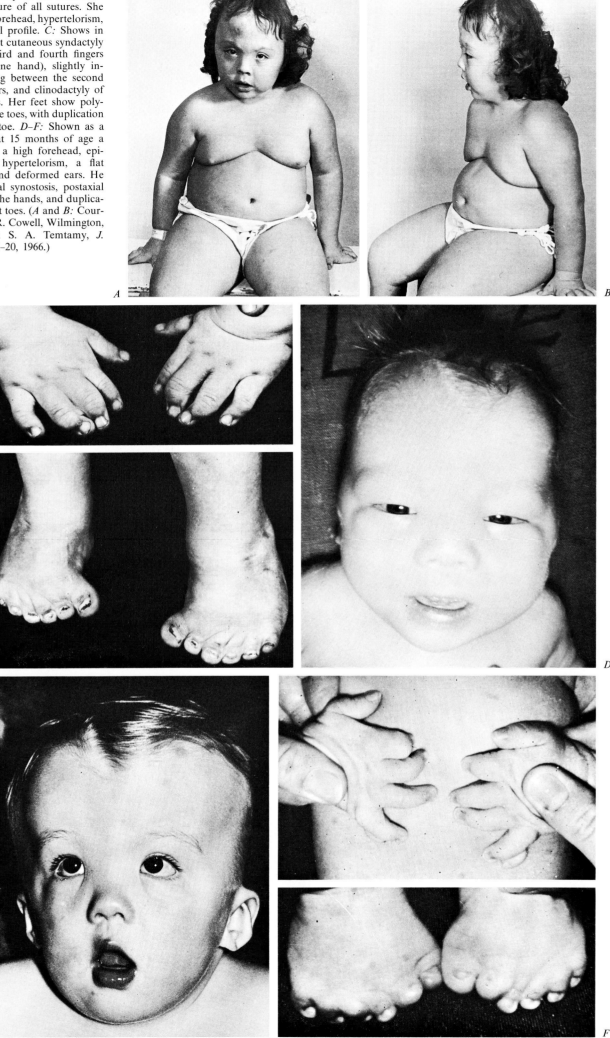

Plate VI-7. *A* and *B:* This obese girl had a craniectomy as an infant for premature closure of all sutures. She still has a high forehead, hypertelorism, and a flat facial profile. *C:* Shows in the same patient cutaneous syndactyly between the third and fourth fingers (corrected in one hand), slightly increased webbing between the second and third fingers, and clinodactyly of the fifth fingers. Her feet show polysyndactyly of the toes, with duplication of the second toe. *D–F:* Shown as a newborn and at 15 months of age a child who had a high forehead, epicanthic folds, hypertelorism, a flat nasal bridge, and deformed ears. He also had sagittal synostosis, postaxial polydactyly of the hands, and duplication of the great toes. (*A* and *B:* Courtesy of Dr. H. R. Cowell, Wilmington, Del. *C:* From S. A. Temtamy, *J. Pediatr.,* **69:**111–20, 1966.)

Cloverleaf Skull
(Kleeblattschädel Syndrome)

Infants with a trilobed skull, hydrocephalus, proptosis, and shortened limbs have been designated by Holtermüller and Wiedemann [1] as having the Kleeblattschädel syndrome. The term *cloverleaf skull*, an American translation, was suggested by Comings [2]. By 1971 over 25 patients with this syndrome had been described [3–5]. It has been suggested that the patients with this syndrome may be a heterogeneous group [5].

Physical Features

HEAD: The skull shape at birth is trilobed because of upward and lateral bulging in the areas of the sagittal and squamosal sutures. This is the result of two factors: first, increased intracranial pressure due to congenital hydrocephalus; and second, coronal, lambdoid, squamous, and sagittal suture synostosis (*Figures A, C, D, E, and F*).

FACE: The most striking features are the high, wide forehead, proptosis, and a downward, posterior displacement of the ears. Hypertelorism, a downward palpebral slant, and divergent strabismus are usually present (*Figures A, C, D, and E*). The nasal bridge is flat and the nose has a beaked appearance in profile.

EYES: The eyes often protrude (*Figures C and D*) and have corneal ulcerations.

LIMBS: Shortening of the arms and legs has been reported in most of the patients [3,4]. Ankylosis of the elbows, knees, shoulders, and hips has often been noted.

Nervous System

These patients are usually severely retarded. The cause of the hydrocephalus is not known; extraventricular obstruction by a small foramen magnum has been suggested [1,3]. One patient had aqueductal stenosis [4].

Pathology

The only description of postmortem findings [3] noted that in one patient all cerebral ventricles were dilated, the meninges were thickened, and the cerebellum was smaller than normal.

Laboratory Studies

Skull x-rays (*Figure B*) show premature fusion of the coronal and lambdoid sutures, absence of the lateral portion of the orbits and the squamosal bones, and underdevelopment of the maxilla and zygoma. Patients with short limbs have short, wide long bones with metaphyseal flaring [2,3]. One reported patient [3] had multiple vertebral anomalies. Another had flaring of the metaphyses and decreasing interpedicular distances in the lower lumbar spine [4]. Chromosome and amino acid studies have revealed no abnormalities.

Treatment and Prognosis

The life expectancy of these patients is not known. Some have died in the first months of life [1–3]; one patient was reported at age 14 years [4]. Early corrective surgery for the craniosynostosis and hydrocephalus is recommended, but the effect of this on the intelligence and survival of these patients is not known.

Genetics

In one report [5] there were two similarly affected siblings, each of whom had severe shortening of the limbs.

Differential Diagnosis

1. A tower skull, proptosis, maxillary hypoplasia, a beaklike nose, and hydrocephalus are features of patients with Apert's syndrome, but they are distinguished by the presence of syndactyly of the hands and feet and the absence of lateral protrusion of the skull (see page 222).
2. A tower skull, proptosis, and maxillary hypoplasia are features of patients with Crouzon's disease, but they do not have hydrocephalus or lateral protrusion of the skull (see page 230).
3. A large head and short limbs are features of patients with achondroplasia, but these patients do not have craniosynostosis and have generalized head enlargement at birth (see page 260).

References

1. Holtermüller, K., and Wiedemann, H. R. Kleeblattschädel Syndrom. *Med. Monatsschr.*, **14**:439–46, 1960.
2. Comings, D. E. The Kleeblattschädel syndrome—a grotesque form of hydrocephalus. *J. Pediatr.*, **67**:126–29, 1965.
3. Angle, C. R., McIntire, M. S., and Moore, R. C. Cloverleaf skull: Kleeblattschädel-deformity syndrome. *Am. J. Dis. Child.*, **114**:198–202, 1967.
4. Feingold, M., O'Connor, J. F., Berkman, M., and Darling, D. B. Kleeblattschädel syndrome. *Am. J. Dis. Child.*, **118**:589–94, 1969.
5. Partington, M. W., Gonzalez-Crussi, F., Khakee, S. G., and Wollin, D. G. Cloverleaf skull and thanatothorphoric dwarfism. Report of four cases, two in the same sibship. *Arch. Dis. Child.*, **46**:656–64, 1971.

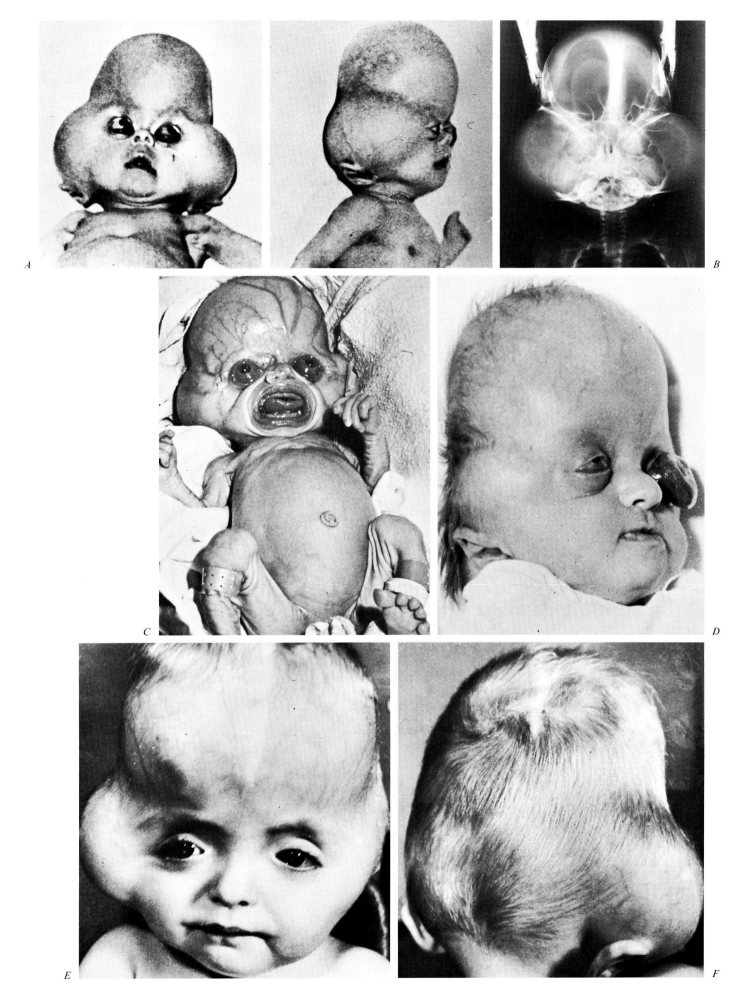

Plate VI-8. *A* and *B:* An infant with a trilobed skull and proptosis. The pneumoencephalogram showed marked ventricular dilatation. Note the absence of recognizable bony orbits. *C:* This 2-month-old infant had hydrocephalus, protrusion of both eyes, and flexion contractures of the fingers, elbows, knees, hips, and shoulders. *D:* A 9-day-old infant with prolapse of one eye, a beaklike nose, and marked upward growth of the skull. *E* and *F:* A 16-month-old boy with asymmetric squamosal protrusion, hypertelorism, a downward palpebral slant, and posterior displacement of both ears. (*A* and *B:* From K. Holtermüller and H. R. Wiedemann, *Med. Monatsschr.,* **14:**439–46, 1960. *C:* From D. E. Comings, *J. Pediatr.,* **67:**126–29, 1965. *D* and *F:* Courtesy of Dr. C. R. Angle, Omaha, Neb. *E:* From C. R. Angle *et al., Am. J. Dis. Child.,* **114:**198–202, 1967.)

Craniotelencephalic Dysplasia

In 1958 Daum, LeBeau, and Minuit [1] described an infant with protrusion of the frontal bone, craniosynostosis, an encephalocele, and mental retardation. A patient with a similar appearance, but no encephalocele, was described by Jabbour and Taybi [2] in 1964 and the term *craniotelencephalic dysplasia* was suggested.

The first reported infant [1] had brachycephaly due to craniosynostosis and a frontal encephalocele which contained most of the frontal lobe. The child had no vision and was considered retarded in her psychomotor development. There were no skeletal anomalies. An outgrowth of the frontal bone was removed, and the encephalocele and craniosynostosis were repaired.

The second child [2] had a hard midline mass that protruded forward in the middle of the frontal squamosa, a midline hemangioma, and hypotelorism (*Figures A and B*). There were no other deformities. Skull x-rays showed closure of the coronal, metopic, and the anterior portion of the sagittal sutures, a short anterior fossa, and a vertical slope of the middle fossa (*Figures C and D*). The intraorbital distance was 9 mm, which is below normal. Craniectomy was performed in the first weeks of life. At age 36 months her developmental age was 18 months. Chromosome studies revealed no abnormalities.

A third infant [3] with similar skull deformity, encephalocele, and mental retardation is shown in *Figures E and F*.

Genetics

None of these children had any similarly affected relatives.

Differential Diagnosis

1. Protrusion in the area of the anterior fontanel, microcephaly, and mental retardation may occur in patients with premature closure of several sutures, but these children are differentiated by the absence of a midfrontal bony protuberance (see page 220).
2. A prominent midforehead ridge extending down to the glabella is a feature of patients with premature fusion of the metopic suture, but they do not have as large a frontal protrusion, a short anterior fossa, or mental retardation (see page 218).

References

1. Daum, S., LeBeau, J., and Minuit, P. Dysplasie télencéphalique avec excroissance de l'os frontal. *Sem. Hop. Paris,* **34**:1893–96, 1958.
2. Jabbour, J. T., and Taybi, H. Craniotelencephalic dysplasia. *Am. J. Dis. Child.,* **108**:627–32, 1964.
3. Hogan, G. R. Personal communication, 1969.

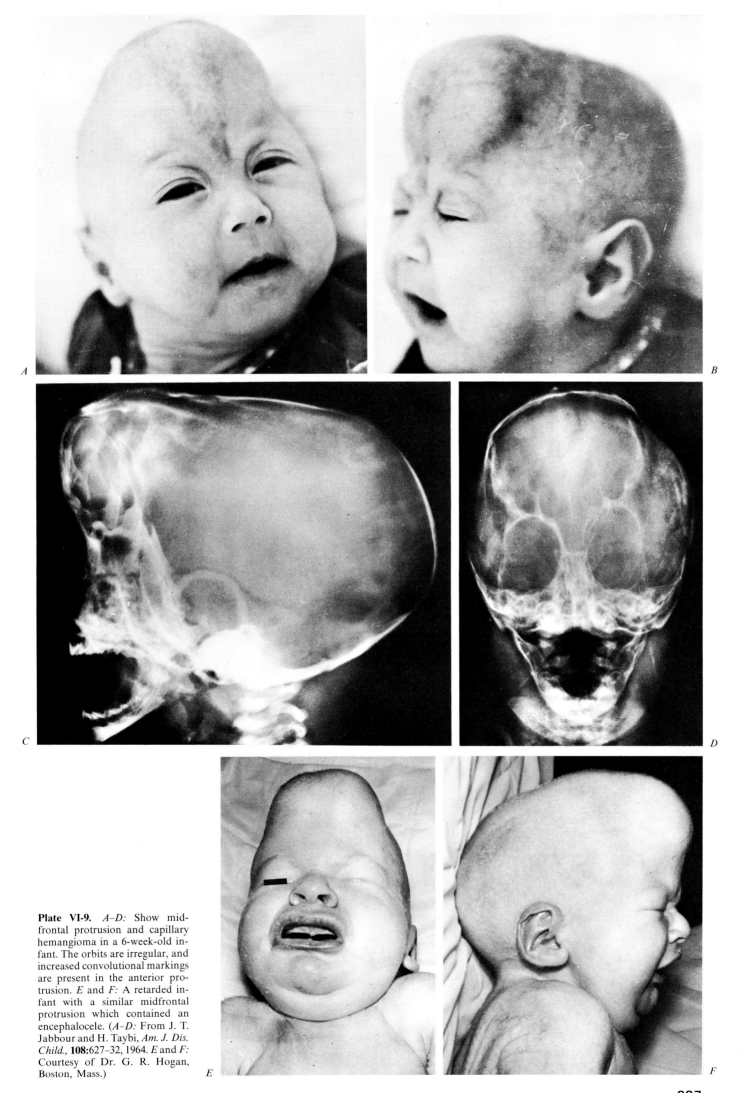

Plate VI-9. *A–D:* Show midfrontal protrusion and capillary hemangioma in a 6-week-old infant. The orbits are irregular, and increased convolutional markings are present in the anterior protrusion. *E* and *F:* A retarded infant with a similar midfrontal protrusion which contained an encephalocele. (*A–D:* From J. T. Jabbour and H. Taybi, *Am. J. Dis. Child.,* **108:**627–32, 1964. *E* and *F:* Courtesy of Dr. G. R. Hogan, Boston, Mass.)

Syndrome of Acrocephalosyndactyly, Absent Digits, and Cranial Defects

In 1969 Herrmann, Pallister, and Opitz [1,2] reported a 7-year-old boy with an unusual craniosynostosis syndrome, characterized by acrocephaly, syndactyly, brachydactyly, absent digits, and a large cranial defect. They considered this case unique.

Physical Features

HEAD: He had a tall, bitemporally flattened head both at birth and when older. His occiput was also flattened (*Figure B*).

FACE: The eyes were widely spaced, and were prominent because of the shallow orbits. The supraorbital ridges were very hypoplastic. His chin was small. The ears were small, posteriorly rotated, and had incompletely formed helices (*Figure B*).

MOUTH: His palate was highly arched.

CHEST: His chest was asymmetric.

GENITALIA: Neither testis was palpable.

LIMBS: He had limited extension and rotation of each elbow (*Figure A*). The fingers of each hand were short; the second to fourth had cutaneous syndactyly to the distal interphalangeal joints and to a lesser degree between the fourth and fifth fingers (*Figure C*). There was only one digit on each foot, each of which originated from the medial aspect and pointed inward (*Figure D*).

HEIGHT AND WEIGHT: His size had always been below the third percentile.

Nervous System

This boy had been living in an institution for the mentally retarded since the age of 9 months. His IQ was estimated as 62. He grunted and pointed to objects when he wanted something.

Laboratory Studies

He had a large defect (7 cm) in the posterior parietal area (*Figures E and F*). Ossification defects up to 2.5 cm in size were also seen in the frontal bone (*Figure F*). The ethmoid sinuses were prominent; the mastoid sinuses were poorly developed, which may have been related to his recurrent middle ear infections. Contrast studies when he was 1 year old suggested that he had a pericardial cyst or hernia. At 7 years of age the epiphyses of the radial heads were not present; the ossification of the carpal bones was normal for his age. He had small proximal phalanges of the thumbs and small or absent middle phalanges of fingers 2–5 (*Figure C*). Each foot had four metacarpals (*Figure D*). Chromosome analysis showed no abnormalities.

Genetics

No member of his family had any similar structural malformations.

Differential Diagnosis

1. Acrocephaly, hypertelorism, cranial defects, and absent toes were features of the child with the amethopterin embryopathy reported by Milunsky and coworkers [3] (see page 134). Their patient did not have syndactyly and brachydactyly of his hands. There was no known history of exposure to aminopterin, amethopterin, or any other teratogens in the present case [4].

2. Acrocephaly, hypertelorism, ear deformities, and syndactyly are features of patients with Carpenter's syndrome, but they also have polydactyly and do not have cranial defects or absent digits (see page 232).

References

1. Herrmann, J., Pallister, P. D., and Opitz, J. M.   Craniosynostosis and craniosynostosis syndromes. *Rocky Mt. Med. J.,* **66**(5):45–56, 1969.
2. Herrmann, J., and Opitz, J. M.   An unusual form of acrocephalosyndactyly. *Birth Defects: Original Article Series,* Vol. V, No. 3, March, 1969, pp. 39–42. Williams & Wilkins Co., Baltimore.
3. Milunsky, A., Graef, J. W., and Gaynor, M. F., Jr.   Methotrexate-induced congenital malformations, with a review of the literature. *J. Pediatr.,* **72**:790–95, 1968.
4. Opitz, J. M.   Personal communication, 1969.

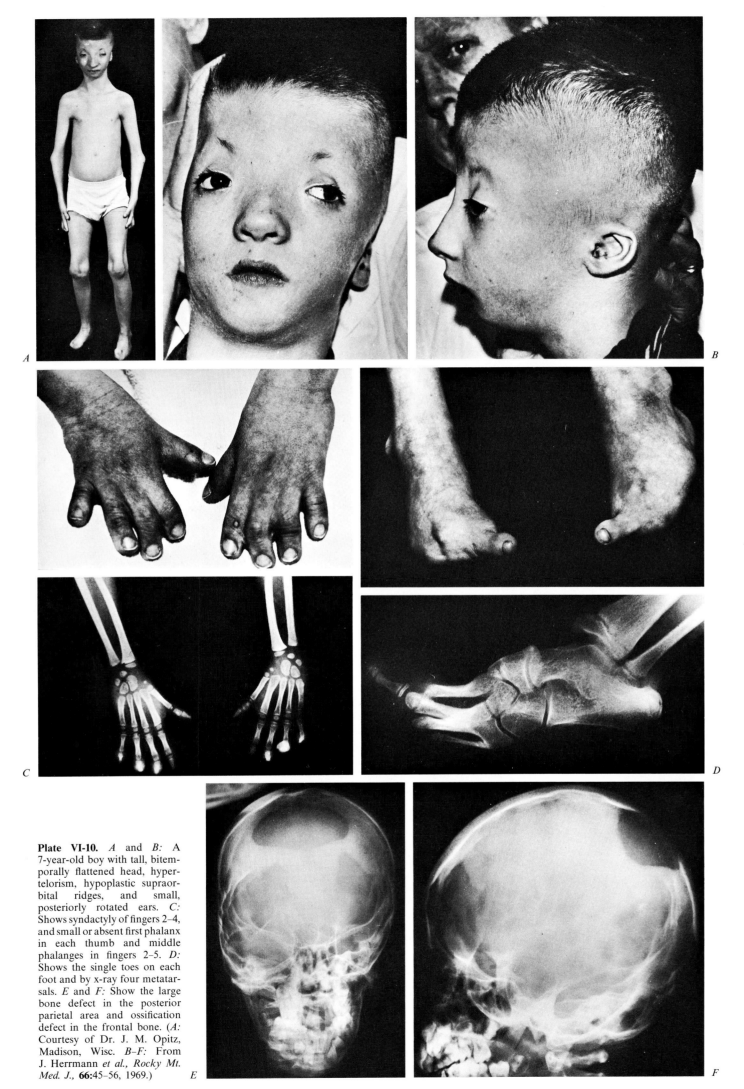

Plate VI-10. *A* and *B:* A 7-year-old boy with tall, bitemporally flattened head, hypertelorism, hypoplastic supraorbital ridges, and small, posteriorly rotated ears. *C:* Shows syndactyly of fingers 2–4, and small or absent first phalanx in each thumb and middle phalanges in fingers 2–5. *D:* Shows the single toes on each foot and by x-ray four metatarsals. *E* and *F:* Show the large bone defect in the posterior parietal area and ossification defect in the frontal bone. (*A:* Courtesy of Dr. J. M. Opitz, Madison, Wisc. *B–F:* From J. Herrmann *et al., Rocky Mt. Med. J.,* **66:**45–56, 1969.)

Syndrome of Acrocephaly, Cleft Lip and Palate, Radial Aplasia, and Absent Digits

In 1969 Herrmann, Pallister, and Opitz [1] reported an 11-year-old boy of Indian-white descent with severe skull, facial, and limb anomalies. No other similarly affected individuals have been reported.

Physical Features

HEAD: He had microbrachycephaly due to craniosynostosis of portions of the coronal, sagittal, and lambdoid sutures (*Figures B and D*).

FACE: Hypertelorism, a deviated nasal septum, and repaired cleft lip were present (*Figure B*).

EARS: The helices of both ears were thin and misshapen.

MOUTH: He had a cleft palate, malpositioned upper and lower incisors, and a low and widely curved mandible.

CHEST: The shoulders and thorax were narrow, and there was a slight depression of the lower sternum.

GENITALIA: The scrotum was small. Neither testis was palpable.

LIMBS: The ulnae were short and the radii were absent. There were three fingers and metacarpals. His hands were held in a severe valgus position (*Figures A and C*). He had congenital dislocation of the hips and ankylosis of the knees, and moved around by sliding on the floor. The tibia and femur were short. His feet were held in a marked varus position. The third and fourth toes were hypoplastic.

Nervous System

This boy could feed himself, but did not speak. He communicated by making sounds and grimaces. His muscle strength was good. His IQ was estimated to be 27.

Laboratory Studies

X-rays showed a steep base of the skull, fusion of the carpal bones, absence of the fibula and radius, and dysplasia of the femoral head and neck. The femoral shaft was relatively narrow (*Figures C, E, and F*). Chromosome studies were normal.

Genetics

No other family member was similarly affected.

Differential Diagnosis

1. Shortened limbs and cleft lip and palate are features of infants with the syndrome of tetraphocomelia, cleft lip and palate, and genital hypertrophy, but they do not have craniosynostosis (see page 344).
2. Infants with the syndrome of phocomelia, flexion deformities, and facial anomalies have hypertelorism, absent radii and digits, and ear deformities, but they also have silvery-blond hair, eye anomalies, and capillary hemangiomas of the face and no cleft lip or palate (see page 340).

Reference

1. Herrmann, J., Pallister, P. D., and Opitz, J. M. Craniosynostosis and craniosynostosis syndromes. *Rocky Mt. Med. J.,* **66**(5):45–56, 1969.

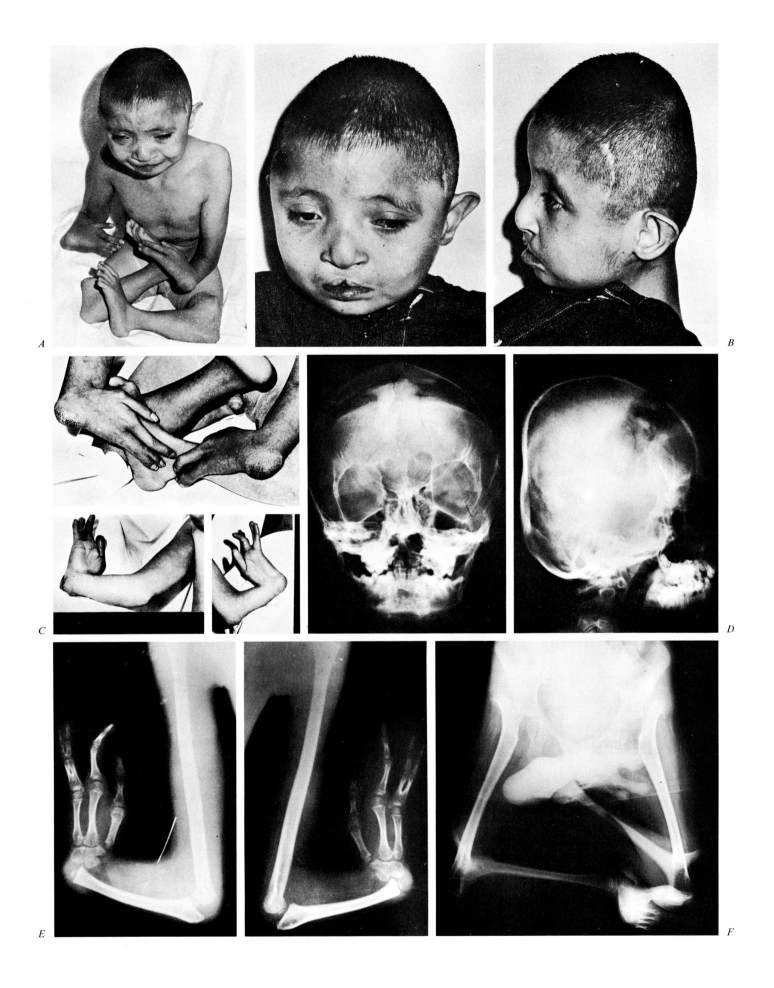

Plate VI-11. *A–C:* An 11-year-old boy with repaired cleft lip, hypertelorism, tower-shaped skull, deformed ears, absent radii, and only three fingers on each hand. His hips and knees were ankylosed and he stayed in this position. *D–F:* X-rays show the flat occiput, increased vertical diameter of the cranium, dislocated hips, short ulnae, and one bifid digit in each hand. (*A, B, D–F:* From J. Herrmann *et al., Rocky Mt. Med. J.,* **66:**45–56, 1969. *C:* Courtesy of Dr. J. M. Opitz, Madison, Wisc.)

241

Eye Anomaly Syndromes
Anophthalmia, X-Linked

In 1963 Hoefnagal, Keenan, and Allen [1] reported a family with X-linked anophthalmia in which there were four affected males—two brothers, a maternal uncle, and a cousin. Only the male cousin, who died shortly after birth, had multiple congenital anomalies in addition to anophthalmia. A family in which three brothers had bilateral anophthalmia was briefly described by Joseph [2a]; this might be another example of X-linked recessive anophthalmia. No other families with X-linked anophthalmia have been reported, although one sporadic case with similar features has been described [2].

Physical Features

HEAD: All were microcephalic [1–3].

EYES: In each of the patients the eyeballs were clinically absent and the orbit cavities were small, shallow, and lined with conjunctiva. The palpebral fissures were smaller than normal (*Figures B, C, D, E, and F*). The lids were sunken and closed, but could be partially opened voluntarily.

BACK: One patient had slight kyphosis and scoliosis [2].

LIMBS: Two patients [1,2], including the infant with multiple anomalies [1], had equinovarus deformities. One also had a congenital flexion contracture of an index finger [1].

GROWTH AND DEVELOPMENT: The sexual development at puberty was normal. Two males were moderately obese [1,3].

Nervous System

All of the patients had slow psychomotor development during childhood and subnormal intelligence. One had spastic diplegia (*Figure A*). All of the patients could taste and smell normally.

Pathology

The infant whose birth weight was 3 pounds and who died shortly after birth had atresia of the ileum and bilateral absence of the kidneys [1]. Careful neuropathologic studies were done on the adult male with bilateral anophthalmia and no positive family history [2]. These showed a total absence of the eyeballs, optic nerves, chiasm, and optic tracts. The central visual pathways were incompletely developed, which may have been the result of the absence of the retinal elements and their projection fibers. He also had small circular defects in the parietal portion of the calvarium, an anomaly of the circle of Willis and absence of the right middle lobe of the lung.

Laboratory Studies

X-rays showed small orbits and small optic foramina. An electroencephalogram showed an almost complete absence of occipital alpha rhythm with no change produced by photic stimulation [1]. Chromosome studies on two of these patients showed no abnormalities.

Genetics

X-linked recessive inheritance is suggested in the family reported by Hoefnagel and coworkers [1].

Differential Diagnosis

1. Microphthalmia and anophthalmia are features of many patients with the chromosome 13 trisomy, but complete absence of both eyes is uncommon (see page 164).
2. Congenital bilateral anophthalmia has also been reported in two female infants, including one whose parents were cousins [3]. No additional anomalies were noted.
3. Patients with cryptophthalmos have no palpebral openings, and often no eyebrows, but do have much of the posterior portion of the globe and can perceive light. They may also have syndactyly and a variety of facial, genital, and renal anomalies (see page 274).

References

1. Hoefnagel, D., Keenan, M. E., and Allen, F. H., Jr. Heredofamilial bilateral anophthalmia. *Arch. Ophthalmol. (Chicago)*, **69**:760–64, 1963.
2. Haberland, C., and Perou, M. Primary bilateral anophthalmia. *J. Neuropathol. Exp. Neurol.*, **28**:337–51, 1969.
2a. Joseph, R. A pedigree of anophthalmos. *Br. J. Ophthalmol.*, **41**:541–43, 1957.
3. Goco, R. V. Personal communication, 1970.
4. Hesselberg, C. Congenital bilateral anophthalmia. *Acta Ophthalmol. (Kbh.)*, **29**:183–89, 1951.

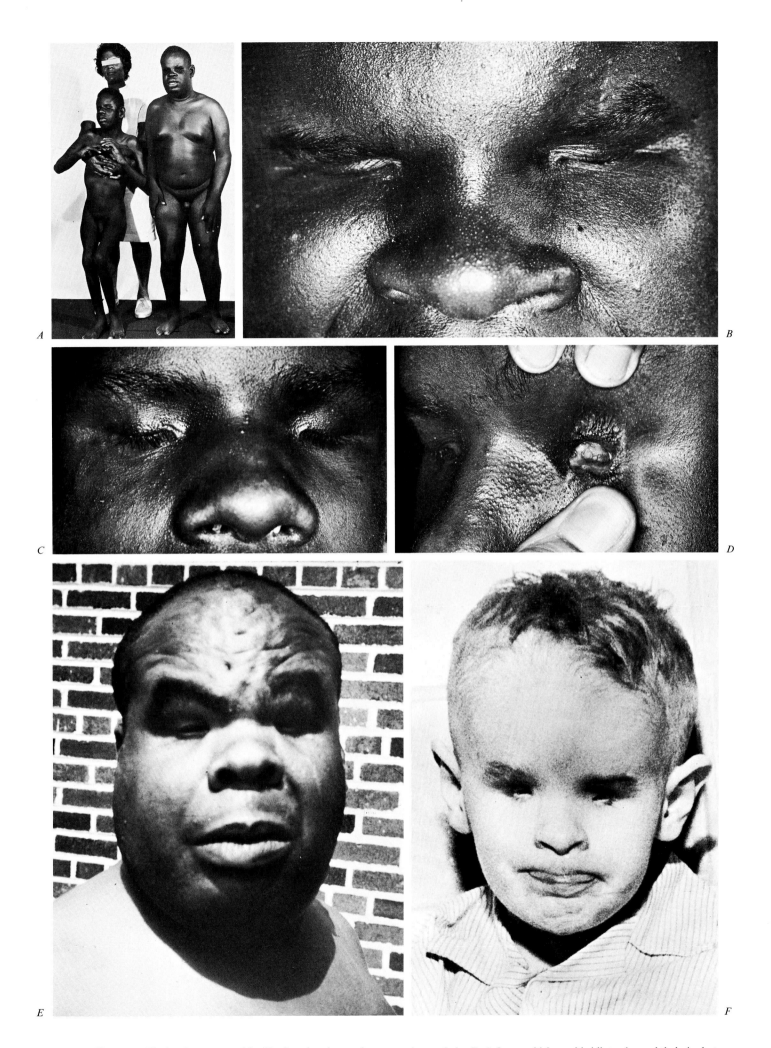

Plate VI-12. *A–D:* The brothers reported by Hoefnagel and coworkers [1], shown at the ages of 13 and 17. The younger one was unable to stand because of severe spasticity. Close-up views show the presence of eyebrows and eyelashes and narrow palpebral fissures. *E:* The 33-year-old uncle of the first two boys with similar facial features and microcephaly. *F:* A 9-year-old boy with bilateral anophthalmia, but a negative family history. He too had narrow palpebral fissures and normal eyebrows and eyelashes. (*E:* Courtesy of Dr. R. V. Goco, Laurel, Md. *F:* From C. Haberland and M. Perou, *J. Neuropathol. Exp. Neurol.,* **28:**337–51, 1969.)

Norrie's Disease

In 1927 Norrie [1] described a type of congenital blindness which he called atrophia oculi congenita. Warburg [2–4] subsequently studied 35 patients in 6 families in Sweden and Denmark and reviewed 106 similar patients from other countries. She showed that a retinal malformation is the primary ocular abnormality. Four affected families have been described in the United States [5–9].

Physical Features

EYES: Most patients never have any vision. Some infants have appeared to have some light perception during the first year and to be able to see large objects. The earliest signs of eye diseases are white vascularized masses behind clear lenses. These retrolental opacities may be visible at birth or not until after a few days or weeks. The eyes are initially normal in size, and the cornea and lens are clear (*Figure A*). Later, the globes become small and shrunken (phthisis bulbi). Lens and corneal opacities develop (*Figures B, C, D, and E*). Both eyes do not always have the same appearance (*Figure D*). Some infants also develop glaucoma.

LIMBS: Shortened distal phalanges have been reported in some affected males in two families [5,9], but it is not certain that this is a feature of Norrie's disease.

Nervous System

In Warburg's study of 35 patients, 20 were considered mentally retarded, 9 severely and 11 to a moderate degree [4]. She noted that the mental development was often normal in the preschool years, but later mental deterioration occurred. Many of the older patients no longer spoke or dressed themselves, became withdrawn, sometimes had outbursts of anger, and hallucinated. In this study 11 men had decreased hearing, the degree of loss ranging from total to a minor deafness that could be overcome with a hearing aid. The hearing loss is considered progressive and is usually not evident until adulthood. It is attributed to cochlear degeneration, but this has not been well established.

Pathology

One enucleated eye showed absence of the rods, cones, and ganglion cells of the retina. The interior of the eye was filled with excessive proliferation of ciliary and retinal pigment epithelium [2] (*Figure F*). In other instances rosettes of rods and cones were found in the retina. Only a few autopsies have been performed, and no neuropathologic changes have been consistently observed [2–4].

Laboratory Studies

Chromosome and amino acid screening tests have shown no abnormalities.

Treatment and Prognosis

There is no treatment for the retinal malformation. Hearing aids may be helpful to some patients. Some patients remain self-sufficient throughout their lifetime, and others become progressively more withdrawn and uncommunicative.

Genetics

X-linked recessive. No abnormalities have been demonstrated in carrier females.

Differential Diagnosis

1. A similar retrolental opacity can be caused by retrolental fibroplasia, retinoblastoma, and congenital toxoplasmosis (see page 124).
2. X-linked recessive microphthalmia, cataract, and mental retardation have been reported by Cuendet [10], but these patients did not have normal-looking eyes at birth, phthisis bulbi, or hearing loss.
3. Corneal opacities, cataracts, glaucoma, and X-linked recessive inheritance are features of infants with Lowe's syndrome, but their cataracts and glaucoma are usually noted soon after birth and they also have hypotonia and aminoaciduria (see page 248).

References

1. Norrie, G. Causes of blindness in children. Twenty-five years' experience of Danish institutes for the blind, *Acta Ophthalmol. (Kbh.)*, **5**:357–86, 1927.
2. Warburg, M. Norrie's disease. A new hereditary bilateral pseudotumor of the retina. *Acta Ophthalmol. (Kbh.)*, **39**:757–72, 1961.
3. Warburg, M. Norrie's disease: a congenital progressive oculo-acoustico-cerebral degeneration. *Acta Ophthalmol. (Kbh.)*, Suppl. 89, pp. 1–147, 1966.
4. Warburg, M. Norrie's disease. *J. Ment. Defic. Res.*, **12**:247–51, 1968.
5. Stephens, F. E. A case of sex-linked microphthalmia. *J. Hered.*, **38**:306–10, 1947.
6. Hansen, A. C. Norrie's disease. *Am. J. Ophthalmol.*, **66**:328–32, 1968.
7. Nance, W. E., Hara, S., Hansen, A., Elliott, J., Lewis, M., and Chown, B. Genetic linkage studies in a Negro kindred with Norrie's disease. *Am. J. Hum. Genet.*, **21**:423–29, 1969.
8. Blodi, F. C., and Hunter, W. S. Norrie's disease in North America. *Doc. Ophthalmol.*, **26**:434–50, 1969.
9. Holmes, L. B. Norrie's disease: an X-linked syndrome of retinal malformation, mental retardation, and deafness. *J. Pediatr.*, **79**:89–92, 1971.
10. Cuendet, J. F. La microphtalmie compliquée. *Ophthalmologica*, **141**:380–85, 1961.

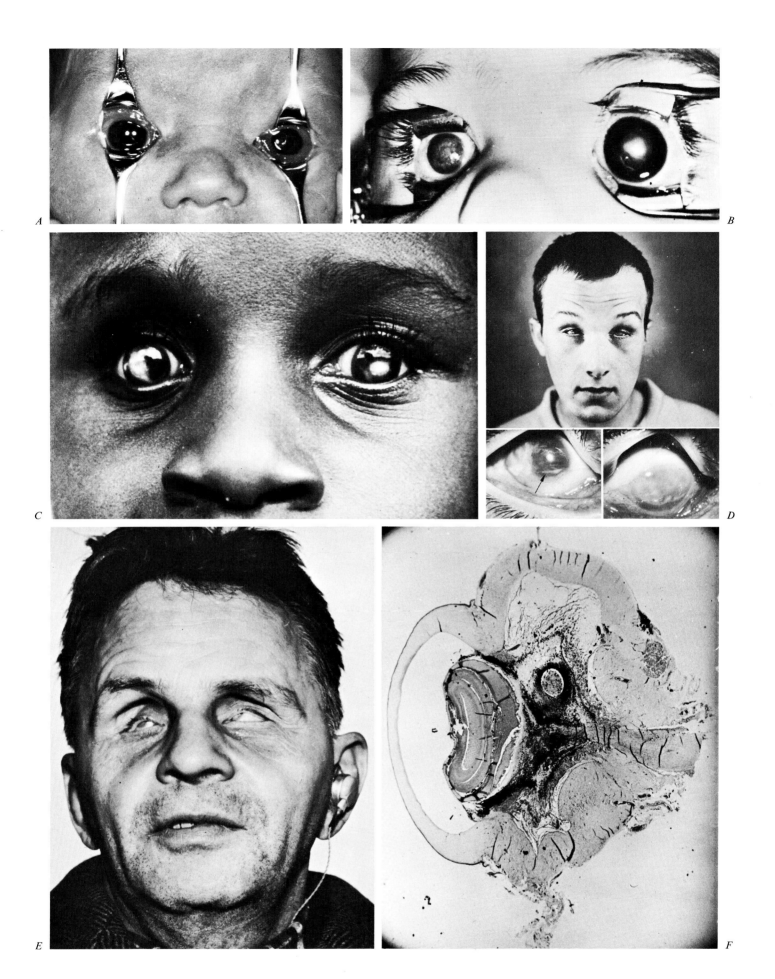

Plate VI-13. *A:* Shows with retractors during anesthesia the eyes of a 7-day-old boy which were normal in size, had a clear cornea and lens, but also had a large retrolental opacity. The cause of the unusual pupil size was not apparent. *B:* Shows the eyes of a 3-year-old boy, the right having an opaque cornea and the left a large retrolental mass. *C:* Shows bilateral corneal opacities, cataracts, and a divergent squint in a boy from the first reported U.S. family. *D:* The 22-year-old uncle of the infant in *A.* He has small, shrunken eyes and normal intelligence. His right eye shows a band keratopathy (*arrow*) and cataract; the anterior chamber of his left eye is opacified by extruded lens material. *E:* A Scandinavian man with shrunken eyes, hearing loss, and normal intelligence. *F:* Cross section of an infant's phthisical eye, showing retinal hypoplasia, proliferation of the vitreous, folding of the sclera, detachment of the ciliary body, and opacification of the lens. (*A:* From L. B. Holmes, *J. Pediatr.,* **79:**89–92, 1971; courtesy of Dr. A. H. Fradkin, Galveston, Texas. *B* and *E:* From M. Warburg, *Acta Ophthalmol.* [*Kbh.*], (Suppl.) **89:**1–147, 1966. *C:* Courtesy of Dr. W. E. Nance, Indianapolis, Ind. *D* [*bottom, left*]: From L. B. Holmes, *J. Pediatr.,* **79:**89–92, 1971. *D* [*bottom, right*]: From L. B. Holmes, *N. Engl. J. Med.,* **284:**367–68, 1971; courtesy of Dr. A. H. Fradkin, Galveston, Texas. *F:* From M. Warburg, *Acta Ophthalmol.* [*Kbh.*], **39:**757–72, 1961.)

245

Oculocerebral Syndrome with Hypopigmentation

In 1967 Cross, McKusick, and Breen [1] reported four siblings with an oculocerebral syndrome characterized by hypopigmentation, ocular anomalies, spasticity, athetosis, and mental retardation. These children were members of a genetic isolate, the Old Order Amish. This was thought to be a new genetic disorder.

Physical Features

EYES: At birth the children had small, cloudy, vascularized corneas (*Figures B and E*). Ectropion of the lower lids was present in one or both eyes (*Figure C*). The palpebral fissures were narrow, the globes were small, and the eyes had a sunken appearance and exhibited coarse nystagmus. The iris and retina could not be seen.

MOUTH: The teeth were widely spaced. The palate was narrow and high-arched.

GENITALIA: Both males had undescended testes.

SKIN AND HAIR: Hair and skin pigment was absent at birth. Two children had a few darkly pigmented strands of hair at 2 and 3 years of age. The hair shafts were abnormally fragile. The oldest child had several darkly pigmented nevi.

HEIGHT AND WEIGHT: The two younger children were at or below the third percentile for height and weight. Their 12-year-old sister had more severe growth retardation.

Nervous System

None of the three living children had ever attained any normal developmental milestones; the fourth child was stillborn. Involuntary writhing movements of the limbs began when each child was a few months old. When examined at 12, 3, and 2 years of age the children had spontaneous slow, writhing movements of the hands, fingers, and toes. There were no apparent dystonic movements or fasciculations. The limbs were severely spastic, and deep tendon reflexes were markedly exaggerated. In response to slight stimulation the younger children showed an extremely brisk startle reflex with extension of the arms and flexion of the lower extremities (*Figure D*). The older child had flexion contractures of the shoulders, elbows, hips, and knees (*Figure A*). Grasp and sucking reflexes were present bilaterally.

Laboratory Studies

The hair shafts were abnormally thin. Hair bulbs contained less than the normal amount of pigment. Incubation of the hair bulbs with tyrosine did not produce the normal intensity of pigmentation. Electroencephalograms, chromosome studies, and amino acid chromatography of the urine revealed no abnormalities.

Treatment and Prognosis

The oldest child died at the age of 15 years 10 months [2].

Genetics

Autosomal recessive inheritance is most likely because of the consanguinity of the parents.

Differential Diagnosis

1. Patients with the syndrome of microphthalmos, corneal opacity, mental retardation, and spasticity have normal pigmentation (see page 250).
2. Spastic diplegia and severe mental retardation are features of the Sjögren-Larsson syndrome, but these patients also have ichthyosis and congenital cataracts (see page 370).
3. Corneal clouding and mental retardation are features of the oculocerebrorenal syndrome of Lowe, but these children have striking hypotonia, cataracts, glaucoma, and a generalized aminoaciduria (see page 248).
4. A new oculocerebral syndrome including microcornea, myopia, optic atrophy, facial anomalies, microcephaly, and mental retardation in four siblings was described in 1971 by Kaufman and coworkers [3].

References

1. Cross, H. E., McKusick, V. A., and Breen, W. A new oculocerebral syndrome with hypopigmentation. *J. Pediatr.*, **70**:398–406, 1967.
2. Cross, H. E. Personal communication, 1969.
3. Kaufman, R. L., Rimoin, D. L., Prensky, A. L., and Sly, W. S. An oculocerebrofacial syndrome. *Birth Defects: Original Article Series,* Vol. VII, No. 1, pp. 135–38. Williams & Wilkins Co., Baltimore, 1971.

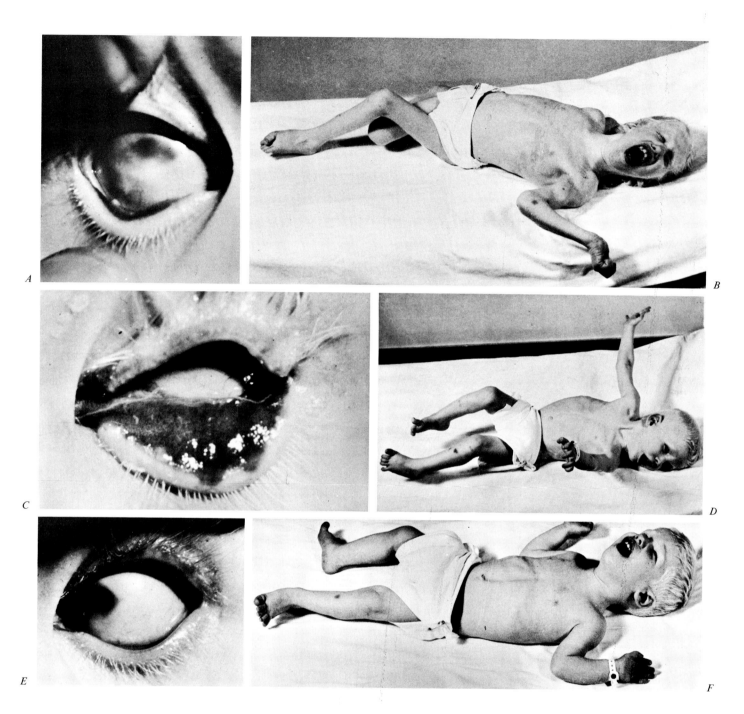

Plate VI-14. *A–C:* The oldest child at 12 years of age, showing severe flexion contractures, growth retardation, and white hair. Her eyes show in *B* an ectropion of the lower lid and a poorly visualized cornea (the darkened area in *A* just below the upper lid). *D:* The 3-year-old boy showing an exaggerated Moro reflex. *E:* An eye of this boy turned medially with the irregular border of the cornea partially visible in the darkened area. *F:* The 2-year-old boy who also had small eyes, cloudy corneas, and a prompt, exaggerated Moro reflex in response to sudden stimuli. (*A–F:* From H. E. Cross *et al., J. Pediatr.,* **70:**398–406, 1967.)

Oculocerebrorenal Syndrome of Lowe (Lowe's Syndrome)

In 1952 Lowe, Terrey, and MacLachlan [1] described three unrelated male infants with congenital glaucoma, hypotonia, mental retardation, and abnormalities of renal function. Seventy cases were reviewed in 1968 [2].

Physical Features

FACE: The affected infants have a high, prominent forehead (*Figures A, B, and E*).

EYES: Most patients have cataracts at birth and develop glaucoma in the first few months of life (*Figure D*). The cataracts, which are white and opaque, may be nuclear or located on either the anterior or posterior surface of the lens. The cause of the glaucoma is not known. It usually is refractory to surgical treatment and leads to blindness [2]. The pupils usually are miotic and do not respond to mydriatics. Some patients have posterior synechiae between the lens and iris. Pigmentary degeneration in the region of the macula has also been observed [3].

GENITALIA: Most patients have undescended testes.

LIMBS: The oldest living patient (*Figures C and D*) developed acute arthritis involving fingers, wrists, elbows, ankles, and knees at age 26 years.

HEIGHT: The height is usually below the third percentile of normal.

Nervous System

Marked muscular hypotonia is present in the newborn and persists throughout infancy (*Figure E*). During this time deep tendon reflexes cannot be elicited, although they may be elicited in older patients. All reported patients have been mentally retarded, usually to a severe degree. Some patients are hyperexcitable and will suddenly scream for no apparent reason. Seizures are uncommon.

Pathology

The reported pathologic changes have been nonspecific and variable. Some brains have shown no abnormalities, while others have shown changes such as cerebellar atrophy, encephalitislike porencephaly, and hydrocephalus. Muscle biopsies have shown disuse atrophy with variation in the size of the muscle fibers and an increase in fat and connective tissue. The frequency and types of renal abnormalities vary with age. The first change is dilatation of the tubules and the presence of proteinaceous casts. By the age of 5 to 6 years there is focal involvement of the renal parenchyma with fibrotic or hyalinized glomeruli, thickened basement membranes, tubular atrophy, and interstitial fibrosis. No specific eye pathology has been observed; some authors have reported congenital anomalies of the canal of Schlemm [2].

Laboratory Studies

A generalized aminoaciduria develops in the first few weeks of life. The amount of amino acid excreted shows a wide daily variation. Proteinuria is also present; the protein is a beta-globulin. Some patients have intermittent glucosuria; some have deficient renal ammonia production. Metabolic acidosis and rickets develop in the first year of life in many patients (*Figure F*). Organic aciduria is greatest in those with severe bone disease. Chronic renal insufficiency develops in some patients who have acidosis and rickets [2]. The jejunal mucosa of two patients showed partially defective transport of lysine and arginine [3]. Studies on six males showed normal peripheral nerve conduction times; specimens of sural nerve had a normal appearance by electron microscopy and normal chemical composition by gas liquid chromatography [6].

Treatment and Prognosis

Treatment of the glaucoma usually is ineffective and blindness develops. Patients with metabolic acidosis and rickets respond to treatment with alkali supplement and vitamin D. The principal cause of death in infancy is chronic renal insufficiency. The average life expectancy is not known, but some patients have survived to adulthood (*Figure C*).

Genetics

X-linked recessive. It has been suggested that the carrier female could be detected by the presence of lens opacities and the production of an aminoaciduria in response to an oral ornithine load. However, studies of the parents of three affected males, including two of those initially reported by Lowe and coworkers [1], showed no consistent findings in either the lens or the urinary amino acid response [5].

Differential Diagnosis

1. Muscular hypotonia, glaucoma or cataracts, a high and broad forehead, and proteinuria are features of patients with the cerebrohepatorenal syndrome, but they are differentiated by having stippled epiphyses, joint contractures, renal cortical cysts, increased serum iron, and an autosomal recessive mode of inheritance (see page 270).
2. Marked hypotonia is also a feature of infants with Down's syndrome (see page 150), XXXXY syndrome (see page 190), cretinism (see page 10), and the Prader-Willi syndrome (see page 48), but each is readily distinguished by other physical features and laboratory studies.

References

1. Lowe, C. U., Terrey, M., and MacLachlan, E. A. Organic aciduria, decreased renal ammonia production, hydrophthalmos and mental retardation. A clinical entity. *Am. J. Dis. Child.,* **83:**164–84, 1952.
2. Abbassi, V., Lowe, C. U., and Calcagno, P. L. Oculo-cerebro-renal syndrome. A review. *Am. J. Dis. Child.,* **115:**145–68, 1968.
3. Walton, D. S. Personal communication, 1969.
4. Bartsocas, C. S., Levy, H. L., Crawford, J. D., and Thier, S. O. A defect in intestinal amino acid transport in Lowe's syndrome. *Am. J. Dis. Child.,* **117:**93–95, 1969.
5. Holmes, L. B., McGowan, B. L., and Efron, M. L. Lowe's syndrome: a search for the carrier state. *Pediatrics,* **44:**358–64, 1969.
6. Snyder, R. D., Appenzeller, O., Pinkerton, D., and Kornfeld, M. Myogenic component of hypotonia in the oculo-cerebro-renal syndrome. (Abstract.) IVth International Congress of Human Genetics, Paris, 1971.

Plate VI-15. *A–D:* The three patients originally reported by Lowe and coworkers [1]. The two infants show similar high, wide foreheads, and muscle hypotonia. The third patient (D. M. in the original report) at 24 years had a prominent forehead, thin muscles in his legs, and flat, externally rotated feet. He had bilateral corneal opacities and cataracts and had no vision. *E* and *F:* An 8-month-old infant with glaucoma, cataracts, muscle hypotonia, and sagging subcutaneous tissue on his arms and legs. At 6 months his x-rays showed irregular epiphyses due to rickets. (*B:* From C. U. Lowe *et al., Am. J. Dis. Child.,* **83:**164–84, 1952.)

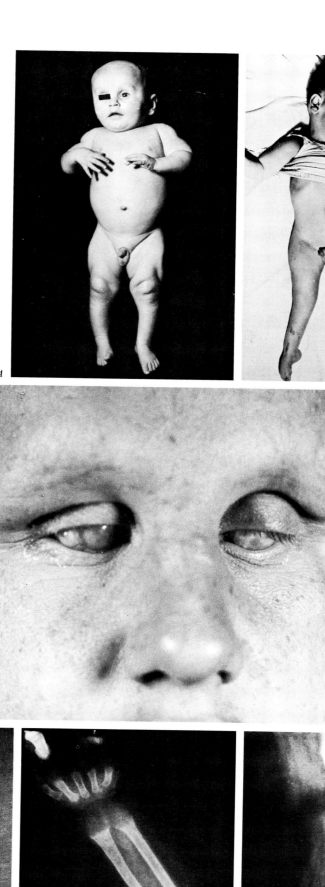

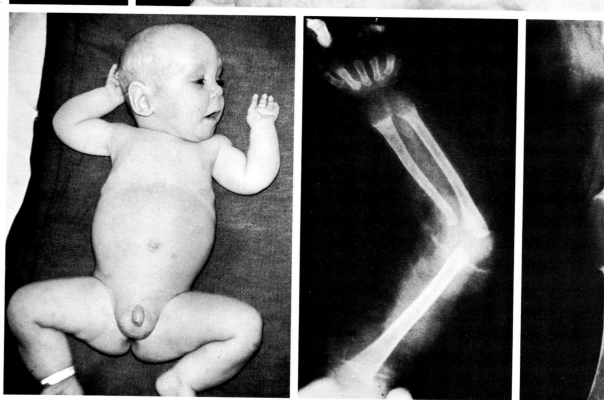

Syndrome of Microphthalmos, Corneal Opacity, Mental Retardation, and Spasticity

In 1965 Pinsky, DiGeorge, Harley, and Baird [1] reported three sisters with microphthalmos, corneal opacities, severe mental retardation, and spastic diplegia. This was the first report of the familial occurrence of this combination of abnormalities.

Physical Features

HEAD: Two of the children were microcephalic. The third had an enlarged head.

FACE: The bridge of the nose was broad and flat. One child had a unilateral cleft lip and cleft palate.

EYES: All three children had small eyes and corneal opacities (*Figures A, B, D, and E*), which varied in appearance from diffuse and generalized to faint and streaky. The slit-lamp examination of one child showed that all layers of the cornea were affected and in another child that only the inner half of the cornea was involved. One child had a spindle-shaped pupil on the right (*Figure B*) and an eccentric pupil on the left (*Figure A*). Two of the children had nystagmus and strabismus.

Nervous System

All three children had severely retarded mental and motor development. All began to have seizures in the first months of life. Each had strikingly hyperactive deep tendon reflexes in the arms and legs. Scissoring of the legs was common (*Figure F*). One child at 2 years of age lay continuously in an opisthotonic position with her tongue protruding, her legs extended and adducted, and her thumbs tightly clenched across her palms (*Figure C*). The oldest child sat without support at 8 months and had learned to walk by the age of 39 months.

Pathology

A corneal biopsy in one child showed changes closely resembling lattice dystrophy of the cornea.

Laboratory Studies

Electroencephalograms showed spike and wave patterns in all three children. No intracranial calcifications were seen on the skull x-rays. Screening tests for congenital toxoplasmosis, syphilis, and cytomegalovirus infections and for amino acid, mucopolysaccharide, and chromosomal abnormalities were negative.

Genetics

This syndrome was presumed to be hereditary, but the mode of inheritance is not known. Possibly relevant to the children's disease is the fact that their mother had unilateral microphthalmos and a partial posterior embryotoxon.

Differential Diagnosis

1. Corneal opacities, spasticity, and mental retardation are features of patients with the oculocerebral syndrome with hypopigmentation, but they lack skin and hair pigment (see page 246).
2. Spastic diplegia and severe mental retardation are features of patients with the Sjögren-Larsson syndrome, but they also have ichthyosis and congenital cataracts (see page 370).
3. Corneal opacities are part of the syndrome of elbow contractures, corneal opacities, pointed nose, and mental retardation (see page 324).
4. Corneal opacities and mental retardation are features of patients with the oculocerebrorenal syndrome of Lowe (see page 248) and infants with the cerebrohepatorenal syndrome (see page 270), but patients with either of these disorders also have marked hypotonia, a high forehead, and other distinguishing features.

Reference

1. Pinsky, L., DiGeorge, A. M., Harley, R. D., and Baird, H. W., III. Microphthalmos, corneal opacity, mental retardation and spastic cerebral palsy. An oculocerebral syndrome. *J. Pediatr.*, **67**:387–98, 1965.

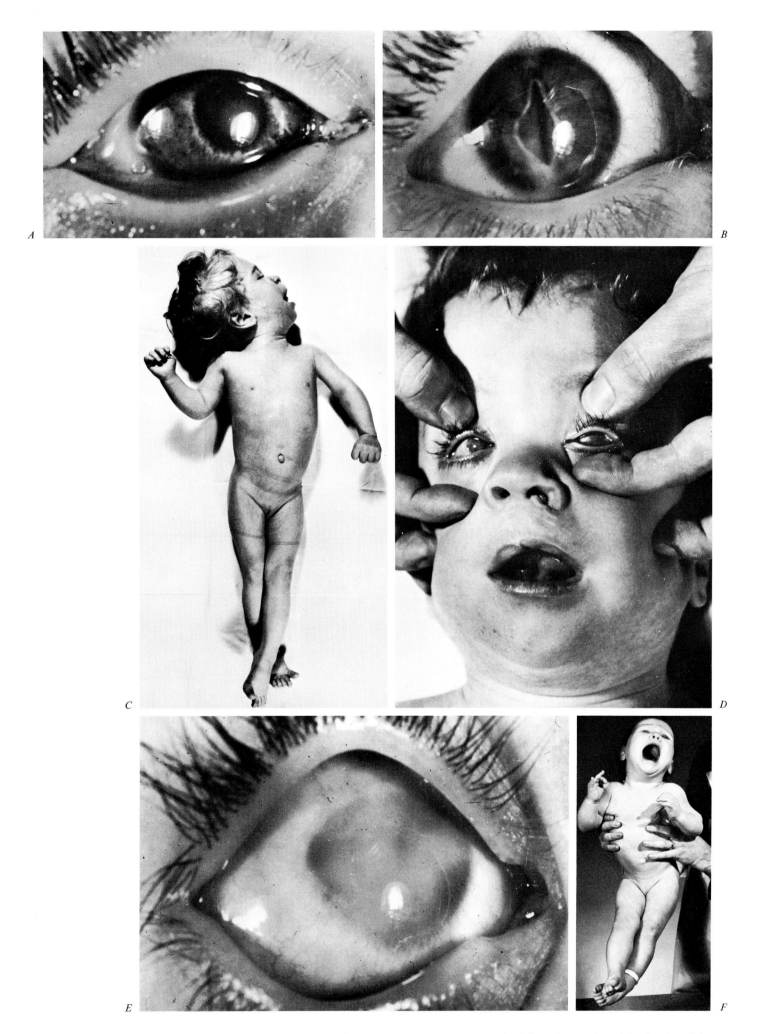

Plate VI-16. *A* and *B:* The left and right eyes of the first of three affected siblings at 2¾ years of age. Both eyes were small and corneal opacities covered the lower portion of each pupil. The left pupil was eccentric inferiorly. The right pupil was spindle shaped. *C–E:* The second child at 2 years of age. She had diffuse, dense corneal opacities, a repaired cleft lip, and opisthotonic posturing with scissoring of the legs and clasped thumbs. *F:* The third child at 1 year of age, when she already had scissoring of her legs and faint, streaky corneal opacities. (*A–F:* From L. Pinsky *et al., J. Pediatr.,* **67:**387–98, 1965.)

Syndrome of Trichomegaly and Retinal Degeneration

In 1965 Oliver and McFarlane [1] reported a child with long eyelashes and eyebrows, retinal degeneration, and short stature. A second similarly affected child was reported in 1967 [2], and a third in 1971 [2a].

Physical Features

EYES: All three children had long eyelashes and eyebrows, a finding noted in the first child at birth. The eyelashes measured 40 mm or more (*Figure A*), but were sparse (*Figure E*). Their eyebrows were bushy and met in the midline. All three children had very poor vision, which was attributed to their diffuse retinal pigmentary degeneration (*Figures B and F*).

HAIR: Two children had sparse scalp hair [2,2a] and one also had alopecia areata (*Figure C*) [2].

HEIGHT AND WEIGHT: The first patient weighed only 1.8 kilograms at birth after a term pregnancy and 13.4 kilograms at 8 years 2 months [1,3]. The second patient weighed 2.5 kilograms at birth and was always small for her age (*Figure D*). The third patient weighed 2.0 kilograms at birth; at 5 years he weighed 10 kilograms and was 86.2 cm tall.

Nervous System

The first patient had slow psychomotor development. His IQ at $2\frac{1}{2}$ years was 68 and subsequently was 52 [1,3]. The second patient had normal intelligence. The third had a developmental age of 3 to $3\frac{1}{2}$ years when 5 years old.

Laboratory Studies

Only the first reported child had any endocrinologic deficiencies. At $2\frac{1}{2}$ years of age her protein-bound iodine was 2.4 μg/100 ml, and the radioactive iodine uptake by the thyroid after stimulation was only 11 percent [1]. When restudied at 8 years of age [3], she had normal T_3 and thyroxine levels, but again had a low (6 to 11 percent) radioactive iodine uptake after thyroid stimulation. Both the metapyron test of adrenocorticotropic hormone reserve and the serum growth hormone levels after both insulin-induced hypoglycemia and arginine stimulation showed an impaired response. The bone age was only 15 months at age 64 months. The third child had a retarded bone age [2a]. The second patient had a biopsy of the skin of the scalp which showed alopecia areata. All patients had normal chromosome karyotypes.

Differential Diagnosis

1. Long eyelashes and eyebrows and short stature are features of patients with de Lange's syndrome, but they are distinguished by their facial features and skeletal anomalies (see page 276).
2. Excessive growth of eyelash and brow hair may be an isolated familial characteristic [4].

References

1. Oliver, G. L., and McFarlane, D. C.   Congenital trichomegaly with associated pigmentary degeneration of the retina, dwarfism, and mental retardation. *Arch. Ophthalmol. (Chicago)*, **74**:169–71, 1965.
2. Cant, J. S.   Ectodermal dysplasia. *J. Pediatr. Ophthalmol.*, **4** (No. 4):13–17, 1967.
2a. Corby, D. G., Lowe, R. S., Jr., Haskins, R. C., and Hebertson, L. M.   Trichomegaly, pigmentary degeneration of the retina, and growth retardation. A new syndrome originating in utero. *Am. J. Dis. Child.*, **121**:344–45, 1971.
3. McKim, J. S.   Personal communication, 1970.
4. Gray, H.   Trichomegaly or movie lashes. *Stanford Med. Bull.*, **2**:157–58, 1944.

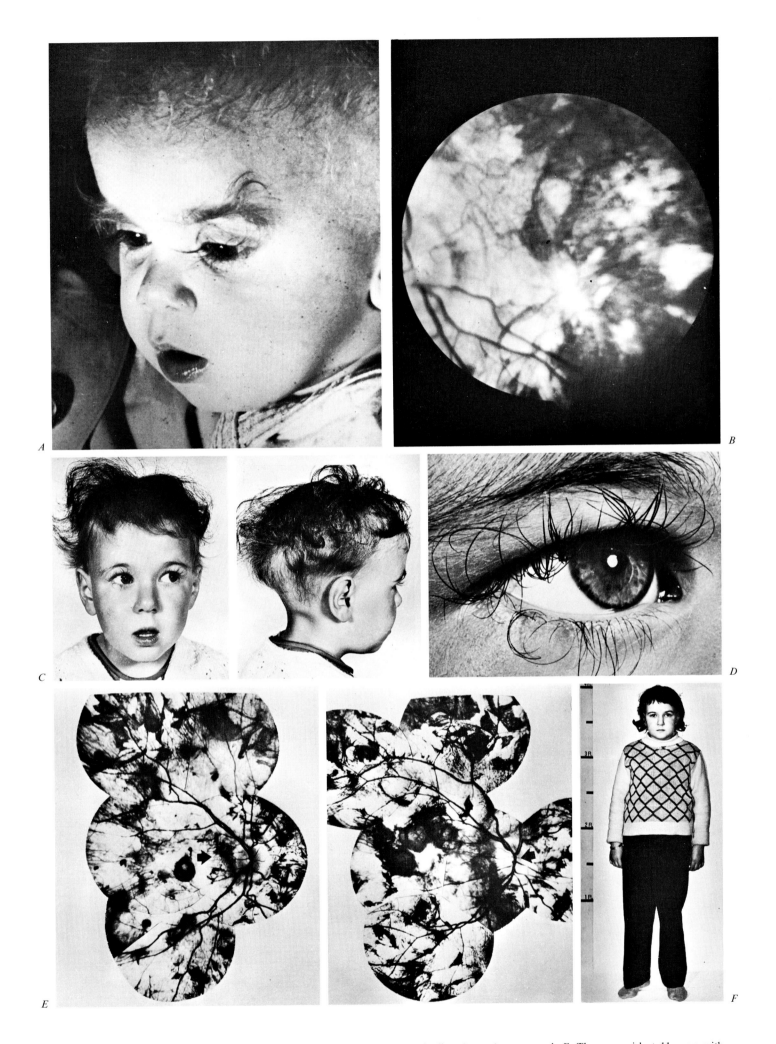

Plate VI-17. *A* and *B:* Show the long eyelashes and eyebrows, sparse scalp hair, and retinal degeneration in a 30-month-old child. *C–E:* A 4-year-old girl with patchy alopecia of her scalp, long sparse eyelashes, and retinal degeneration. Composite photographs of both optic fundi (*E*) illustrate extent of retinal degeneration; retinal vessels and optic discs (*arrows*) are normal. *F:* The same girl at 11 years with shortness of stature. She had normal intelligence. (*A* and *B:* From G. L. Oliver and D. C. McFarlane, *Arch. Ophthalmol.* [*Chicago*], **74:**169–71, 1965. *C–E:* From J. S. Cant, *J. Pediatr. Ophthalmol.,* **4** [No. 4]:13–17, 1967. *F:* Courtesy of Dr. J. S. Cant, Glasgow, Scotland.)

Neurologic Syndromes
Congenital Sensory Neuropathy with Anhidrosis

Insensitivity to pain has been reported in association with hysteria, spinal cord anomalies, degenerative peripheral neuropathies, and congenital sensory neuropathies. Within this large, heterogeneous group of conditions a specific disorder seems distinguishable, a congenital sensory neuropathy associated with diminished sweating, episodes of unexplained fever, and mental retardation. Eight affected children have been reported [1–6].

Physical Features

EYES: Lacrimation in response to frustration is normal.

MOUTH: Because these patients cannot feel pain, ulceration of the mouth and scars from biting the tongue and lips are common (*Figures A and B*). Two patients had aplasia of the dental enamel [4,6].

LIMBS: Multiple fractures from trauma result in deformities, because the fractures are not noticed and thus the injured area is not adequately immobilized for healing (*Figures E and F*).

SKIN: During warm weather, the skin is warm and dry due to the absence of sweating. Scars from self-inflicted bites may be present on the fingers and arms. Chronic sores are common on the hands, feet, and pressure points, such as the buttocks (*Figures C and D*).

HAIR: Sparseness of the hair in some areas of the scalp was noted in one family [4].

Nervous System

The sensory loss is universal. Pain perception and any physiologic response to painful stimuli are absent. Temperature and touch perception are impaired. The deep tendon reflexes are diminished in most patients. One child had encopresis and enuresis [6]. All of the reported patients had subnormal intelligence; the IQ estimates ranged between 40 and 80 [1–6].

Pathology

Skin biopsies show normal sweat glands. In two studies [4,5] nerve biopsies showed normal dermal nerve networks and myelinization. A postmortem study of the nervous system of one patient, who died when his temperature reached 110°F, showed spinal cord abnormalities. Thinly myelinated sensory fibers of the dorsal nerve roots were absent and the dorsolateral fasciculus (Lissauer's tract) could not be identified [3].

Laboratory Studies

There is no axon flare in response to intradermal histamine. Sweat is not produced in response to thermal or emotional stimuli, electrical stimulation, or intradermal pilocarpine and mecholyl [4,5]. However, the simultaneous injection of acetylcholine and epinephrine resulted in local sweating at a low rate in one patient [5]. Pneumoencephalography showed mild dilatation of the ventricles in three patients [5]. Chromosome studies have shown no abnormalities.

Treatment and Prognosis

Careful attention must be paid to the early detection and adequate treatment of trauma and febrile illnesses. A hot environment must be avoided.

Genetics

Except for two brothers in one family [2], no similarly affected family members have been reported.

Differential Diagnosis

1. Insensitivity to pain, self-mutilating activity, and defective temperature control are features of patients with familial dysautonomia, but they also have hyperhidrosis, impaired lacrimation and corneal hypesthesia, and lack of tongue papillae (see page 256).

2. Self-inflicted injuries and mental retardation are features of patients with the Lesch-Nyhan syndrome, but they also have athetosis, hyperuricemia, a defect in purine biosynthesis, and self-mutilation, rather than injuries of which they are unaware. Their sensation of pain is normal (see page 30).

References

1. Gillespie, J. B., and Perucca, L. G.   Congenital generalized indifference to pain (congenital analgia). *Am. J. Dis. Child.,* **100:**124–26, 1960.
2. Swanson, A. G.   Congenital insensitivity to pain with anhydrosis. A unique syndrome in two male siblings. *Arch. Neurol. (Chicago),* **8:**299–306, 1963.
3. Swanson, A. G., Buchan, G. C., and Alvord, E. C., Jr.   Absence of Lissauer's tract and small dorsal root axons in familial, congenital, universal insensitivity to pain. *Trans. Am. Neurol. Assoc.,* **88:**99–103, 1963.
4. Pinsky, L., and DiGeorge, A. M.   Congenital familial sensory neuropathy with anhidrosis. *J. Pediatr.,* **68:**1–13, 1966.
5. Vassella, F., Emrich, H. M., Kraus-Ruppert, R., Aufdermaur, F., and Tönz, O.   Congenital sensory neuropathy with anhidrosis. *Arch. Dis. Child.,* **43:**124–30, 1968.
6. Brown, J. W., and Podosin, R.   A syndrome of the neural crest. *Arch. Neurol. (Chicago),* **15:**294–301, 1966.

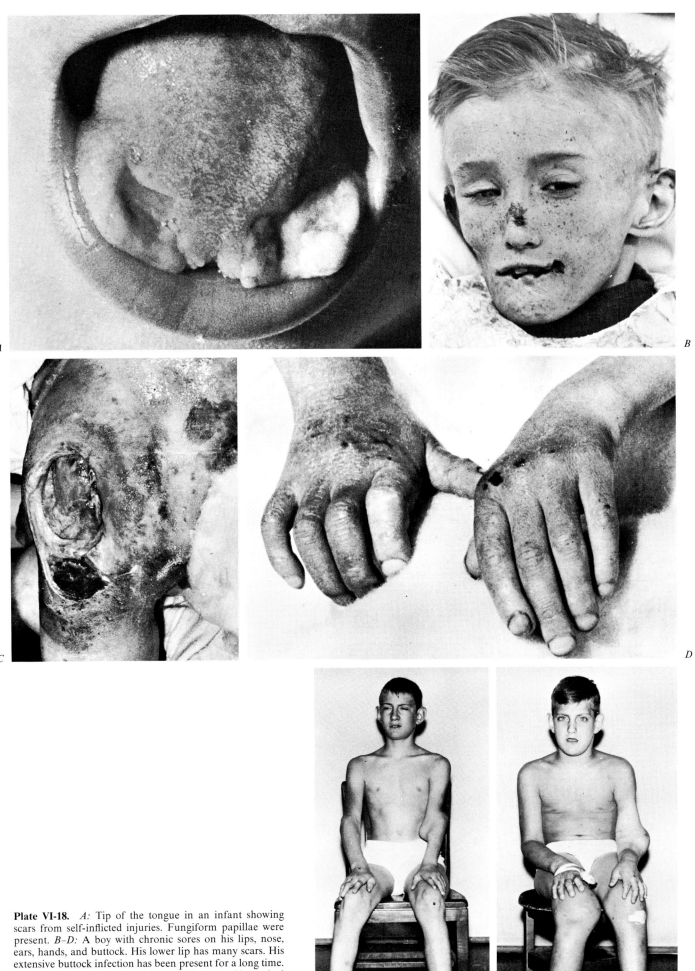

Plate VI-18. *A:* Tip of the tongue in an infant showing scars from self-inflicted injuries. Fungiform papillae were present. *B–D:* A boy with chronic sores on his lips, nose, ears, hands, and buttock. His lower lip has many scars. His extensive buttock infection has been present for a long time. *E* and *F:* Two brothers aged 12 and 10 years with marked deformities of the elbows, knees, and ankles, as a result of inadequate immobilization and healing of numerous fractures. (*A:* Reprinted From F. Vassella, *Arch. Dis. Child.,* **43:**124, 1968, by permission of author and editor. *B* and *C:* From B. Kirman and J. Bicknell, *Dev. Med. Child Neurol.,* **10:**57–63, 1968. *D:* Courtesy of Dr. B. H. Kirman, Epsom, Surrey, England. *E* and *F:* From A. G. Swanson, *Arch. Neurol.* [*Chicago*], **8:**299–306, 1963.)

Familial Dysautonomia
(Riley-Day Syndrome)

In 1949 Riley, Day, Greeley, and Langford [1] described five children who had deficient lacrimation and whose reaction to mild anxiety was characterized by hypotension, excessive sweating, drooling, and blotchy skin. It has since been shown that these patients had a complex genetic neurophysiologic abnormality. Over 200 affected families have been identified, almost all being Jews of eastern European extraction (Ashkenazi). The incidence of familial dysautonomia in American Jews has been estimated as between 1 in 10,000 and 1 in 20,000 births [2].

Physical Features

FACE: Many patients have a frozen apprehensive face with an empty look and minimal grimacing. The face is thin and frequently asymmetric. Hypertelorism is often noted [3].

EYES: Although most patients' eyes appear moist, all have diminished tear production. Myopia, exotropia, corneal hypesthesia, and corneal ulcerations and opacities (*Figure A*) are common. Anisocoria and tortuosity of retinal vasculature have also been reported [4].

MOUTH: Both the fungiform papillae, which are pinhead-sized red projections normally concentrated on the tip of the tongue (*Figures C and D*), and the vallate papillae, which are normally present on the posterior portion of the tongue, are usually absent. In one study [3] a few patients had either isolated fungiform or normal circumvallate papillae.

BACK: Kyphoscoliosis is common (*Figure B*).

LIMBS: Some patients develop neuropathic arthropathy of the knee, shoulder, or elbow.

SKIN: When excited, these patients develop erythematous blotches over any part of the body, except the palms and soles. The blotches begin as small red macules. Within a few seconds they increase in number, size, and intensity, and become confluent and dark red.

HEIGHT: These patients are often undersized.

Nervous System

Many neurologic and physiologic abnormalities have been observed: difficulty in swallowing, excessive sweating and salivation, defective lacrimation, postural hypotension, paroxysmal hypertension, relative insensitivity of the respiratory control mechanism to carbon dioxide excess and to oxygen deficit, reduced sensitivity to pain, absent gag reflex and deep tendon reflexes, ataxia, and poor sucking, chewing, and speech. Emotional lability is common.

Several patients have had subnormal intelligence, but it is not clear whether this is a primary feature of the disease or due to damage from recurrent anoxia and high fevers. An extensive psychometric evaluation [5] of 25 affected children and 10 of their normal siblings indicated significant mental impairment. The overall average was dull normal intelligence, but their normal siblings had above average intelligence. Some of the affected patients had a moderate degree of mental retardation while others had above average intelligence. In another study [3], 19 of 23 patients had psychomotor retardation.

Pathology

Sensory nerves and organs, nerve fibers, and autonomic nerve plexuses have a normal anatomic distribution; histochemical staining shows cholinesterase is present [6]. Demyelination of the posterior columns of the spinal cord was observed in 3 of 10 autopsied cases [7]. An extreme paucity of subcutaneous sensory nerves was found in a 1-year-old with no taste buds. He also had reduced neuron populations in sensory and autonomic ganglia [8].

Laboratory Studies

Taste perception and discrimination are markedly deficient. The intradermal injection of histamine produces little pain or erythema (*Figure E*). The instillation of 2.5 percent methacholine into the conjunctival sac causes a miotic pupillary response (*Figure F*). The ratio of homovanillic acid to vanillylmandelic acid in the urine is elevated. The concentrations of epinephrine and norepinephrine in the adrenal glands of three children were higher than normal [9]. Plasma levels of dopamine-β-hydroxylase, the enzyme that converts dopamine to norepinephrine, has been shown to be significantly decreased in patients with familial dysautonomia. Weinshilboum *et al.* [9a] found that 6 of 26 had no detectable activity of this enzyme and that the mothers of only these 6 had decreased activity. These two groups, based on different levels of enzyme activity, may indicate that there are different genetic abnormalities that cause familial dysautonomia.

Treatment and Prognosis

Of 200 affected patients in one study [2], more than 50 had died by the age of 10 years. Pulmonary infection, following regurgitation and aspiration, is a common cause of death in both infants and older children.

Genetics

Autosomal recessive. The frequency of the gene in American Jews is estimated as 1:100 at the highest; thus, the frequency of the heterozygous individual is 1:50 [2].

Differential Diagnosis

1. Areflexia, absence of the fungiform papillae of the tongue, and a lack of overflow tearing are features of patients with the pupillotonia-areflexia syndrome, but they have hypohidrosis, are sensitive to pain, and do not have postural hypotension [10].
2. Insensitivity to pain, recurrent febrile episodes, diminished tearing, and a diminished response to histamine are features of patients with the syndrome of congenital sensory neuropathy with anhidrosis, but these patients have diminished sweating and have normal tongue papillae (see page 254).

References

1. Riley, C. M., Day, R. L., Greeley, D. M., and Langford, W. S. Central autonomic dysfunction with defective lacrimation. I. Report of five cases. *Pediatrics*, **3**:468–78, 1949.
2. McKusick, V. A., Norum, R. A., Farkas, H. J., Brunt, P. W., and Mahloudji, M. The Riley-Day syndrome—observations on genetics and survivorship. An interim report. *Israel J. Med. Sci.*, **3**:372–79, 1967.
3. Moses, S. W., Rotem, Y., Jagoda, N., Talmor, N., Eichhorn, F., and Levin, S. A clinical, genetic and biochemical study of familial dysautonomia in Israel. *Israel J. Med. Sci.*, **3**:358–71, 1967.
4. Goldberg, M. F., Payne, J. W., and Brunt, P. W. Ophthalmologic studies of familial dysautonomia. *Arch. Ophthalmol.* (*Chicago*), **80**:732–43, 1968.
5. Sak, H. G., Smith, A. A., and Dancis, J. Psychometric evaluation of children with familial dysautonomia. *Am. J. Psychiatry*, **124**:682–87, 1967.
6. Winkelmann, R. K., Bourlond, A., and Smith, A. A. Nerves in the skin of a patient with familial dysautonomia (Riley-Day syndrome). *Pediatrics*, **38**:1060–62, 1966.
7. Fogelson, M. H., Rorke, L. B., and Kaye, R. Spinal cord changes in familial dysautonomia. *Arch. Neurol.* (*Chicago*), **17**:103–108, 1967.
8. Pearson, J., Finegold, M. J., and Budzilovich, G. The tongue and taste in familial dysautonomia. *Pediatrics*, **45**:739–45, 1970.
9. Smith, A. A., and Dancis, J. Catecholamine release in familial dysautonomia. *N. Engl. J. Med.*, **277**:61–64, 1967.
9a. Weinshilboum, R. M., and Axelrod, J. Reduced plasma dopamine-β-hydroxylase activity in familial dysautonomia. *N. Engl. J. Med.*, **285**:938–42, 1971.
10. Esterly, N. B., Cantolino, S. J., Alter, B. P., and Brusilow, S. W. Pupillotonia, hyporeflexia and segmental hypohidrosis: autonomic dysfunction in a child. *J. Pediatr.*, **73**:852–59, 1968.

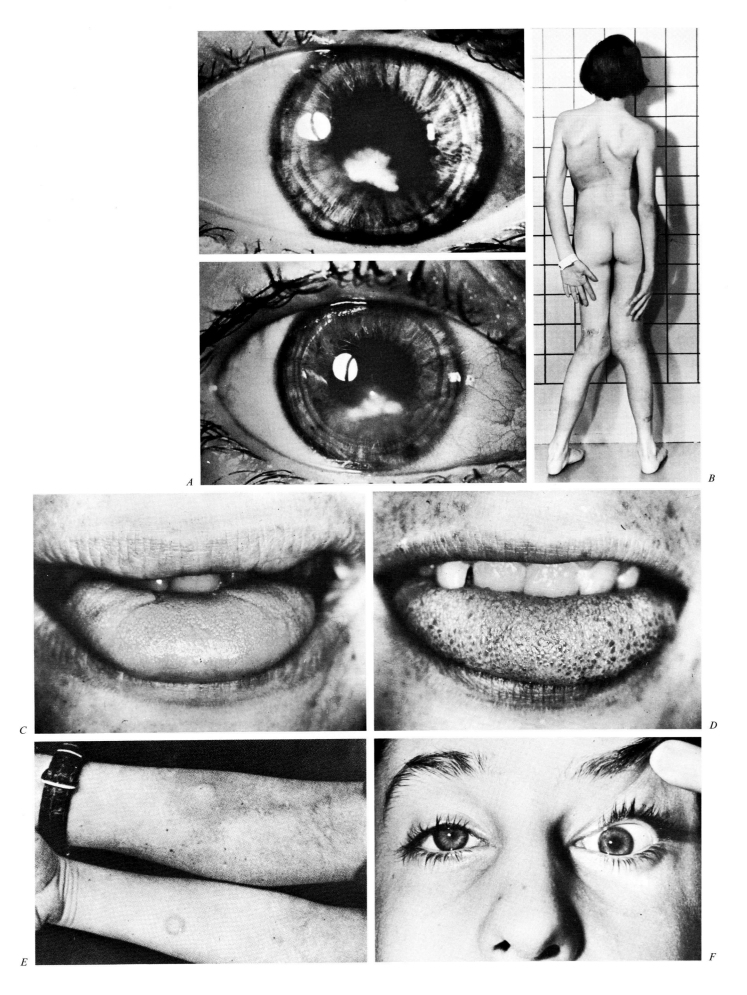

Plate VI-19. *A:* Two examples of scars from corneal ulceration. *B:* A 12-year-old girl with kyphoscoliosis and a neuropathic arthropathy of the knees. *C:* Shows the lack of fungiform papillae on the tip of the tongue. *D:* Tip of the tongue of a normal child. The pinhead-sized dark spots are fungiform papillae. *E:* The response to intradermal histamine in a normal individual (*above*) and his dysautonomic sister (*below*). The normal response is a wheal with a large axon flare around it. The dysautonomic response is a similar wheal, but only a narrow erythematous areola. *F:* Shows a very small pupil in the right eye 30 minutes after the instillation of 2.5 percent methacholine drops, suggesting an excessive sensitivity to this drug. (*A, B,* and *F:* From M. F. Goldberg *et al., Arch. Ophthalmol.* [*Chicago*], **80:**732–43, 1968. *C* and *D:* From A. A. Smith *et al., Science,* **147:**1040–41, 1965; copyright 1965 by the American Association for the Advancement of Science. *E:* From A. A. Smith and J. Dancis, *J. Pediatr.,* **63:**889–94, 1963.)

Happy Puppet Syndrome

In 1965 Angelman [1] described three unrelated children with similar facial appearances who had ataxic jerky movements and paroxysms of laughter. Two similar patients were described in 1967, and the term *happy puppet* was suggested because of the behavior and gait [2]. A sixth patient was reported in 1972 [3].

Physical Features

HEAD: All of the patients were microcephalic and most had a flat occiput.

FACE: They had a similar facial appearance. Widely spaced eyes and prognathism were the most striking features (*Figures A, B, C, and D*).

EYES: One girl had optic nerve pallor and gradually lost her vision [1]. Three patients had a deficiency of iris and choroid pigment [1,2].

Nervous System

All five children were subject to easily provoked and prolonged paroxysms of laughter (*Figures E and F*) and had a tendency to protrude their tongues for long periods of time (*Figures A and C*). As infants, they had muscular hypotonia and slow psychomotor development. When older, their gait was stiff and jerky. Voluntary arm movements were incoordinate. In some patients the hypotonia persisted in association with hyperactive deep tendon reflexes. All patients had seizures and marked mental deficiency, and none ever learned to speak.

Laboratory Studies

Abnormal electroencephalographic changes, primarily spike and slow wave activity, were present before, during, and after the paroxysms of laughter, tongue protrusion, and seizures [1]. No hypsarrhythmic pattern was present [2]. Pneumoencephalograms showed dilated ventricles. Studies of chromosomes and amino acids showed no abnormalities.

Treatment and Prognosis

The seizures were difficult to control. The patients needed custodial care.

Genetics

This syndrome has not occurred in more than one member of a sibship.

References

1. Angelman, H. "Puppet" children. A report on three cases. *Dev. Med. Child Neurol.*, **7**:681–88, 1965.
2. Bower, B. D., and Jeavons, P. M. The "happy puppet" syndrome. *Arch. Dis. Child.*, **42**:298–302, 1967.
3. Berg, J. M., and Pakula, Z. Angelman's ("happy puppet") syndrome. *Am. J. Dis. Child.*, **123**:72–74, 1972.

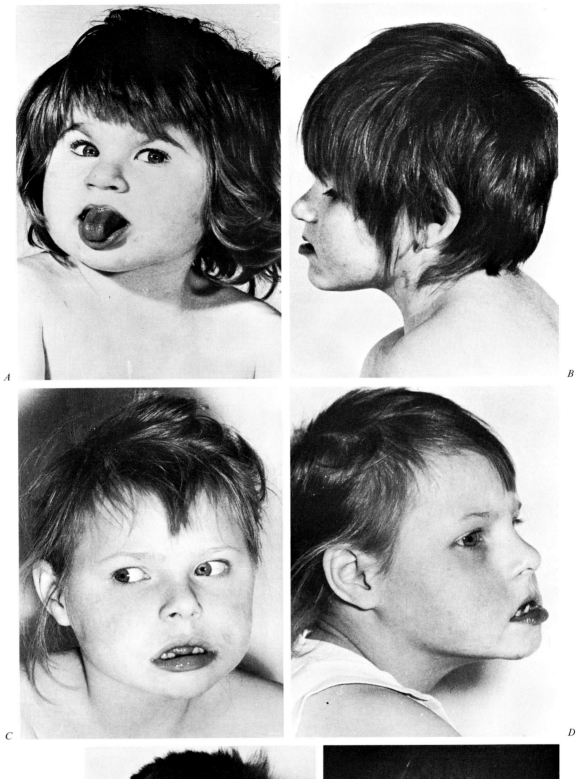

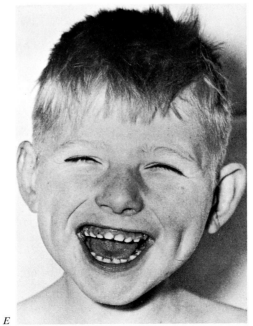

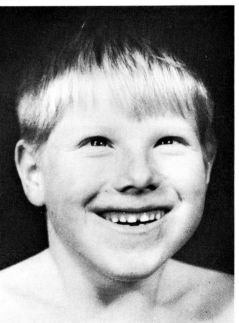

Plate VI-20. *A:* A 3-year-old girl who had fits of uncontrollable laughter and would stick out her tongue for long periods of time. *B:* The same girl at 5½ years, showing her protruding chin. At this time she was deaf and blind, and continued to have paroxysms of laughter. *C* and *D:* A 5-year-old girl shown when she was having a seizure and when protruding her chin. *E:* Shows an 8-year-old boy laughing. He was often in an almost convulsive state of laughter; the laughter often preceded and followed his seizures. *F:* A 7-year-old boy who also was continuously smiling, laughing, and sticking out his tongue. (*A–E:* From H. Angelman, *Dev. Med. Child Neurol.,* 7:681–88, 1965. *F:* Courtesy of Dr. P. M. Jeavons, Birmingham, England.)

Skeletal Diseases
Achondroplasia

Achondroplasia is the best-known form of chondrodystrophy. The basic defect may be a quantitive decrease in the rate of endochondral ossification [1]. Because of this the tubular bones in the limbs are short and broad.

Physical Features

HEAD: The membranous bones in the skull grow normally, but the cartilaginous bones of the base of the skull grow slowly. As a result of this, the infant has compensatory enlargement of the cranial vault and bulging of the forehead (*Figures A and C*). During the first year of life the head size is always above average, but the growth rate is parallel to the normal. After infancy the disproportionate head size is less striking [2,3]. Hydrocephalus with an accelerating increase in head size is uncommon.

FACE: The bridge of the nose is flattened or appears depressed in comparison with the prominent brow, reflecting the slow growth of the cartilaginous bone.

EYES: Optic atrophy has been reported in some of the patients with marked hydrocephalus.

CHEST: The thoracic cage is relatively small in the anteroposterior diameter because of slow growth of the ribs. Beading of the costochondral junction may be evident in infants due to the cupped appearance of the anterior ends of the ribs.

BACK: Infants have mild kyphosis at the thoracolumbar junction associated with muscular hypotonia (*Figure B*). Once a child has learned to walk the lumbar spine is held straight and the sacrum is rotated posteriorly (*Figure D*).

LIMBS: Shortening of the limbs, especially in the proximal portion, is evident at all ages (*Figures A and E*). Associated with the shortening in infants is a greater number of skin folds (*Figure A*). The shortening is most evident in the humerus. The proximal and middle phalanges of the fingers are short and broad, and the fingers form a radiating or spoke-wheel pattern, rather than lying in parallel (*Figures A and B*). The fingers of the adult are not strikingly short [2] (*Figure E*).

HEIGHT: The length of the infant and the height of the adult are well below average. In one series [4] the average height of 15 adult males was 4 feet 2½ inches (129 cm) (range 3 feet 10 inches to 4 feet 7 inches) and the average height of 26 females was 4 feet (123 cm) (range 3 feet 6 inches to 4 feet 4 inches).

Nervous System

Because of the large head and short limbs, the age at reaching early motor milestones is often below the average for normal infants. Because of this delay in development, many infants with achondroplasia are evaluated for mental retardation. Opinions differ as to whether or not there is an increased incidence of mental retardation [3,5]. One study of 16 patients showed that 5 had subnormal intelligence [5]. The enlargement of the head is often associated with mild dilatation of the ventricles, as demonstrated by pneumoencephalography, but there are no other signs of increased intracranial pressure. Occasionally an infant will have hydrocephalus due to extraventricular obstruction by a small foramen magnum. High cervical cord compression by the small foramen magnum which leads to quadriparesis, and sometimes death, has also been reported [3]. Patients with anteriorly wedged vertebral bodies have a high incidence of spinal cord compression [2].

Pathology

Biopsies of chondroosseous junctions [1] have shown that endochondral ossification is regular and well organized. A review [6] of the neuropathology of 40 patients with achondroplasia showed that 10 had primary megalencephaly and 20 had internal hydrocephalus. Some of the patients with excessive brain weight had additional cerebral anomalies. However, most of these patients were deceased newborns and it is possible that they had thanatophoric dwarfism [7], not achondroplasia.

Laboratory Studies

Diagnostic features of achondroplasia that are readily detected in the x-rays of patients of all ages are (1) the lack of the normal increase in interpediculate distance from upper lumbar to lower lumbar vertebrae (*Figure F*); (2) square iliac bones with a short sacrosciatic notch; (3) increased angulation of the spine at the lumbosacral junction that may be associated with vertebral hypoplasia and anterior wedging; (4) thickened, widened, and cupped epiphyses of the ribs and long bones; (5) greater shortening of the humerus in comparison with the bones of the forearm; and (6) a large calvarium and a decrease in the size of the base of the skull caused by fusion of the sphenooccipital synchondrosis [2] (*Figure C*).

Treatment and Prognosis

Many patients do not survive fetal life or early infancy. The cause of death may be cervical cord compression in some instances, but often remains unknown. The infant with an enlarged head requires careful observation to make certain that the head size continues to parallel normal skull growth. The occasional infant with obstructive hydrocephalus is treated with a ventriculoatrial shunt [3]. Any growing child with one or more hypoplastic vertebral bodies should have some type of external bracing to minimize the progression of the kyphosis. If signs of spinal cord compression develop, extensive laminectomy, possibly combined with fusion, is advisable before irreversible changes occur [2]. Osteotomies of the lower extremities are sometimes performed to improve function.

Genetics

Autosomal dominant.

Differential Diagnosis

Short-limbed dwarfism is a feature of patients with hypochondroplasia [8], achondrogenesis, thanatophoric dwarfism [7], Conradi's disease (see page 272), the Ellis-van Creveld syndrome (see page 280), the syndrome of dyschondroplasia, facial anomalies and polysyndactyly (see page 322), and the cloverleaf skull syndrome (see page 234). Each is distinguished by the associated physical features and radiologic findings.

References

1. Rimoin, D. L., Hughes, G. N., Kaufman, R. L., Rosenthal, R. E., McAlister, W. H., and Silberberg, R. Endochondral ossification in achondroplastic dwarfism. *N. Engl. J. Med.*, **283**:728–35, 1970.
2. Langer, L. O., Jr., Baumann, P. A., and Gorlin, R. J. Achondroplasia. *Am. J. Roentgenol.*, **100**:12–26, 1967.
3. Cohen, M. E., Rosenthal, A. D., and Matson, D. D. Neurological abnormalities in achondroplastic children. *J. Pediatr.*, **71**:367–76, 1967.
4. Langer, L. O., Jr. Personal communication, 1969.
5. Morris, J. V., and MacGillivray, R. C. The mental capacity in achondroplasia. *J. Ment. Sci.*, **99**:547–56, 1953.
6. Dennis J. P., Rosenberg, H. S., and Alvord, E. C., Jr. Megalencephaly, internal hydrocephalus and other neurological aspects of achondroplasia. *Brain*, **84**:427–45, 1961.
7. Kaufman, R. L., Rimoin, D. L., McAlister, W. H., and Kissane, J. M. Thanatophoric dwarfism. *Am. J. Dis. Child.*, **120**:53–57, 1970.
8. Walker, B. A., Murdoch, J. L., McKusick, V. A., Langer, L. O., and Beals, R. K. Hypochondroplasia. *Am. J. Dis. Child.*, **122**:95–104, 1971.

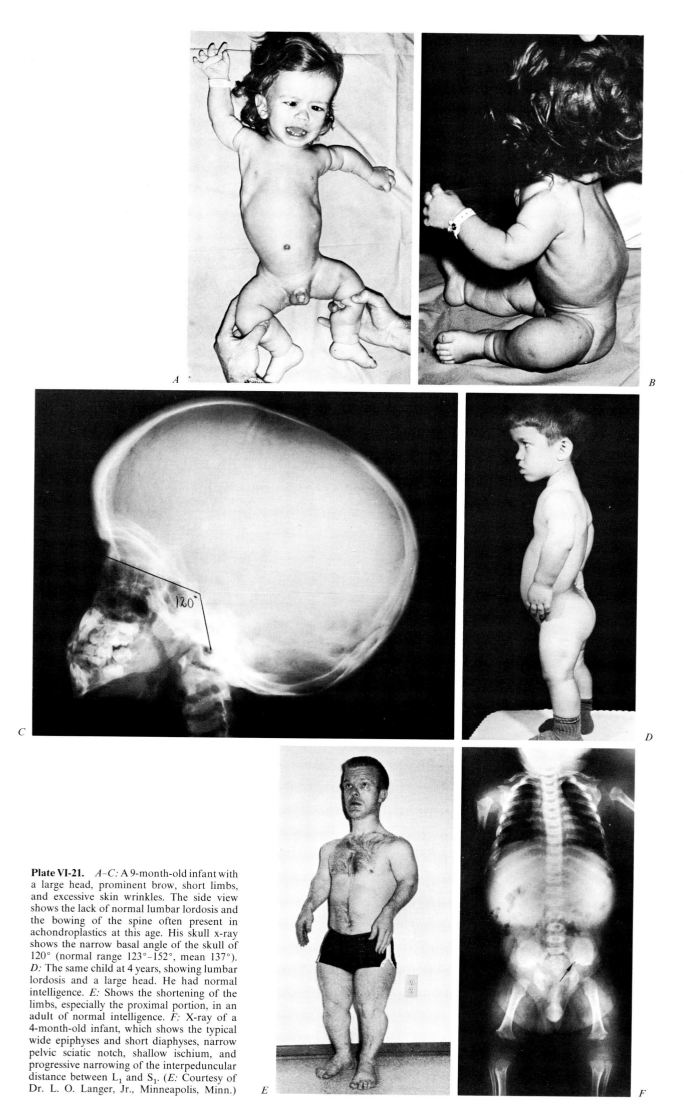

Plate VI-21. *A–C:* A 9-month-old infant with a large head, prominent brow, short limbs, and excessive skin wrinkles. The side view shows the lack of normal lumbar lordosis and the bowing of the spine often present in achondroplastics at this age. His skull x-ray shows the narrow basal angle of the skull of 120° (normal range 123°–152°, mean 137°). *D:* The same child at 4 years, showing lumbar lordosis and a large head. He had normal intelligence. *E:* Shows the shortening of the limbs, especially the proximal portion, in an adult of normal intelligence. *F:* X-ray of a 4-month-old infant, which shows the typical wide epiphyses and short diaphyses, narrow pelvic sciatic notch, shallow ischium, and progressive narrowing of the interpeduncular distance between L_1 and S_1. (*E:* Courtesy of Dr. L. O. Langer, Jr., Minneapolis, Minn.)

261

Engelmann's Disease
(Progressive Diaphyseal Dysplasia)

In 1929 Engelmann [1] described an 8-year-old boy with leg pains, a waddling gait, poor muscular development, and dense bones. A review [2] in 1961 noted that 52 patients had been reported, and another review [3] in 1964 listed only 23 reported cases, a difference that is indicative of the varied clinical criteria for the diagnosis and the range of severity of the signs and symptoms. The cause is not known, but the disorder is considered a progressive diaphyseal dysplasia.

Physical Features

HEAD: A few patients have marked head enlargement with prominence of the forehead and a small face (*Figures A and D*).

FACE: Proptosis (due to small orbits), a flat nasal bridge, and prominent jaw are features of some patients (*Figures A and D*). In a review [2] of 52 patients, 6 had proptosis.

ABDOMEN: A few patients have hepatosplenomegaly.

BACK: The more severely affected individuals develop exaggerated lumbar lordosis and thoracic kyphosis.

LIMBS: The most severely affected also have relatively long, thin arms and small hands and feet (*Figure D*). The lower legs develop a full, rounded appearance while the thighs remain slender (*Figure A*). Many patients develop genu valgum, a valgus deformity of the ankles and pes planus.

HEIGHT AND WEIGHT: Thinness and short stature occur in the more severely affected patients.

GROWTH AND DEVELOPMENT: A delay in puberty and deficient secondary sexual characteristics, including diminished or absent pubic, axillary, and facial hair, are frequently observed.

Nervous System

Leg pains and a waddling gait may be evident in the first year of life. Severely affected patients have small and weak muscles throughout life. Deep tendon reflexes are often hyperactive. Optic pallor and nerve deafness develop in some patients with severe sclerosis of the calvarium, apparently due to progressive narrowing of the foramina of the optic and acoustic nerves. In one patient followed for 15 years progressive signs of hearing loss, blurred vision, vertigo, loss of taste and smell, and a neuropathy in the legs developed during his late twenties [3a]. The intelligence of most reported patients is not indicated. Five out of 52 patients have been considered to have subnormal intelligence, including the patient reported by Engelmann [1,2].

Pathology

There is fusiform enlargement of the diaphyseal area of the long bones. The cortex appears thick and the marrow space is greatly reduced (*Figure B*). The affected bone contains few haversian systems. Instead, there is an excessive amount of cancellous bone of an abnormal pattern and a decrease in the compact bone structure. Similar changes may be found in the membranous bones of the skull. In an autopsy of one child [4] with marked head enlargement, deafness, and hepatosplenomegaly, the only abnormal findings were the diaphyseal dysplasia and dysplastic changes in the middle ear ossicles.

Laboratory Studies

The x-ray changes vary with the severity of the clinical findings and are more marked in patients with muscle weakness. The first changes are seen in the long bones, most often in the tibia. There is an increase in the density and width of the diaphysis, usually in the middle third (*Figures B and E*). As the involvement spreads toward the metaphyses, the width of the shaft increases and the marrow cavity is encroached upon by both periosteal and endosteal new bone. Finally, the whole bone has a dense amorphous appearance and its diameter is almost uniform throughout its length. The areas of the skull most often involved are the anterior and middle fossae (*Figures C and F*). A few patients have involvement of the facial bones [2].

Treatment and Prognosis

Treatment of four children [5,6] with corticosteroids produced a remission of their clinical symptoms, and in one child [5] an improvement in the radiologic appearance of the bones.

Genetics

Autosomal dominant.

Differential Diagnosis

1. Dense bones and a large head with prominent eyes and frontal bossing are features of patients with pycnodysostosis, but the increased bone density is present throughout all parts of the bones, not just the diaphysis (see page 266).
2. Dense bones and cranial nerve palsies are also features of patients with infantile osteopetrosis, but they also have hepatosplenomegaly and severe anemia, and the bone density is generalized (see page 264).
3. Osteosclerosis of the skull and long bones, optic atrophy, and deafness are features of patients with generalized leontiasis ossea, but they also have an elevated alkaline phosphatase, involvement of the metaphysis, and a wide mandible [7].
4. Congenital stenosis of medullary spaces in the diaphyseal portion of tubular bones and calvaria associated with dwarfism and hypocalcemic tetany has been described by Kenny and Linarelli [8], but these patients had decreased width of the diaphysis.

References

1. Engelmann, G. Ein Fall von Osteopathia hyperostotica (sclerotisans) multiplex infantilis. *Fortschr. Roentgenstr.,* **39**:1101–1106, 1929.
2. Lennon, E. A., Schechter, M. M., and Hornabrook, R. W. Engelmann's disease. Report of a case with a review of the literature. *J. Bone Joint Surg.,* **43B**:273–84, 1961.
3. Clawson, D. K., and Loop, J. W. Progressive diaphyseal dysplasia. (Engelmann's disease). *J. Bone Joint Surg.,* **46A**:143–50, 1964.
3a. Trunk, G., Newman, A., and Davis, T. E. Progressive and hereditary diaphyseal dysplasia. *Arch. Intern. Med.,* **123**:417–22, 1969.
4. Cohen, J., and States, J. D. Progressive diaphyseal dysplasia. Report of a case with autopsy findings. *Lab. Invest.,* **5**:492–508, 1956.
5. Royer, P., Vermeil, G., Apostolides, P., and Engelmann, F. Maladie d'Engelmann. Resultat du traitement par la prednisone. *Arch. Fr. Pediatr.,* **24**:693–702, 1967.
6. Allen, D. T., Saunders, A. M., Northway, W. H., Jr., Williams, G. F., and Schafer, I. A. Corticosteroids in the treatment of Engelmann's disease: progressive diaphyseal dysplasia. *Pediatrics,* **46**:523–31, 1970.
7. Van Buchem, F. S. P., Hadders, H. N., Hansen, J. F., and Woldring, M. G. Hyperostosis corticalis generalisata. *Am. J. Med.,* **33**:387–97, 1962.
8. Kenny, F. M., and Linarelli, L. Dwarfism and cortical thickening of tubular bones: transient hypocalemia in a mother and son. *Am. J. Dis. Child.,* **111**:201–207, 1966.

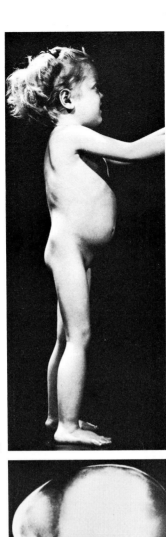
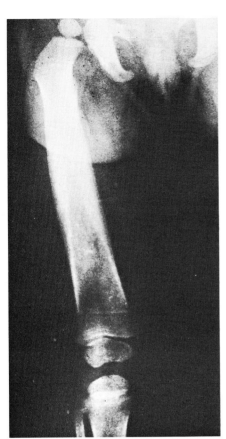
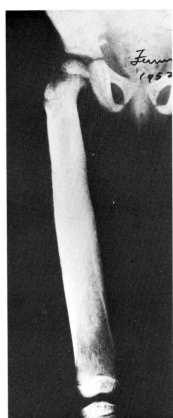
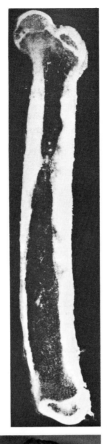

A

B

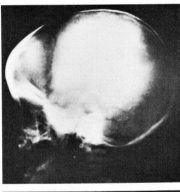

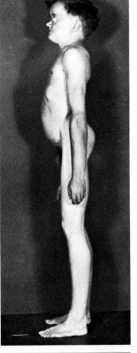

Plate VI-22. *A:* A 4-year-old girl with a prominent jaw, protuberant abdomen, slender thighs, and full legs. *B:* X-rays of the right femur of this girl at 13 months and at almost 6 years of age show progressive diaphyseal thickening. The longitudinal section of this femur at autopsy at 7 years of age shows marked thickening of the cortex. *C:* Skull x-rays of this patient at 13 months and at 5 years show the progressive widening of the sutures and thickening of all cranial bones. *D–F:* A 34-year-old man of normal intelligence who had proptosis, a prominent brow, long thin limbs, and increased lumbar lordosis. His forearm muscles are small, and the width of the bones is increased. The x-rays show marked thickening of the radius, ulna, humerus, cranium, and mandible. (*A–C:* From J. Cohen and J. D. States, *Lab. Invest.,* **5:**492–508, 1956; © 1956, International Academy of Pathology. *D–F:* From E. A. Lennon *et al., J. Bone Joint Surg.,* **43B:**273–84, 1961.)

C

D

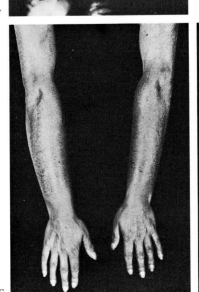
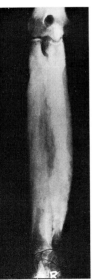
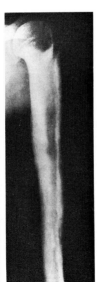
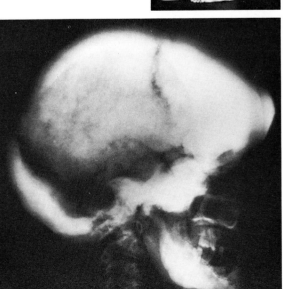

E

F

Osteopetrosis, Infantile Form

Osteopetrosis is a rare disease characterized by a generalized increase in bone density. It is attributed to an overproduction of poorly formed bone structure [1]. There are at least two types, the infantile and adult forms. The infantile form not only is evident in infancy but is rapidly progressive and fatal. More than 50 affected infants have been reported [1–3]. It has recently been suggested [4,5] that retinal degeneration may also be a feature of the infantile form of osteopetrosis.

Physical Features

HEAD: The head becomes progressively larger than normal, and the brow more prominent during the first year of life.

EYES: Retinal degeneration has been noted in four patients [4,5] (*Figure B*).

ABDOMEN: Liver and spleen enlargement is present in most infants [1].

LIMBS: Genu valgum is sometimes present.

LENGTH: Linear growth is usually less than normal.

Nervous System

Optic atrophy was present in 78 percent of the infants in a review of 50 cases [1]. These patients often develop cranial nerve palsies, which are manifested by ptosis, facial palsies, and deafness (*Figures A and E*). Mental retardation is frequently noted—22 percent in one review [1]. However, it is difficult to be certain of the intelligence of these infants, many of whom have marked sensory deprivation.

Pathology

The bones are well calcified. The cortex is thick and there is little or no marrow space (*Figure C*). Both membranous and endochondral bones are affected. There is a deficiency of osteoclasts, an excessive amount of calcified cartilage, and a lack of remodeling of bone during growth. As a result of excessive endochondral bone formation, the bone foramina through which some of the cranial nerves pass fail to enlarge during growth, leading to slow destruction of these nerves [3]. Fractures (*Figure C*) are frequent but heal rapidly. Because of the lack of adequate bone marrow space, extramedullary hematopoiesis persists and is the basis for the hepatosplenomegaly. The ocular pathology findings in one 3-month-old child included degeneration of the rods and cones and the outer nuclear area, atrophy and gliosis of the ganglion cell layer, and atrophy of the optic nerves [4]. It is thought that the retinal degeneration is a primary process in osteopetrosis and is not due to the bone overgrowth [4,5].

Laboratory Studies

All bones are symmetrically involved with a diffuse sclerotic process. Medullary canals and trabecular patterns are usually absent (*Figures C, D, and F*). Plasma levels of calcium, phosphorus, and alkaline phosphatase are usually normal. Red blood cell survival becomes progressively shorter due to destruction by the enlarged spleen.

Treatment and Prognosis

There is no effective treatment. Transfusions are necessitated by the progressive anemia. Splenectomy improves red blood cell survival. Most infants die from either anemia or secondary infection in the first months or years of life [1].

Genetics

Autosomal recessive [1–3].

Differential Diagnosis

1. Increased bone density, frequent fractures, a large head, and prominent brow are also features of patients with pycnodysostosis, but they have shortened distal phalanges and an open anterior fontanel and a lack of either hepatosplenomegaly or cranial nerve palsies (see page 266).

2. Increased bone density and cranial nerve palsies are features of patients with Engelmann's disease, but they have a diaphyseal dysplasia and usually do not have hepatosplenomegaly (see page 262).

References

1. Johnston, C. C., Jr., Lavy, N., Lord, T., Vellios, F., Merritt, A. D., and Deiss, W. P., Jr. Osteopetrosis. A clinical, genetic, metabolic, and morphologic study of the dominantly inherited, benign form. *Medicine,* **47:**149–67, 1968.
2. Tips, R. L., and Lynch, H. T. Malignant congenital osteopetrosis resulting from a consanguineous marriage. *Acta Paediatr.,* **51:**585–88, 1962.
3. Dent, C. E., Smellie, J. M., and Watson, L. Studies in osteopetrosis. *Arch. Dis. Child.,* **40:**7–15, 1965.
4. Keith, C. G. Retinal atrophy in osteopetrosis. *Arch. Ophthalmol. (Chicago),* **79:**234–41, 1968.
5. Walton, D. S. Personal communication, 1970.

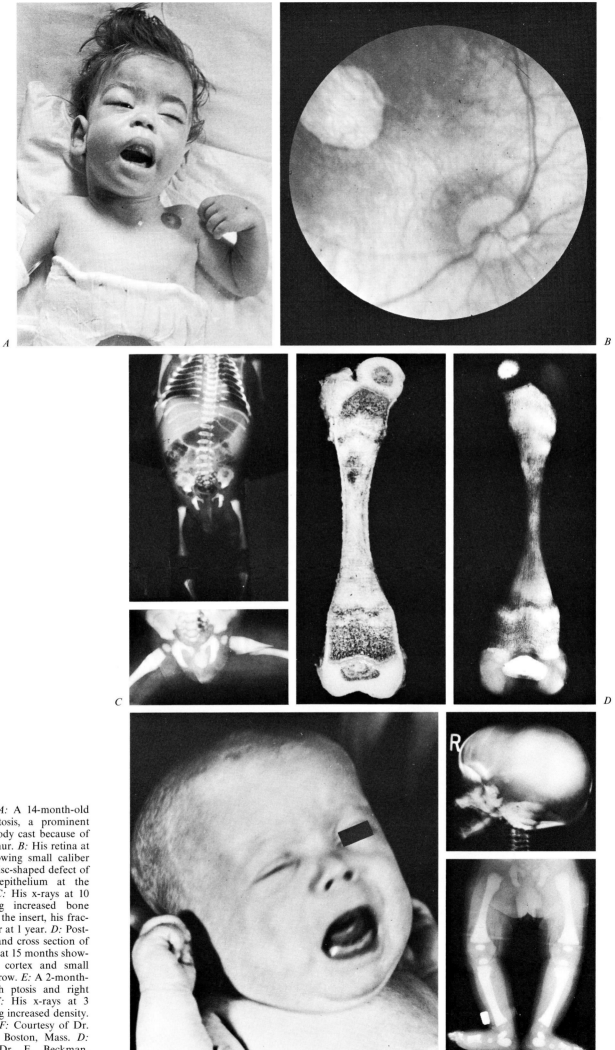

Plate VI-23. *A:* A 14-month-old infant with ptosis, a prominent brow, and a body cast because of a fractured femur. *B:* His retina at 12 months showing small caliber vessels and a disc-shaped defect of the pigment epithelium at the macula area. *C:* His x-rays at 10 weeks showing increased bone density and, in the insert, his fractured left femur at 1 year. *D:* Postmortem x-ray and cross section of his right femur at 15 months showing the dense cortex and small amount of marrow. *E:* A 2-month-old infant with ptosis and right facial palsy. *F:* His x-rays at 3 months showing increased density. (*B, C, E,* and *F:* Courtesy of Dr. D. S. Walton, Boston, Mass. *D:* Courtesy of Dr. E. Beckman, Boston, Mass.)

Pycnodysostosis

In 1962 Maroteaux and Lamy [1] described a new syndrome consisting of short stature, increased bone density, a large head with open fontanels and sutures, and a predisposition to fracture. Pycnodysostosis, meaning dense and defective bones, was suggested as an appropriate name for this syndrome. Thirty-two previously reported patients were considered by Elmore to have this disease [2], although many were originally described as having atypical forms of other diseases. In 1968, 73 cases were reviewed [3]. In 1971 Sugiura reported 6 new cases and 20 more previously described in the Japanese literature [3a].

Physical Features

HEAD: The head is large with frontal and sometimes parietal bossing. The cranial sutures and the anterior fontanel remain open into adulthood.

FACE: The face is small in comparison to the head. The facial bones are underdeveloped and the chin is small. The eyes are often proptosed. The nose is parrotlike in appearance [3] (*Figures A, C, and E*).

MOUTH: The deciduous teeth persist into adulthood, resulting sometimes in a double row of teeth. The permanent teeth may be unerupted or deformed and malaligned. The palate is narrow and high-arched.

BACK: Some patients have scoliosis and kyphosis.

LIMBS: Both the arms and legs are shortened. The joints are hypermobile. The fingers and toes often have short terminal phalanges. The nails may be brittle and soft.

HEIGHT: The average adult height is less than 5 feet. The range was 53 to 60 inches (134 to 152 cm) in one review [3].

Nervous System

Mental retardation has been described in 7 of 34 cases [2,4,5].

Pathology

Bone biopsies in three patients [6–8] showed persistent islands of osteochondroid, poorly formed haversian spaces and the presence of marrow in the medullary cavity.

Laboratory Studies

Bone density is increased in the entire skeleton (*Figure D*). The facial bones are hypoplastic, the mandible has an obtuse angle, and the paranasal sinuses are poorly pneumatized. The medullary canals of the long bones are present but poorly formed. The distal phalanges (*Figure B*) and the acromial ends of the clavicle are poorly developed. The ungual tufts of the distal phalanges are often missing. The pelvis shows coxa valga and shallow acetabula. Persistent transverse fractures often occur in the middle of the affected long bones [2,3,9]. Studies in one patient showed a reduction both in bone formation and in resorption [5]. Two patients have had different chromosomal abnormalities, both of which were probably coincidental findings [5,6].

Treatment and Prognosis

Fractures may occur at any age from only mild trauma. They occur most often in the legs, but also frequently involve the mandible and clavicle.

Genetics

Autosomal recessive [2,3].

Differential Diagnosis

1. A large head with frontal bossing and prominent eyes and dense bones are features of some patients with Engelmann's disease, but they have progressive bone involvement that begins in the diaphysis and results in increased width of the long bones (see page 262).

2. Open fontanels, aplasia of the clavicles, underdevelopment of the facial bones, and persistence of deciduous teeth are features of cleidocranial dysostosis, but those affected are distinguished by normal stature and an absence of generalized bone density [10].

3. Generalized bone density is a feature of patients with the infantile form of osteopetrosis, but they have cranial nerve palsies, normal phalanges, and retinal degeneration, and develop hepatosplenomegaly and severe anemia (see page 264).

References

1. Maroteaux, P., and Lamy, M. Deux observations d'une affection osseuse condensante: la pycnodysostose. *Arch. Fr. Pediatr.,* **19:**267–74, 1962.
2. Elmore, S. M. Pycnodysostosis: a review. *J. Bone Joint Surg.,* **49-A:**153–62, 1967.
3. Sedano, H. D., Gorlin, R. J., and Anderson, V. E. Pycnodysostosis. Clinical and genetic considerations. *Am. J. Dis. Child.,* **116:**70–77, 1968.
3a. Sugiura, Y. Pycnodysostosis in Japan. Report of 6 cases and a review of Japanese literature. (Abstract.) IVth International Congress of Human Genetics, Paris, 1971, p. 172.
4. Giedion, A., and Zachmann, M. Pyknodysostose. *Helv. Paediatr. Acta,* **21:**612–21, 1966.
5. Lacey, S. H., Eyring, E. J., and Shaffer, T. E. Pycnodysostosis: a case report of a child with associated trisomy X. *J. Pediatr.,* **77:**1033–38, 1970.
6. Elmore, S. M., Nance, W. E., McGeen, B. J., Engel-deMontmollin, M., and Engel, E. Pycnodysostosis, with a familial chromosome anomaly. *Am. J. Med.,* **40:**273–82, 1966.
7. Krabbe, K. H. Les formes atypiques de la dysostose cléido-cranienne (dysostose cranienne sans dysostose claviculaire). *Folia Psychiatr. Neurol. Neurochir. Neerlandica,* **53:**328–33, 1950.
8. Plamer, P. E. S. Case report. Osteopetrosis with multiple epiphyseal dysplasia. *Br. J. Radiol.,* **33:**455–57, 1960.
9. Dusenberry, J. F., Jr., and Kane, J. J. Pycnodysostosis. Report of three new cases. *Am. J. Roentgenol.,* **99:**717–23, 1967.
10. Forland, M. Cleidocranial dysostosis. A review of the syndrome and report of a sporadic case with hereditary transmission. *Am. J. Med.,* **3:**792–99, 1962.

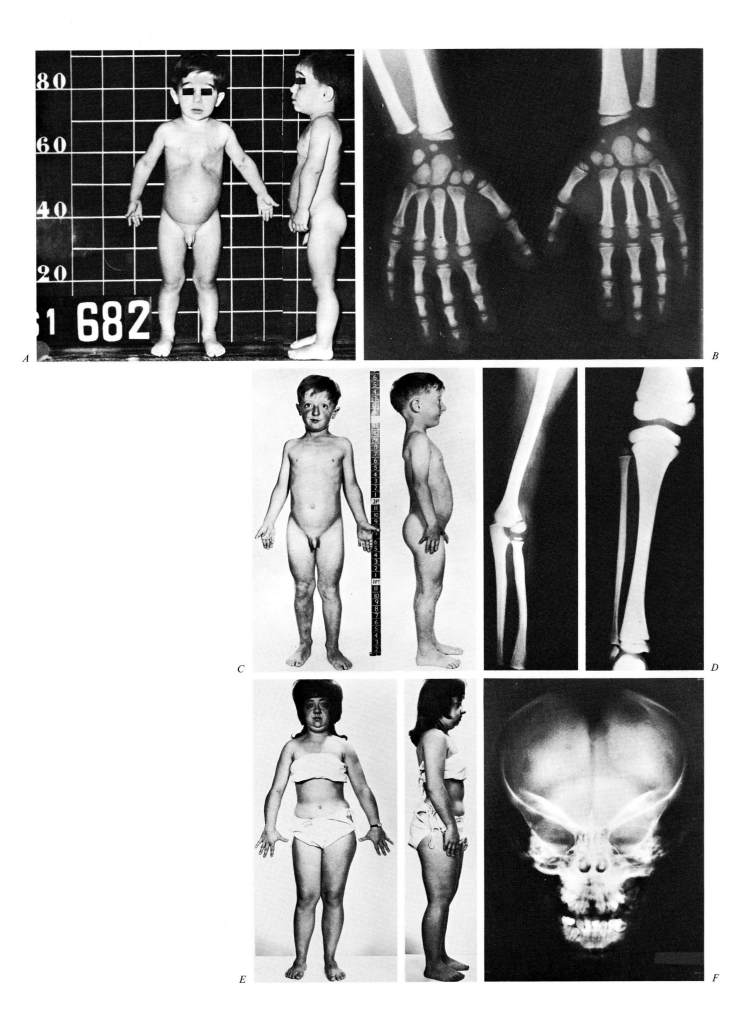

Plate VI-24. *A* and *B:* A 4-year-old boy with a prominent brow and occiput. He also has pectus carinatum, but this is not typical of this disease. His hand x-ray shows increased bone density and short distal phalanges. This boy, like the other patients shown on this page, had normal intelligence. *C* and *D:* A 7-year-old boy with short distal phalanges. X-rays of his arm and leg show increased density and poorly formed medullary spaces. *E* and *F:* A 15-year-old girl with proptosis, open sutures and fontanels, and frontal bossing. The skull x-ray shows open sutures and lack of pneumatization of the sinuses. (*A* and *B:* From P. Maroteaux and M. Lamy, *Presse Med.,* **70:**999–1002, 1962. *C* and *D:* Reprinted from S. E. Shuler, *Arch. Dis. Child.,* **38:**620, 1963, by permission of the author and editor. *E* and *F:* From S. M. Elmore *et al., Am. J. Med.,* **40:**273–82, 1966.)

Syndrome of Peripheral Dysostosis, Nose Hypoplasia, and Mental Retardation

Individuals with short, wide hands and feet and cone-shaped epiphyseal ossification centers have been reported for many years. The radiologic appearance prompted the term *peripheral dysostosis*. Several patients with peripheral dysostosis were also found to have nasal hypoplasia and subnormal intelligence [1–5]. This is now considered a specific clinical syndrome; at least 20 patients have been reported.

Physical Features

HEAD: Most patients have a flat occiput.

FACE: The nose is short and flat and the nostrils are anteverted; the bridge of the nose is flat. The philtrum is long. Epicanthal folds are often present. The maxilla is hypoplastic and the chin is prominent [5] (*Figures A, B, and E*).

LIMBS: The fingers and toes are often short and stubby at birth. The nails are short and broad. Because of the short bones the skin on the digits appears to be bulging out (*Figures C and D*).

HEIGHT: These patients are below normal in length at birth and have marked shortness of stature as adults [4,5].

GROWTH AND DEVELOPMENT: A few patients as adults have had inadequate development of their secondary sexual characteristics [2,3,5].

Nervous System

Most reported patients have had mild to moderate mental retardation. Some patients may be slow in learning to walk because of difficulty in balancing on their small feet [4,5].

Laboratory Studies

The metacarpals, metatarsals, and phalanges are short and broad. Almost all epiphyses in the hands and feet are deformed and fuse prematurely (*Figures C and D*). The distal radius and ulna are often hypoplastic. The nasal bones are either hypoplastic (*Figure F*) or absent entirely [5]. The bone age is usually advanced for the chronologic age. Studies of thyroid, pituitary, and adrenal function have shown no abnormalities [4].

Treatment and Prognosis

Because of the premature cessation of epiphyseal growth, the relative shortness of the fingers and toes becomes more pronounced with age. Eventually the patients have difficulty with manual skills. Arthritis often develops in the hands, feet, and other areas [5].

Genetics

None of the reported patients has had any similarly affected relatives.

Differential Diagnosis

1. Short stature and short digits, metacarpals, and metatarsals are due to premature closure of epiphyses and are also features of patients with pseudohypoparathyroidism, but they also have a diminished response to parathormone, have cataracts, subcutaneous ossification, and obesity, and do not have nose hypoplasia (see page 50).
2. Peripheral dysostosis is also a feature of the trichorhinophalangeal syndrome, but these patients have thin, scant hair and a pear-shaped nose [6].
3. Anteverted nostrils and advanced bone age are features of the two boys with the syndrome of marked acceleration of skeletal maturation and facial anomalies, but they did not have nose hypoplasia or peripheral dysostosis (see page 330).

References

1. Cohen, P., and van Creveld, S. Peripheral dysostosis. *Am. J. Roentgenol.*, **84:**499–505, 1960.
2. Maroteaux, P., and Malamut, G. L'acrodysostose. *Presse Med.*, **76:**2189–92, 1968.
3. Gideon, A. Die periphere Dysostose (PD)—ein Sammelbegriff. *Fortschr. Geb. Roentgenstr. Nuklearmed.*, **110:**507–24, 1969.
4. Garces, L. Y., Blank, E., Drash, A. L., and Kenny, F. M. Peripheral dysostosis: investigation of metabolic and endocrine functions. *J. Pediatr.*, **74:**730–37, 1969.
5. Robinow, M., Pfeiffer, R. A., Gorlin, R. J., McKusick, V. A., Renuart, A. W., Johnson, G. F., and Summitt, R. L. Acrodysostosis. A syndrome of peripheral dysostosis, nasal hypoplasia, and mental retardation. *Am. J. Dis. Child.*, **121:**195–203, 1971.
6. Giedion, A. Das tricho-rhino-phalangeal Syndrom. *Helv. Paediatr. Acta*, **21:**475–82, 1966.

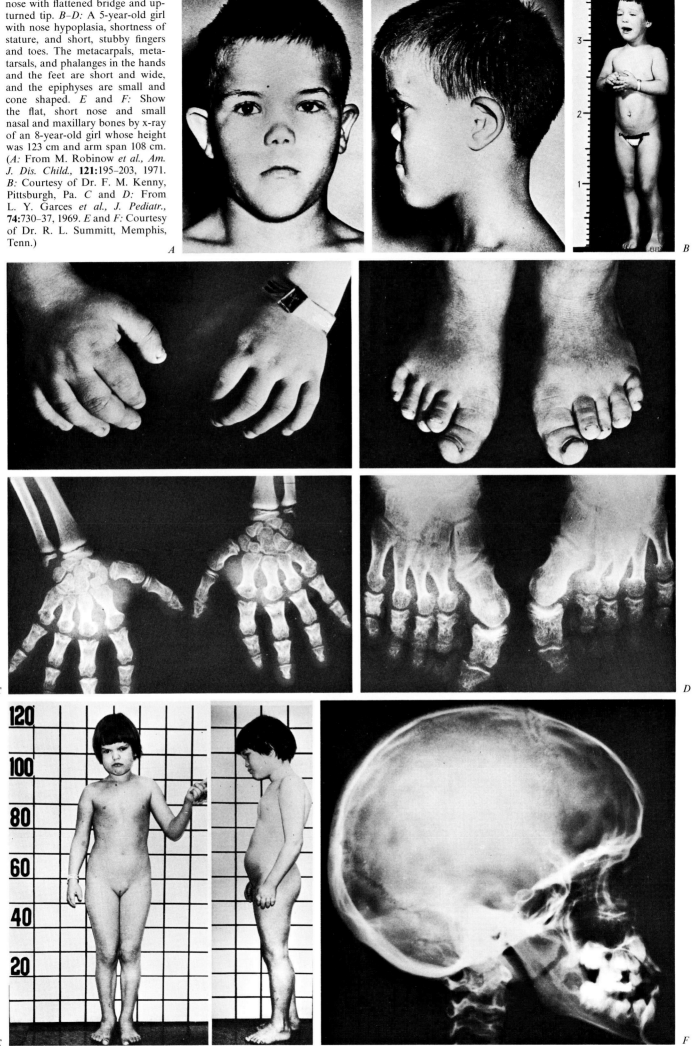

Plate VI-25. *A:* Shows the short nose with flattened bridge and up-turned tip. *B–D:* A 5-year-old girl with nose hypoplasia, shortness of stature, and short, stubby fingers and toes. The metacarpals, meta-tarsals, and phalanges in the hands and the feet are short and wide, and the epiphyses are small and cone shaped. *E* and *F:* Show the flat, short nose and small nasal and maxillary bones by x-ray of an 8-year-old girl whose height was 123 cm and arm span 108 cm. (*A:* From M. Robinow *et al., Am. J. Dis. Child.,* **121:**195–203, 1971. *B:* Courtesy of Dr. F. M. Kenny, Pittsburgh, Pa. *C* and *D:* From L. Y. Garces *et al., J. Pediatr.,* **74:**730–37, 1969. *E* and *F:* Courtesy of Dr. R. L. Summitt, Memphis, Tenn.)

A

B

C

D

E

F

Syndromes with Multiple Congenital Malformations
Cerebrohepatorenal Syndrome

In 1964 Bowen, Lee, Zellweger, and Lindenberg [1] described a female infant with marked hypotonia, glaucoma, corneal opacities, epicanthal folds, a high forehead, flexion contractures of the fingers, and stippled patellae and digit epiphyses. A deceased male sibling had similar features and also hypospadias.* Subsequently, more than 15 infants with many of these same features have been described [2–7], and are thought to have the same disorder. Because brain, liver, and kidney abnormalities are usually present, the condition has been called the cerebrohepatorenal syndrome [3].

Physical Features

HEAD: The fontanels and sutures are usually widely patent at birth. However, two children had sagittal craniosynostosis [3].

FACE: All of the reported infants have had a similar facial appearance with a high, prominent forehead, hypertelorism, epicanthal folds, and shallow supraorbital ridges. The chin is small and the cheeks are full (*Figures A, C, D, E, and F*).

EYES: Corneal clouding, glaucoma, and cataracts have been present in several infants [1,3,4,7]. Deficient and scattered retinal pigment was described in one patient [4].

EARS: The ears are often malrotated. The helices may be malformed or overfolded.

MOUTH: The palate is usually narrow and high-arched.

ABDOMEN: The liver is often enlarged.

GENITALIA: Three males were cryptorchid [2,4,5] and another had hypospadias [1]. One female had an enlarged clitoris [1].

LIMBS: Congenital flexion contractures of the fingers and knees, ulnar deviation of the hands and fingers, and clubfoot deformity have been present in several patients (*Figure F*).

Nervous System

All of the reported patients had severe muscular hypotonia (*Figures D, E, and F*). They show little psychomotor development. Some patients have seizures.

Pathology

The brain usually shows extensive abnormalities, most often of the cerebral cortex [8]. One showed hypoplasia of the cerebellar hemispheres [1]. Two siblings had macrogyria, polymicrogyria, and a sudanophilic leukodystrophy [3]. One child had a small brain, normal-sized ventricles, and a 3-cm cyst in the cerebral cortex [4]. Another child had a large brain, dilated ventricles, macrogyria and polymicrogyria, diffuse heteropias in the cortex and cerebellum, and a leukoencephalomyelopathy [5,6]. Renal cortical cysts have been found in all patients. No consistent liver abnormality has been observed. Some patients have had a diffuse interstitial fibrosis of the liver. In one family [5] heavy iron deposits were found in the liver, kidney, and bone marrow of one child. The brother had a striking increase in the serum iron and total body iron levels. In another family [4] the patient did not have increased amounts of hemosiderin in the liver or bone marrow, but had an elevated serum iron level. Several patients have had congenital heart disease, especially septal defects and patent ductus arteriosus.

*The affected patients in the second family discussed in this report [1] are thought to have an entirely different syndrome of multiple anomalies.

Laboratory Studies

Stippling of the patellae and ribs and punctate calcification near the acetabulum have been described [1,4,6,7,8] (*Figure B*), but are not always present.

Treatment and Prognosis

Severe hypotonia and failure to thrive persist throughout the short lives of these patients. Most require nasogastric tube feedings. Many have intestinal hemorrhages associated with hypoprothrombinemia, which responds to vitamin K. Pneumonia is a frequent cause of death. The oldest living child is 18 months old [9].

Genetics

An autosomal recessive mode of inheritance is suggested, because in several sibships two or more infants have been affected [1–6].

Differential Diagnosis

1. Hypotonia, epicanthal folds, and malformed ears are features of infants with Down's syndrome, but they do not have glaucoma or corneal opacities, flexion contractures, or liver enlargement (see page 150).

2. Glaucoma, cataracts, hypotonia, and cryptorchidism are features of patients with the oculocerebrorenal syndrome of Lowe, which is an X-linked recessive disorder. However, they also have an aminoaciduria, and do not have flexion contractures; only males are affected (see page 248).

3. Hypotonia and mental retardation are features of infants with the Prader-Labhart-Willi syndrome, but they do not have eye anomalies, liver enlargement, or flexion contractures (see page 48).

4. Congenital stippled epiphyses of any endochondral bone, joint contractures, and cataracts are features of patients with Conradi's disease, but they also have short limbs, their epiphyseal calcifications are more widespread, and they do not have hypotonia (see page 272).

References

1. Bowen, P., Lee, C. S. N., Zellweger, H., and Lindenberg, R. A familial syndrome of multiple congenital defects. *Johns Hopkins Med. J.,* **114:**402–14, 1964.
2. Smith, D. W., Opitz, J. M., and Inhorn, S. L. A syndrome of multiple developmental defects including polycystic kidneys and intrahepatic biliary dysgenesis in 2 siblings. *J. Pediatr.,* **67:**617–24, 1965.
3. Passarge, E., and McAdams, A. J. Cerebro-hepato-renal syndrome. A newly recognized hereditary disorder of multiple congenital defects including sudanophilic leukodystrophy, cirrhosis of the liver, and polycystic kidneys. *J. Pediatr.,* **71:**691–702, 1967.
4. Punnett, H. H., and Kirkpatrick, J. A., Jr. A syndrome of ocular abnormalities, calcification of cartilage, and failure to thrive. *J. Pediatr.,* **73:**602–606, 1968.
5. Vitale, L., Opitz, J. M., and Shahidi, N. T. Congenital and familial iron overload. *N. Engl. J. Med.,* **280:**642–45, 1969.
6. Opitz, J. M., ZuRhein, G. M., Vitale, L., Shahidi, N. T., Howe, J. J., Chou, S. M., Shanklin, D. R., Sybers, H. D., Dood, A. R., and Gerritsen, T. The Zellweger syndrome (cerebro-hepato-renal syndrome). *Birth Defects: Original Article Series,* Vol. V, No. 2, February, 1969, pp. 144–60. Williams & Wilkins Co., Baltimore.
7. Jan, J. E., Hardwick, D. F., Lowry, R. B., and McCormick, A. Q. Cerebro-hepato-renal syndrome of Zellweger. *Am. J. Dis. Child.,* **119:**274–77, 1970.
8. Poznanski, A. K., Nosanchuk, J. S., Baublis, J., and Holt, J. F. The cerebro-hepato-renal syndrome (CHRS) (Zellweger's syndrome). *Am. J. Roentgenol. Radium Ther. Nucl. Med,* **109:**313–22, 1970.
9. Passarge, E. Personal communication, 1970.

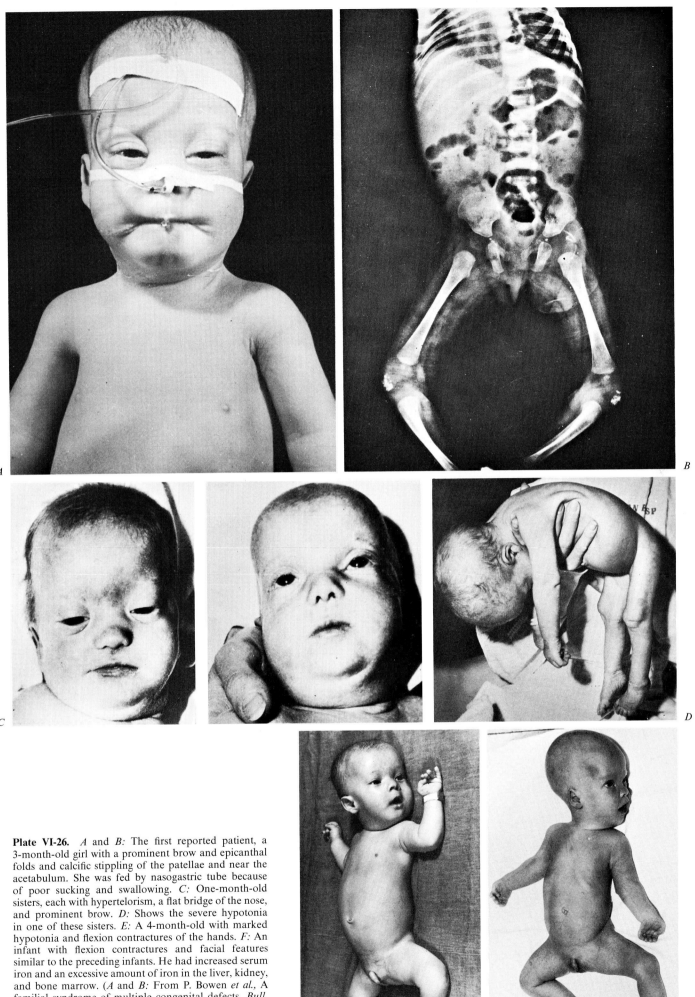

Plate VI-26. *A* and *B:* The first reported patient, a 3-month-old girl with a prominent brow and epicanthal folds and calcific stippling of the patellae and near the acetabulum. She was fed by nasogastric tube because of poor sucking and swallowing. *C:* One-month-old sisters, each with hypertelorism, a flat bridge of the nose, and prominent brow. *D:* Shows the severe hypotonia in one of these sisters. *E:* A 4-month-old with marked hypotonia and flexion contractures of the hands. *F:* An infant with flexion contractures and facial features similar to the preceding infants. He had increased serum iron and an excessive amount of iron in the liver, kidney, and bone marrow. (*A* and *B:* From P. Bowen *et al.,* A familial syndrome of multiple congenital defects, *Bull. Johns Hopkins Hosp., Med. J.,* **114:**402–14, 1964; Courtesy of The Johns Hopkins Press. *C* and *D:* From E. Passarge and A. J. McAdams, *J. Pediatr.,* **71:**691–702, 1967. *E:* From H. H. Punnett and J. A. Kirkpatrick, *J. Pediatr.,* **73:**602–606, 1968. *F:* From L. Vitale *et al.,* *N. Engl. J. Med.,* **280:**642–45, 1969.)

Conradi's Disease (Chondrodystrophia Calcificans Congenita; Congenital Stippled Epiphyses)

In 1914 Conradi [1] reported a newborn female with the condition which he called chondrodystrophia fetalis hypoplastica. Since then more than 100 patients have been described [2–7]. This experience has shown that this syndrome, which is referred to by a variety of descriptive terms, includes many different features, such as craniofacial anomalies, short limbs, cataracts, skin manifestations, and stippled epiphyses. In 1971 Spranger, Opitz, and Bidder [7a] showed that there are at least two distinct phenotypes which probably reflect different genetic abnormalities. Each will be described briefly.

I. Conradi-Hünermann Type

Physical Features

FACE: The forehead is prominent and the bridge of the nose is flat. The eyes are widely separated, and there is an upward palpebral slant.

EYES: Cataracts were present in 18 percent of the 65 patients reviewed by Spranger and coworkers [7a].

NECK: The neck is short.

LIMBS: Contractures, especially of large joints, were noted in 27 percent of the patients [7a]. Several had a clubfoot deformity.

SKIN: Dry, scaly, and atrophic skin is frequently described. These skin changes, called atrophoderma follicularis, may persist into adulthood [4] (Figure E). Often associated with this is loss of scalp hair due to cicatricial alopecia [4] (Figure D).

HEIGHT: The affected newborn is short. The adult height varies between 130 cm and normal [7a].

Nervous System

Mental retardation is rarely present [7a].

Pathology

Mucoid degeneration, cystic spaces, and calcification are present in the epiphyseal cartilage [3,7a]. There is invasion of fibrous tissue and bone formation irregularly scattered in the epiphyseal areas. Endochondral bone is usually normal.

Laboratory Studies

In infancy there are punctate calcifications in the vertebral column (Figure F) epiphyses, flat and round bones, and occasionally in the larynx and trachea [7a]. The tubular bones are mildly shortened, often asymmetrically. The vertebral bodies are irregularly deformed; scoliosis is common (Figure C). The epiphyses are flattened, irregular, and small. The metaphyses are normal.

Treatment and Prognosis

Some patients have died in early infancy, usually from infection. Those who survive the first three months of life are likely to live to adulthood.

Genetics

Possibly autosomal dominant [7a].

II. Rhizomelic Type

Physical Features

HEAD: Microcephaly is usually present.

EYES: Cataracts are found in all infants in whom a careful examination is performed [7a].

LIMBS: There is severe shortening of both the upper arm and the thighs (Figure A).

HEIGHT: Many, but not all, infants are short at birth. In one review [7a] the mean length at birth was 48.2 cm. Thereafter the linear growth is usually below normal.

Nervous System

Mental retardation usually present.

Pathology

The endochondral bone formation is grossly abnormal. The maturation of cartilage cells is severely disturbed. The epiphyseal cartilage appears friable; there are areas of degenerating cartilage which are partly ossified and partly resorbed.

Laboratory Studies

The humerus and femur both show marked symmetrical shortening, capping of the metaphyses, and disturbed ossification. Epiphyseal and extraepiphyseal calcifications are usually severe. There is a coronal cleft of the lateral aspects of the vertebrae.

Treatment and Prognosis

Of 36 infants 24 died in the first year with infection usually the presumed cause of death [7a]. Survival beyond the first few years of life is uncommon.

Genetics

Autosomal recessive.

Differential Diagnosis

1. Chondrodystrophy and hair and dental anomalies are features of patients with the Ellis–van Creveld syndrome, but they also have cardiac anomalies, polydactyly, and gingivolabial frenula (see page 280).
2. Shortening of the proximal portion of the limbs and a flat nasal bridge are also features of patients with achondroplasia, but they do not have cataracts or stippled epiphyses (see page 260).
3. Stippled epiphyses and a flat nasal bridge are features of patients with cretinism (see page 10) and patients with the cerebrohepatorenal syndrome (see page 270).
4. A hypoplastic nasal bridge and short stature are features of patients with the syndrome of peripheral dysostosis, nose hypoplasia, and mental retardation, but they also have short digits and do not have stippled epiphyses (see page 268).
5. Infants who had stippled epiphyses and as adolescents had roentgen findings of multiple epiphyseal dysplasia have been described by Silverman [8].

References

1. Conradi, E. Vorzeitiges Auftreten von Knochen-und eigenartigen Verkalkungskernen bei Chondrodystrophia fötalis hypoplastica. Histologische und Röntgenuntersuchungen. Jahrbuch Kinderheilk, 80:86–97, 1914.
2. Melnick, J. C. Chondrodystrophia calcificans congenita. Chondrodysplasia epiphysialis punctata, stippled epiphyses. Am. J. Dis. Child., 110:218–25, 1965.
3. Tasker, W. G., Mastri, A. R., and Gold, A. P. Chondrodystrophia calcificans congenita (dysplasia epiphysalis punctata). Recognition of the clinical picture. Am. J. Dis. Child., 119:122–27, 1970.
4. Comings, D. E., Papazian, C., and Schoene, H. R. Conradi's disease. Chondrodystrophia calcificans congenita, congenital stippled epiphyses. J. Pediatr., 72:63–69, 1968.
5. Armaly, M. F. Ocular involvement in chondrodystrophia calcificans congenita punctata. Arch. Ophthalmol. (Chicago), 57:491–502, 1957.
6. van Balen, A. Th. M., and Santens, P. Chondrodystrophia calcificans congenita. J. Pediatr. Ophthalmol., 5:151–56, 1968.
7. Fraser, F. C., and Scriver, J. B. A hereditary factor in chondrodystrophia calcificans congenita. N. Engl. J. Med., 250:272–77, 1954.
7a. Spranger, J. W., Opitz, J. M., and Bidder, U. Heterogeneity of chondrodysplasia punctata. Humangenetik, 11:190–212, 1971.
8. Silverman, F. N. Dysplasies épiphysaires: entité protéiforme. Ann. Radiol., 4:833–67, 1961.

Plate VI-27. *A* and *B:* A 7-month-old infant with the rhizomelic type of Conradi's disease. He has a large head, cataracts, depressed nasal bridge, short arms and legs, and stiff joints. *C–F:* This 15-year-old girl with the Conradi-Hünermann type of this disease had cataracts, a saddle-nose deformity, severe kyphoscoliosis, and a short right leg. Her hair was coarse and she had cicatricial alopecia. On her forearm she had follicular atrophoderma. Spinal x-ray taken at 5 days of age showed multiple punctate calcific densities at the epiphyseal junctions. (*A* and *B:* From A. Th. M. van Balen and P. Santens, *J. Pediatr. Ophthalmol.,* **5:**151–56, 1968. *C–F:* From D. E. Comings *et al., J. Pediatr.,* **72:**63–69, 1968.)

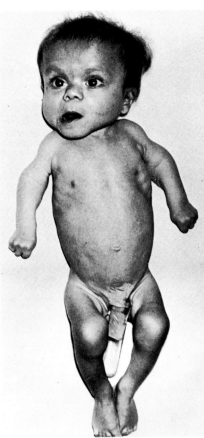

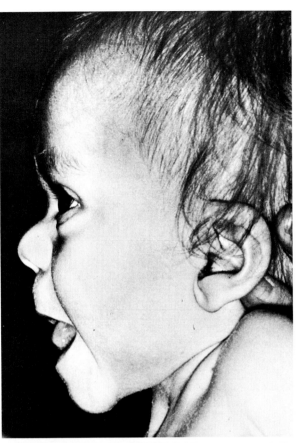

A

B

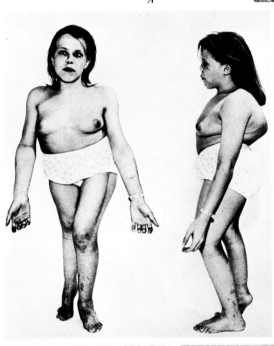

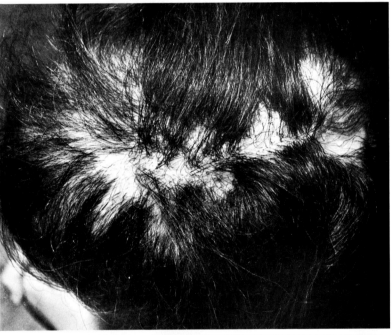

C

D

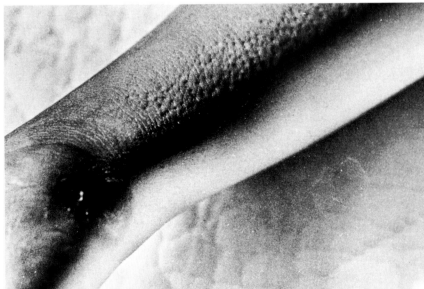

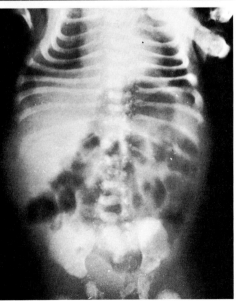

E

F

Cryptophthalmos Syndrome

The term *cryptophthalmos,* which means "hidden eye," was first used in 1872 by Zehender and Manz [1] to describe a patient born with skin covering the eyes. While the absence of the palpebral fissures is the most striking anomaly, these patients also have other facial, genitourinary, and skeletal anomalies. The incidence of this syndrome is not known. Fifty cases were reviewed in 1966 [2].

Physical Features

FACE: The absence of the palpebral fissure may be bilateral (*Figure A*) or unilateral (*Figure F*); in one series [3] of 39 patients the deformity was unilateral in 17 and bilateral in 22. The supraorbital ridge is always flattened on the side where the palpebral fissure is absent. Deformities of the nose, such as a lateral cleft of the nostril and a broad bridge of the nose, were present in 10 of 39 patients in this series [3]. The hairline may extend from the temporal area toward the orbit (*Figures A and B*).

EYES: On the side with no palpebral fissures there are no eyelids and no eyelashes, and the lacrimal ducts may be absent or malformed [4]. Small eyeballs are usually palpable beneath the skin covering. Although these globes have severe anomalies of the anterior portion, the posterior portion may remain functional. This may explain why many patients with bilateral absence of the palpebral fissures can perceive light and some can even distinguish colors [5]. Several patients have had orbitopalpebral cysts [2] which have the appearance of a protrusion in the region of the globe. Patients with unilateral cryptophthalmos usually have severe ocular anomalies, such as symblepharon (*Figure F*) on the side with the palpebral fissure.

EARS: Many patients have ear deformities, the most common being abnormally shaped pinnae and atretic external auditory canals (*Figures B and D*). Malformed middle ear ossicles have also been reported. A striking finding in a few patients is that the skin of the pinnae is continuous with the scalp [5,6].

MOUTH: A high palate arch is common; cleft lip and palate are occasionally present. Often there are deformed teeth and tongue anomalies, such as tongue-tie (*Figure C*).

THROAT: In many patients the larynx is small.

CHEST: A few patients have had a shieldlike chest with widely spaced nipples [4,7].

ABDOMEN: Ventral and umbilical hernias (*Figure C*) and separation of the symphysis pubis may be present.

GENITALIA: Males often have either mild or severe hypospadias and cryptorchidism. Females may have enlargement of the clitoris and fusion of the labia.

LIMBS: Syndactyly was present in 16 of 39 patients in one series [3]. The syndactyly usually involves both the hands and the feet. The number of digits fused may vary from only two to all five (*Figures C and E*).

Nervous System

Subnormal intelligence has been considered to be relatively frequent [8]. One recently reported patient [5] had an IQ of 74. A brother and sister on whom no intelligence testing was performed were considered to be mentally retarded [6]. Hearing loss is common, especially in patients with external ear deformities. The frequency of this deficit has not been established.

Pathology

Cerebral defects and meningomyelocele have been reported [2]. The most common internal anomalies are kidney malformations, which include hydronephrosis and bilateral and unilateral renal agenesis. Primitive mesentery of the small bowel, bicornuate uterus, and malformed fallopian tubes have been present in some patients [4].

Laboratory Studies

Skull x-rays in one patient [5] showed a calcified dislocated lens in one eye, asymmetry of the frontal sinuses, and calcification of the falx cerebri [5]. Chromosome studies in several patients have shown no abnormalities.

Treatment and Prognosis

Marked improvement in hearing following middle ear reconstructive surgery has been observed in one patient [11].

Genetics

Autosomal recessive inheritance seems likely in view of the high incidence of consanguinity [2] and multiple affected siblings [4–7].

Differential Diagnosis

1. Anomalies of the face, ears, limbs, and external genitalia are also features of Potter's syndrome of bilateral renal agenesis, but these patients do not have cryptophthalmos [12].
2. Severe microphthalmia, renal dysgenesis, cryptorchidism, syndactyly, and dental anomalies are features of the microphthalmia syndrome first described by Lenz [13], but these patients do not have cryptophthalmos.
3. Renal dysgenesis, deformed ears, hearing loss, and genital anomalies are features of the patients with the autosomal recessive syndrome reported by Winter and coworkers [14], but they did not have cryptophthalmos.

References

1. Zehender, W. Eine Missgeburt mit hautüberwachsenen Augen oder Kryptophthalmus. *Klin. Monatsbl. Augenheilkd.,* **10**:225–49, 1872.
2. Ehlers, N. Cryptophthalmos with orbito-palpebral cyst and microphthalmos. *Acta Ophthalmol.,* **44**:84–94, 1966.
3. Otradovec, J., and Janovský, M. O Kryptoftalmu. *Cesk. Oftalmol.,* **18**:128–38, 1962.
4. Fraser, G. R. Our genetical "load." A review of some aspects of genetical variation. *Ann. Hum. Genet.,* **25**:387–415, 1962.
5. Ide, C. H., and Wollschlaeger, P. B. Multiple congenital abnormalities associated with cryptophthalmia. *Arch. Ophthalmol. (Chicago),* **81**:638–44, 1969.
6. Ashley, L. M. Bilateral anophthalmos in a brother and sister. *J. Hered.,* **38**:174–76, 1947.
7. Gupta, S. P., and Saxena, R. C. Cryptophthalmos. *Br. J. Ophthalmol.,* **46**:629–32, 1962.
8. François, J. Syndrome malformatif avec cryptophtalmie. *Acta Genet. Med. Gemellol.,* **18**:18–50, 1969.
9. Fraser, G. R. XX chromosomes and renal agenesis. *Lancet,* **1**:1427, 1966.
10. Sugar, H. S. The cryptophthalmos-syndactyly syndrome. *Am. J. Ophthalmol.,* **66**:897–99, 1968.
11. Fraser, G. R. Personal communication, 1969.
12. Passarge, E., and Sutherland, J. M. Potter's syndrome. Chromosome analysis of three cases with Potter's syndrome or related syndromes. *Am. J. Dis. Child.,* **109**:80–84, 1965.
13. Lenz, W. Recessiv-geschlechtsgebundene Mikrophthalmie mit multiplen Missbildungen. *Z. Kinderheilkd.,* **77**:384–90, 1955.
14. Winter, J. S. D., Kohn, G., Mellman, W. J., and Wagner, S. A familial syndrome of renal, genital, and middle ear anomalies. *J. Pediatr.,* **72**:88–93, 1968.

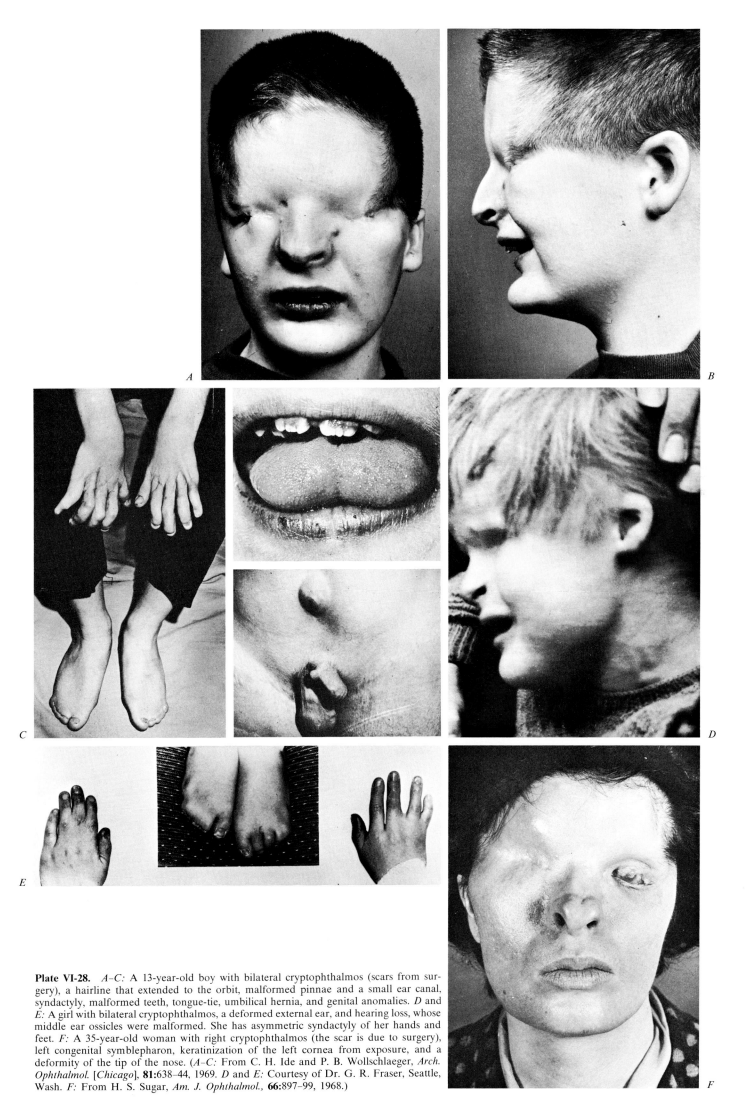

Plate VI-28. *A–C:* A 13-year-old boy with bilateral cryptophthalmos (scars from surgery), a hairline that extended to the orbit, malformed pinnae and a small ear canal, syndactyly, malformed teeth, tongue-tie, umbilical hernia, and genital anomalies. *D* and *E:* A girl with bilateral cryptophthalmos, a deformed external ear, and hearing loss, whose middle ear ossicles were malformed. She has asymmetric syndactyly of her hands and feet. *F:* A 35-year-old woman with right cryptophthalmos (the scar is due to surgery), left congenital symblepharon, keratinization of the left cornea from exposure, and a deformity of the tip of the nose. (*A–C:* From C. H. Ide and P. B. Wollschlaeger, *Arch. Ophthalmol.* [*Chicago*], **81:**638–44, 1969. *D* and *E:* Courtesy of Dr. G. R. Fraser, Seattle, Wash. *F:* From H. S. Sugar, *Am. J. Ophthalmol.,* **66:**897–99, 1968.)

de Lange Syndrome

In 1933 Cornelia de Lange [1] described two infants with brachycephaly, hypertrophy of the brows and lashes, small hands and feet, micromelia, and syndactylism of the feet. By 1970 248 patients had been reported [2]. It has been shown that this syndrome includes craniofacial deformities, increased amount of body hair, and a variety of skeletal malformations. An estimate of the incidence of this syndrome is 1:30,000 to 1:50,000 livebirths [2].

Physical Features

Head: These patients are microcephalic and have a flat occiput.

Face: There is pronounced hirsutism of the face with bushy eyebrows which join above the nose (synophrys). The eyes are often widely spaced. The palpebral fissures often slant downward. Some patients have a wide medial canthus [3]. The nose is small and the nostrils are anteverted. The philtrum is longer than average. The lips are thin and the corners of the mouth curve downward. The chin is small (*Figures A, B, C, E, and F*).

Eyes: The eyelashes are long and curly. Many ocular anomalies have been described, the most common being narrow palpebral fissures, strabismus, ptosis, nystagmus, eccentric pupils, microphthalmia, and optic atrophy [2,3].

Ears: The ears are usually well differentiated but low-set.

Mouth: The teeth erupt late and are smaller than normal [4]. The palate is often narrow. Cleft palate has been noted in over 10 percent of the patients [2].

Neck: The neck is usually short.

Voice: Usually infants, and sometimes older individuals, have a low, growling voice.

Chest: The nipples are small.

Genitalia: The penis and scrotum are usually small and the testes undescended. Some patients also have hypospadias. The external genitalia of females are also considered hypoplastic.

Limbs: The arms are usually shortened. The hands and feet are small. Inability to fully extend the elbows and knees is common. The spectrum of anomalies ranges from thin, tapering digits and clinodactyly to micromelia, phocomelia and oligodactyly (*Figure E*), and ectrodactyly (*Figure C*). About 20 percent of the reported patients have had one of these severe malformations [2]. The most frequent abnormality of the thumb is shortening and proximal placement. Syndactyly between the second and third toes is common.

Dermatoglyphics: Simian creases are common. The dermal ridges of the hypothenar areas of the palms and soles are hypoplastic.

Skin: Hirsutism is usually present on the forehead, upper lip, back, and forearms (*Figures A, D, and F*). The hair may be coarse and dry [2]. Many patients have pronounced vascular lability and cutis marmorata [5].

Height and Weight: Most infants have a low birth weight for term gestation and their length at birth is also below normal. The height and weight of both children and adults is usually below the third percentile of normal [2].

Growth and Development: The weight gain in infancy is poor. Adolescent males and females usually develop normal secondary sexual characteristics, and menstruation in females is normal [4].

Nervous System

All are mentally retarded. Most reported patients have intelligence quotients of less than 50, but some have only been mildly retarded [6]. Increased muscle tone is common in infancy. Some older patients are spastic. Convulsions of various types have been noted in about 10 percent of the reported patients [2]. Self-mutilation has been observed [6a].

Pathology

A variety of abnormalities have been reported. The brain and many other organs are quite small for the age of the child. Cerebral convolutional abnormalities, demyelinization, and many different cardiac, intestinal, and genitourinary anomalies have been described [4]. Among 250 reported patients 15 percent had cardiac anomalies and another 12 percent had a heart murmur; there is no specific malformation that is predominant [6b].

Laboratory Studies

The most common x-ray findings are in the arms and hands: hypoplasia of the metacarpals and middle phalanges [1], clinodactyly, hypoplasia and subluxation of the radial head, and retarded epiphyseal development in all bones. Low acetabular angles of the pelvis and short sternum have also been noted [7]. While recurrent infections are often described, studies of the serum immunoglobulins of 16 patients between 3 and 46 years of age did not show any abnormalities [8]. A normochromic normocytic anemia is often present. While a variety of endocrinologic abnormalities have been reported, none has been consistently present [2]. Most patients have normal chromosomes; several different abnormalities have been reported, but they are considered coincidental findings.

Treatment and Prognosis

Many infants have difficulty in swallowing and develop aspiration pneumonia, which is a common cause of death.

Genetics

In a study of 54 families [6] the recurrence rate among siblings was estimated as between 2.2 and 5.1 percent. Based on this recurrence risk, polygenic inheritance was suggested. Later, additional data were interpreted as more compatible with autosomal recessive inheritance [9].

Differential Diagnosis

1. Synophrys and hirsutism are features of patients with the Rubinstein-Taybi syndrome, but they also have a prominent nose, downward palpebral slant, and large thumbs and great toes (see page 306).
2. A short nose with anteverted nostrils, cryptorchidism, and hypospadias are features of patients with the Smith-Lemli-Opitz syndrome, but they also have a broad upper alveolar ridge and ptosis and do not have synophrys or hirsutism (see page 312).
3. Brachycephaly, hirsutism, long eyelashes, and a small chin were features of the three siblings with the new mental retardation reported by Scott and coworkers [10].

References

1. de Lange, C. Sur un type nouveau de dégénération (Typus Amstelodamensis). *Arch. Méd. Enfants*, **36**:713–19, 1933.
2. Berg, J. M., McCreary, B. D., Ridler, M. A. C., and Smith, G. F. *The De Lange Syndrome.* Pergamon Press, Oxford, 1970, p. 127.
3. Nicholson, D. H., and Goldberg, M. F. Ocular abnormalities in the de Lange syndrome. *Arch. Ophthalmol. (Chicago)*, **76**:214–20, 1966.
4. McArthur, R. G., and Edwards, J. H. de Lange syndrome: report of 20 cases. *Can. Med. Assoc. J.*, **96**:1185–98, 1967.
5. Abraham, J. M., and Russell, A. de Lange syndrome. A study of nine examples. *Acta Paediatr. Scand.*, **57**:339–53, 1968.
6. Pashayan, H., Whelan, D., Guttman, S., and Fraser, F. C. Variability of the de Lange syndrome: report of 3 cases and genetic analysis of 54 families. *J. Pediatr.*, **75**:853–58, 1969.
6a. Shear, C. S., Nyhan, W. L., Kirman, B. H., and Stern, J. Self-mutilative behavior as a feature of the de Lange syndrome. *J. Pediatr.*, **78**:506–509, 1971.
6b. Syamasundar Rao, P., and Sissman, N. J. Congenital heart disease in the de Lange syndrome. *J. Pediatr.*, **79**:674–77, 1971.
7. Lee, F. A., and Kenny, F. M. Skeletal changes in the Cornelia de Lange syndrome. *Am. J. Roentgenol.*, **100**:27–39, 1967.
8. Bartsocas, C. S., Crawford, J. D., and Littlefield, J. W. Immunoglobulins in de Lange syndrome. *Lancet*, **2**:733–34, 1968.
9. Motl, M. L., and Opitz, J. M. Studies of malformation syndromes XXVA. Phenotypic and genetic studies of the Brachmann-de Lange syndrome. *Hum. Hered.*, **21**:1–16, 1971.
10. Scott, C. R., Bryant, J. I., and Graham, C. B. A new craniodigital syndrome with mental retardation. *J. Pediatr.*, **78**:658–63, 1971.

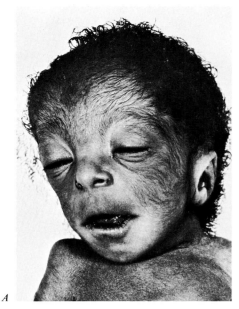 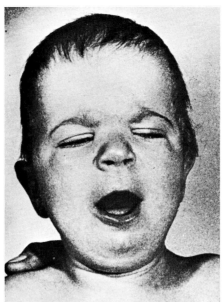 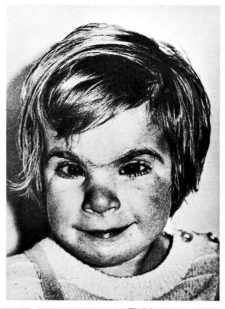

A

B

Plate VI-29. *A:* A 3-day-old Negro infant with marked facial hirsutism, a long philtrum, and malformed ears. *B:* A child at 9 and 22 months of age showing the development of synophrys. *C* and *D:* A newborn with unilateral ectro-dactyly and marked hirsutism. *E:* A 4-year-old girl with synophrys, anteverted nostrils, absence of digits on all limbs, and bilateral forearm deformities. *F:* A 9-year-old girl with short stature, increased lumbar lordosis, pectus ex-cavatum, and hirsutism that was most marked on her back. (*A:* From M. J. Thorburn, *Am. J. Obstet. Gynec.,* **89:**828–29, 1964. *B:* Courtesy of Dr. E. Passarge, Hamburg, Germany. *E:* Courtesy of Dr. B. Hagberg, Uppsala, Sweden.)

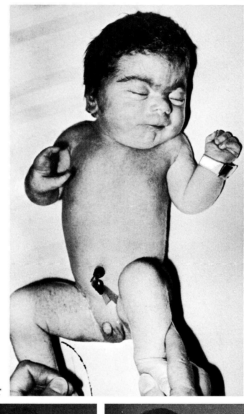 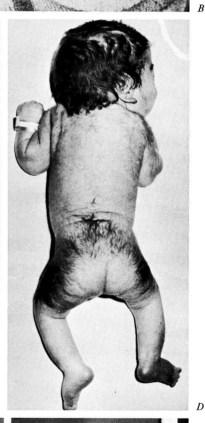

C

D

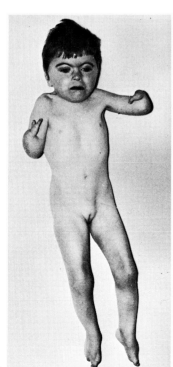 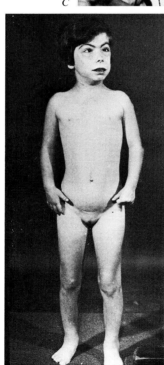 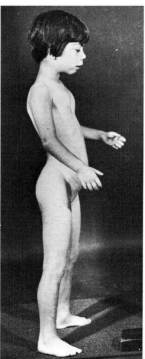 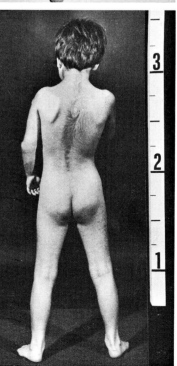

E

F

Dysmorphogenesis of Joints, Brain, and Palate

In 1968 Aase and Smith [1] described two infants who had multiple joint contractures at birth, cleft palate, and the Dandy-Walker malformation of the fourth ventricle. Their father also had joint contractures at birth, and it was suggested that he had less severe manifestations of the same multiple anomaly syndrome present in his children. This syndrome had not been previously described.

Physical Features

HEAD: The first child, a female, had a head circumference of 36.5 cm (90th percentile) at birth, and her head size increased rapidly during the first few weeks of life. The second child, a male, developed massive, generalized head enlargement during fetal life, requiring decompression before vaginal delivery (*Figures A and B*).

FACE: The father had a high forehead and bilateral ptosis (*Figure C*).

EARS: Both the second child and the father had ear deformities. The father's ears protruded.

MOUTH: Both infants had a cleft palate. The father had a narrow palate.

BACK: The male infant had thoracic scoliosis. The father had lumbar scoliosis, which was secondary to unequal leg length.

LIMBS: All three had contractures of the hips, knees, elbows, wrists, and fingers at birth (*Figures A and B*). One child also had bilateral congenital dislocation of the hips, and the father had a unilateral equinus deformity of the foot. When 26 years old, the father had flexion contractures of all fingers (*Figure D*), mild limitation of extension of the elbows, and mild flexion contractures of the hips and knee.

DERMATOGLYPHICS: One infant had hypoplastic dermal ridges. The father had whorls on nine fingers and no distal flexion creases on any of his fingers.

Nervous System

One child was hydrocephalic and stillborn. The other developed hydrocephalus rapidly after birth and was quite de-bilitated when she died at 6 weeks of age. The father was intelligent. His only neurologic abnormalities were a marked limitation of lateral gaze and strabismus.

Pathology

The first child had gross dilatation of the fourth ventricle, absence of the midportion of the cerebellum, and deformity of the medulla, as in the Dandy-Walker malformation; there also was an early neuroblastoma in one adrenal gland. The second child also had a Dandy-Walker malformation, in addition to multiple small interventricular septal defects, a single ossification center of the sternum, and a single umbilical artery.

Laboratory Studies

Chromosome analyses of the father and the second child showed no abnormalities.

Genetics

Autosomal dominant inheritance was presumed in this family.

Differential Diagnosis

1. Infants with X-linked aqueductal stenosis (see page 200), hydranencephaly (see page 204), and the Dandy-Walker syndrome (see page 202) may develop massive hydrocephalus during fetal life, but they have neither congenital joint contractures nor cleft palate.
2. Congenital flexion contractures and a large head were features of the infants with the syndrome of cryptorchidism, chest deformities, contractures, and arachnodactyly, but they did not have cleft palate or hydrocephalus (see page 332).

Reference

1. Aase, J. M., and Smith, D. W. Dysmorphogenesis of joints, brain, and palate: a new dominantly inherited syndrome. *J. Pediatr.*, **73**:606–609, 1968.

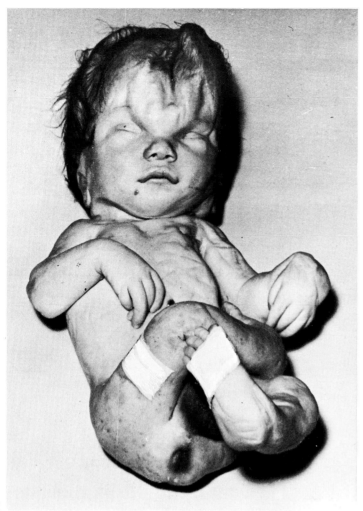

A

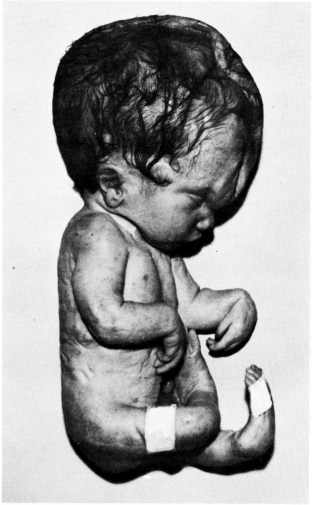

B

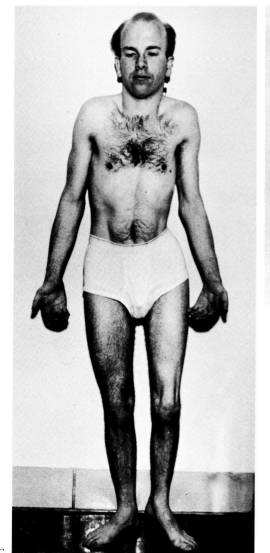

C

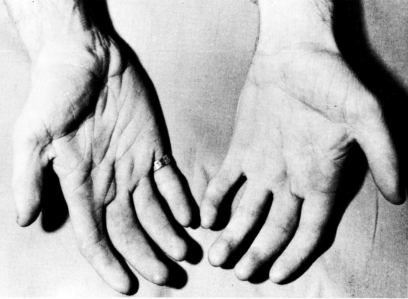

D

Plate VI-30. *A* and *B:* A stillborn male infant with hydrocephalus due to aqueductal stenosis, shortening and flexion contracture of all extremities, dislocation of both hips, and complete cleft palate. *C* and *D:* The father, who had bilateral ptosis, limitation of lateral gaze, congenital flexion contractures of the fingers, elbows, and knees, shortening of the left leg, and normal intelligence. (*A:* Courtesy of Dr. J. M. Aase, Seattle, Wash. *B–D:* From J. M. Aase and D. W. Smith, *J. Pediatr.,* **73:**606–609, 1968.)

Ellis–van Creveld Syndrome (Chondroectodermal Dysplasia)

In 1940 Ellis and van Creveld [1] described three infants with chondrodystrophy, polydactyly, and dysplasia of the hair, teeth, and nails. Two of them also had congenital heart disease. By 1968 over 100 patients [2] had been reported, including 52 persons in a religious isolate, the Old Order Amish [3].

Physical Features

FACE: The upper lip is usually short and is fused by multiple frenula to the maxillary gingiva in the region of the incisors (*Figure B*).

MOUTH: Teeth may erupt before birth or in the first weeks of life; these teeth are usually lost prematurely. The secondary dentition may never appear. The teeth are usually small, irregularly spaced, and either conical or bicuspid with deep fissures (*Figure C*). The enamel is hypoplastic in some patients.

GENITALIA: Mild epispadias was noted in several males in the Amish kindreds [3].

LIMBS: Polydactyly is one of the most common features. The extra digit, which is always present on the hands and sometimes on the feet as well, is usually well formed and may be functional (*Figure B*). It is always postaxial—i.e., located on the ulnar or fibular side. Adults cannot make a tight fist because the proximal phalanges are relatively long compared to the others. The limbs are short, primarily in the distal portion (*Figures A and F*). Genu valgum, due to hypoplasia of the lateral aspect of the proximal tibia, is common.

HAIR: Some patients have thin and sparse hair.

NAILS: The nails are usually small and scaly, and on some digits they may be completely absent (*Figure B*).

HEIGHT: The length at birth and throughout life is below the third percentile of normal. The height of the Amish adults ranged from $42\frac{3}{4}$ to $60\frac{1}{2}$ inches (110 to 154 cm) [3].

Nervous System

The incidence of mental retardation is difficult to establish. In one review of 36 patients, 4 were mentally retarded [4]. The patient shown in *Figures C and D* is severely retarded. The experience with 52 affected Amish patients, however, leads to the suggestion that mental deficiency is not a part of this syndrome [3].

Pathology

Congenital heart disease occurs in 50 to 60 percent of the patients. The most common cardiac anomalies are single atrium and endocardial fusion defect [2]. Pulmonary and bronchial cartilage hypoplasia have also been described. The neuropathologic examination of two siblings showed poor development of the gyri with atrophy of the vermis and hydrocephalus in one and thinning of the corpus callosum [4a]. The phalanges of these two patients showed the changes typical of this disorder, which are uneven epiphyseal lines, a decreased number of cartilage cells in the cartilage plate and a disorganized columnar arrangement of the chondrocytes.

Laboratory Studies

Fusion of the hamate and capitate bones of the wrist is common. The middle phalanges are short and the distal phalanges are hypoplastic (*Figure E*).

Treatment and Prognosis

Cardiopulmonary diseases are the most common cause of death. In the study of the 52 Amish patients, it was found that over half were dead within the first 6 months of life; 3 were stillborn, 20 died within the first 2 weeks of life, and a total of 30 died within the first 6 months [3].

Genetics

Autosomal recessive.

Differential Diagnosis

1. Sparse scalp hair, a short philtrum, partial cleft upper lip, and frenula obliterating the super gingivolabial sulcus are features of patients with the oral-facial-digital syndrome (type I), but they also have frenula on the lower alveolar ridge, a lobulated tongue, are always females, and are not dwarfed (see page 300).
2. Polydactyly and short middle and distal phalanges may occur in patients with asphyxiating thoracic dystrophy [5], but they do not have either abnormal nails and teeth or frenula of the upper lip.
3. Gingivolabial frenula, short stature, and polydactyly are features of the two siblings with the syndrome of dyschondroplasia, facial anomalies, and polysyndactyly, but they also had syndactyly and did not have hair, teeth, or nail abnormalities (see page 322).
4. Patients with achondroplasia also have short-limbed dwarfism, but the shortening is more in the proximal portion and they do not have polydactyly or ectodermal defects (see page 260).

References

1. Ellis, R. W. B., and van Creveld, S. A syndrome characterized by ectodermal dysplasia, polydactyly, chondro-dysplasia and congenital morbus cordis. Report of three cases. *Arch. Dis. Child.,* 15:65–84, 1940.
2. Lynch, J. I., Perry, L. W., Takakuwa, T., and Scott, L. P., III. Congenital heart disease and chondroectodermal dysplasia. Report of two cases, one in a Negro. *Am. J. Dis. Child.,* 115:80–87, 1968.
3. McKusick, V. A., Egeland, J. A., Eldridge, R., and Krusen, D. E. Dwarfism in the Amish. 1. The Ellis-van Creveld syndrome. *Johns Hopkins Med. J.,* 115:306–36, 1964.
4. Ellis, R. W. B., and Andrew, J. D. Chondroectodermal dysplasia. *J. Bone Joint Surg. (Br.),* 44B:626–36, 1962.
4a. Blackburn, M. G., and Belliveau, R. E. Ellis-van Creveld syndrome. A report of previously undescribed anomalies in two siblings. *Am. J. Dis. Child.,* 122:267–70, 1971.
5. Langer, L. O., Jr. Thoracic-pelvic-phalangeal dystrophy. *Radiology,* 91:447–56, 1968.

Plate VI-31. *A* and *B:* An 8-month-old infant with a narrow thorax, short arms and legs, postaxial polydactyly, and small or absent nails. Turning up his lip revealed multiple frenula. *C* and *D:* Show in a retarded patient conical and irregularly spaced teeth, short fibula and ulna, and hypoplasia of the lateral half of the proximal tibial epiphysis. *E:* Shows the broad fifth metacarpal, small distal phalanges, and fusion of carpal bones. *F:* One of the patients originally reported by Ellis and van Creveld shown at the ages of 4, 17, and 28 years. Normal heights for these ages are shown for comparison. (*A* and *B:* From J. I. Lynch *et al., Am. J. Dis. Child.,* **115:**80–87, 1968. *E:* Courtesy of Dr. P. Maroteaux, Paris, France. *F:* From W. H. deHaas and W. deBoer, *Arch. Interam. Rheumat.,* **8:**197–218, 1965.)

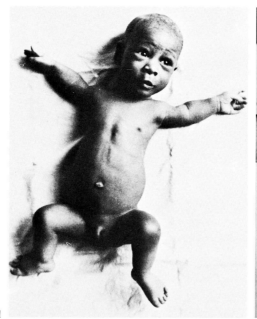

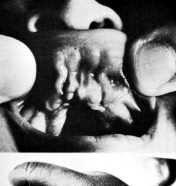

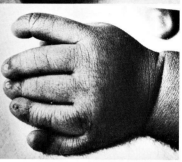

A

B

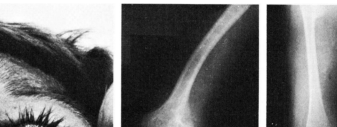

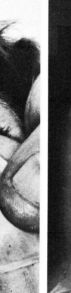

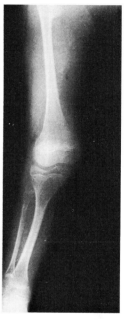

C

D

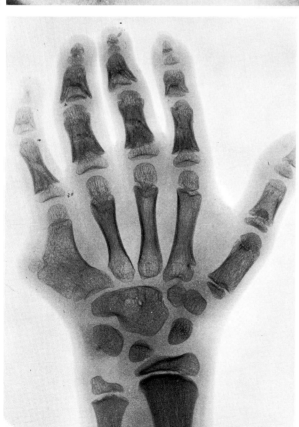

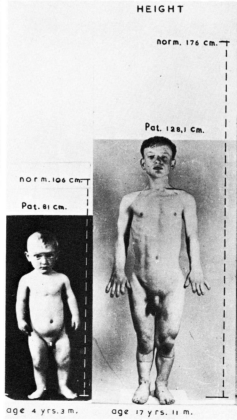

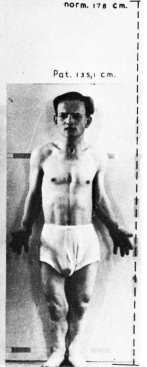

HEIGHT

norm. 176 cm.

norm. 178 cm.

Pat. 135,1 cm.

Pat. 128,1 cm.

norm. 106 cm.

Pat. 81 cm.

age 4 yrs. 3 m.

age 17 yrs. 11 m.

age 28 yrs. 7 m.

E

F

281

Fanconi's Anemia

In 1927 Fanconi [1] described three brothers with a disorder that was characterized by pancytopenia, brown hyperpigmentation, genital hypoplasia, and microcephaly. Subsequently, more than 150 patients have been reported [2,3]. It has been shown that this syndrome also includes skeletal and renal anomalies, short stature, chromosomal abnormalities, and a predisposition to malignancies.

Physical Features

HEAD: Fifty-one out of 129 patients in one review [3] were microcephalic.

EYES: Twenty-eight patients had strabismus [2,3]. Microphthalmia is occasionally noted.

GENITALIA: In the study of 74 males, 26 had hypogenitalism and 12 were cryptorchid [3].

LIMBS: Skeletal anomalies, especially radial forearm deformities, are very common. Of 129 patients, 48 had hypoplasia or aplasia of the thumb, 15 had hypoplasia or aplasia of the radius (*Figures A, B, and C*), 12 had syndactyly, and 33 had a reduced number of carpal bones [3]. Another frequent finding is absence of the radial pulse.

SKIN: Hyperpigmentation, which is the most frequent physical finding, was present in 99 of 129 patients [2,3]. It appears within the first few years of life. The skin lesions may be large or small, and have a patchy distribution. The neck, axilla, groin, and trunk are usually involved (*Figures A and D*).

WEIGHT: The birth weight for term infants is often below normal; 20 out of 36 patients [2,3] weighed less than 2500 g.

HEIGHT: Short stature, usually below the third percentile, is a common feature of this disease.

Nervous System

Twenty-two of 129 patients were mentally retarded; 24 had hyperreflexia, and 9 had a hearing loss [3].

Pathology

Renal anomalies such as unilateral agenesis, hydronephrosis, and horseshoe kidneys are common. A few patients have had congenital heart disease. Several have developed either acute leukemia or solid malignant tumors [4,4a].

Laboratory Studies

Pancytopenia usually develops between 4 and 10 years of age. The chromosomes of most patients show structural abnormalities, such as breaks, gaps, and endoreduplications [4,5] (*Figures E and F*). Skin fibroblasts have been shown to be unusually susceptible to transformation by SV40 oncogenic virus [5a].

Treatment and Prognosis

Testosterone and corticosteroids may produce temporary improvement in the pancytopenia, but it is usually fatal [6]. A few patients have shown remissions of several years following this therapy [7]. The use of oxymetholone [7a] has recently been the preferred treatment.

Genetics

Autosomal recessive. An increased incidence of leukemia has been observed among the relatives of patients with Fanconi's anemia [4,8]. Furthermore, it has been estimated that the individual heterozygous for Fanconi's anemia has a risk of dying from a malignant neoplasm three times greater than normal [8a].

Differential Diagnosis

1. The disorder known as thrombocytopenia with radial aplasia is distinguished by the onset of petechiae in infancy, the predominance of megakaryocyte abnormalities, and the absence of hyperpigmentation [9].
2. A syndrome of congenital hypoplastic anemia associated with triphalangeal thumbs has recently been described, but these patients did not have short stature, mental retardation, or hyperpigmentation [10].
3. Pancytopenia and malignancies are also features of patients with dyskeratosis congenita, but they have different skin lesions and no skeletal anomalies [11].
4. Short stature, chromosome breaks, and a predisposition to leukemia and solid tumors are features of patients with Bloom's syndrome, but they also have dermatitis in sun-exposed areas and do not have hyperpigmentation, microcephaly, or radial anomalies [12].

References

1. Fanconi, G. Familiäre infantile perniziosaartige Anämie (perniziöses Blutbild and Konstitution). *Jahrbuch Kinderheilkd.,* **117:**257–80, 1927.
2. Fanconi, G. Familial constitutional panmyelocytopathy, Fanconi's anemia (F. A.) I. Clinical aspects. *Semin. Hematol.,* **4:**233–40, 247–49, 1967.
3. Gmyrek, D., and Syllm-Rapoport, I. Zur Fanconi-Anämie (F. A.). Analyse von 129 beschriebenen Fällen. *Z. Kinderheilkd.,* **91:**297–337, 1964.
4. Bloom, G. E., Warner, S., Gerald, P. S., and Diamond, L. K. Chromosome abnormalities in constitutional aplastic anemia. *N. Engl. J. Med.,* **274:**8–14, 1966.
4a. Swift, M., Zimmerman, D., and McDonough, E. R. Squamous cell carcinomas in Fanconi's anemia. *J.A.M.A.,* **216:**325–26, 1971.
5. Schroeder, T. M., Anschütz, F., and Knopp, A. Spontane Chromosomen-aberrationen bei familiärer Panmyelopathie. *Humangenetik,* **1:**194–96, 1964.
5a. Todaro, G. J., Green, H., and Swift, M. R. Susceptibility of human diploid fibroblast strains to transformation by SV40 virus. *Science,* **153:**1252–54, 1966.
6. Shahidi, N. T., and Diamond, L. K. Testosterone-induced remission in aplastic anemia of both acquired and congenital types. Further observations in 24 cases. *N. Engl. J. Med.,* **264:**953–67, 1961.
7. McDonald, R., and Mibashan, R. S. Prolonged remission in Fanconi type anemia. *Helv. Paediatr. Acta,* **23:**566–76, 1968.
7a. Allen, D. M., Fine, M. H., Necheles, T. F., and Dameshek, W. Oxymetholone therapy in aplastic anemia. *Blood,* **32:**83–89, 1968.
8. Garriga, S., and Crosby, W. H. The incidence of leukemia in families of patients with hypoplasia of the marrow. *Blood,* **14:**1008–14, 1959.
8a. Swift, M. Fanconi's anaemia in the genetics of neoplasia. *Nature* (*Lond.*), **230:**370–73, 1971.
9. Hall, J. G., Levin, J., Kahn, J. P., Ottenheimer, E. J., van Berkun, K. A. P., and McKusick, V. A. Thrombocytopenia with absent radius. *Medicine,* **48:**411–39, 1969.
10. Aase, J. M., and Smith, D. W. Congenital anemia and triphalangeal thumbs: a new syndrome. *J. Pediatr.,* **74:**471–74, 1969.
11. Bryan, H. G., and Nixon, R. K. Dyskeratosis congenita and familial pancytopenia. *J.A.M.A.,* **192:**203–208, 1965.
12. German, J. Bloom's syndrome. I. Genetical and clinical observations in the first twenty-seven patients. *Am. J. Hum. Genet.,* **21:**196–227, 1969.

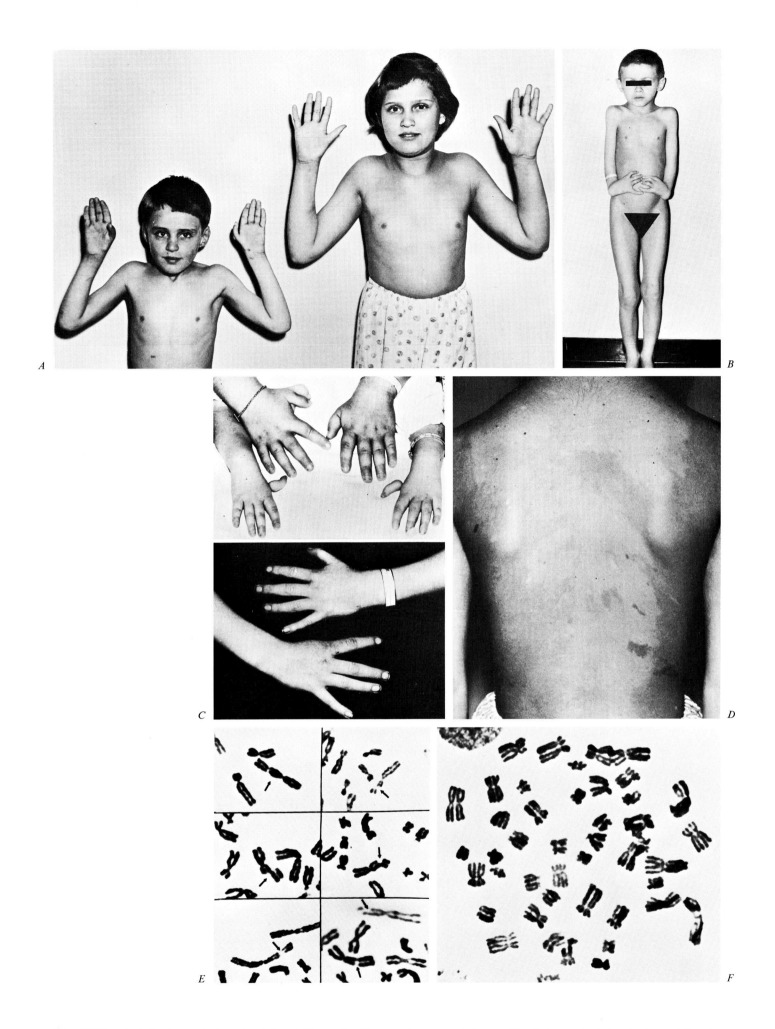

Plate VI-32. *A:* A brother and sister (aged 7 and 11 years) with hyperpigmentation, pancytopenia, thumb anomalies, and normal intelligence. Both of the boy's thumbs were distally placed and hypoplastic. The girl's right hand had a small thumb and thenar muscles. *B:* A boy with absence of both radii and thumbs. *C:* Shows the different types of thumb anomalies in three patients. *D:* Shows the areas of hyperpigmentation on a child's back. *E:* Shows the typical chromosomal abnormalities that occur, including isochromatid breaks (*top right*) and chromatid breaks (*middle*). *F:* Shows a cell with endoreduplication. (*A:* Reprinted from R. McDonald and B. Goldschmidt, *Arch. Dis. Child.,* **35:**367, 1960, by permission of the authors and editor. *B* and *C* [*bottom*]: Courtesy of Dr. L. K. Diamond, San Francisco, Calif. *C* [*top*]–*F:* From D. Hoefnagel *et al., Helv. Paediatr. Acta,* **21:**230–38, 1966.)

Goldenhar's Syndrome
(Oculoauriculovertebral Dysplasia)

In 1952 Goldenhar [1] reported 3 patients who had epibulbar dermoids, auricular appendages, and mandibular anomalies and reviewed 16 previously reported cases. In 1958 the oculovertebral syndrome was described by Weyers and Thier [2]. Later, it was suggested that the patients described in these reports had different features of the same malformation syndrome. The term *oculoauriculovertebral syndrome* was suggested [3]. More than 40 patients were reviewed in 1963 [3]. Experience has shown that affected individuals do not always have anomalies of each anatomic area—i.e., eyes, ears, and vertebrae. None of these anomalies can be considered obligatory in making this diagnosis.

Physical Features

FACE: Some patients have mild facial asymmetry (*Figure A*) and others have severe hemifacial microsomia. In most patients the forehead is prominent, the malar area is hypoplastic, and the chin is small and receding. A few patients have hypoplasia of the alae nasi.

EYES: The epibulbar dermoid or lipodermoid is the most common feature. These lesions are usually located at the corneal-scleral junction of the lateral portion of the eye (*Figures A, B, C, and D*) and are present bilaterally in two thirds of the patients [3]. Colobomas of the upper eyelid are common and usually unilateral. A few patients have other ocular anomalies, such as iris colobomas, microphthalmia, anophthalmia, and optic atrophy [4].

EARS: The preauricular appendages may be single or multiple, unilateral or bilateral. They are usually located just in front of the tragus on a line that can be drawn from the tragus to the angle of the mouth, which is the line of fusion of the maxillary and mandibular processes (*Figures A, C, and E*). Blind fistulas are often found along the same line. Some patients have small or abnormally shaped pinnae.

MOUTH: Unilateral macrostomia, meaning enlargement and lateral extension of one corner of the mouth, is common (*Figures B and C*). On the side with macrostomia there may be a thickened band on the buccal mucosa which extends from the angle of the mouth to the tragus. A few patients have cleft palate, cleft uvula, or tongue anomalies [4].

BACK: Scoliosis due to malformed vertebrae is sometimes present.

Nervous System

Mild mental retardation is occasionally noted. A severe unilateral or bilateral hearing loss has been present in a few reported patients [3].

Pathology

Cardiac, pulmonary, intestinal, and renal anomalies have been found in the few instances where autopsies were performed [5].

Laboratory Studies

X-rays of the spine may show a variety of anomalies, including hemivertebrae, fused or cuneiform vertebrae (*Figure F*), and occipitalization of the atlas. Patients with hemifacial microsomia have x-ray evidence of underdevelopment of the maxilla, zygoma, mandible, and mastoids on the smaller side of the face.

Treatment and Prognosis

The preauricular skin tags and large dermoids require surgical excision. Hearing tests should be performed on all patients.

Genetics

A mode of inheritance has not been established with certainty. Autosomal dominant inheritance was suggested in two reported families [6,7].

Differential Diagnosis

1. Microtia, preauricular skin tags, and malar hypoplasia are features of patients with the Treacher Collins syndrome, but they are distinguished by the absence of dermoids and vertebral anomalies and the fact that their eyelid colobomas are on the lower lids rather than the upper (see page 348).
2. Epibulbar dermoids and upper lid colobomas may be associated with the median cleft face syndrome (see page 294).

References

1. Goldenhar, M. Associations malformative de l'oeil et de l'oreille, en particulier le syndrome dermoid épibulbaire-appendices auriculaires-fistula auris congenita et ses relations avec la dysostose mandibulo-faciale. *J. Genet. Hum.*, **1**:243–82, 1952.
2. Weyers, H., and Thier, C. J. Malformations mandibulo-faciales et d'élimitation d'un syndrome oculo-vertébral. *J. Genet. Hum.*, **7**:143–73, 1958.
3. Gorlin, R. J., Jue, K. L., Jacobsen, U., and Goldschmidt, E. Oculoauriculovertebral dysplasia. *J. Pediatr.*, **63**:991–99, 1963.
4. Sugar, H. S. The oculoauriculovertebral dysplasia syndrome of Goldenhar. *Am. J. Ophthalmol.*, **62**:678–82, 1966.
5. Opitz, J. M., and Faith, G. C. Visceral anomalies in an infant with the Goldenhar syndrome. *Birth Defects: Original Article Series*, Vol. V, No. 2, February, 1969, pp. 104–105. Williams & Wilkins Co., Baltimore.
6. Summitt, R. L. Familial Goldenhar syndrome. *Birth Defects: Original Article Series*, Vol. V, No. 2, February, 1969, pp. 106–109. Williams & Wilkins Co., Baltimore.
7. Herrmann, J., and Opitz, J. M. A dominantly inherited first arch syndrome. *Birth Defects: Original Article Series*, Vol. V, No. 2, February, 1969, pp. 110–12. Williams & Wilkins Co., Baltimore.

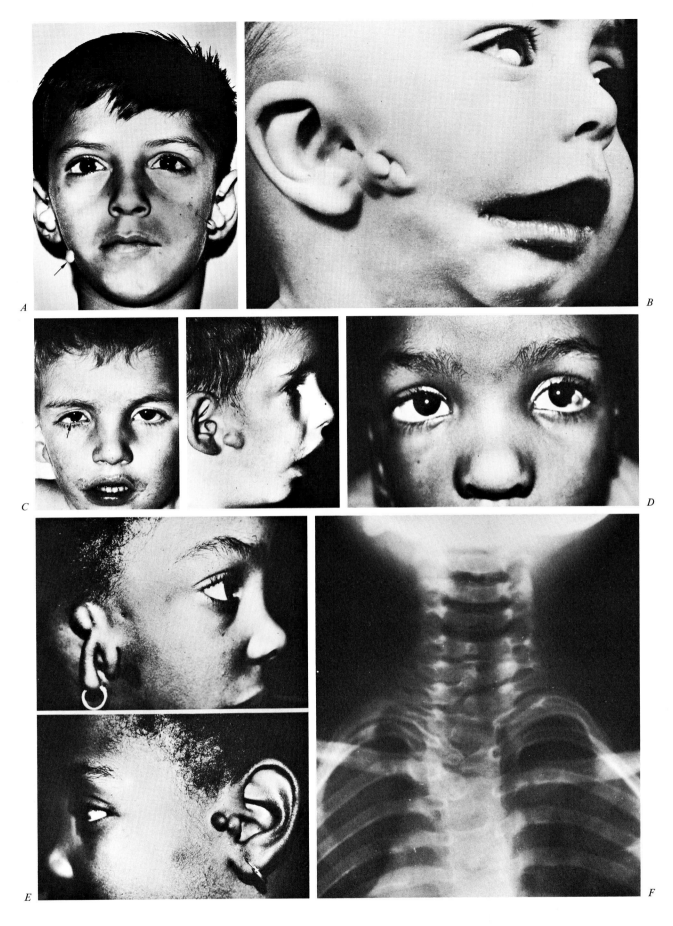

Plate VI-33. *A:* A boy with facial asymmetry, bilateral dermoids and skin appendages (*arrows*), which are located in front of his ears and near the corners of his mouth. He has no vertebral anomalies. His intelligence is normal. *B:* A boy with lateral extension of the right corner of his mouth (macrostomia), preauricular tags and fistula, and a unilateral dermoid. *C:* A boy with mild macrostomia on the same side as his preauricular appendage and dermoid (*arrow*). He has vertebral anomalies and congenital heart disease. *D–F:* A 4-year-old girl with microtia on one side, a preauricular tag and a dermoid on the other, and multiple vertebral anomalies. (*A:* From L. J. Van Riet, *J. Pediatr. Ophthalmol.,* **6:**150–52, 1969. *B:* From W. C. Grabb *et al., Plast. Reconstr. Surg.,* **36:**485–508, 1965. *D–F:* From D. Pieroni, *J. Pediat. Ophthalmol.,* **6:**16–18, 1969.)

285

Hallermann-Streiff Syndrome (Oculomandibulodyscephaly with Hypotrichosis)

Hallermann in 1948 [1] and Streiff in 1950 [2] described patients with unusual craniofacial abnormalities and recognized that these patients represented a specific syndrome. More than 60 cases have been reported [3–7].

Physical Features

HEAD: The brow and parietal areas are prominent (*Figures A, B, C, D, and E*) and the occiput is flat. The sutures and the anterior and posterior fontanels remain open for many years, at least 20 years in one patient [4]. The head circumference is usually normal.

FACE: In the newborn the tip of the nose is small and has a beaked appearance (*Figure A*). Older patients have a long nose with a thin tip, which when combined with the small chin forms a parrotlike profile (*Figures D and F*). The malar and zygomal areas appear hypoplastic. The mouth and chin are small.

EYES: Most patients have microphthalmia and bilateral congenital cataracts. In a review [7] of 60 cases, 57 had cataracts and 45 microphthalmia. Spontaneous rupture and resorption of cataracts have been reported [3,4]. Retinal degeneration has also been described [5]. In addition to poor vision, nystagmus and strabismus are common.

EARS: The ears are low-set.

MOUTH: Teeth are often present at birth. Some teeth are congenitally absent, especially the upper incisors. The deciduous and permanent teeth erupt irregularly and are often malformed. The ability to open the mouth may be severely limited by temporomandibular joint abnormalities [5]. The palate is narrow.

GENITALIA: The penis is small, and the testicles are usually small and undescended.

LIMBS: The joints are often hyperextensible, especially the knees.

SKIN: The skin of the face and scalp is thin and tense, with many small blood vessels visible.

HAIR: The hair is thin and sparse with areas of baldness. Eyebrows and eyelashes are thin.

HEIGHT: Both children and adults are short.

Nervous System

Mental retardation was present in several reported children and adults [3,5]. In one review, 10 of 60 patients were mentally retarded [7].

Pathology

No brain abnormalities were found in two autopsies. One patient had no testicular tissue [5].

Laboratory Studies

Skull x-rays show wide sutures, a thin calvarium, small orbits, hypoplasia of the nasal, maxillary, and zygomatic bones and the mandibular rami, malposition of the temporomandibular joints and gracile tubular bones [6]. Chromosomal studies have revealed no abnormalities.

Genetics

None of the reported patients had any similarly affected family members.

Differential Diagnosis

1. A thin nose, microphthalmia, and hypotrichosis are also features of patients with the oculodentodigital syndrome [8], but they have digit anomalies and normal stature, and do not have either cataracts or micrognathia.
2. Short stature, a beaked nose, and mental retardation are features of patients with Cockayne's syndrome (see page 82), but they also have a light-sensitive dermatitis and a progressive neurologic disorder.
3. Micrognathia and malar hypoplasia are features of patients with the Treacher Collins syndrome, but they also have ear anomalies and lower eyelid colobomas (see page 348).
4. Persistent open fontanels, premature eruption of teeth, and malar bone hypoplasia are features of patients with cleidocranial dysostosis, a generalized disorder of bone [9], but these patients do not have cataracts, micrognathia, a prominent nose, or hypotrichosis.

References

1. Hallermann, W. Vogelgesicht und Cataracta congenita. *Klin. Monatsbl. Augenheilkd.*, **113**:315–18, 1948.
2. Streiff, E. B. Dysmorphie mandibulo-faciale (tête d'oiseau) et altérations oculaires. *Ophthalmologica*, **120**:79–83, 1950.
3. Francois, J. A new syndrome. Dyscephalia with bird face and dental anomalies, nanism, hypotrichosis, cutaneous atrophy, microphthalmia and congenital cataract. *Arch. Ophthalmol. (Chicago)*, **60**:842–62, 1958.
4. Falls, H. F., and Schull, W. J. Hallermann-Streiff syndrome. A dyscephaly with congenital cataracts and hypotrichosis. *Arch. Ophthalmol. (Chicago)*, **63**:409–20, 1960.
5. Hoefnagel, D., and Benirschke, K. Dyscephalia mandibulo-oculo-facialis (Hallermann-Streiff syndrome). *Arch. Dis. Child.*, **40**:57–61, 1965.
6. Caspersen, I., and Warburg, M. Hallermann-Streiff syndrome. *Acta Ophthalmol. (Kbh.)*, **46**:385–90, 1968.
7. Suzuki, Y., Fujii, T., and Fukuyama, Y. Hallermann-Streiff syndrome. *Dev. Med. Child Neurol.*, **12**:496–506, 1970.
8. Kurlander, G. J., Lavy, N. W., and Campbell, J. A. Roentgen differentiation of the oculodentodigital syndrome and the Hallermann-Streiff syndrome in infancy. *Radiology*, **86**:77–86, 1966.
9. Forland, M. Cleidocranial dysostosis. A review of the syndrome and report of a sporadic case, with hereditary transmission. *Am. J. Med.*, **33**:792–99, 1962.

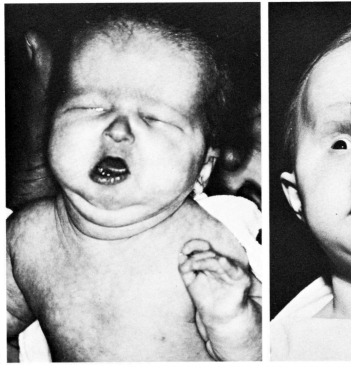

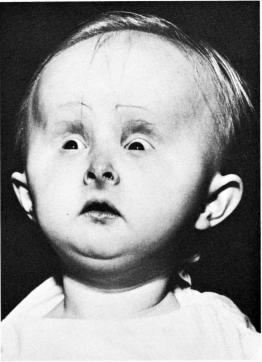

Plate VI-34. *A:* A 3-week-old female with a small thin nose and a very small chin. She also had several teeth, microphthalmia, and cataracts. *B:* A 1-year-old girl weighing 5.3 kg with prominent frontal and parietal eminences, sparse hair, eyebrows, and eyelashes, low-set ears, microphthalmia, and a small chin. *C* and *D:* A 6½-year-old male with a prominent nose, small chin, and posteriorly rotated ears. *E* and *F:* A 33-year-old man with microphthalmia, microcornea, a long nose, and small chin. He was 61 inches (156 cm) tall. (*A:* From G. J. Kurlander *et al., Radiology,* **86:**77–86, 1966. *B* and *D:* Reprinted from D. Hoefnagel and K. Benirschke, *Arch. Dis. Child.,* **40:**57–61, 1965, by permission of the authors and editor. *C:* Courtesy of Dr. D. Hoefnagel, Hanover, N.H. *E* and *F:* From J. Jancar, *J. Ment. Defic. Res.,* **10:**255–59, 1966.)

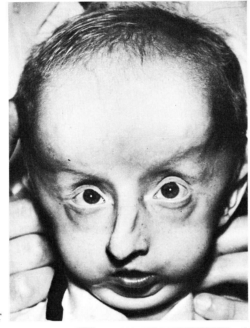

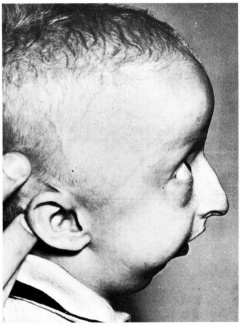

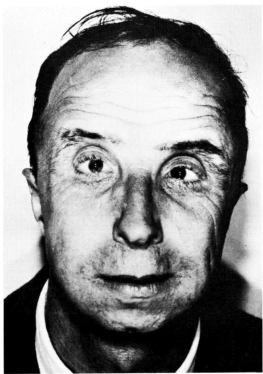

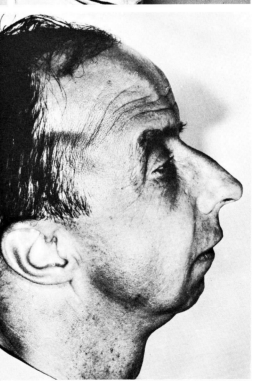

Laurence-Moon Syndrome
(Laurence-Moon-Biedl-Bardet Syndrome)

In 1866 Laurence and Moon [1] described four siblings with retinitis pigmentosa, three of whom had subnormal intelligence and two were obese. Polydactyly was not mentioned in this report, but subsequent descriptions of other patients by Bardet [2], Biedl [3], and others indicated that polydactyly, hypogenitalism, and hypogonadotropic hypogonadism are also features of this disorder [2–7]. Two hundred seventy-three affected patients were reviewed in 1958 [4].

Physical Features

FACE: Some patients have hypertelorism and an upward slant of the palpebral fissures.

EYES: Pigmentary retinal dystrophy is one of the most common features (*Figure E*). Widespread retinal degeneration with early involvement of the macula is the most frequent finding. The term *progressive cone-rod degeneration* more accurately describes this retinal abnormality [8], rather than the term *retinitis pigmentosa,* which is often used in reference to this syndrome. Night-blindness, nystagmus, and poor visual acuity are secondary to macular involvement. Optic atrophy may be present and is usually associated with extreme atrophy of the retina and choroid. Attenuation of retinal vessels is often marked. Cataracts are present in some patients [4,6].

BREASTS: Females with evidence of hypogonadism have no breast development.

GENITALIA: The external genitalia are often, but not always, infantile in appearance in adult-age individuals.

LIMBS: Digit anomalies occurred in 75 percent of 273 cases in one review [4]. Polydactyly on the ulnar side of the hands and the fibular side of the foot (i.e., postaxial polydactyly) is the most common anomaly. It is usually bilateral and may affect all four limbs, or only the hands or feet (*Figures C and D*).

HEIGHT: Short stature is only occasionally present [4,6].

WEIGHT: Obesity is first evident in infancy. In general, the excessive fat is most evident on the chest, abdomen, and hips (*Figures A, B, and F*).

Nervous System

The frequency of subnormal intelligence was about 80 percent in the review of 273 patients [4]. Several patients had a hearing deficiency.

Pathology

Very few postmortem studies have been performed, and no consistent neuropathologic abnormality has been found.

The testicular biopsy in one patient showed an absence of Leydig cells and a deficiency of germ cells [7].

Laboratory Studies

The urinary gonadotropin levels are far below normal in those adults without normal secondary sexual characteristics. Chromosomal studies have shown no abnormalities.

Treatment and Prognosis

The life expectancy is normal.

Genetics

Autosomal recessive.

Differential Diagnosis

1. Obesity, mental retardation, hypogenitalism, and polydactyly are features of Carpenter's syndrome. However, these patients also have a peculiar face, acrocephaly, and syndactyly, and do not have retinal degeneration. Several patients with Carpenter's syndrome have been erroneously reported as examples of the Laurence-Moon syndrome (see page 232).
2. Obesity, mental retardation, and hypogenitalism are also features of patients with the Prader-Labhart-Willi syndrome, but they do not have polydactyly or retinal degeneration (see page 48).
3. Obesity, hypogenitalism, postaxial polydactyly, and mental deficiency are features of patients with Biemond's syndrome, but they also have iris colobomas, hypospadias, and hydrocephalus [9].

References

1. Laurence, J. Z., and Moon, R. C. Four cases of "retinitis pigmentosa," occurring in the same family, and accompanied by general imperfections of development. *Ophthalmic Review,* **2:**32–41, 1866.
2. Bardet, G. Sur un syndrome d'obésité congénitale avec polydactylie et rétinite pigmentaire. These de Paris, 1920.
3. Biedl, A. Berichte uber Krankheitsfalle und Behandlungsverfahren. Über das Laurence-Biedlsche Syndrom. *Med. Klin.,* **29:**839–40, 1933.
4. Bell, J. The Laurence-Moon syndrome. *The Treasury of Human Inheritance,* Vol. 5, Part 3, Cambridge University Press, Cambridge, England, 1958, pp. 51–69.
5. Ciccarelli, E. C., and Vesell, E. S. Laurence-Moon-Biedl syndrome. Report of an unusual family. *Am. J. Dis. Child.,* **101:**519–24, 1961.
6. Galindo, J., and Junker, H. The Laurence-Moon-Biedl syndrome. *J. Maine Med. Assoc.,* **57:**230–36, 1966.
7. Reinfrank, R. F., and Nichols, F. L. Hypogonadotrophic hypogonadism in the Laurence-Moon syndrome. *J. Clin. Endocrinol. Metab.,* **24:**48–53, 1964.
8. Bisland, T. The Laurence-Moon-Biedl syndrome. *Am. J. Ophthalmol.,* **34:**874–84, 1951.
9. Biemond, A. Het syndroom van Laurence-Biedl en cen aanverwant, nieuw syndroom. *Ned. Tijdschr. Geneeskd.,* **78:**1801–1809, 1934.

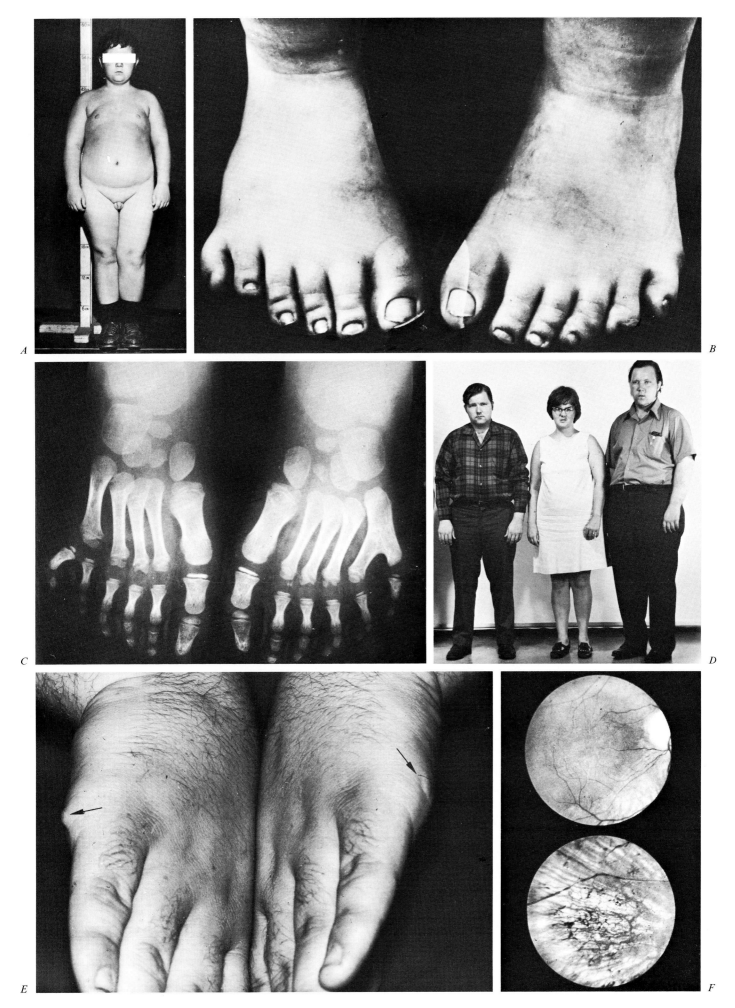

Plate VI-35. *A:* A 9-year-old obese boy. *B* and *C:* His foot showing fibular polydactyly and broad fifth metatarsals, one of which is bifid. *D:* This boy as an adult (*right*) with his affected brother and sister. All were obese, had retinal degeneration, polydactyly, and subnormal intelligence. *E:* The lateral view of the hands of the same patient as an adult showing (*arrows*) the scars from the removal of the extra fingers. *F:* The retina of the right eye of this man showing mild pigmentary changes in the macula (*top*) and more marked depigmented areas interspersed in the equatorial area (*bottom*). (*A–C:* From E. C. Ciccarelli and E. S. Vesell, *Am. J. Dis. Child.*, **101**:519–24, 1961. *F:* Courtesy of Retina Associates, Boston, Mass.)

Leprechaunism (Donohue's Syndrome)

In 1948 Donohue [1] described an emaciated female with an elfin appearance who was thought to represent a previously undescribed syndrome of multiple endocrine abnormalities. A similarly affected sibling was born a few years later and had the same facial features, i.e., large, wide-set eyes, long, low-set ears, and hirsutism, which prompted the term leprechaunism for this syndrome [2]. Since that time at least eight more infants with the same general appearance and a wide variety of congenital anomalies and pathologic abnormalities have been described, including the first of the two patients reported by Evans [3–8].

Physical Features

HEAD: The head appears large relative to the small, emaciated body.

FACE: At birth the peculiar appearance is evident. The nose is broad with flaring nostrils. The eyes appear large and widely spaced. The lips are thick and the chin is receding. The skin is loose and wrinkled due to the lack of subcutaneous fat (*Figures A, B, C, D, E, and F*).

EARS: The ears are large, low-set, and posteriorly rotated.

BREASTS: In both newborn and older infants the mammary tissue and the nipples are abnormally prominent [1–3,7].

ABDOMEN: Inguinal hernias and diastasis recti are a common finding.

GENITALIA: Enlargement of the clitoris and the labia majora and minora has been described in several females [1–4]. One female also had posterior fusion of the labia minora [6]. Cryptorchidism was present in both of the reported males [5,7].

LIMBS: The hands and feet are large in proportion to the limbs (*Figures B, D, and F*). The nails are hypoplastic. One child had camptodactyly of the third, fourth, and fifth fingers of both hands, short distal phalanges of the fifth fingers, and absent nails on the fifth fingers and toes [6]. Another child had talipes cavus bilaterally [8].

SKIN: Over the entire body the subcutaneous tissue is sparse, and the skin is loose and wrinkled (*Figures B, C, D, E, and F*).

HAIR: An abundance of hair over the face and the entire body was noted in six patients from three families [2,4,8] (*Figures E and F*).

HEIGHT AND WEIGHT: The length and weight at birth were below normal for the gestational age of all but one of the infants [5]. Throughout life the weight gain and linear growth rate are subnormal.

Nervous System

At birth these patients have generalized muscular hypotonia. Their psychomotor development is very poor.

Pathology

No consistent abnormalities were observed in five postmortem examinations. Excessive hepatic glycogen and pancreatic islet hyperplasia were reported in four patients [2,4]. One child had absence of the corpus callosum, hydromelia of the spinal cord, pyloric stenosis, eventration of the diaphragm, and a bicornuate uterus [6]. The brain of one child was two thirds the normal weight and had intense nonspecific subependymal fibrillary gliosis [7]. An infant with a decreased muscle mass had evidence of denervation atrophy in a muscle biopsy [8]. All of the children had evidence of poor development of the thymolymphatic system, but this may be a nonspecific finding. Four of the five females had premature ovarian follicular maturation.

Laboratory Studies

Hepatic glycogen and enzyme studies in one child were normal, but the child did have a prolonged elevation of blood sugar after glucose loading [6]. One of two affected siblings had no rise in blood glucose following an oral load; the other sibling had a normal response [8]. Carbohydrate and lipid studies in another patient were normal [5]. The level of the 17-ketosteroids in the urine is normal. The bone age is retarded. Chromosome studies revealed no abnormalities in four patients [5,6,8]. One child had an abnormal C-group chromosome [7].

Treatment and Prognosis

Six of the eight patients died in the first six months of life. All had difficulty with feeding and frequent regurgitation of food.

Genetics

The occurrence of leprechaunism in siblings in three families [2,4,8] and the presence of consanguinity in two families [2,8] suggest autosomal recessive inheritance. The C-group chromosome abnormality found in one patient [7] may have been coincidental.

Differential Diagnosis

A lack of subcutaneous tissue, prominent eyes, short stature, and relatively large hands and feet are features of Cockayne's syndrome, but children with this disease look normal at birth (see page 82).

References

1. Donohue, W. L. Dysendocrinism. *J. Pediatr.,* **32:**739–48, 1948.
2. Donohue, W. L., and Uchida, I. Leprechaunism. A euphemism for a rare familial disorder. *J. Pediatr.,* **45:**505–19, 1954.
3. Evans, P. R. Leprechaunism. *Arch. Dis. Child.,* **30:**479–83, 1955.
4. Kálló, A., Lakatos, I., and Szijártó, L. Leprechaunism (Donohue's syndrome). *J. Pediatr.,* **66:**372–79, 1965.
5. Dekaban, A. Metabolic and chromosomal studies in leprechaunism. *Arch. Dis. Child.,* **40:**632–36, 1965.
6. Summitt, R. L., and Favara, B. E. Leprechaunism (Donohue's syndrome): a case report. *J. Pediatr.,* **74:**601–10, 1969.
7. Ferguson-Smith, M. A., Hamilton, W., Ferguson, I. C., and Ellis, P. M. An abnormal metacentric chromosome in an infant with leprechaunism. *Ann. Genet.,* **11:**195–200, 1968.
8. Der Kaloustian, V. M., Kronfol, N. M., Takla, R., Habash, A., Khazin, A., and Najjar, S. S. Leprechaunism. A report of two new cases. *Am. J. Dis. Child.,* **122:**442–45, 1971.

Plate VI-36. *A* and *B:* A 7-month-old male with prominent eyes, epicanthal folds, large ears, sparse subcutaneous tissue, and equinovarus foot deformity. He weighed only 4.5 kg. *C* and *D:* A 4-month-old female with a similar appearance who weighed 2.4 kg. *E* and *F:* Two sisters who weighed only 1700 and 1850 g at birth and died at 3 and 6 weeks of age. The first had marked facial hirsutism. The second had disproportionately large hands and feet, wrinkled skin, and prominent labia majora and clitoris. (*A* and *B:* Reprinted from A. Dekaban, *Arch. Dis. Child.,* **40:**632–36, 1965, by permission of the author and editor. *C* and *D:* From R. L. Summitt and B. E. Favara, *J. Pediatr.,* **74:**601–10, 1969. *E* and *F:* From A. Kálló *et al., J. Pediatr.,* **66:**372–79, 1965.)

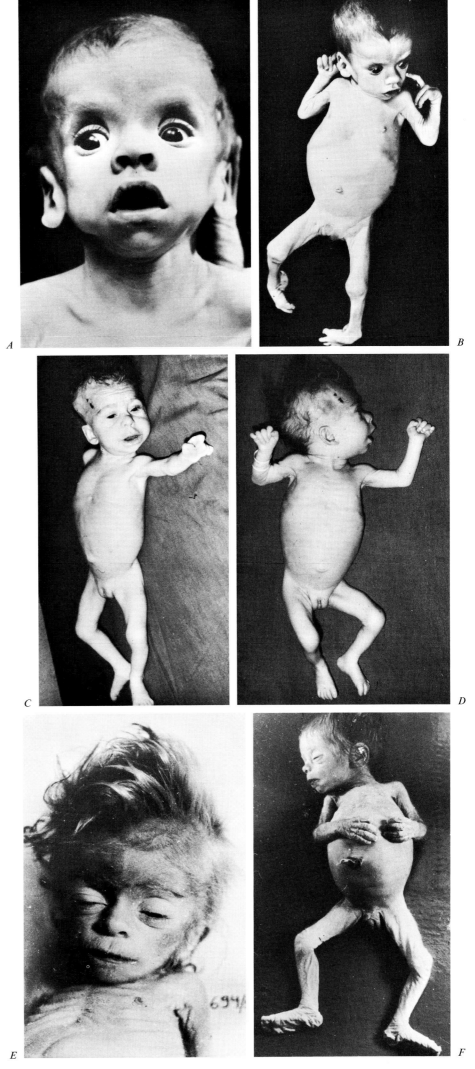

Meckel Syndrome (Dysencephalia Splanchnocystica, Gruber Syndrome)

In 1822 Meckel [1] described a brother and sister with a complex group of congenital anomalies, including microcephaly with an occipital encephalocele, cleft palate, postaxial hexadactyly or heptadactyly, and polycystic kidneys. Patients with this syndrome were also described by several other authors, including Gruber [2], who used the descriptive title of dysencephalia splanchnocystica, and Battaglia and Locatelli [3]. This diagnosis was recently introduced to Anglo-American physicians by Opitz and Howe [4] in their description of one infant in 1969. Several other recent reports [5–9] described infants who probably had the Meckel syndrome. In 1971 19 more affected infants were reported [10–12].

Physical Features

HEAD: These patients have microcephaly, with the forehead sloping back sharply (*Figures A and C*). Usually there is also an occipital encephalocele (*Figures B, D, and E*); in a review [11] of 51 patients 41 had an encephalocele. Some patients have premature fusion of cranial sutures. Anencephaly was present in 2 of 10 infants in another review [12].

FACE: The eyes may be narrowly spaced. The chin is small. A few patients have had a single nostril [4].

EYES: Many patients have eye anomalies, such as microphthalmia, anophthalmia, and colobomas [4,5,8,12].

EARS: The ears are often malformed.

MOUTH: Cleft lip and/or palate was present in 29 of 51 infants [11]. One infant had multiple gingival frenula and a bifid tongue [6].

GENITALIA: A variety of genital anomalies have been reported, including hypoplastic phallus, severe hypospadias, and cryptorchidism [4,8,9] (*Figure C*). Out of 51 patients 22 had small or ambiguous genitalia [11].

LIMBS: Thirty-three of 49 infants had postaxial polydactyly of the hands and/or feet; 12 had clubfeet [10] (*Figure F*).

Pathology

In general, these patients had various types of cerebral and cerebellar dysgenesis, encephaloceles, lung hypoplasia, genital anomalies, and polycystic kidneys. There are varying degrees of arhinencephaly. There may be absent olfactory bulbs and optic nerves, microgyria, and malformations of the brainstem and basal ganglia. Often there is absence of the pituitary in association with hypoplasia of the thyroid, absent or hypoplastic adrenals, and abnormal gonads. The kidneys usually show cysts which range in size from small to very large. Other renal anomalies that have been noted include horseshoe kidneys and hypoplasia [11]. In one series of 10 infants [12] all had either hepatic fibrosis with bile duct proliferation or polycystic liver. Cardiac anomalies are occasionally present.

Laboratory Studies

Chromosomal studies in the most recently described patients have been normal.

Treatment and Prognosis

All infants are either stillborn or die shortly after birth.

Genetics

Autosomal recessive [10,11].

Differential Diagnosis

1. Microcephaly, eye anomalies, cleft palate, and polydactyly are features of patients with the chromosome 13 trisomy, but they do not have occipital encephaloceles or pseudohermaphroditism in males (see page 164).
2. Microcephaly, cleft lip and palate, forebrain anomalies, and endocrine deficiencies are features of infants with holotelencephaly with cleft lip, but they do not have encephalocele, polydactyly, or polycystic kidneys (see page 208).
3. Male pseudohermaphroditism, polydactyly, and multiple minor facial anomalies are features of children with the Smith-Lemli-Opitz syndrome, but they do not usually have encephaloceles or clubfeet and do have a distinctive facies with anteverted nostrils and a thick alveolar ridge (see page 312).

References

1. Meckel, J. F. Beschreibung zweier, durch sehr ähnliche Bildungsabweichungen entstellter Geschwister. *Dtsch. Arch. Physiol.*, **7**:99–172, 1822.
2. Gruber, G. B. Beiträge zur Frage "gekoppelter" Missbildungen (Akrocephalo-Syndactylie und Dysencephalia splanchnocystica). *Beitr. Pathol. Anat.*, **93**:459–76, 1934.
3. Battaglia, S., and Locatelli, L. Malattia di Gruber e Giordano (dysencephalia splanchnocystica). *Folia Hered. Pathol.*, **5**:259–76, 1956.
4. Opitz, J. M., and Howe, J. J. The Meckel syndrome (dysencephalia splanchnocystica, the Gruber syndrome). *Birth Defects: Original Article Series*, Vol. V, No. 2, February, 1969, pp. 167–79. Williams & Wilkins Co., Baltimore.
5. Marshall, R., Newnham, R. E., Rawstron, J. R., Ellis, J. R., and Stevens, L. J. Features of 13–15 trisomy syndrome with normal karyotype. *Lancet*, **1**:556, 1964.
6. Tucker, C. C., Finley, S. C., Tucker, E. S., and Finley, W. H. Oral-facial-digital syndrome, with polycystic kidneys and liver: pathological and cytogenetic studies. *J. Med. Genet.*, **3**:145–47, 1966.
7. Walbaum, R., Dehaene, Ph., and Duthoit, F. Polydactylie familiale avec dysplasie neuro-cranienne. *Ann. Genet.*, **10**:39–41, 1967.
8. Miller, J. Q., and Selden, R. F. Arhinencephaly, encephalocele, and 13–15 trisomy syndrome with normal chromosomes. *Neurology (Minneap.)*, **17**:1087–91, 1967.
9. Simopoulos, A. P., Brennan, G. G., Alwan, A., and Fidis, N. Polycystic kidneys, internal hydrocephalus and polydactylism in newborn siblings. *Pediatrics*, **39**:931–34, 1967.
10. Mecke, S., and Passarge, E. Encephalocele, polycystic kidneys, and polydactyly as an autosomal recessive trait simulating certain other disorders: the Meckel syndrome. *Ann. Genet.*, **14**:97–103, 1971.
11. Hsia, Y. E., Bratu, M., and Herbordt, A. Genetics of the Meckel syndrome (dysencephalia splanchnocystica). *Pediatrics*, **48**:237–47, 1971.
12. Fried, K., Liban, E., Lurie, M., Friedman, S., and Reisner, S. H. Polycystic kidneys associated with malformations of the brain, polydactyly, and other birth defects in newborn sibs. A lethal syndrome showing the autosomal-recessive pattern of inheritance. *J. Med. Genet.*, **8**:285–90, 1971.

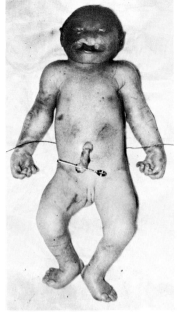

A

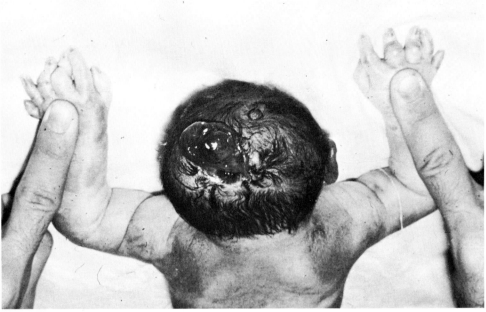

B

Plate VI-37. *A* and *B:* A newborn with cleft lip, absence of nasal cartilage, microcephaly, occipital encephalocele, polydactyly, and clubfeet. *C* and *D:* A similarly affected newborn who had arhinencephaly and polycystic kidneys. *E:* Identical twins with a median cleft upper lip and large encephalocele. *F:* A 3-day-old infant with microcephaly, a small occipital defect, micrognathia, polydactyly of the hands and feet, and valgus foot deformity. (*A, B,* and *E:* Y. E. Hsia *et al., Pediatrics,* **48:**237–47, 1971. *C* and *D:* From J. Q. Miller and R. F. Selden, *Neurology* [*Minneap.*], **17:**1087–91, 1967. *F:* From J. M. Opitz and J. J. Howe, *Birth Defects: Original Article Series,* Vol. V, No. 2, February, 1969, pp. 167–79. Williams & Wilkins Co., Baltimore.)

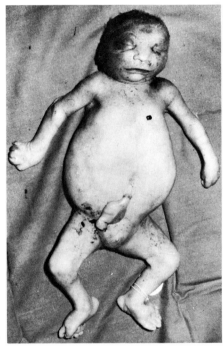

C

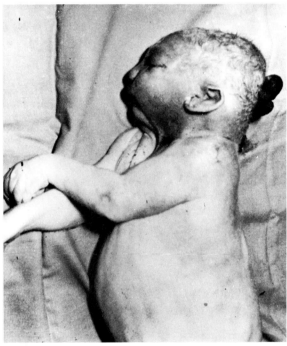

D

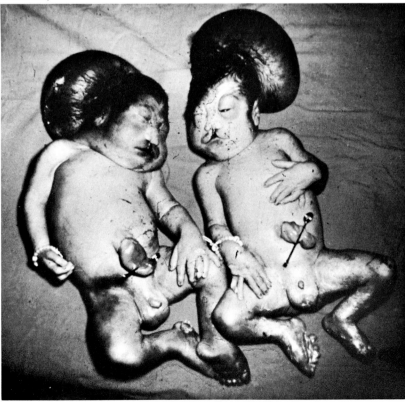

E

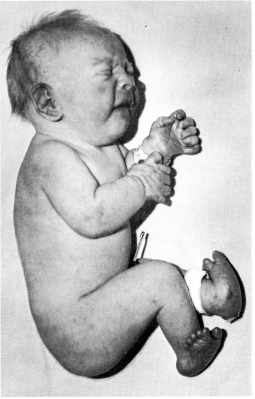

F

Median Cleft Face Syndrome

In 1924 Greig [1] proposed the term *ocular hypertelorism* to describe the cranial deformity that produced an increased distance between the eyes. Reports by others who saw Greig's patient indicate that she also had a slightly cleft nose [2]. Individuals with hypertelorism and a cleft nose have been shown to have many abnormalities in the median portion of the face, most of which are the result of defective fusion of midline structures. The name *median cleft face syndrome* has been proposed as most descriptive of these fusion defects. More than 70 patients have been described [2–5].

Physical Features

HEAD: The head circumference is normal.

FACE: The interorbital distance is increased, and the medial canthi are displaced laterally. The midline cleft may involve the tip of the nose, as well as the premaxilla and palate. Some patients have only a broad nose with a midline depression, while others have widely separated nostrils and absence of portions of the nasal cartilage (*Figures A, B, C, D, E, and F*). A low V-shaped frontal hairline (*Figure C*) is common. Midline frontal lipomas, dermoids, and teratomas have been reported in a few patients. A heteropic anterior fontanel with a pulsatile brain palpable through a midline cranial defect has also been reported [3].

EYES: Strabismus is common. Two of our patients have had epibulbar dermoids and one had a cleft of the upper eyelid (*Figures A, B, and C*).

MOUTH: Some patients have absence of the entire prolabium and premaxilla, as well as a midline cleft of the hard and soft palate. A median cleft of the lower lip is rare. A midline sinus tract above the lip has been reported [4] (*Figure C*).

Nervous System

Visual acuity is normal. Three patients cited in a review [2] of 25 were mildly retarded in psychomotor development and 2 were severely retarded.

Laboratory Studies

Some patients have a cranium bifidum occultum frontalis, which is visible in the midline on the skull x-ray. This is covered with dura and periosteum and may close completely after a few years. Individuals with a wide nasal cleft also have a wide cleft between the bony orbits, maxillary bones and ethmoids, and may also have a median frontal osseous bar. The skull size, clinoid processes, and sella turcica are usually normal [6].

Treatment and Prognosis

When possible, early surgical repair of the fusion defects is indicated. Unfortunately most patients still have an abnormal appearance after surgery.

Genetics

Most patients have no similarly affected relatives. However, in several families autosomal dominant inheritance has been evident [4,7,8].

Differential Diagnosis

1. Hypertelorism and a wide forehead are features of some patients with Crouzon's disease, but they are distinguished by the absence of any midline clefts and the presence of craniosynostosis, proptosis, and an underdeveloped maxilla (see page 230).
2. A broad nose and a median cleft lip and palate are features of patients with the oral-facial-digital (OFD I) syndrome, but they do not have hypertelorism and do have multiple oral and digital anomalies and sparse hair (see page 300).
3. Hypertelorism, wide forehead, and deformed nose are features of patients with the Chotzen syndrome, but they are distinguished by the absence of any midline clefts and the presence of craniosynostosis and syndactyly (see page 226).
4. A broad nose with a bifid tip is also a feature of patients with the Mohr syndrome (OFD II), but they also have oral anomalies, a hearing loss, preaxial polysyndactyly, and autosomal recessive inheritance [8].
5. Hypertelorism and a broad bridge of the nose are features of patients with craniometaphyseal dysplasia, but they have overgrowth of the frontal and nasal bones, and have a normal tip of the nose and no midline fusion defects [8].

References

1. Greig, D. M. Hypertelorism. A hitherto undifferentiated congenital craniofacial deformity. *Edinburgh Med. J.,* **31**:560–93, 1924.
2. DeMyer, W. The median cleft face syndrome. *Neurology (Minneap.),* **17**:961–71, 1967.
3. Rosasco, S. A., and Massa, J. L. Frontonasal syndrome. *Br. J. Plast. Surg.,* **21**:244–49, 1968.
4. Francesconi, G., and Fortunato, G. Median dysraphia of the face. *Plast. Reconstr. Surg.,* **43**:481–91, 1969.
5. Sedano, H. O., Cohen, M. M., Jr., Jirasek, J., and Gorlin, R. J. Frontonasal dysplasia. *J. Pediatr.,* **76**:906–13, 1970.
6. Kurlander, G. J., DeMyer, W., and Campbell, J. A. Roentgenology of the median cleft face syndrome. *Radiology,* **88**:473–78, 1967.
7. Montford, T. Hereditary hypertelorism without mental deficiency. *Arch. Dis. Child.,* **4**:381–84, 1929.
8. Cohen, M. M., Jr., Sedano, H. O., Gorlin, R. J., and Jirásek, J. E. Frontonasal dysplasia (median cleft face syndrome): comments on etiology and pathogenesis. *Birth Defects: Original Article Series,* Vol. VII, No. 7, June 1971, pp. 117–19. Williams & Wilkins Co., Baltimore.
9. Rimoin, D. L., and Edgerton, M. T. Genetic and clinical heterogeneity in the oral-facial-digital syndrome. *J. Pediatr.,* **71**:94–102, 1967.
10. Millard, D. R., Jr., Maisels, D. O., Barstone, J. H. F., and Yates B. W. Craniofacial surgery in craniometaphyseal dysplasia. *Am. J. Surg.,* **113**:615–21, 1967.

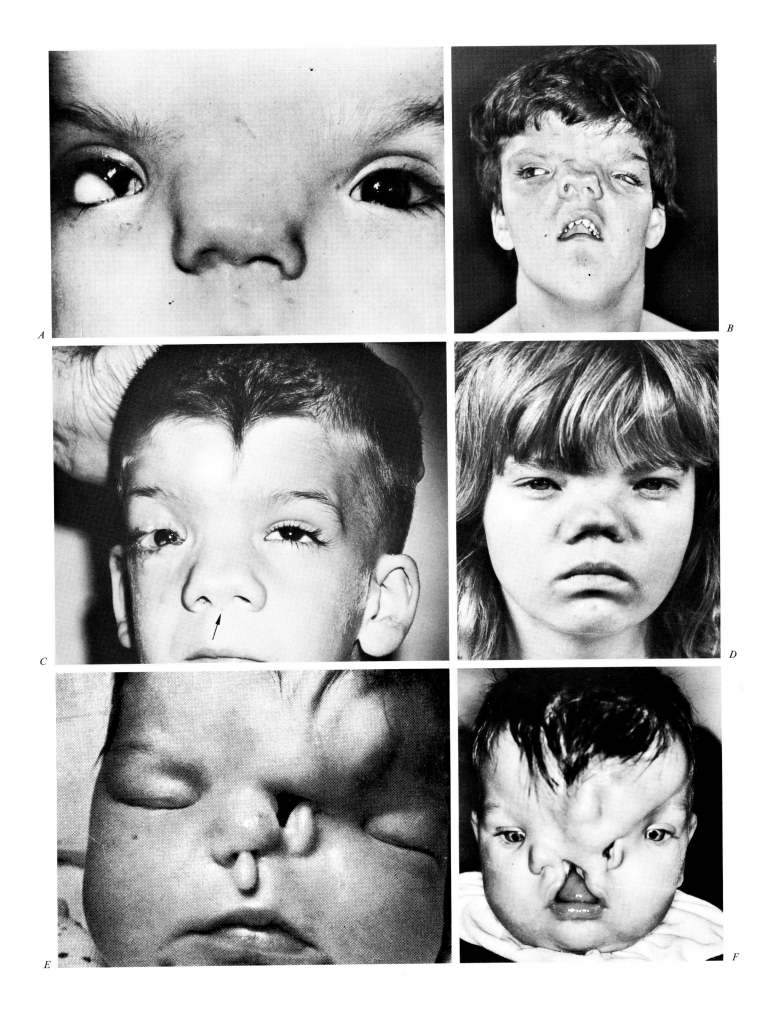

Plate VI-38. *A* and *B:* An infant with hypertelorism, a broad nose, and an epibulbar dermoid. At 14 years she has a marked cleft in the tip of the nose and divergent strabismus. *C:* This boy has a V-shaped forelock and a midline sinus tract (*arrow*). An upper lid coloboma had been repaired and an epibulbar dermoid removed. He has normal intelligence. *D:* A 16-year-old girl with mild hypertelorism and a broad, cleft nose. *E:* A 3-day-old infant with a frontal bone defect, absence of some nasal cartilage, and a skin appendage. *F:* An infant with marked defect in midline fusion with a median cleft lip and widely separated nostrils. (*E:* From S. A. Rosasco and J. L. Massa, *Brit. J. Plast. Surg.,* **21:**244–49, 1968. *F:* From W. DeMyer, *Neurology* [*Minneap.*], **17:**961–71, 1967.)

Möbius Syndrome
(Congenital Facial Diplegia)

Although the association of congenital facial diplegia, skeletal deformities, and muscle defects had been previously described, Möbius has been credited for having recognized it as an independent entity in 1888 [1]. Individuals with the Möbius syndrome may have a variety of cranial nerve and muscle abnormalities, the most common of which is congenital facial diplegia. More than 125 patients have been reported [2,3].

Physical Features

FACE: At birth the affected infant has no facial expression when crying. The eyes remain open during sleep because of the weakness of the orbicularis oculi muscles. As the child grows older, drooling and a lack of expression when laughing or smiling (*Figure A*) are prominent features. Because the paralysis is present at birth, older affected individuals do not exhibit the sagging of the subcutaneous tissue or the contractures that follow acquired facial paralysis.

EYES: Some patients have ptosis. A convergent squint is common.

EARS: Deformities of the ear occurred in 8 of 61 patients [2]. Three patients had a hearing loss, two of whom also had an external ear deformity.

MOUTH: Atrophy of a portion of the tongue is common (*Figure D*).

LIMBS: Approximately a quarter to a third of the patients have associated skeletal or muscle deformities [2,4]. In a study [2] of 61 patients, 19 had a clubfoot deformity, 13 had hand anomalies, and 8 had a deficiency of the pectoralis muscle. Syndactyly is the most common hand anomaly; it may be unilateral or bilateral, and is often associated with shortening and flexion deformities of the fingers (*Figure F*).

Nervous System

Bilateral abducens paralysis is the most characteristic feature of this syndrome. The oculomotor nerve may also be involved, but internal ophthalmoplegia has never been observed. Some patients apparently have horizontal gaze paralysis; they substitute the near reflex to achieve lateral gaze by use of a convergence ocular movement [5]. Bell's phenomenon is present (*Figures B and C*). Nystagmus is uncommon. Vision is normal and diplopia is usually not a symptom. The paralysis of the face is almost always bilateral (*Figures A, B, and C*), but may be unilateral (*Figure E*). Often the lower portion of the face is affected less severely than the upper portion. Facial, tongue, and soft palate weakness combine to produce a speech impairment. Difficulty with swallowing is a major problem in infants [4]. While most of the patients have normal intelligence, a review of 61 patients listed 6 as suffering from "mental defect" [2].

Pathology

Autopsy studies of the brain and peripheral nerves have been performed on a small number of patients. In some the cranial nerve nuclei have been small, and the number of cells in each nucleus has been below normal. In other patients the nerves and nerve nuclei have been normal. In general, no evidence of inflammation or degeneration has been found [2,4]. Studies in a 48-day-old infant revealed almost total absence of the facial muscles [6]. However, the facial nerve and its nucleus were normal. The only other abnormality found in that patient was hypoplasia of the cerebellum. Absence of the trochlear abducens, facial, and accessory nerves was found in each of identical twin infants [6a].

Laboratory Studies

Electromyograms of the frontalis and orbicularis oculi muscles in a father and son showed no response [3]. Electromyograms of the facial and external rectus muscles in another patient showed only a few motor unit potentials [4]. These muscles had no visible contraction on response to electrical stimulation.

Treatment and Prognosis

The eyes must be protected against exposure keratitis. Because of the difficulty with swallowing and the risk of aspiration, gastrostomy feedings may be necessary. The muscle weaknesses that are present at birth remain unchanged throughout childhood and adult life.

Genetics

A few families have been reported in which both a parent and child are affected, including father and son [2–4,6]. This suggests an autosomal dominant mode of inheritance.

Differential Diagnosis

1. Ptosis, difficulty in swallowing, and a lack of facial expressions are also features of patients with myotonic dystrophy (see page 106) and neonatal myasthenia gravis. The former is distinguished by testing for muscle dystonia and the latter by a Tensilon test.
2. Limitation of abduction of the eye is a feature of Duane's syndrome [8], but this disorder is not associated with other skeletal and muscle anomalies or mental retardation.
3. A deficiency of the pectoralis major and a small syndactylous hand on the same side feature a localized anomaly known as Poland's syndrome. It is not associated with any neurologic abnormalities [9].
4. Ptosis and deficient extraocular movements are features of patients with ocular myopathy, but they do not have muscle weakness at birth. In addition, there is a cephalocaudal progression of the muscle involvement [10].
5. Three unrelated children reported by Hanson and Rowland [11] had congenital facial diplegia and later developed a muscular dystrophy similar to the facioscapulohumeral type.

References

1. Möbius, P. Ueber angeborene doppelseitige Abducens-Facialis-Lahmung. *Munch. Med. Wochenschr.,* **35:**91–94, 108–11, 1888.
2. Henderson, J. L. The congenital facial diplegia syndrome: clinical features, pathology and aetiology. *Brain,* **62:**381–403, 1939.
3. Masaki, S., and Yada, G. A familial occurrence of congenital bilateral facial nerve palsy—Möbius syndrome. *Otolaryngology (Tokyo),* **41:**633–39, 1969.
4. Van Allen, M. W., and Blodi, F. C. Neurologic aspects of the Möbius syndrome. A case study with electromyography of the extraocular and facial muscles. *Neurology (Minneap.),* **10:**249–59, 1960.
5. Hicks, A. M. Congenital paralysis of lateral rotators of eyes with paralysis of muscles of face. *Arch. Ophthalmol. (Chicago),* **30:**38–42, 1943.
6. Pitner, S. E., Edwards, J. E., and McCormick, W. F. Observations on the pathology of the Möbius syndrome. *J. Neurol. Neurosurg. Psychiatry,* **28:**362–74, 1965.
6a. Hanissian, A. S., Fuste, F., Hayes, W. T., and Duncan, J. M. Möbius syndrome in twins. *Am. J. Dis. Child.,* **120:**472–75, 1970.
7. Krüger, K. E., and Friedrich, D. Familiäre kongenitale Motilitätsstörungen der Augen. *Klin. Monatsbl. Augenheilkd.,* **142:**101–17, 1963.
8. Alexander, C. M. Bilateral Duane's retraction syndrome. *Am. J. Ophthalmol.,* **60:**907–10, 1965.
9. Resnick, E. Congenital unilateral absence of the pectoral muscles often associated with syndactylism. *J. Bone Joint Surg.,* **24:**925–28, 1942.
10. Schotland, D. L., and Rowland, L. P. Muscular dystrophy. Features of ocular myopathy, distal myopathy, and myotonic dystrophy. *Arch. Neurol.,* **10:**433–45, 1965.
11. Hanson, P. A., and Rowland, L. P. Möbius syndrome and facioscapulohumeral muscular dystrophy. *Arch. Neurol.,* **24:**31–39, 1971.

Plate VI-39. *A:* A girl trying to smile, but unable to do so because of facial diplegia. *B:* A 3½-year-old boy with open mouth, no facial expression, and visible sclera as his eyes roll upward and back (normal Bell's phenomenon) when he attempts to close his eyelids. *C* and *D:* A boy with bilateral facial diplegia who was more successful at closing his eyes. However, he had marked difficulty with speaking. His tongue was furrowed and atrophied, especially on the left side. Both this boy and the first patient had normal intelligence. *E* and *F:* A 29-year-old man with unilateral facial palsy, deafness, and hand deformities. He had syndactyly and camptodactyly of the left hand, clinodactyly and camptodactyly of the right hand, and short nails bilaterally. (*B:* From R. L. Sogg, *Arch. Ophthalmol.* [*Chicago*], **65:**16–19, 1961.)

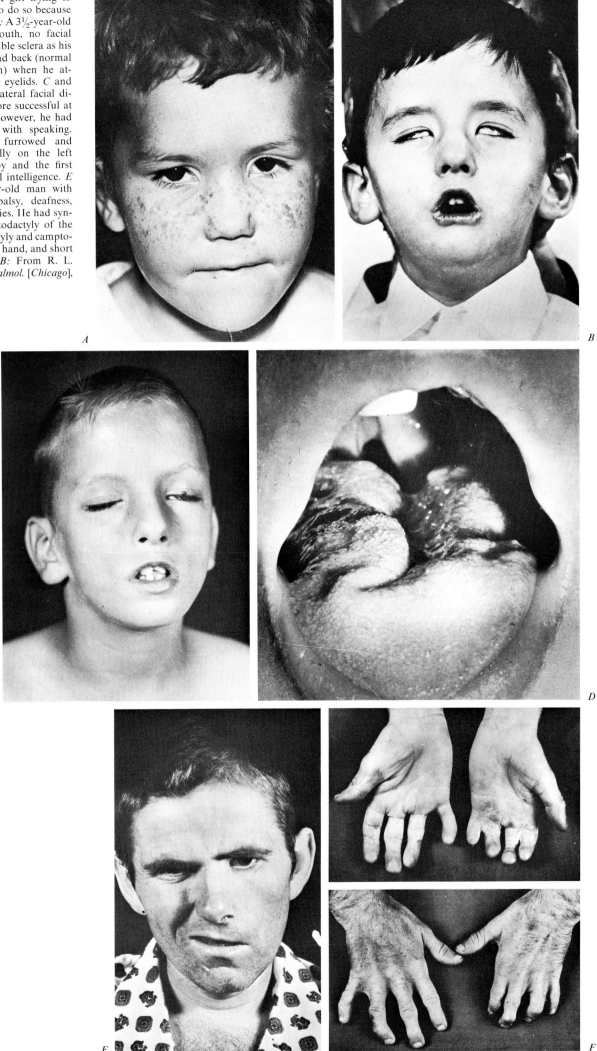

A

B

C

D

E

F

Noonan's Syndrome

In 1963 Noonan and Ehmke [1] reported nine male and female patients with valvular pulmonic stenosis, short stature, hypertelorism, ptosis, skeletal anomalies, and mental retardation. While these patients had some features of the XO (Turner's) syndrome, it was evident that they had many distinguishing physical features, as well as normal chromosomes. Later, it was suggested [2,3] that the males and females who had been previously reported as having the Turner's syndrome phenotype in association with normal chromosomes were probably examples of the syndrome described by Noonan and Ehmke. To emphasize that the phenotypic features are not identical with those of Turner's syndrome, that both males and females may be affected, and that there is no gross chromosomal abnormality, the name *Noonan's syndrome* has been suggested. More than 100 males with Noonan's syndrome, as well as many females, have now been reported [2–6,6a,6b].

Physical Features

FACE: In the evaluation of 43 patients, hypertelorism was found in 26, a downward palpebral slant in 30, ptosis in 14, epicanthal folds in 13, and a small chin in 25 (*Figures A, B, C, D, and E*) [6a].

EARS: The ears are often slanted posteriorly.

MOUTH: A narrow palate and a cleft uvula are common findings. Many patients have dental anomalies and malocclusion.

NECK: Some patients have webbing of the neck (*Figures A, C, D, and F*); others have a short, broad neck with excessive skin folds.

CHEST: In a study of 43 patients, 34 had pectus carinatum deformity of the upper sternum and excavatum of the lower sternum (*Figures A and B*).

BREASTS: The breast development and the appearance of the nipples are usually normal.

GENITALIA: Cryptorchidism is common in the males.

BACK: Scoliosis, kyphosis, and vertebral anomalies are present in some patients.

LIMBS: Clinodactyly and cubitus valgus are common. Several reported patients had congenital lymphedema of the hands and feet (*Figure E*). The nails are short and poorly developed.

DERMATOGLYPHICS: A distally placed axial triradius, a high incidence of arches, and a low ridge count are the most common findings [5].

HAIR: The hair is often coarse [6a].

HEIGHT: Most of the patients are below the tenth percentile in height [4].

GROWTH AND DEVELOPMENT: Some females have a delayed onset of menarche. Among 16 females the average age at menarche was 13.5 years [6a].

Nervous System

The intelligence of the reported patients has ranged from normal to severe mental retardation. Thirty of 43 patients in one study were mentally retarded [6a]. A few infants have had muscular hypotonia [4].

Pathology

No testicular abnormalities have been consistently observed. While germinal hypoplasia is often noted, the biopsies are from either prepubescent or cryptorchid gonads, which means that the findings are not necessarily abnormal.

Laboratory Studies

The incidence of congenital heart disease is not known, but the most common abnormality found at cardiac catheterization or surgery is valvular pulmonary stenosis [4]. A variety of other cardiac anomalies have also been reported.

Genetics

Polygenic inheritance has been suggested because many of the physical features of Noonan's syndrome have also been found in the parents and siblings of the affected [2–4] (*Figures B and C*). Fully affected male and female siblings have also been reported, including one family with parental consanguinity [6]. Direct male-to-male inheritance has been observed, which would rule out X-linked inheritance [7]. Autosomal dominant inheritance has also been suggested [6b].

Differential Diagnosis

1. Females with the XO (Turner's) syndrome may have ptosis, neck webbing, cubitus valgus, and lymphedema, but they are usually distinguished in adolescence by sexual infantilism, severe short stature, and normal intelligence (see page 178). Patients with Turner's syndrome do not usually have hypertelorism, pectus excavatum and carinatum, and pulmonary stenosis, while these anomalies are common in patients with Noonan's syndrome.
2. Neck webbing, short stature, lymphedema, and mental retardation have also been reported in patients with the 18p− syndrome (see page 162).
3. Hypertelorism, pulmonary stenosis, and genital anomalies are features of patients with the multiple lentigenes syndrome [8].

References

1. Noonan, J. A., and Ehmke, D. A. Associated noncardiac malformations in children with congenital heart disease. *J. Pediatr.,* **63**:468–70, 1963.
2. Kaplan, M. S., Opitz, J. M., and Gosset, F. R. Noonan's syndrome. *Am. J. Dis. Child.,* **116**:359–66, 1968.
3. Summitt, R. L. Turner syndrome and Noonan's syndrome. *J. Pediatr.,* **74**:155–56, 1969.
4. Noonan, J. A. Hypertelorism with Turner phenotype. *Am. J. Dis. Child.,* **116**:373–80, 1968.
5. Nora, J. J., and Sinha, A. K. Direct familial transmission of the Turner phenotype. *Am. J. Dis. Child.,* **116**:343–50, 1968.
6. Abdel-Salam, E., and Temtamy, S. A. Familial Turner phenotype. *J. Pediatr.,* **74**:67–72, 1969.
6a. Wilroy, R. S., and Summitt, R. L. The Noonan syndrome—a study of 43 patients. (Abstract.) IVth International Congress of Human Genetics, Paris, 1971, p. 189.
6b. Baird, P. A., and De Jong, B. P. Noonan's syndrome (XX and XY Turner phenotype) in three generations of a family. *J. Pediatr.,* **80**:110–14, 1972.
7. Nora, J. J., and Sinha, A. K. Direct male-to-male transmission of the XY Turner phenotype? *Lancet,* **1**:250–51, 1970.
8. Gorlin, R. J., Anderson, R. C., and Blaw, M. Multiple lentigenes syndrome: complex comprising multiple lentigenes, electrocardiographic conduction abnormalities, ocular hypertelorism, pulmonary stenosis, abnormalities of genitalia, retardation of growth, sensorineural deafness and autosomal dominant hereditary pattern. *Am. J. Dis. Child.,* **117**:652–62, 1969.

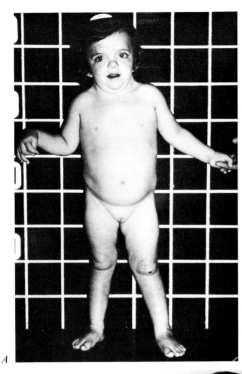

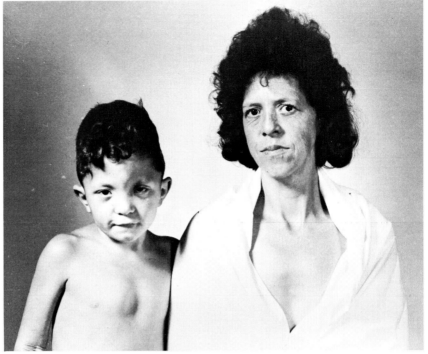

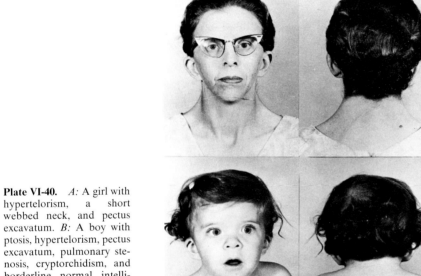

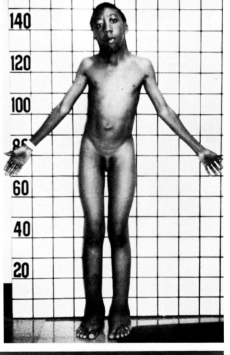

Plate VI-40. *A:* A girl with hypertelorism, a short webbed neck, and pectus excavatum. *B:* A boy with ptosis, hypertelorism, pectus excavatum, pulmonary stenosis, cryptorchidism, and borderline normal intelligence shown with his mother, who had a similar chest deformity and delayed onset of puberty. *C:* An infant and her mother who both had hypertelorism, webbing of the neck, a low hairline, pulmonary stenosis, and clinodactyly. Both had normal intelligence. *D:* A boy with ptosis, webbed neck, and marked lymphedema of both legs. *E:* A tall, retarded boy with marked neck webbing and cubitus valgus. *F:* A mildly retarded boy with neck webbing, cubitus valgus, situs inversus, cardiac septal defects, cryptorchidism, and clinodactyly. (*A* and *D:* Courtesy of Dr. R. L. Summitt, Memphis, Tenn. *B:* From J. A. Noonan, *Am. J. Dis. Child.,* **116:**373–80, 1968. *C:* From J. J. Nora and A. K. Sinha, *Am. J. Dis. Child.,* **116:**343–50, 1968. *E:* From L. J. Jackson and S. Lefrak, *Birth Defects: Original Article Series,* Vol. V, No. 5, May, 1969, pp. 36–38. Williams & Wilkins Co., Baltimore.)

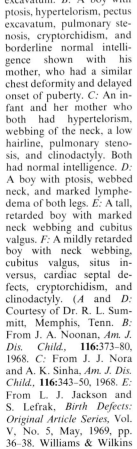

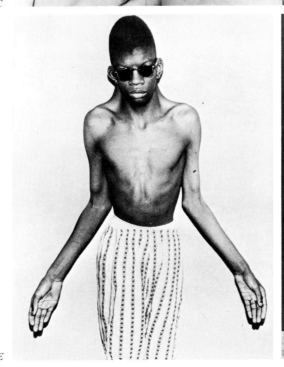

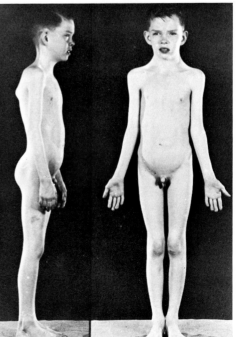

299

Oral-Facial-Digital Syndrome
(OFD I Syndrome)

In 1954 Papillon-Léage and Psaume [1] described a syndrome of abnormal frenula, cleft tongue and palate, median cleft of the upper lip, hypoplasia of the nasal alar cartilages, digit anomalies, and mental retardation. More than 80 affected individuals have been reported, almost all of whom have been females [2–4].

Physical Features

FACE: The striking features are a midline cleft of the upper lip, a broad nasal bridge, and lateral displacement of the medial canthi. The tip of the nose is often short and thin, due to hypoplasia of the alar cartilages. In profile the brow is prominent, there is no frontonasal angle, and the midportion of the face appears flattened (*Figures A and B*).

MOUTH: These patients have thick frenula (*Figure C*), and usually clefts in the alveolar ridges as well (*Figure D*). These thickened bands and clefts eradicate the mucobuccal fold and are often associated with the absence of teeth, especially the lower lateral incisors. The tip of the tongue may be split into 2, 3, or 4 parts; small firm, whitish or yellow tumors are often present on the ventral surface of the tongue between the lobules (*Figures D and F*). The palate may be cleft laterally by deep grooves in addition to a complete and asymmetric cleft in the soft palate. Other anomalies include supernumerary canine teeth, mucous membrane fistulas of the lower lip, and tongue-tie.

LIMBS: These patients often have anomalies of the fingers, less frequently of the toes. The most common anomalies are clinodactyly, syndactyly (*Figure E*), brachydactyly, and polydactyly.

DERMATOGLYPHICS: A high incidence of whorls on the digits has been reported [4].

SKIN: Milia on the face is common in infants.

HAIR: The scalp hair is often sparse and coarse (*Figure A*).

Nervous System

One third to one half of the patients have had subnormal intelligence, usually to a mild degree. In one study [4], three affected sisters had significantly lower intelligence than their three unaffected sisters, although all six were mildly retarded. In another study [5] of twelve affected female relatives, four had mental deficiency; one of these four was a child with hydranencephaly and another had hydrocephalus and a large porencephalic cyst.

Pathology

The tumors on the tongue are hamartomas, containing fibrous stroma, clusters of mucous glands, and smooth muscle. There are few data on the neuropathology of these patients. One infant [6] had microgyria, porencephaly, a tiny cerebellum, and a fourth ventricle cyst.

Laboratory Studies

Skull x-rays show a steep anterior fossa and a hypoplastic mandible. The tubular bones of the hands and feet are irregular, short, and thick. The tubular bones often show osteoporosis. Chromosomal abnormalities have been present in a few patients, but these have been considered coincidental.

Genetics

This syndrome is thought to be inherited either as a dominant X-linked trait, lethal in males, or as a sex-limited autosomal dominant. The complete clinical syndrome has been described in a 46,XY male [7], as well as a 47,XXY male [8].

Differential Diagnosis

1. Oral, facial, and digital anomalies may occur in patients with the Mohr (OFD II) syndrome, but they also have a broad, bifid tip of the nose, normal hair, bilateral polysyndactyly of the great toe, and loss of hearing. The Mohr syndrome affects both males and females and is inherited as an autosomal recessive trait [9].
2. Alar hypoplasia, digital anomalies, and absence of teeth are features of the oculodentodigital syndrome, but these patients are distinguished by having microphthalmia and enamel hypoplasia, and by not having either tongue clefts or hypertrophied frenula [10].
3. Loss of the mucobuccal fold, absence of teeth, thin and sparse hair, and polydactyly are features of patients with the Ellis–van Creveld syndrome, but they have no other oral anomalies, have severe dwarfism, and both males and females may be affected (see page 280).

References

1. Papillon-Léage, Mme., and Psaume, J. Une malformation héréditaire de la muqueuse buccale, brides et freins anormaux: généralités. *Rev. Stomatatol. Chir. Maxillofac.,* **55**:209–27, 1954.
2. Gorlin, R. J., and Psaume, J. Orodigitofacial dysostosis—a new syndrome. A study of 22 cases. *J. Pediatr.,* **61**:520–30, 1962.
3. Koberg, W., and Schettler, D. Papillon-Léage-Psaume syndrome (Vier kasuistische Beiträge zur Dysostosis orodigitofacialis). *Z. Kinderheilkd.,* **96**:147–62, 1966.
4. Doege, T. C., Campbell, M. M., Bryant, J. S., and Thuline, H. C. Mental retardation and dermatoglyphics in a family with the oral-facial-digital syndrome. *Am. J. Dis. Child.,* **116**:615–22, 1968.
5. Ruess, A. L., Pruzansky, S., Lis, E. F., and Patau, K. The oral-facial-digital syndrome: a multiple congenital condition of females with associated chromosomal abnormalities. *Pediatrics,* **29**:985–95, 1962.
6. Co-Te, P., Dolman, C. L., Tischler, B., and Lowry, R. B. Oral-facial-digital syndrome. A case with necropsy findings. *Am. J. Dis. Child.,* **119**:280–83, 1970.
7. Mandell, F., Ogra, P. L., Horowitz, S. L., and Hirschhorn, K. Oral-facial-digital syndrome in a chromosomally normal male. *Pediatrics,* **40**:63–68, 1967.
8. Wahrman, J., Berant, M., Jacobs, J., Aviad, I., and Ben-Hur, N. The oral-facial-digital syndrome. A male-lethal condition in a boy with 47/XXY chromosomes. *Pediatrics,* **37**:812–21, 1966.
9. Rimoin, D. L., and Edgerton, M. T. Genetic and clinical heterogeneity in the oral-facial-digital syndromes. *J. Pediatr.,* **71**:94–102, 1967.
10. Reisner, S. H., Kott, E., Bornstein, B., Salinger, H., Kaplan, I., and Gorlin, R. J. Oculodentodigital dysplasia. *Am. J. Dis. Child.,* **118**:600–607, 1969.

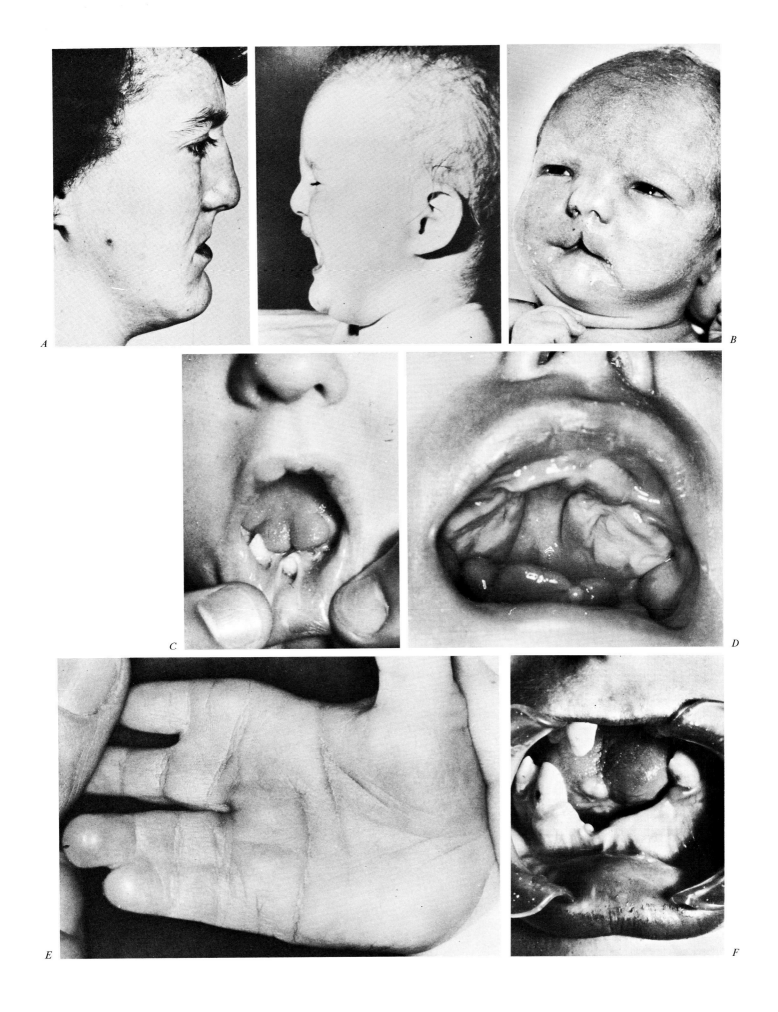

Plate VI-41. *A:* Profile views of a mother and daughter showing short nose and upper lip. The infant also had sparse hair. *B:* An infant with a median cleft lip and hypertelorism. *C:* Shows in a child a trifurcated tip of the tongue and multiple thickened frenula associated with absence of teeth. *D* and *E:* Show in a female infant clefts in the tongue and alveolar ridge, a small nodule on the tip of the tongue, and syndactyly of fingers 2–3 and 4–5. *F:* Shows absent teeth and a hamartoma on the tip of the tongue. (*A* and *F:* From T. C. Doege *et al.*, *N. Engl. J. Med.*, **271:**1073–80, 1964. *B:* From V. W. Fuhrmann and F. Vogel, *Monatsschr. Kinderheilkd.*, **108:**20–25, 1960. *C:* Courtesy of Dr. R. J. Gorlin, Minneapolis, Minn. *D* and *E:* From T. C. Doege *et al.*, *Am. J. Dis. Child.*, **116:**615–22, 1968.)

301

Otopalatodigital Syndrome
(OPD Syndrome)

In 1962 Taybi [1] described a boy with multiple congenital anomalies, short stature, mild mental retardation, and a generalized abnormality of bone. Three brothers with similar physical features were described in 1967 [2–4], and it was suggested that this syndrome be called the otopalatodigital syndrome. Six more individuals, including two females, have been subsequently reported [5–7].

Physical Features

HEAD: The brow and occiput are prominent, and the anteroposterior length is increased (*Figures A, C, D, and F*).

FACE: All of the reported patients have had a similar "pugilistic" appearance, which is characterized by a prominent forehead, widely spaced eyes, a downward palpebral slant, and a broad bridge of the nose. The corners of the mouth are turned downward, and the mouth is often held open (*Figures A, C, and D*).

EARS: The ear canals are small. Exploratory tympanotomy in two boys showed abnormally shaped ossicles [4].

MOUTH: All have had either a cleft soft palate or a submucous cleft palate. The teeth are maloccluded and some are congenitally absent. Two boys had lip pits [6].

CHEST: Each of the children has had pectus excavatum and a small chest.

LIMBS: The most striking feature is the long, curved second and third toes in comparison with the short, broad great toe. Two patients had syndactyly between the second and third digits [1,2] (*Figures B and E*). The space between the first and second digits is increased in both the hands and the feet. The thumbs are short and broad. The distal phalanges of the other fingers are short. Several patients have had limitation of extension and supination at the elbow; two had dislocation of the head of the radius [1,2]. One patient had congenital dislocation of the hips [1].

HEIGHT: The height of four of the boys was below the tenth percentile of normal [1–4].

Nervous System

The IQ estimates of the first four patients ranged between 74 and 90 [1,2]; two others were mildly retarded [6]. All had a bilateral conductive hearing loss of 30 to 70 decibels at most frequencies and had nasal speech.

Laboratory Studies

Skull x-rays on three brothers did not confirm the presence of hypertelorism [2]. In this family the supraorbital ridge was prominent, the frontal bone thick, and the paranasal sinuses poorly pneumatized. The nasion-sella-basion angle was almost 90°. The middle ear ossicles were thickened. The facial bones were small. The mandible was small and had a more obtuse angle than normal. In two boys the proximal radius was hypoplastic in association with posterior dislocation of the radial head. There were many changes in the hands, including

capitate-hamate fusion and clinodactyly. Some of the epiphyses in the toes had an abnormal shape and irregular partial fusion. Coxa valga and mild bowing of the femoral shaft were present. The iliac bones were small and had a decreased flare. The neural arches were not completely fused in several vertebrae [3]. Endocrine function, chromosome, amino acid, and mucopolysaccharide studies have shown no abnormalities.

Treatment and Prognosis

Two boys had no improvement in their hearing after tympanotomy [4].

Genetics

Dominant inheritance was suggested by the occurrence of this syndrome in a woman and her two sons [6]. X-linked inheritance was suggested by its occurrence in two half-brothers whose mother was mildly retarded but normal in appearance [7]. An affected female with unaffected parents has also been reported [5], which indicates that X-linked recessive inheritance is unlikely.

Differential Diagnosis

1. A prominent nose, downward palpebral slant, and broad thumbs and great toes are also features of patients with the Rubinstein-Taybi syndrome, but they do not have long curved digits and they do have microcephaly, hirsutism, and more severe mental retardation (see page 306).
2. A prominent brow and occiput, small facial bones, and short fingers and toes are also features of patients with pycnodysostosis, but they also have a generalized increase in bone density and do not have a "pugilistic" appearance (see page 266).
3. A prominent nose and hypertelorism are features of patients with the telecanthus-hypospadias syndrome (see page 346), the 4p− syndrome (see page 174), and the 5p− syndrome (see page 170).

References

1. Taybi, H. Generalized skeletal dysplasia with multiple anomalies. *Am. J. Roentgenol.*, **88**:450–57, 1962.
2. Dudding, B. A., Gorlin, R. J., and Langer, L. O. The oto-palato-digital syndrome. *Am. J. Dis. Child.*, **113**:214–21, 1967.
3. Langer, L. O., Jr. The roentgenographic features of the oto-palato-digital (OPD) syndrome. *Am. J. Roentgenol.*, **100**:63–70, 1967.
4. Buran, D. J., and Duvall, A. J., III. The oto-palato-digital (OPD) syndrome. *Arch. Otolaryngol.*, **5**:394–99, 1967.
5. Jäger, M., and Refior, H. J. Ein Knochendysplasie-Syndrom. *Z. Orthop.*, **105**:196–208, 1968.
6. Aase, J. M. Oto-palato-digital syndrome. *Birth Defects: Original Article Series,* Vol. V, No. 3, March, 1969, pp. 43–44. Williams & Wilkins Co., Baltimore.
7. Turner, G. Inheritance of the oto-palato-digital syndrome. *Am. J. Dis. Child.,* **119**:377, 1970.
8. Gall, J. C., Jr., Stern, A. M., Poznanski, A. K., Garn, S. M., Weinstein, E. D., and Hayward, J. R. Oto-palato-digital syndrome: Comparison of clinical and radiographic manifestations in males and females. *Am. J. Hum. Genet.,* **24**:24–36, 1972.

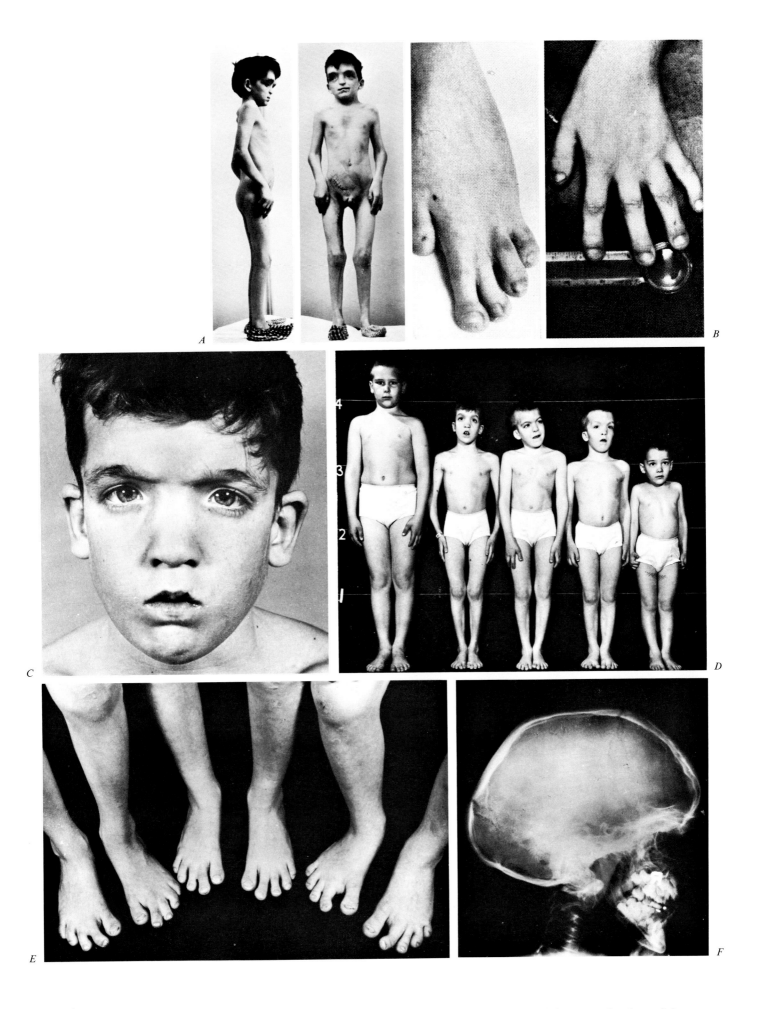

Plate VI-42. *A:* A 9-year-old boy with marked prominence of the supraorbital ridge, hypertelorism, downward eye slant, pectus excavatum, and limited elbow extension. *B:* Shows this boy's wide distal phalanges and short great toe with hypoplasia of the nail. *C* and *D:* An 8-year-old boy with a prominent bridge of the nose and supraorbital ridges and a downward palpebral slant. He is also shown (*second from left*) with two affected (*third and fourth from left*) and two normal brothers (*at ends*). *E:* The three affected brothers' feet show prominence of the distal phalanges, syndactyly, medial curvature of the second toe, and shortening of the great toe. *F:* Shows the typical skull changes: the prominent supraorbital ridge, thick base of the anterior fossa, prominent occiput, small facial bones, a small mandible with an obtuse angle, and poor pneumatization of the mastoids. (*A* and *B:* From H. Taybi, *Am. J. Roentgenol.,* **88:**450–57, 1962. *C–F:* B. A. Dudding *et al., Am. J. Dis. Child.,* **113:**214–21, 1967.)

303

Pierre Robin Syndrome

The association of micrognathia, cleft palate, and glossoptosis has been described by many authors over the past hundred years. The designation as the Pierre Robin syndrome is a result of the articles written by Pierre Robin [1] between 1923 and 1934 on this subject. Micrognathia is the primary developmental anomaly, and glossoptosis is secondary to the posterior displacement of the attachment of the genioglossi muscles to the hypoplastic mandible. More than 150 patients have been reported [2–10]. However, patients with this syndrome may be a heterogeneous group with several etiologies.

Physical Features

FACE: The very small, receding chin is evident at birth (*Figures A and E*). The bridge of the nose is often flat.

EYES: In a study [2] of 39 patients, 13 had a positive history of ocular abnormalities. Eye examinations were done on 15 patients, and major eye lesions were found in 9, including esotropia in 6 and glaucoma in 2.

EARS: The ears are low-set.

MOUTH: Due to poor support by the hypoplastic, receding mandible, the tongue falls backward into the pharynx obstructing the epiglottis. This prevents normal inspiration and causes respiratory distress, cyanosis, and difficulties with feeding. Most patients have a cleft hard and soft palate. Occasionally only a high-arched palate or a cleft uvula is present.

LIMBS: Eight of 39 patients in one review [2] had many different limb anomalies, including clubfoot, short or absent digits, and syndactyly.

Nervous System

In this study [2] of 39 patients, 2 had mild mental retardation and 8 had marked mental retardation, including 2 children with microcephaly and 1 with hydrocephalus. Three had a significant hearing loss. In another study [3] of 13 patients, 7 were retarded and 8 were microcephalic. In a review of 44 patients [4], mental deficiency was considered infrequent.

Pathology

Congenital heart disease is often present; it was noted in 14 of 120 patients [2–5].

Treatment and Prognosis

There are two major problems in the newborn: respiratory distress caused by glossoptosis, and the aspiration of feedings. The glossoptosis can usually be managed by placing the patient in the prone position. In general, surgical tongue fixation is done for the patient with moderately severe airway obstruction. Tracheotomy is reserved for those patients who do not respond to tongue fixation, because of the difficulties encountered in removing the tracheotomy in these infants. Feeding gastrostomies are recommended. In some patients the chin may be of nearly normal size by age 1 to 2 years (*Figures A, B, C, D, E, and F*); in others the micrognathia persists [6]. Correction of the cleft palate is usually postponed until the patient is more than 2½ years old because of the difficulties in endotracheal intubation for anesthesia [7]. The leading causes of death are aspiration and congenital heart disease.

Genetics

Three families have been reported in which there were affected siblings [8–10].

Differential Diagnosis

1. Two brothers originally reported by Smith and Stowe [2] may have a distinctive syndrome that includes cleft soft palate, micrognathia, arachnodactyly, joint hyperextensibility, and retinal detachment [11].
2. Another similar but distinct syndrome complex [12] includes cleft palate, micrognathia, talipes equinovarus, atrial septal defect, and persistence of the left superior vena cava. X-linked recessive inheritance has been suggested for this syndrome.
3. Micrognathia and cleft palate are features of patients with Hanhart's syndrome, type III, but these patients also have peromelia [13].
4. Micrognathia, low-set ears, cleft palate, and congenital heart disease are features of some patients with the 18 trisomy syndrome (see page 164) and the pseudotrisomy 18 syndrome (see page 336).
5. Micrognathia, cleft palate, and microcephaly are features of patients with the Smith-Lemli-Opitz syndrome, but they have anteverted nostrils, a broad alveolar ridge, and genital anomalies (see page 312).
6. Micrognathia, cleft palate, and neonatal respiratory difficulty are features of infants with camptomelic dwarfism, but they also have a skeletal dysplasia [14].

References

1. Robin, P. Glossoptosis due to atresia and hypotrophy of the mandible. *Am. J. Dis. Child.*, **48**:541–47, 1934.
2. Smith, J. L., and Stowe, F. R. The Pierre Robin syndrome (glossoptosis, micrognathia, cleft palate). A review of 39 cases with emphasis on associated ocular lesions. *Pediatrics*, **27**:128–33, 1961.
3. Sacrez, R., Francfort, J.-J., Gigonnet, J.-M., Beauvais, P., and Boll, G. A propos de la débilite intellectuelle et d'anomalies associées a la triade symptomatique du syndrome de Pierre Robin. *Ann. Pediatr.*, **14**:28–33, 1967.
4. Dennison, W. M. The Pierre Robin syndrome. *Pediatrics*, **36**:336–41, 1965.
5. Crow, M. L., Holder, T. M., McCoy, F. J., and Chandler, R. A. The use of temporary gastrostomy to prevent aspiration in Pierre Robin syndrome. *Plast. Reconstr. Surg.*, **35**:494–503, 1965.
6. Randall, P., Krogman, W. M., and Jahina, S. Pierre Robin and the syndrome that bears his name. *Cleft Palate J.*, **2**:237–46, 1965.
7. Hoffman, S., Kahn, S., and Seitchik, M. Late problems in the management of the Pierre Robin syndrome. *Plast. Reconstr. Surg.*, **35**:504–11, 1965.
8. Sachtleben, P. Zur Pathogenese und Therapie des Pierre-Robin-Syndroms. *Arch. Kinderheilkd.*, **171**:55–63, 1964.
9. Shah, C. V., Pruzansky, S., and Harris, W. S. Cardiac malformations with facial clefts. With observations on the Pierre Robin syndrome. *Am. J. Dis. Child.*, **119**:238–44, 1970.
10. Schimke, R. N. The Pierre Robin syndrome in sibs. *Birth Defects: Original Article Series*, Vol. V, No. 2, February, 1969, pp. 222–23. Williams & Wilkins Co., Baltimore.
11. Smith, W. K. Pierre Robin syndrome in brothers. *Birth Defects: Original Article Series*, Vol. V, No. 2, February, 1969, pp. 220–21. Williams & Wilkins Co., Baltimore.
12. Gorlin, R. J., Cervenka, J., Anderson, R. C., Sauk, J. J., and Bevis, W. D. Robin's syndrome. A probably X-linked recessive subvariety exhibiting persistence of left superior vena cava and atrial septal defect. *Am. J. Dis. Child.*, **119**:176–78, 1970.
13. Garner, L. D., and Bixler, D. Micrognathia, an associated defect of Hanhart's syndrome, types II and III. *Oral Surg.*, **27**:601–606, 1969.
14. Gardner, L. I., Assemany, S. R., and Neu, R. L. Syndrome of multiple osseous defects with pretibial dimples. *Lancet*, **2**:98, 1971.

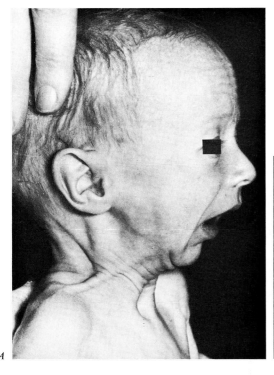

A

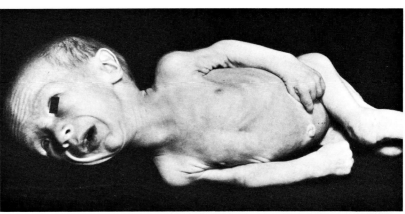

B

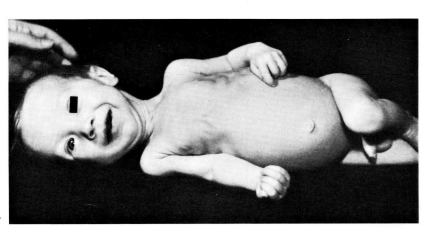

C

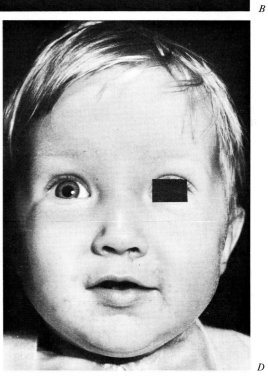

D

Plate VI-43. *A* and *B:* A 3-week-old infant with marked respiratory embarrassment, micrognathia, and cleft palate. *C:* This infant was carefully fed by tube and spoon, but at 7 months of age still weighed only 8 pounds. *D:* By 13 months he was asymptomatic and his mandible had reached almost normal proportions. His intelligence was normal. *E:* Shows an infant whose tongue has been sutured to prevent airway obstruction from glossoptosis. *F:* Same child at about age 2 years with less severe micrognathia. (*A–D:* From W. M. Dennison, *Pediatrics,* **36:**336–41, 1965. *E* and *F:* Courtesy of Dr. J. L. Smith, Miami, Fla.)

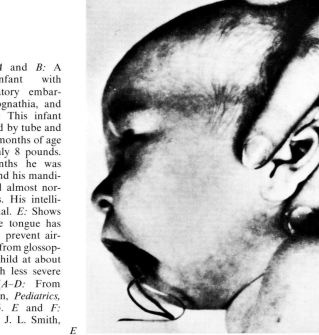

E

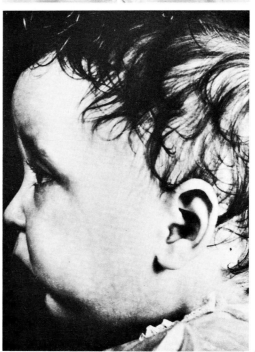

F

Rubinstein-Taybi Syndrome

In 1963 Rubinstein and Taybi [1] reported seven children with broad thumbs and toes, facial abnormalities, and mental retardation. Subsequently, this was found to be a common syndrome. By 1968 more than 100 patients had been reported [2].

Physical Features

HEAD: Many of these patients are microcephalic.

FACE: Hypertelorism, a downward palpebral slant, heavy eyebrows, a beaked nose with the nasal septum extending below the alae nasi, mild retrognathia, and a grimacing smile are common facial features (*Figures A, D, E, and F*). Ptosis and deviation of the nasal septum are present in some patients.

EYES: The most common eye abnormalities are strabismus, refractive errors, cataracts, and obstructed nasolacrimal canals [3].

MOUTH: The palate is narrow and high-arched.

GENITALIA: Most of the males have undescended testes.

LIMBS: Broad terminal phalanges of the thumbs and great toes are the most common limb anomalies (*Figures B, E, and F*). Other digits are often larger than normal. The enlargement may include the entire digit or only the distal phalanx. The nails of the enlarged digits are usually short, flat, and wide. In many patients the thumb and great toe are deviated radially. Duplication of the great toe, but not the thumb, has been observed. Clinodactyly and overlapping digits are less common digital abnormalities [2].

DERMATOGLYPHICS: The most distinctive feature is a high frequency of pattern formations in the thenar first interdigital area. A few patients have double patterns on the tip of the thumbs or the fifth fingers [4].

SKIN: Capillary hemangiomas are common on the forehead (*Figure A*), back of the neck, and lower back (*Figure B*).

HAIR: Many patients have an excessive amount of dark hair over the entire body (*Figure B*).

HEIGHT: Most patients are below the third percentile of normal in height.

WEIGHT: Out of 80 patients [2], 17 had a birth weight of 2500 g or less.

Nervous System

All of the reported patients have been mentally retarded, but there has probably been a bias in ascertainment. Of 89 patients [2], 74 had intelligence quotients of less than 50. Hypotonia, lax ligaments, and hyperextensible joints are common. The gait is usually stiff. Seizures had occurred in 11 of 47 patients. Deep tendon reflexes were hyperactive in 37 of 71 [2].

Pathology

Few autopsies have been reported and no consistent pathologic changes have been observed. Absence of the corpus callosum was present in several of the patients studied either by pneumoencephalography or at autopsy [2,5]. Congenital heart disease has been present in several patients.

Laboratory Studies

X-rays show that the broad digits are associated with enlargement of the phalanges. Many skeletal anomalies are frequently observed: enlarged foramen magnum, parietal foramina, flat acetabular angles, flared ilia, and vertebral and rib anomalies. The bone age is often retarded. The anterior fontanel is large and late in closing [2].

Treatment and Prognosis

Difficulties with feeding and recurrent infections are common during infancy. The life expectancy of these patients is not known, but many survive to adulthood.

Genetics

There is no evidence of simple mendelian inheritance. Polygenic inheritance is suggested by the presence of some features of this syndrome among the relatives of affected patients [3].

Differential Diagnosis

1. A prominent nose and a downward palpebral slant are features of the Treacher Collins syndrome, but these patients are distinguished by having lower lid colobomas, ear deformities, normal digits, and usually normal intelligence (see page 348).

2. Broad thumbs and great toes are features of patients with Apert's syndrome (see page 222) and Pfeiffer's syndrome (see page 228), but they also have craniosynostosis, syndactyly, and a different facial appearance.

3. Microcephaly, short stature, and a prominent nose are features of patients with Seckel's bird-headed dwarfism (see page 308) and Cockayne's syndrome (see page 82).

4. Broad thumbs and toes are features of the patients with the frontodigital syndrome [7], but they also have frontal bossing, a bony sagittal ridge, normal intelligence, and sometimes syndactyly and polydactyly.

References

1. Rubinstein, J. H., and Taybi, H. Broad thumbs and toes and facial abnormalities. *Am. J. Dis. Child.,* **105:**588–608, 1963.
2. Rubinstein, J. H. The broad thumbs syndrome—progress report 1968. *Birth Defects: Original Article Series,* Vol. V, No. 2, February, 1969, pp. 25–41. Williams & Wilkins Co., Baltimore.
3. Roy, F. H., Summitt, R. L., Hiatt, R. L., and Hughes, J. G. Ocular manifestations of the Rubinstein-Taybi syndrome. *Arch. Ophthalmol. (Chicago),* **79:**272–78, 1968.
4. Padfield, C. J., Partington, M. W., and Simpson, N. E. The Rubinstein-Taybi syndrome. *Arch. Dis. Child.,* **43:**94–101, 1968.
5. Neuhaüser, G., and Schulze, H. Das Rubinstein-Taybi Syndrom. Klinische und pneumencephalographische Befunde. *Z. Kinderheilkd.,* **103:**90–108, 1968.
6. Taybi, H., and Rubinstein, J. H. Broad thumbs and toes, and unusual facial features. *Am. J. Roentgenol.,* **93:**362–66, 1965.
7. Marshall, R. E., and Smith, D. W. Frontodigital syndrome: a dominantly inherited disorder with normal intelligence. *J. Pediatr.,* **77:**129–33, 1970.

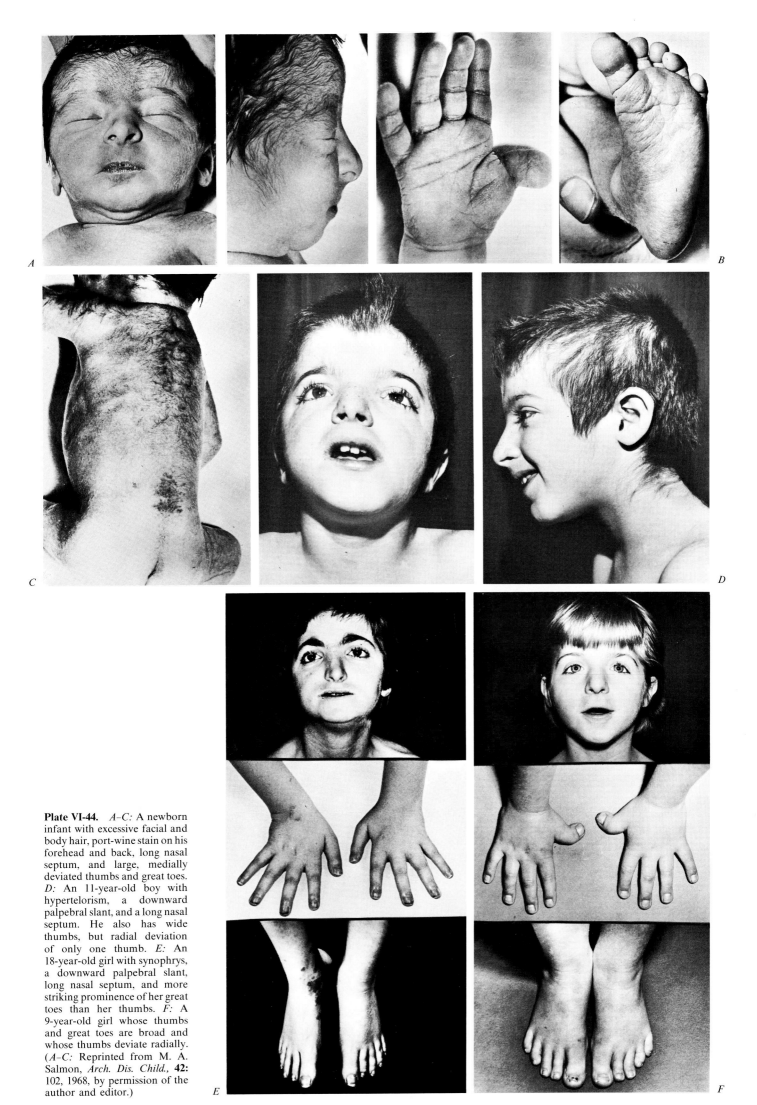

Plate VI-44. *A–C:* A newborn infant with excessive facial and body hair, port-wine stain on his forehead and back, long nasal septum, and large, medially deviated thumbs and great toes. *D:* An 11-year-old boy with hypertelorism, a downward palpebral slant, and a long nasal septum. He also has wide thumbs, but radial deviation of only one thumb. *E:* An 18-year-old girl with synophrys, a downward palpebral slant, long nasal septum, and more striking prominence of her great toes than her thumbs. *F:* A 9-year-old girl whose thumbs and great toes are broad and whose thumbs deviate radially. (*A–C:* Reprinted from M. A. Salmon, *Arch. Dis. Child.,* **42:** 102, 1968, by permission of the author and editor.)

Seckel's Bird-Headed Dwarfism

In 1960 Seckel [1] described two children with extreme microcephaly, short stature, prominent eyes, a beaklike nose, a narrow face, and a small chin. The terms *bird-headed dwarfism* and *nanocephalic dwarfism* were used to describe these features. These patients were thought to represent a specific clinical disorder and 13 similar patients from the earlier literature were cited. Ten patients have subsequently been described as examples of Seckel's bird-headed dwarfism [2–7]. Some of these had only nanocephaly and extremely short stature [2–5]. Others [6,7] had numerous skeletal and urogenital anomalies, as did Seckel's patients. Whether all of these patients represent a single genetic disorder or a heterogeneous group of disorders with only nanocephaly and short stature in common cannot be established at this time.

Physical Features

HEAD: All of the patients had severe microcephaly.

FACE: The nose was prominent, the eyes appeared to be large, the malar area was hypoplastic, and the chin was small (*Figures A, B, C, D, E, and F*). Two siblings [6] had hypertelorism and facial asymmetry (*Figure F*).

EARS: The ears were simple and had no lobe.

MOUTH: The palate was narrow and high-arched. Some patients had small, hypoplastic, and absent teeth [1,6]. One patient [6] had a cleft lip and palate.

BACK: One of three siblings [7] had kyphoscoliosis.

LIMBS: Many different skeletal anomalies, including medial curvature of the second, fourth, and fifth fingers, short digits, syndactyly of the toes, absence of the thumb, dislocation of the elbow, hip, knee, and ankle, and a clubfoot deformity, were noted in three of the reports [1,6,7].

GENITALIA: The males had cryptorchidism and a small penis and scrotum. One female had a large clitoris [5]. Others had small labia [6] and a single cloacal opening [7].

HAIR: Two adult patients had very scant body and scalp hair [7].

HEIGHT: All of the patients were very short at birth and throughout their lives (*Figures C, D, and E*).

WEIGHT: The birth weights were below five pounds and the patients remained slender.

GROWTH AND DEVELOPMENT: During infancy feeding was difficult and the weight gain was slow. The two reported adult females had menstrual periods until they were 45 and 51 years old [7].

Nervous System

Some of the patients were severely retarded, had limited speech, and were unable to care for themselves [6,7]. Others had intelligence quotients between 70 and 80 [1–3,5].

Pathology

Autopsies were performed on two patients [7]. Both showed a small cerebrum with simplified convolutional patterns. Each had a small kidney, which in one was ectopic.

Laboratory Studies

Numerous ossification abnormalities have been observed. The bone age is consistently below the chronologic age. Two siblings had premature closure of cranial sutures, prominent digital markings, facial asymmetry, and hypertelorism. They also had normal fasting plasma levels of growth hormone [6,6a]. Measurements of urinary keto- and hydroxysteroids, protein-bound iodine, and amino acids have been normal. No chromosomal abnormalities have been identified.

Treatment and Prognosis

The three reported adults died at 75, 58, and 55 years of age [7].

Genetics

In three families [3,6,7] there were affected siblings, which suggests that the disorder is due to an autosomal recessive mutant gene.

Differential Diagnosis

1. Low birth weight for term gestation, short stature, a narrow face, and clinodactyly are features of patients with the Silver-Russell syndrome, but they have a normal nose and often have hemihypertrophy (see page 310).
2. Patients with "true" or "pure" microcephaly have a small cranium and short stature, but do not have the prominent nose and eyes that are features of Seckel's bird-headed dwarfism (see page 196).
3. A prominent nose, small chin, and microcephaly are features of patients with the Rubinstein-Taybi syndrome (see page 306) and Cockayne's syndrome (see page 82).

References

1. Seckel, H. P. G.   *Bird-headed Dwarfs.* S. Karger, Basel/New York; Charles C Thomas, Publisher, Springfield, Ill., 1960.
2. Mann, T. P., and Russell, A.   Study of a microcephalic midget of extreme type. *Proc. R. Soc. Med.,* **52:**1024–27, 1959.
3. Black, J.   Low birth weight dwarfism. *Arch. Dis. Child.,* **36:**633–44, 1961.
4. de la Cruz, F. F.   Bird-headed dwarf: a case report. *Am. J. Ment. Defic.,* **68:**54–62, 1963.
5. Szalay, G. C.   Intrauterine growth retardation versus Silver's syndrome. *J. Pediatr.,* **64:**234–40, 1964.
6. Harper, R. G., Orti, E., and Baker, R. K.   Bird-headed dwarfs (Seckel's syndrome). *J. Pediatr.,* **70:**799–804, 1967.
6a. Hillman, J. C., Hammond, J., Noé, O., and Reiss, M.   Endocrine investigations in deLange's and Seckel's syndromes. *Am. J. Ment. Defic.,* **73:**30–33, 1968.
7. McKusick, V. A., Mahloudji, M., Abbott, M. H., Lindenberg, R., and Kepas, D.   Seckel's bird-headed dwarfism. *N. Engl. J. Med.,* **277:**279–86, 1967.

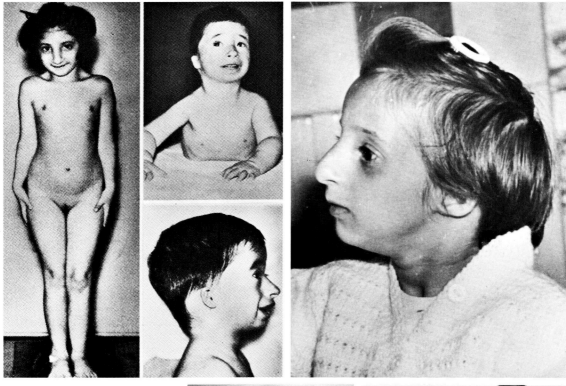

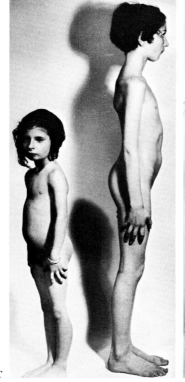

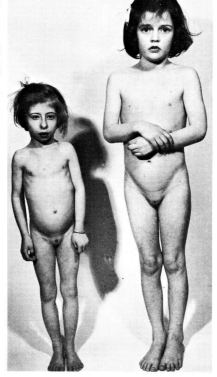

Plate VI-45. *A:* The two patients originally reported by Seckel. *B:* A 2-year-old girl with a prominent nose and small head (circumference $13\frac{1}{4}$ in. [34 cm]) who weighed $3\frac{1}{2}$ pounds [1.5 kg] at birth. *C* and *D:* Two sisters, aged $8\frac{9}{12}$ and 7 years, with prominent noses and small chins. Each is shown with a normal girl of the same age. *E:* A 22-year-old girl who had a shrunken left eye, large nose, and normal breast development. *F:* A 6-year-old brother (*left*) and 3-year-old sister, each with multiple skeletal anomalies, including dislocation of the radius, which caused them to keep their elbows flexed. (*A:* From H. P. G. Seckel, *Bird-headed Dwarfs,* S. Karger, Basel/New York; Charles C Thomas, Publisher, Springfield, Ill., 1960. *B:* From T. P. Mann and A. Russell, *Proc. Roy. Soc. Med.,* **52:**1024-27, 1959. *C* and *D:* Reprinted from J. Black, *Arch. Dis. Child.,* **36:**633, 1961, by permission of author and editor. *E:* Copyright © 1963, American Association on Mental Deficiency; reprinted by permission of the *Am. J. Ment. Defic. F:* From R. G. Harper *et al., J. Pediatr.,* **70:**799-804, 1967.)

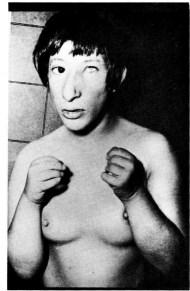

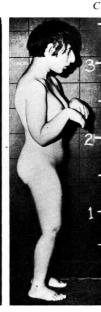

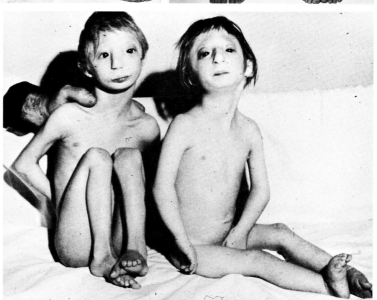

Silver-Russell Syndrome
(Silver's Syndrome, Russell's Dwarf)

In 1953 Silver, Kiyasu, George, and Deamer [1] reported two children with a syndrome of congenital hemihypertrophy, short stature, and elevated urinary gonadotropins. In 1954 Russell [2] described five children with intrauterine dwarfism, craniofacial dysostosis, short arms, and other anomalies. Silver [3] considered two of the patients (cases III and V) described by Russell as similar to his patients. Black [4] used the term *Russell-Silver dwarf* to describe a patient. However, Szalay [5] and Tanner and Ham [6] have suggested that the two syndromes are similar, but not identical. The term *Silver-Russell syndrome* is used here because it is likely that the patients reported by Silver and at least two of those reported by Russell represent a specific multiple anomaly syndrome. More than 50 patients have been described [1–10].

Physical Features

HEAD: The term *pseudohydrocephalus* refers to the appearance of head enlargement in a child with a small face and body, but a normal head circumference. This is an occasional feature of the Silver-Russell syndrome [2,5,10].

FACE: The face has a triangular appearance with a broad forehead and a narrow chin. The lips are thin and the corners of the mouth turn downward (*Figures A, D, and E*). Ptosis is occasionally present.

GENITALIA: Unilateral or bilateral cryptorchidism is common in males.

BACK: A few patients have scoliosis, including some with vertebral anomalies [3,4].

LIMBS: Clinodactyly is present in most patients (*Figure F*). About one third have incomplete syndactyly between the second and third toes [3] (*Figure F*). Three fourths of Silver's patients had asymmetry of the body [3]. The asymmetry is usually evident in infancy. It may involve one entire side of the body (*Figures A, B, and C*) or only part of one limb. The smaller side is considered to be undergrown.

SKIN: Some patients have cafe au lait spots. Excessive sweating has been noted [10].

HEIGHT AND WEIGHT: At birth these infants are usually small for their gestational age. Throughout childhood their linear growth rate and weight gain are parallel to, but below, the third percentile for normal children. The eventual stature as adults is not known. The 21-year-old twins reported by Rimoin [11] were 58 and 60 in. tall.

GROWTH AND DEVELOPMENT: Ten of the 29 patients reviewed by Silver [3] had abnormalities of sexual development, usually precocious sexual development and an elevated level of urinary gonadotropins at a time when significant excretion of gonadotropins does not normally occur. A delayed onset of puberty has been noted in several patients.

Nervous System

Few data are available on the intelligence of these patients, but it was the impression of Silver [3] that significant mental deficiency occurs more often than in normal children. Others [10] have noted that early motor development may be delayed because of muscle weakness, but mental capabilities are usually normal.

Pathology

The autopsy of one patient [5] showed a normal central nervous system. Both adrenal glands were very small, but normal in histologic appearance.

Laboratory Studies

Delay in closure of the anterior fontanel and epiphyseal maturation has been found in many patients. The elevation of urinary gonadotropins has been found in both males and females, but these patients do not necessarily exhibit precocious sexual maturation. One reported child with precocious puberty had elevated serum and urine gonadotropins [7]. Two infants had fasting hypoglycemia [10]. Some, but not all, infants have had elevated growth hormone levels [10].

Genetics

The mothers in two families had similar, but milder, features [9,10]. In another family siblings were affected [8].

Differential Diagnosis

1. A triangular face with a narrow chin, ptosis, clinodactyly, and short stature are also features of the XO (Turner's) syndrome (see page 178).
2. Low birth weight for gestational age, a large head (due to a prominent occiput), micrognathia, and clinodactyly are features of the 18 trisomy syndrome (see page 156).
3. A triangular face, downturned corners of the mouth and body asymmetry have been features of three reported patients with diploid-triploid mosaicism [12].

References

1. Silver, H. K., Kiyasu, W., George, J., and Deamer, W. C. Syndrome of congenital hemihypertrophy, shortness of stature and elevated urinary gonadotropins. *Pediatrics,* **12**:368–76, 1953.
2. Russell, A. A syndrome of "intra-uterine" dwarfism recognizable at birth with cranio-facial dysostosis, disproportionately short arms, and other anomalies (5 examples). *Proc. R. Soc. Med.,* **47**:1040–44, 1954.
3. Silver, H. K. Asymmetry, short stature, and variations in sexual development. *Am. J. Dis. Child.,* **107**:495–515, 1964.
4. Black, J. Low birth weight dwarfism. *Arch. Dis. Child.,* **36**:633–44, 1961.
5. Szalay, G. C. Pseudohydrocephalus in dwarfs: the Russell dwarf. *J. Pediatr.,* **63**:622–33, 1963.
6. Tanner, J. M., and Ham, T. J. Low birthweight dwarfism with asymmetry (Silver's syndrome): treatment with human growth hormone. *Arch. Dis. Child.,* **44**:231–43, 1969.
7. Curi, J. F. J., Vanucci, R. C., Grossman, H., and New, M. Elevated serum gonadotropins in Silver's syndrome. *Am. J. Dis. Child.,* **114**:658–61, 1967.
8. Callaghan, K. A. Asymmetrical dwarfism, or Silver's syndrome, in two male siblings. *Med. J. Aust.,* **2**:789–92, 1970.
9. Fuleihan, D. S., Der Kaloustian, V. M., and Najjar, S. S. The Russell-Silver syndrome: report of three siblings. *J. Pediatr.,* **78**:654–57, 1971.
10. Gareis, F. J., Smith, D. W., and Summitt, R. L. The Russell-Silver syndrome without asymmetry. *J. Pediatr.,* **79**:775–81, 1971.
11. Rimoin, D. L. The Silver syndrome in twins. *Birth Defects: Original Article Series,* Vol. V, No. 2, 1969, p. 183. Williams & Wilkins Co., Baltimore.
12. Jenkins, M. E., Eisen, J., and Seguin, F. Congenital asymmetry and diploid-triploid mosaicism. *Am. J. Dis. Child.,* **122**:80–84, 1971.

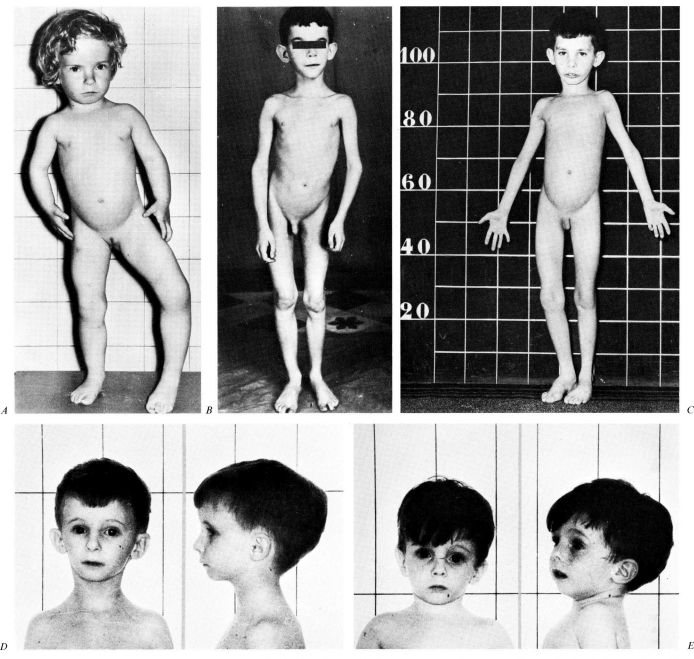

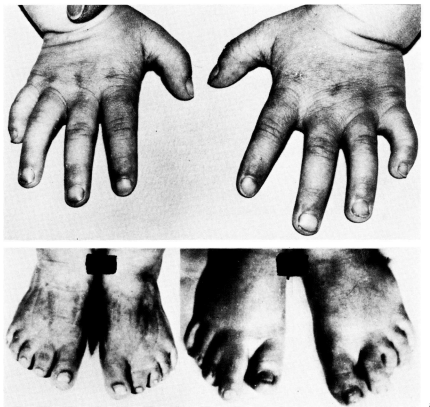

Plate VI-46. *A:* A 4½-year-old girl with striking asymmetry of her arms and legs, down-turned corners of the mouth, and a small chin. *B:* An 8½-year-old boy with short stature (101 cm), asymmetry of the body, exaggerated lumbar lordosis, and a pelvic tilt because of the differing length of his legs. *C:* A 10-year-old boy with short stature, mild body asymmetry, a small chin, and clinodactyly. *D* and *E:* Two boys with similar facial features, a triangular-shaped face, a small chin and mouth, and down-turned corners of the mouth. The patients shown in *B, C,* and *D* had normal intelligence. *F:* The most common skeletal anomalies, clinodactyly of the fifth finger and mild syndactyly of toes 2–3. (*A:* From P. E. Ferrier and S. A. Ferrier, *J. Pediatr.,* **70:**438–40, 1967. *B* and *C:* From A. Rossier and J. C. Job, *Ann. Pediatr.* [*Paris*], **11:**639–45, 1964. *D* and *E:* Reprinted from J. M. Tanner and T. J. Ham, *Arch. Dis. Child.,* **44:**231, 1969, by permission of the authors and editor. *F* [*top*]: Courtesy of Dr. P. E. Ferrier, Seattle, Wash. *F* [*bottom*]: From H. K. Silver, *Am. J. Dis. Child.,* **107:**495–515, 1964.)

Smith-Lemli-Opitz Syndrome

In 1964 Smith, Lemli, and Opitz [1] described three unrelated boys with mental retardation and a similar pattern of anomalies of the facial features, limbs, and genitalia. More than 40 children with this syndrome have been reported [2–8].

Physical Features

HEAD: These patients are microcephalic.

FACE: A broad, short nose with upturned nares, a wide medial canthus, epicanthic folds, ptosis, and a small chin are the most common facial characteristics (*Figures A, B, and F*).

EYES: Many patients have strabismus. A few have bilateral cataracts.

EARS: The ears are usually either posteriorly rotated or low-set.

MOUTH: Most patients have a broad maxillary alveolar ridge with an arched palate (*Figures B and F*). In a review of 40 patients there were 15 with a cleft palate [8].

NECK: The neck is short.

SHOULDERS: The shoulders are narrow.

GENITALIA: Thirty-nine of the 40 reported males have had hypospadias, chordee, and usually undescended testes [8] (*Figure C*). The reported females have had no abnormalities of the external genitalia.

LIMBS: Out of 40 reported patients [8], 30 had cutaneous syndactyly between the second and third toes (*Figure D*). In a review of 23 patients [5] 5 had polydactyly. Less common anomalies are clubfoot, metatarsus adductus, dislocation of the hip, and short digits.

SKIN: A deep pit anterior to the anus was noted in four of seven patients [2].

DERMATOGLYPHICS: Most patients have an increased incidence of whorls on the digits, a high ridge count, and transverse palmar creases.

HEIGHT AND WEIGHT: These patients are usually below average at birth and remain subnormal.

Nervous System

The activity of the fetus is below normal. At birth the infants have a poor suck and muscular hypotonia. These patients become progressively more spastic after the first months of life. Most are severely retarded.

Pathology

In the few autopsies that have been performed, no neuropathologic abnormalities have been observed. Two infants were found to have congenital pyloric stenosis and one had a hypoplastic thymus [1]. Another infant had an endocardial cushion defect, patent ductus arteriosus, three accessory spleens, and a Meckel's diverticulum [8]. A testis biopsy in a 20-year-old boy with hypogonadotropic hypogonadism showed normal tubules, most of which had no spermatogonia [7].

Laboratory Studies

Pneumoencephalography showed dilatation of the ventricles and a small cerebellum in one patient [2]. Several different renal anomalies have been reported, but none is consistently present. Eight out of 40 patients were thought to have a cardiac defect [8]. Chromosomal, amino acid, and serum immunoglobulins studies have revealed no abnormalities.

Treatment and Prognosis

Frequent irritability, difficulty with feeding, and regurgitation are common problems in infancy. Some patients have pyloric stenosis. Of 13 patients in one review, 5 died before 14 months of age, the cause of death being various types of infections and heart failure [2].

Genetics

Autosomal recessive. There was a slight predominance of males in the first 23 patients reported [5], but this may be a reflection of the fact that the diagnosis can be made more easily in males because most of them have hypospadias and cryptorchidism.

Differential Diagnosis

1. Micrognathia, positioning of the flexed index finger over the middle finger, cryptorchidism, and failure to thrive are also features of 18 trisomy (see page 156).

2. Ptosis, epicanthic folds, and mental retardation are features of Noonan's syndrome (see page 298).

3. Anteverted nostrils are features of patients with deLange's syndrome (see page 276) and the syndrome of microcephaly, snub nose, livedo reticularis, and low-birth-weight dwarfism (see page 334).

4. Upturned nares, a broad bridge of the nose, hypotonia in infancy, short stature and mental retardation are features of the syndrome reported by Lowry and coworkers [9], but the affected patients did not have a broad alveolar ridge, cleft palate, or cardiac or genital anomalies, furthermore autosomal dominant inheritance seemed likely.

References

1. Smith, D. W., Lemli, L., and Opitz, J. M. A newly recognized syndrome of multiple congenital anomalies. *J. Pediatr.,* **64:**210–17, 1964.
2. Park, S. C., Needles, C. F., Dimich, I., and Sussman, L. Congenital heart disease in an infant with the Smith-Lemli-Opitz syndrome. *J. Pediatr.,* **73:**896–902, 1968.
3. Zucker, J. M., Job, J. C., and Rossier, A. Une nouvelle variété de nanisme intra-utérin dystrophique: le syndrome de Smith, Lemli et Opitz. *Sem. Hop. Paris,* **43:**2409–11, 1967.
4. Schumacher, H. Das Smith-Lemli-Opitz-Syndrom. *Z. Kinderheilkd.,* **105:**88–98, 1969.
5. Dallaire, L. Syndrome of retardation with urogenital and skeletal anomalies (Smith-Lemli-Opitz syndrome): clinical features and mode of inheritance. *J. Med. Genet.,* **6:**113–20, 1969.
6. Opitz, J. M., Zellweger, H., Shannon, W. R., and Ptacek, L. J. The RSH syndrome. *Birth Defects: Original Article Series,* Vol. V, No. 2, February, 1969, pp. 43–52. Williams & Wilkins Co., Baltimore.
7. Hoefnagel, D., Wurster, D., Pomeroy, J., and Benz, R. The Smith-Lemli-Opitz syndrome in an adult male. *J. Ment. Defic. Res.,* **13:**249–57, 1969.
8. Robinson, C. D., Perry, L. W., Barlee, H., and Mella, G. W. Smith-Lemli-Opitz syndrome with cardiovascular abnormality. *Pediatrics,* **47:**844–47, 1971.
9. Lowry, B., Miller, J. R., and Fraser, F. C. A new dominant gene mental retardation syndrome. Association with small stature, tapering fingers, characteristic facies, and possible hydrocephalus. *Am. J. Dis. Child.,* **121:**496–500, 1971.

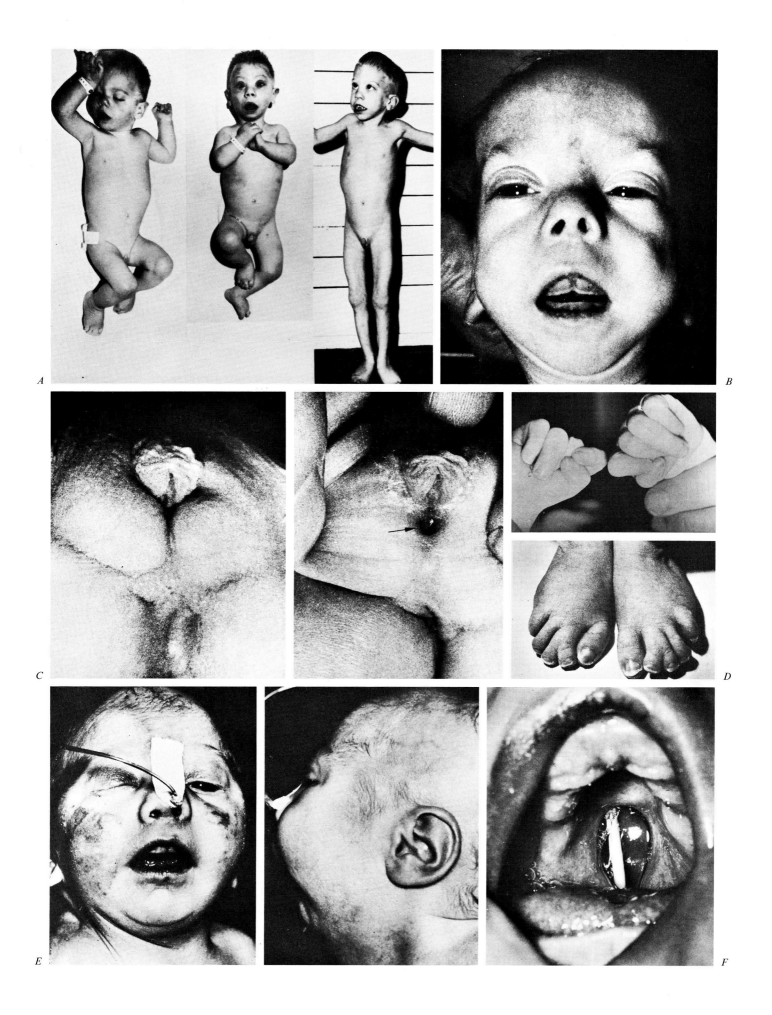

Plate VI-47. *A:* The first three reported patients. Each had a similar facial appearance, hypospadias, and limb anomalies. *B–D:* A newborn with ptosis of both eyes, a short nose with anteverted nares, and a prominent broad maxillary alveolar ridge. His index fingers overlap the middle fingers, and both feet show cutaneous syndactyly between the second and third toes. He has a perineal urethral opening (*arrow*), chordee, and bifid scrotum. *E* and *F:* A newborn female with ptosis and a small chin. The nasogastric tube was used for feeding,

because of her poor sucking and swallowing. The open-mouth view shows the broad alveolar ridge and cleft soft palate. (*A:* From D. W. Smith *et al., J. Pediatr.,* **64:**210–17, 1964. *B* and *D:* From S. C. Park *et al., J. Pediatr.,* **73:**896–902, 1968. *C:* Courtesy of Dr. L. Sussman, New York, N.Y. *E* [*right*]: From R. B. Lowry *et al., J. Pediatr.,* **72:**859–61, 1968. *E* and *F* [*left*]: Courtesy of Dr. R. B. Lowry, Vancouver, British Columbia, Canada.)

313

Syndrome of Absent Fifth Fingernails and Toenails, Short Distal Phalanges, and Lax Joints

In 1970 Coffin and Siris [1] described three unrelated girls with short distal phalanges of the fingers and toes, absent nails on the fifth fingers and toes, lax joints, and marked retardation of linear growth and psychomotor development. Many other skeletal anomalies were also present. This was thought to be a new syndrome. A fourth affected female was reported later in the same year [2].

Physical Features

HEAD: Three were microcephalic [1].

FACE: Each had a wide nose and mouth and thick lips. Two had bushy eyebrows (*Figures A, B, and C*).

MOUTH: One girl had a cleft palate.

ABDOMEN: One girl had an umbilical hernia and bilateral inguinal hernias.

LIMBS: The fingers and toes were short. In addition to absence of the fifth fingernails and toenails, the other nails were small. One child had no nail on either her thumbs or great toes [2]. Three patients also had clinodactyly of the fifth fingers. Each had marked laxity of all joints and unilateral or bilateral dislocation of the head of the radius.

SKIN: Two had sparse scalp hair (*Figures A and B*) and two had hirsutism of the back and extremities.

HEIGHT AND WEIGHT: They were all well below the third percentile of normal. Their birth weights were normal.

Nervous System

Three girls were severely retarded and lived in a state institution. Their intelligence quotients were estimated to be less than 30. One had seizures in infancy [1]. The fourth sat at 9 months and walked, but had no speech at 19 months of age [2].

Pathology

The only autopsy showed a middle cerebral artery infarct and a Dandy-Walker malformation. This child also had an aberrant pulmonary vein which entered the right atrium [1].

Laboratory Studies

Radiographic findings in three girls included absent terminal phalanges in the fifth fingers and toes (*Figures D and F*), small terminal phalanges in the other digits, small middle phalanges in the fingers (*Figure D*), small or absent patella, mild coxa valga, and retarded bone ages. Two girls also had

six lumbar vertebrae and two had a short sternum [1]. The fourth patient at age 13 months had no terminal phalanges in the fifth fingers, hypoplastic terminal phalanges of the fifth toes and coxa valga [2].

Thyroid, amino acid, mucopolysaccharide, and chromosomal studies showed no abnormalities.

Treatment and Prognosis

All three patients had recurrent respiratory infections in infancy and two had feeding difficulties [1].

Genetics

None of the four girls had any similarly affected family members.

Differential Diagnosis

1. Senior [3] reported 6 children who have this same syndrome. His patients were short at birth, had small nails on one or more toes, short middle phalanges of the fifth digits, broad noses, and mild intellectual impairment.

2. Hypoplastic nails are features of patients with the nail-patella syndrome, but they have ischial horns, absent or hypoplastic patellae, and nephritis and do not have short digits, lax joints, or mental retardation [4].

3. Coarse facial features, short fingers and toes, and small nails were also features of the two infants with the syndrome of micromelia and coarse facial features, but they did not have absence of the fifth digit nails (see page 334).

4. Short fingers and absent or hypoplastic nails have been described in patients with familial absence of the middle phalanges [2], but they have normal height and intelligence and duplicated distal phalanx of the thumbs.

References

1. Coffin, G. S., and Siris, E. Mental retardation with absent fifth fingernail and terminal phalanx. *Am. J. Dis. Child.,* **119**:433–39, 1970.
2. Bartsocas, C. S., and Tsiantos, A. K. Mental retardation with absent fifth fingernail and terminal phalanx. *Am. J. Dis. Child.,* **120**:493–94, 1970.
3. Senior, B. Impaired growth and onychodysplasia. Short children with tiny toenails. *Am. J. Dis. Child.,* **122**:7–9, 1971.
4. Lucas, G. L., and Opitz, J. M. The nail-patella syndrome. Clinical and genetic aspects of 5 kindreds with 38 affected family members. *J. Pediatr.,* **68**:273–88, 1966.
5. Bass, H. N. Familial absence of middle phalanges with nail dysplasia: a new syndrome. *Pediatrics,* **42**:318–23, 1968.

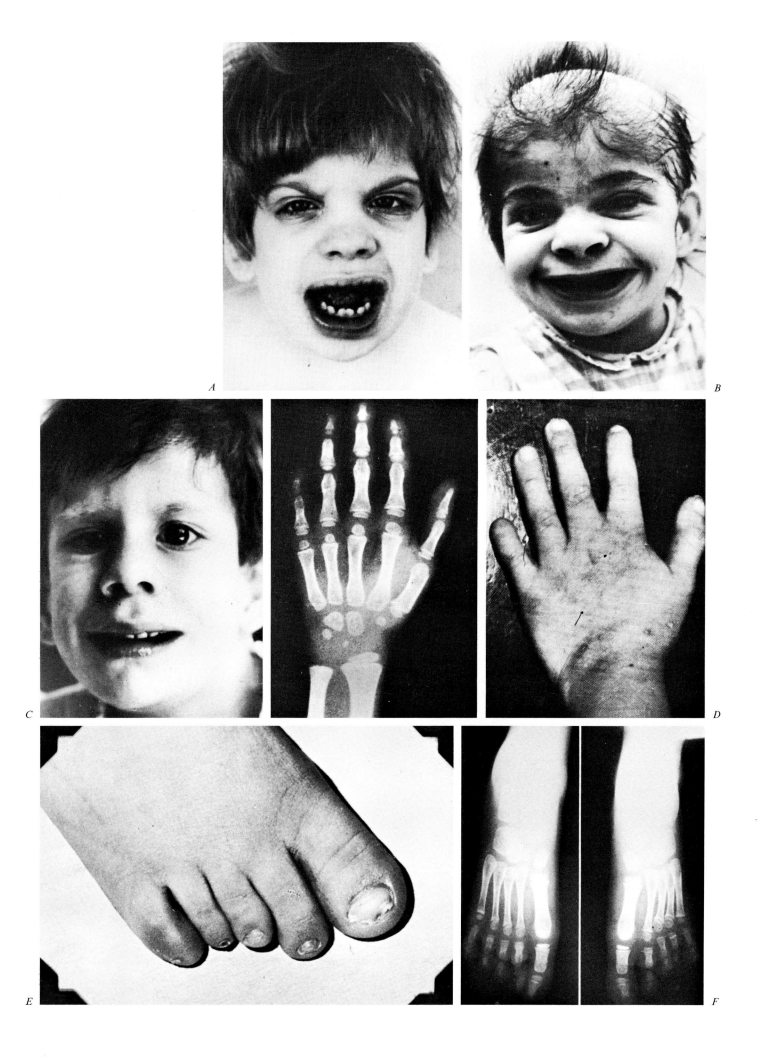

Plate VI-48. *A–C:* The three unrelated girls, aged 6⁷⁄₁₂, 8⁵⁄₁₂, and 7⁵⁄₁₂ years. Each has a wide nose and mouth and thick lips. The first two have bushy eyebrows and sparse scalp hair. *D–F:* The hand and foot of the third girl (case 2) showing no nail on the fifth finger, a tiny nail on the fifth toe, a progressive enlargement of the nail from digits 4 to 1, and absence of the distal phalanges in toes 4–5. (*A–D:* From G. S. Coffin and E. Siris, *Am. J. Dis. Child.,* **119:**433–39, 1970. *E* and *F:* Courtesy of Dr. E. Siris, Eldridge, Calif.)

315

Syndrome of Acromegaloid Features, Hypertelorism, and Pectus Carinatum

In 1966 Coffin, Siris, and Wegienka [1] described two unrelated boys who had many striking facial and skeletal abnormalities, as well as short stature and mental retardation. These patients are thought to represent a previously undescribed clinical syndrome. A third patient was reported in 1969 [2]. A family with possibly seven affected members is now being studied [3].

Physical Features

HEAD: In the first report [1] one boy had microcephaly. The other, who had an enlarged head as an infant, showed frontal and parietal bossing with a normal head circumference (*Figure A*).

FACE: As infants, hypertelorism was the only remarkable facial feature (*Figures A and D*). When studied at 18, 15, and 19 years of age, all three boys had coarse facial features with a broad nose, prognathism, and prominent supraorbital ridges. They also had widely spaced eyes, a downward palpebral slant, epicanthic folds, and a hypoplastic maxilla [1,2] (*Figures B, C, E, and F*).

EARS: All of the patients have had large, low-set, protruding ears.

MOUTH: The upper teeth were crowded and the palate was narrow.

CHEST: One patient had pectus excavatum at birth. He and another patient later had marked pectus carinatum [1] (*Figures C and F*). The third reported patient did not have a deformed sternum [2].

GENITALIA: The first two patients [1] had a normal penis, but small testes. Unilateral cryptorchidism was present in one boy.

BACK: Two patients had thoracic kyphosis [1]. One had a lumbar gibbus deformity [2].

LIMBS: The hands have been described as large, soft, and deviate toward the ulna (*Figures C and F*). The fingers are thick at the base, but taper to narrow tips. All of the joints were lax in one patient, but in another the wrists and elbows had a decreased range of motion [1]. All three patients have had their knees flexed when standing and walking.

SKIN: All patients have had loose skin that stretched easily.

HAIR: They had pubic but not axillary hair.

HEIGHT: The height or reclining length of all patients has been well below the third percentile of normal.

WEIGHT: The birth weights have been normal. The weights of the first two patients were in the third percentile for their ages [1].

Nervous System

All three boys exhibited slow psychomotor development throughout infancy and childhood and were subsequently admitted to institutions for the mentally retarded. The older patient in the first report [1] was placed in an institution at the age of 8 years; he had an IQ of 54 at 10 years and 25 at 18 years. When the younger patient was placed in an institution, his IQ was 44. At 15 years of age his IQ was only 20. Both boys had pleasant dispositions.

Laboratory Studies

Skin and subcutaneous tissue biopsies in the first two patients [1] showed a greatly reduced number of elastic fibers. A biopsy of the iliac crest showed an irregular epiphyseal line and an abnormal arrangement of chondrocytes. Tests of growth hormone, thyroid function, mucopolysaccharides, amino acids, and chromosomes showed no abnormalities. In all three patients x-rays of the hands and wrists showed a slight delay in skeletal maturation and tufting of the terminal phalanges. The paranasal sinuses and maxilla were poorly developed. The first two patients [1] had a short and longitudinally bifid sternum and anterosuperior notch defects and tonguelike anterior protrusions in the lumbar vertebrae. One patient also had a dense and thickened calvarium.

Genetics

Dominant inheritance seems likely. In the first two reported families the mothers had soft hands, wide-set eyes, prominent brows and chins, and short stature. In the family still being studied [3] there are affected individuals in three consecutive generations. As there are no known examples of male-to-male transmission, the mutant gene may be either X-linked or autosomal.

Differential Diagnosis

1. Thoracic kyphosis, prognathism, and small testes are features of patients with the XXXXY syndrome (see page 190).
2. Pectus carinatum and stooped posture are features of the syndrome of blepharophimosis, myotonia, joint stiffness, and progressive skeletal deformities (the Schwartz-Jampel syndrome) [4].
3. Prominent supraorbital ridges, pectus carinatum, and flexed knees were features of the man with frontometaphyseal dysplasia [5], but he had a small chin, arachnodactyly, ankylosis of several joints, and normal intelligence.

References

1. Coffin, G. S., Siris, E., and Wegienka, L. C. Mental retardation with osteocartilaginous anomalies. *Am. J. Dis. Child.*, **112**:205–13, 1966.
2. Martinelli, B., and Campailla, E. Contributo alla conoscenza della sindrome di Coffin, Siris and Wegienka. *G. Psichiat. Neuropatol.*, **3**:449–58, 1969.
3. Siris, E. Personal communication, 1970.
4. Schwartz, O., and Jampel, R. S. Congenital blepharophimosis associated with a unique generalized myopathy. *Arch. Ophthalmol. (Chicago)*, **68**:52–57, 1962.
5. Gorlin, R. J., and Cohen, M. M., Jr. Frontometaphyseal dysplasia. A new syndrome. *Am. J. Dis. Child.*, **118**:487–94, 1969.

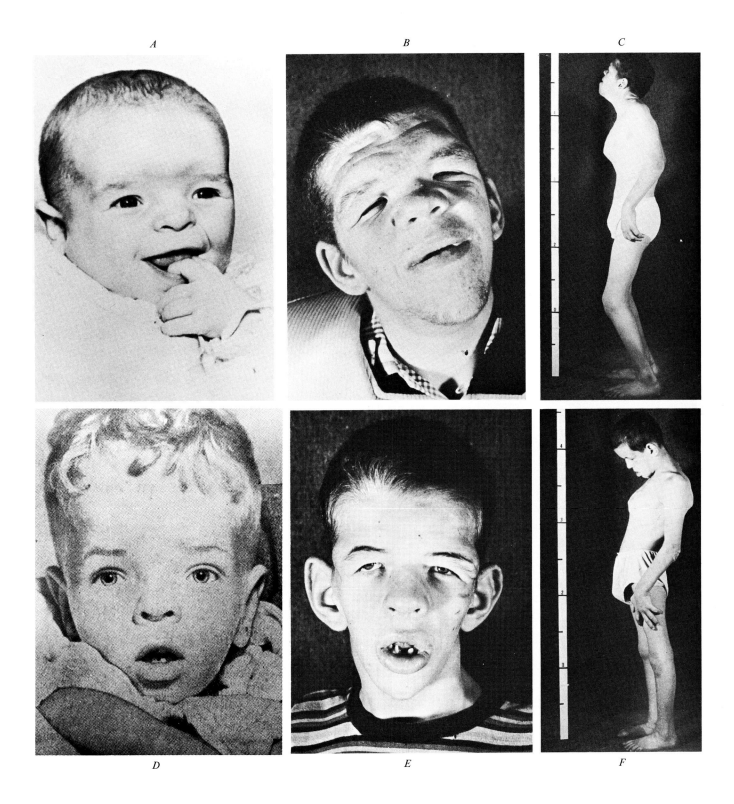

Plate VI-49. *A–C:* Show one patient at 6 months of age and at 18 years. Hypertelorism was evident at both ages. Only when older did he have coarse facial features, large ears, a downward eye slant, and prominent chin and nose. The side view shows the prominence of the lower sternum, the stooped posture, and relatively large hands. *D–F:* The second similar, but unrelated, patient at ages 2 and 15 years. In infancy he had hypertelorism and a rapidly enlarging head. At 15 years he had coarse facial features, pectus carinatum, and large hands. (*A–F:* From G. S. Coffin *et al., Am. J. Dis. Child.,* **112:**205–13, 1966.)

Syndrome of Brain Dysgenesis, Microcephaly, and Skeletal Dysplasia (Cephaloskeletal Dysplasia)

In 1967 Taybi and Linder [1] reported a sister and brother with low birth weight, brain malformations, severe microcephaly, and widespread skeletal abnormalities. This was thought to be a previously undescribed hereditary disorder.

Physical Features

HEAD: Both children had marked microcephaly at birth (head circumference 24.5 cm) (*Figures A and B*).

FACE: The forehead sloped back. The bridge of the nose was flat and the eyes were bulging. The chin was small (*Figure A*).

MOUTH: The boy's palate was highly arched.

LIMBS: Both children had spadelike hands and feet (*Figure A*).

HEIGHT: The girl's length at 1 month of age was 26.5 cm, and the boy's length at 1 year of age was 51 cm.

WEIGHTS: Their birth weights after term gestations were 1125 and 1177 g. The boy at 1 year weighed only 4100 g.

Nervous System

Both children were considered severely retarded.

Pathology

The brains of both children had similar anomalies. They were globular in shape; only the posterior portion of the cerebrum was near normal in size. Gyral abnormalities were evident in all areas (*Figure E*). There was a bilaterally symmetric midline defect involving the parasagittal frontoparietal lobes of the pallidum. The corpus callosum was absent. The lateral ventricles formed one large cavity. The laminar pattern of the cortex was not present. There were numerous islands of heterotopic gray matter scattered through the subcortical white matter. The hippocampus and cerebellum were normal. The costochondral junctions showed irregular alignment of cartilage cells. There was no evidence of bone growth at the metaphysis. There was no cytologic evidence of rickets. The reticuloendothelial cells throughout the body were normal.

Laboratory Studies

The newborn radiograph findings in both children were proportional shortening of all long bones (*Figure F*), irregular metaphyseal margins, concavity of the ends of the short tubular bones in the hands and of the anterior ends of the ribs (*Figure C*), deep intervertebral spaces with a relative decrease in the vertical diameter of the vertebral bodies, and flattening and irregularity of the acetabular roof. X-rays of the boy at 9 and 12 months of age showed severe demineralization of the entire skeleton and indistinct metaphyseal margins (*Figure D*). The boy and two normal siblings had an elevation of urinary acid mucopolysaccharides.

Treatment and Prognosis

The girl died at one month of age and the boy at 12 months.

Differential Diagnosis

In 1971 Neu and coworkers [2] reported three siblings with atrophy of the cerebrum and cerebellum, absent corpus callosum, hypertelorism, micrognathia, congenital flexion deformities, and overlapping fingers. However, they did not have a skeletal dysplasia.

Genetics

Autosomal recessive inheritance is probable as the parents were normal and were first cousins. An earlier deceased sibling of the two patients had had microcephaly, a lumbosacral meningomyelocele, horseshoe kidney deformity, and webbed toes. It was not known if he had the same disorder as the brother and the sister, who were reported in detail.

References

1. Taybi, H., and Linder, D. Congenital familial dwarfism with cephaloskeletal dysplasia. *Radiology,* **89:**275–81, 1967.
2. Neu, R. L., Kajii, T., Gardner, L. I., and Nagyfy, S. F. A lethal syndrome of microcephaly with multiple congenital anomalies in three siblings. *Pediatrics,* **47:**610–12, 1971.

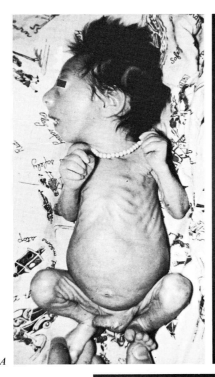

A

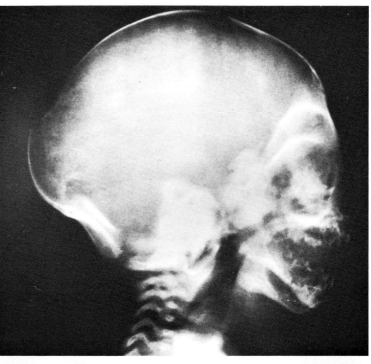

B

Plate VI-50. *A–D:* Show the affected boy with severe microcephaly, bulging eyes, small chin, prominent rib costochondral junctions, and spadelike fingers. His skull x-ray shows open sutures and a small anterior fontanel. The chest x-ray shows cup-shaped costochondral margins. The arm x-ray taken at 12 months shows marked demineralization, indistinct metaphyseal margins, and poor new bone formation along the shaft of the long bones. *E and F:* The brain and x-ray of the girl. The cerebrum shows marked gyral abnormalities. The distal femoral metaphyses are irregular. (*A* and *E:* Courtesy of Dr. H. Taybi, Oakland, Calif. *B–D, F:* From H. Taybi and D. Linder, *Radiology,* **89:**275–81, 1967.)

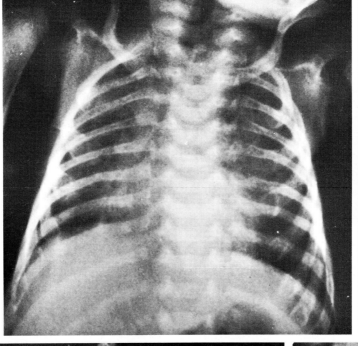

C

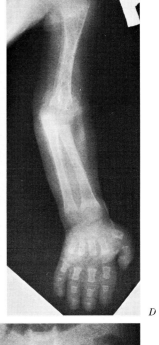

D

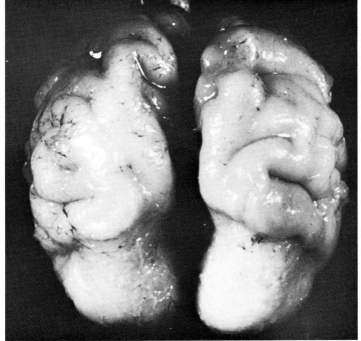

E

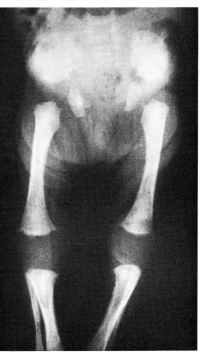

F

Syndrome of Blepharophimosis and Congenital Contractures

In 1966 Marden and Walker [1] reported an infant girl with blepharophimosis and contractures. A second infant, a male, was reported in 1971 [2].

Physical Features

FACE: At birth both had an immobile face, narrow palpebral fissures, depressed nasal bridge, anteverted nostrils, small pursed mouth and small chin (*Figure A*).

EARS: The ears were low-set.

MOUTH: One [1] had a cleft palate and uvula and the other [2] had a highly arched palate.

CHEST: The girl had pectus carinatum. The boy had a shieldlike chest with widely spaced nipples.

BACK: The girl had kyphoscoliosis.

LIMBS: Both infants had marked flexion contractures of the elbows, wrists, hips, knees, and ankles. Arachnodactyly was present only in the girl.

SKIN: The boy had hypertrichosis [2].

WEIGHT: The birth weights were 2600 g [1] and 3550 g [2].

Nervous System

The female infant had decreased deep tendon reflexes and no Moro response [1]. Before her death at 3 months she could not follow objects with her eyes. The boy had thin, hypotonic skeletal muscles and no deep tendon reflexes [2].

Pathology

The girl's brain had a normal appearance; no microscopic studies were performed. The skeletal muscles were atrophic. The kidneys contained microcysts. The inferior vena cava had a common entrance with the superior vena cava into the heart [1]. A muscle biopsy in the boy showed a reduction in the size of scattered muscle fibers [2].

Laboratory Studies

The girl had tall, narrow thoracic and lumbar vertebrae [1]. Pneumoencephalography revealed hypoplasia of the cerebellum and brainstem in the boy [2].

Differential Diagnosis

1. Blepharophimosis and joint stiffness are features of patients with the Schwartz-Jampel syndrome, but they also have myotonia and do not have contractures at birth [3].
2. For a listing of other conditions with congenital contractures see page 78.

References

1. Marden, P. M., and Walker, W. A. A new generalized connective tissue syndrome. Association with multiple congenital anomalies. *Am. J. Dis. Child.*, **112**:225–28, 1966.
2. Fitch, N., Karpati, G., and Pinsky, L. Congenital blepharophimosis, joint contractures, and muscular hypotonia. *Neurology (Minneap.)*, **21**:1214–20, 1971.
3. Mereu, T. R., Porter, I. H., and Hug, G. Myotonia, shortness of stature and hip dysplasia. Schwartz-Jampel syndrome. *Am. J. Dis. Child.*, **117**:470–78, 1969.

Syndrome of Elastic Tissue Deficiency, Corneal Dystrophy, Grimacing, and Mental Retardation

DeBarsy, Moens, and Dierckx [1] in 1968 reported a female infant with a deficient elastic tissue, hypotonia, peculiar movements, and mental retardation. She was thought to represent a new clinical syndrome.

Physical Features

HEAD: Her head size was always below the third percentile.

FACE: As a newborn infant, she looked like an elderly person. Her brow was broad and prominent. Her eyes were widely separated, her palpebral fissures slanted downward, her mouth was small, and her lips were thin (*Figure D*).

EYES: A central opacity was present on each cornea. She had nystagmus when she attempted to fix on an object. The fundi were normal.

EARS: Her ears were low-set and rotated posteriorly (*Figure E*).

SKIN: At 8 days of age her skin was lax and wrinkled, especially in the neck, axillary, and inguinal regions. It was dry, inelastic, and translucent.

HEIGHT AND WEIGHT: She was always below the third percentile of normal in height and weight.

Nervous System

Both mental and motor development were retarded. Muscular hypotonia persisted throughout the first 2 years of life. Her hands were tightly clenched; touching the palm elicited opening of the fist. The deep tendon reflexes were brisk. Starting at about 20 months of age, the child grimaced involuntarily. Later she had abnormal posturing of her body (*Figures D, E, and F*).

Laboratory Studies

Pneumoencephalography showed slight dilatation of the ventricular system and was suggestive of moderate cortical atrophy on one side. The electroencephalogram had a diffuse rapid component, which was considered unusual for the age of 18 months. The anterior fontanel had closed by the age of 22 months, and the bone age was normal. Chromosomal analysis and amino acid screening revealed no abnormalities.

Differential Diagnosis

Patients with cutis laxa, a diffuse elastic tissue disease, may have excessive, inelastic skin at birth. These patients usually have normal intelligence [2].

References

1. DeBarsy, A. M., Moens, E., and Dierckx, L. Dwarfism, oligophrenia and degeneration of the elastic tissue in skin and cornea. A new syndrome? *Helv. Paediatr. Acta*, **23**:305–13, 1968.
2. Goltz, R. W., Hult, A.-M., Goldfarb, M., and Gorlin, R. J. Cutis laxa. A manifestation of generalized elastolysis. *Arch. Dermatol.*, **92**:373–87, 1965.

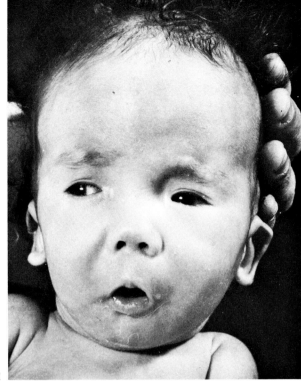

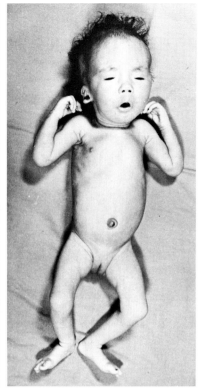

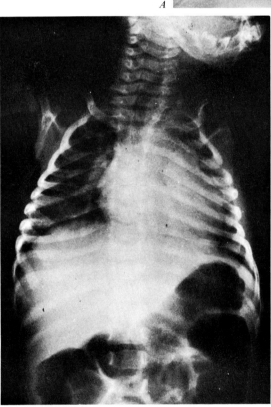

Plate VI-51. *A–C:* A newborn infant with the first of the two syndromes discussed. She had narrow palpebral fissures, a downward palpebral slant, no facial movement, and a small mouth and chin. Less evident in these pictures were the pectus carinatum; contractures of the hips, elbows, and knees; and long, slender digits. The chest x-ray at 10 weeks of age showed a large heart and that the chest was truncated in shape. *D–F:* A 22-month-old infant with the second syndrome. She had facial grimacing and athetoid posturing. Her skin was strikingly lax and she had a prominent brow, hypertelorism, cloudy corneas, and low-set ears. (*A–C:* From P. M. Marden and W. A. Walker, *Am. J. Dis. Child.*, **112:**225–28, 1968. *D–F:* From A. M. deBarsy *et al., Helv. Paediatr. Acta,* **23:**305–13, 1968.)

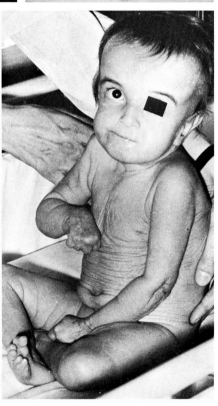

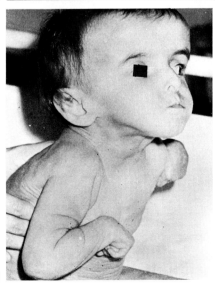

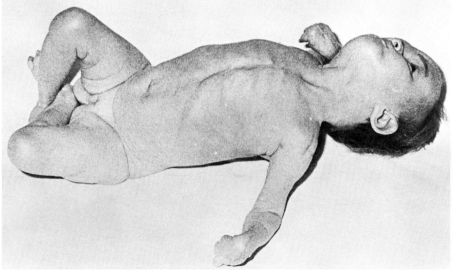

Syndrome of Dyschondroplasia, Facial Anomalies, and Polysyndactyly

In 1969 Opitz, Johnson, McCreadie, and Smith [1] described a sister and brother with a similar pattern of congenital anomalies which was thought to be a new genetic disorder.

Physical Features

HEAD: The male infant had a keel-shaped skull with ridging of the metopic suture (*Figures A, B, and C*). The anterior fontanels were small, but the sutures were open.

FACE: The bridge of the nose of both children was broad and flat. In the boy Brushfield spots, an upward palpebral slant, macrostomia, and micrognathia were noted (*Figure B*).

EARS: The male infant had small pinnae with overfolding of the upper portion of the helix (*Figure C*).

MOUTH: A high-arched palate, thick alveolar ridge and numerous labiogingival frenula were noted in the boy (*Figure B*).

NECK: Both infants had a short neck.

CHEST: Widely spaced nipples, a short sternum, a long xiphisternum, and rib anomalies were described in the male.

GENITALIA: The boy had cryptorchidism.

LIMBS: Both infants had shortening of the arms and legs, genu recurvatum (*Figure A*), postaxial polydactyly of one or both hands, and short digits. The girl had polysyndactyly of the feet. The boy had syndactyly of the feet (*Figure F*), clinodactyly of the index fingers (*Figure E*), and ulnar deviation of the hands.

SKIN: The male infant had marked redundancy of the skin (*Figure D*).

Nervous System

The boy, who survived for 13 weeks, was lethargic and sucked poorly.

Pathology

Autopsy findings in both children were similar and included hepatomegaly, anomalies of the carotid and pulmonary arteries and mesenteric attachment of intestinal tract, patent ductus arteriosus, hypoplastic anterior fossa of the skull with a bone defect over ethmoid sinuses, incomplete development of the tentorium, and extensive fibrosis of the pancreas. In addition, the male infant showed slight platybasia, poor myelinization of the brain, and thin-walled pulmonary arteries.

Laboratory Studies

Skull x-rays of the male showed a bony defect involving the cribriform plate and ethmoid sinus area with complete absence of bone between the inner walls of the orbits superiorly. His chromosomes appeared normal.

Treatment and Prognosis

By the sixth day of life both infants had a serum bilirubin level above 20 mg percent, but the cause was not determined. The girl lived 8 days. The boy died as a result of pneumonia at 13 weeks of age.

Genetics

No other family members had similar anomalies. Autosomal recessive inheritance was presumed.

Differential Diagnosis

1. A flat, broad nose, short limbs, and polysyndactyly are features of patients with Carpenter's syndrome, but they also have craniosynostosis and do not have labiogingival frenula (see page 232).

2. Labiogingival frenula, postaxial polydactyly, and short limbs are features of patients with the Ellis–van Crevald syndrome, but they have dysplastic nails, sparse hair, and cardiac defects, and do not have syndactyly (see page 280).

Reference

1. Opitz, J. M., Johnson, R. C., McCreadie, S. R., and Smith, D. W. The C syndrome of multiple congenital anomalies. *Birth Defects: Original Article Series*, Vol. V, No. 2, February, 1969, pp. 161–66. Williams & Wilkins Co., Baltimore.

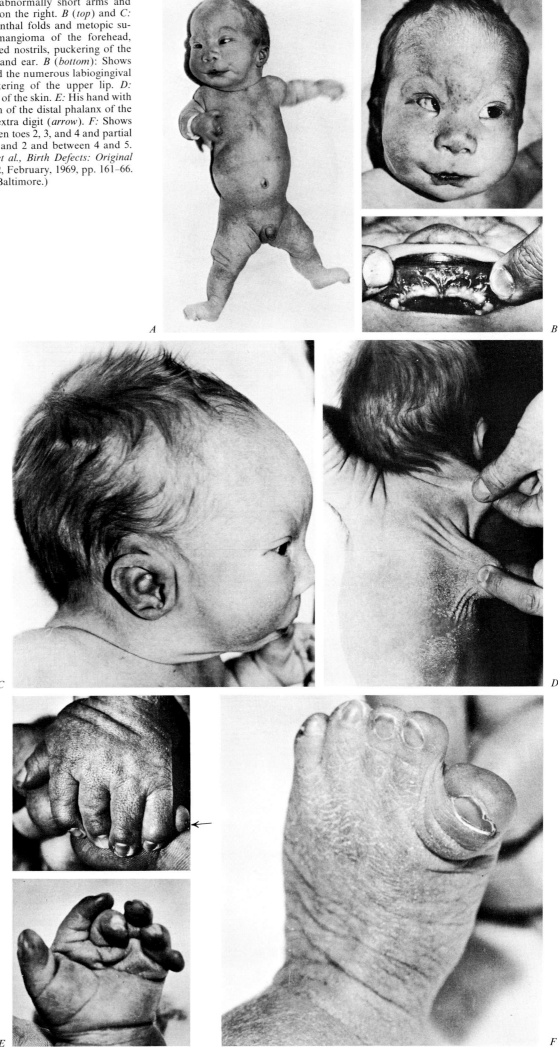

Plate VI-52. *A:* One of the two reported children, at 3 weeks of age. He had abnormally short arms and legs and genu recurvatum on the right. *B* (*top*) and *C:* Show the prominent epicanthal folds and metopic suture, diffuse capillary hemangioma of the forehead, upward eye slant, anteverted nostrils, puckering of the upper lip, and small chin and ear. *B* (*bottom*): Shows the thick alveolar ridge and the numerous labiogingival frenula which cause puckering of the upper lip. *D:* Shows marked redundancy of the skin. *E:* His hand with short digits, ulnar deviation of the distal phalanx of the index finger, and a small extra digit (*arrow*). *F:* Shows complete syndactyly between toes 2, 3, and 4 and partial syndactyly between toes 1 and 2 and between 4 and 5. (*A–F:* From J. M. Opitz *et al., Birth Defects: Original Article Series,* Vol. V, No. 2, February, 1969, pp. 161–66. Williams & Wilkins Co., Baltimore.)

A

B

C

D

E

F

Syndrome of Elbow Contractures, Corneal Opacities, Pointed Nose, and Mental Retardation

In 1966 Mietens and Weber [1] described four siblings with mental retardation and a similar pattern of congenital anomalies. This was thought to be a new hereditary syndrome.

Physical Features

FACE: The prominent features were a small, pointed nose and a depressed bridge of the nose (*Figures A, C, D, and F*).

EYES: Each child had convergent strabismus and corneal opacities, and horizontal and rotary nystagmus were present in all. The corneal opacities were bilateral and produced a diffuse opacification. On slit-lamp examination the opacities appeared to vary in depth in the corneal stroma.

NECK: The shoulders were rounded and the trapezius muscles were prominent (*Figures A and C*).

GENITALIA: The only affected boy had small external genitalia and testes.

LIMBS: Flexion contractures of the elbows were present at birth. Elbow extension was limited to between 70° and 150° in the four children. The forearms were shortened. The only digit anomaly was clinodactyly. One child had congenital dislocation of the hips. The other children held their legs in internal rotation with the knees flexed; the knees could be fully extended by passive movement. The feet were flat and the first metatarsal-phalangeal joint was prominent (*Figure A*).

WEIGHT: One patient had a birth weight of 1300 g after 38 weeks gestation.

HEIGHT: The height was below the tenth percentile of normal.

Nervous System

All four affected members of the family had retarded psychomotor development. The IQ's of the older three patients were estimated to be 70, 81, and 76. The two normal siblings had IQ's of 110 and 117.

Laboratory Studies

X-rays of the arms showed dislocation of the head of the radius and absence of the proximal epiphysis of each radius. Both the radius and the ulna were shorter than normal (*Figures B and E*). X-rays of the skull and lower limbs did not reveal any abnormalities. Chromosomal studies of the father and the affected children showed no abnormalities.

Genetics

As the parents were normal in appearance, but second cousins, autosomal recessive inheritance of a mutant gene was considered likely.

Differential Diagnosis

1. Corneal opacities and a broad bridge of the nose are features of the syndrome of microphthalmos, corneal opacity, mental retardation, and spasticity (see page 250).
2. Limited extension of the elbow due to dislocation of ulnar synostosis of the head of the radius, small testes, and mental retardation are features of males with the XXXY (see page 188) and XXXXY syndromes (see page 190), but they do not have either corneal opacities or a small pointed nose.
3. Four siblings with ocular and facial anomalies and mental retardation were reported by Kaufman and coworkers [2], but they also had microcornea, myopia, an upward eye slant, preauricular skin tags, and micrognathia and did not have corneal opacities or elbow contractures.

References

1. Mietens, C., and Weber, H. A syndrome characterized by corneal opacity, nystagmus, flexion contracture of the elbows, growth failure, and mental retardation. *J. Pediatr.*, **69**:624–29, 1966.
2. Kaufman, R. L., Rimoin, D. L., Prensky, A. L., and Sly, W. S. An oculocerebrofacial syndrome. *Birth Defects: Original Article Series,* Vol. VII, No. 1, February, 1971, pp. 135–38. Williams & Wilkins Co., Baltimore.

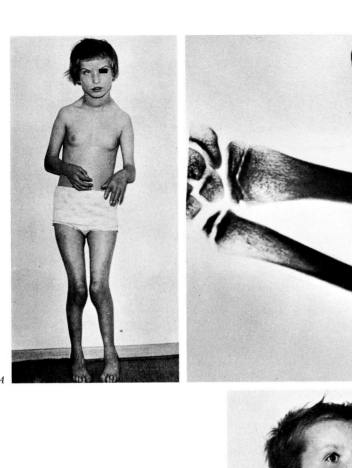

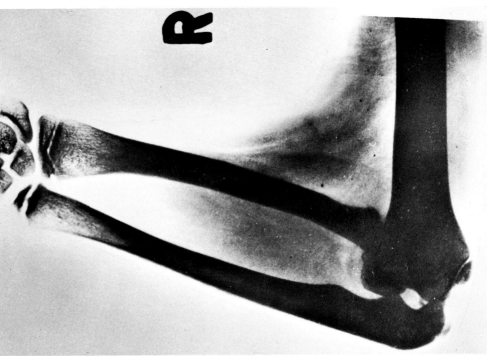

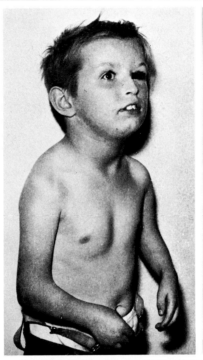

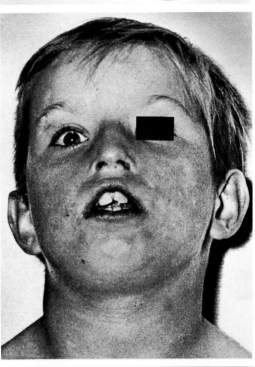

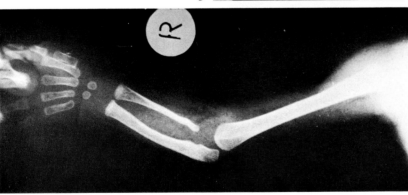

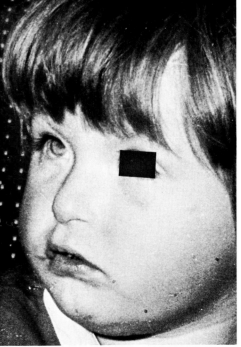

Plate VI-53. *A* and *B:* One of four affected siblings, an 11-year-old girl with a small, pointed nose, convergent strabismus, congenital flexion contractures of her elbows, and bilateral hallux valgus. Her elbow x-ray shows the dislocated head of the radius. She had severe corneal opacities and an IQ of about 70. *C–E:* The 8-year-old brother with a similar facial appearance, corneal opacities, and arm deformities. His x-ray showed absence of the epiphysis in the head of the radius. His IQ was 76. *F:* The youngest affected family member, who has a similar deformity of the tip of her nose. At 5 months of age she had corneal opacities, hypoplasia and dislocation of the proximal radius and dislocation of both hips. (*A* and *C:* From C. Mietens and H. Weber, *J. Pediatr.*, **69:**624–29, 1966. *B, D–F:* Courtesy of Dr. C. Mietens, Würzburg, Germany.)

325

Syndrome of Facial Dysmorphism, Right-Sided Aortic Arch, and Mental Deficiency

In 1968 Strong [1] reported a family in which the mother, two of her daughters, and one son had a peculiar facial appearance, a right-sided aortic arch, and mental deficiency. This was thought to be a new genetic disorder.

Physical Features

HEAD: Two of the children were microcephalic.

FACE: The forehead was broad. The nose was prominent and had a deviated, elongated septum. The mother and the three children all had slight facial asymmetry. The children also had a downward palpebral slant, a flat maxillary area, and a small mouth with downturned corners (*Figures C, D, E, and F*). The mother had a prominent jaw (*Figures A and B*).

EARS: The ears were large and were rotated posteriorly.

HEIGHT AND WEIGHT: The children were between the 10th and 50th percentile of normal in height and weight.

Nervous System

The mother showed psychotic behavior; her IQ was estimated to be 61. All three affected children were thought to have subnormal intelligence, the measured IQ's of the two girls being 86 and 42.

Pathology

Three other siblings had died, but there was no indication that they had the same multiple anomaly syndrome. One premature infant had had the respiratory distress syndrome. A second infant had congenital heart disease and a third had anencephaly.

Laboratory Studies

The right-sided aortic arch was proven at surgery in the boy and by x-ray in the mother and the two girls. All three children had an indentation of the esophagus, which may have been due to a vascular anomaly. Two were thought to have congenital heart disease. Chromosomal studies and urinary amino acid chromatography revealed no abnormalities.

Genetics

Autosomal dominant inheritance is probable in this family.

Differential Diagnosis

A prominent nose, a downward palpebral slant, large posteriorly rotated ears, and microcephaly are features of the Rubinstein-Taybi syndrome, but these patients also have broad thumbs and great toes and short stature (see page 306).

Reference

1. Strong, W. B. Familial syndrome of right-sided aortic arch, mental deficiency, and facial dysmorphism. *J. Pediatr.,* **73**:882–88, 1968.

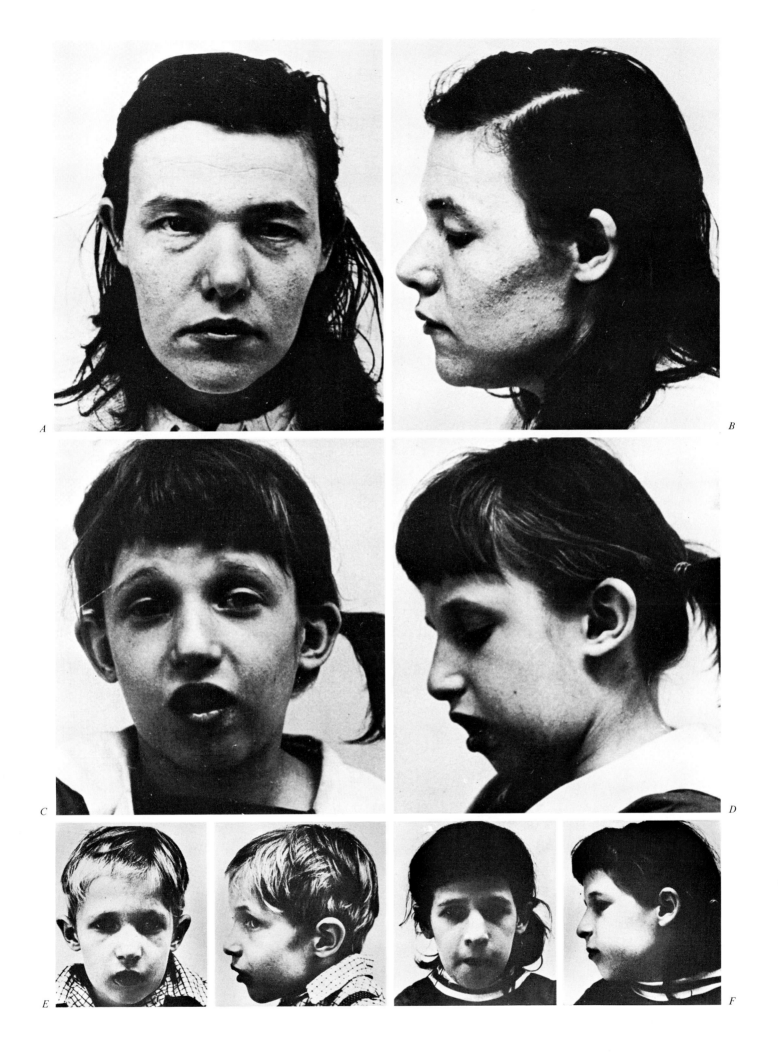

Plate VI-54. *A* and *B:* The mother of the three affected children showing a broad forehead, deviated nasal septum, and facial asymmetry. *C* and *D:* The 8-year-old girl with a beaklike nose, downward palpebral slant, a small mouth, broad forehead, microcephaly, and facial asymmetry. *E* and *F:* The 5-year-old brother and 9-year-old sister of the child above, showing similar facial features. (*A–F:* From W. B. Strong, *J. Pediatr.,* **73:**882–88, 1968.)

327

Syndrome of Malformed, Low-Set Ears and Conductive Hearing Loss

In 1969 Mengel, Konigsmark, Berlin, and McKusick [1] reported six children from two related families who had malformed low-set ears and a conductive hearing loss which was attributed to malformations of the middle ear bones. Three of these patients were also severely retarded. This was thought to be a new genetic disorder.

Physical Features

EARS: All of the patients had deformities of both ears (*Figures A, B, C, D, E, and F*). The mildest was slight overfolding of the helix (*Figure B*) and the most severe was a very small, low-set pinna which was cup-shaped (*Figure F*). An exploratory tympanotomy in one patient showed that only one middle ear ossicle was present; it had the shape of a malleus and was positioned somewhat posteriorly. No incus, stapes, or round window could be seen. It was suggested that middle ear bone malformations were probably responsible for the hearing loss in the other affected children.

MOUTH: Three of the children had a high-arched palate.

GENITALIA: Two of the four affected males had cryptorchidism. All of the males had immature external genitalia, and three also had hypogonadism (*Figure E*).

Nervous System

Three of the six affected children were slow in sitting, walking, and talking. Intelligence tests on four of the patients placed three of them in the severely retarded category and one in the normal range. The degree of retardation could not be correlated with the amount of hearing loss. Neurologic and vestibular examinations were normal in all of the children.

Laboratory Studies

Pure tone audiograms showed four of the children to have a 70- to 80-decibel loss in at least one ear; the other two had more severe losses. Bone conduction testing showed minimally decreased hearing, indicating a conductive loss associated with pathology in the middle ear. Short-increment sensitivity index and recruitment tests were negative, indicating no cochlear damage. Chromosomal studies on two of the males showed no abnormalities.

Treatment and Prognosis

The insertion of a prosthesis in the middle ear of one patient resulted in mild improvement in his hearing.

Genetics

Autosomal recessive. Both families belonged to a Mennonite group in Lancaster County, Pennsylvania, and all of the parents of the affected children could be traced to a common ancestor.

Differential Diagnosis

1. Malformed pinnae and a conductive hearing loss are features of the family described by Wildervanck [2], but their disorder is distinguished by the presence of preauricular tags and pits and its transmission as an autosomal dominant trait.
2. Small pinnae with overfolded helix, conductive hearing loss, and malformed incus and stapes were features of a mother and two sons reported by Wilmot [3], but they were not retarded and did not have hypogonadism. Their disorder was probably due to an autosomal dominant mutant gene.
3. Siblings with microtia, atresia of the external auditory canal, and hearing loss have been reported, but they had normal intelligence and no hypogonadism [4].
4. Ear deformities and a conductive hearing loss are features of patients with the Treacher Collins syndrome, but they also have mandibular and maxillary hypoplasia, a downward palpebral slant, and eyelid colobomas (see page 348).

References

1. Mengel, M. C., Konigsmark, B. W., Berlin, C. I., and McKusick, V. A. Conductive hearing loss and malformed low-set ears, as a possible recessive syndrome. *J. Med. Genet.*, **6**:14–21, 1969.
2. Wildervanck, L. S. Hereditary malformations of the ear in three generations. *Acta Otolaryngol. (Stockh.)*, **54**:553–60, 1962.
3. Wilmot, T. J. Hereditary conductive deafness due to incus-stapes abnormalities and associated with pinnae deformity. *J. Laryngol.*, **84**:469–79, 1970.
4. Ellwood, L. C., Winter, S. T., and Dar, H. Familial microtia with meatal atresia in two sibships. *J. Med. Genet.*, **5**:289–91, 1968.

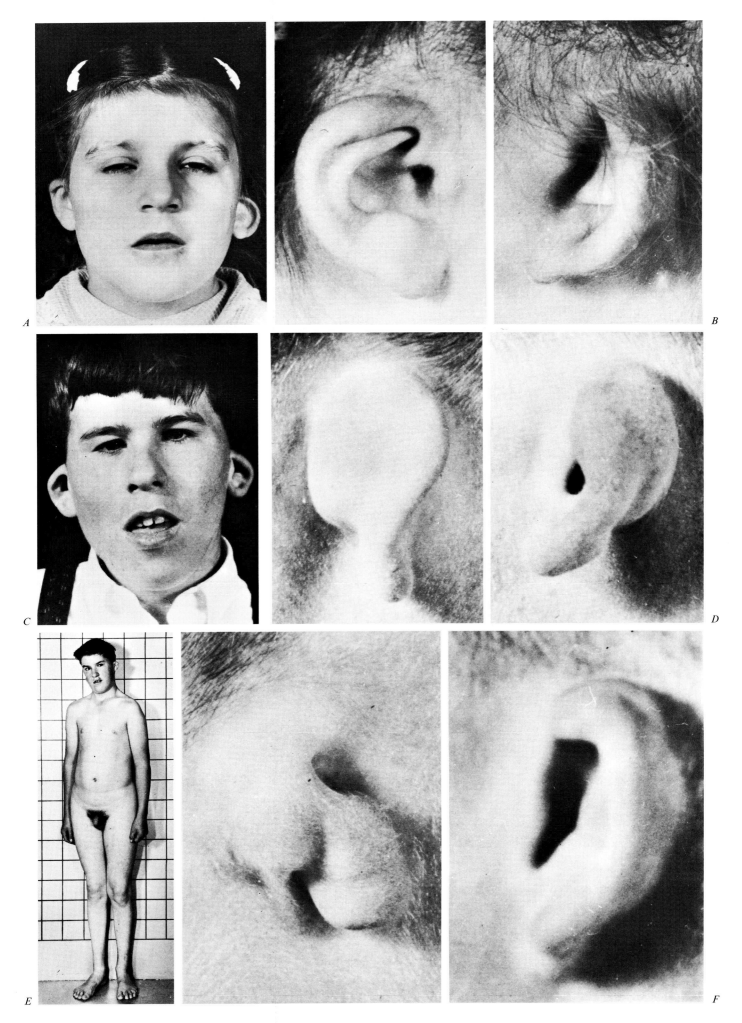

Plate VI-55. *A* and *B:* A 10-year-old girl with malformed ears, one mildly and the other moderately. *C* and *D:* A 6-year-old boy, a distantly related cousin of the first patient, whose ears were small, posteriorly rotated, and had an overfolded upper helix. *E* and *F:* The 18-year-old brother of this boy, who had one very low-set and mal-

formed ear. He was also considered to have hypogonadism. (*A–D* and *F:* From M. C. Mengel *et al., J. Med. Genet.,* **6:**14–21, 1969, by permission of the authors, editor, and publishers. *E:* Courtesy of Dr. B. W. Konigsmark, Baltimore, Md.)

Syndrome of Marked Acceleration of Skeletal Maturation and Facial Anomalies

In 1971 Marshall, Graham, Scott, and Smith [1] reported two unrelated male infants with a syndrome characterized by unusual facial features, relative failure to thrive, and marked acceleration of osseous maturation. This was considered a new clinical entity.

Physical Features

HEAD: One boy had an increased anteroposterior skull diameter (*Figure E*).

FACE: Both boys had bulging eyes, coarse eyebrows, and a turned-up nose (*Figures A and D*).

EYES: Both had blue sclerae.

ABDOMEN: Both had a small umbilical hernia.

LIMBS: By age 10 months one boy had developed a flexion contracture of the distal phalanx of his left fifth finger.

HEIGHT: Their lengths at birth were 50 and 63 cm.

WEIGHT: Their birth weights were 3300 and 4500 g. They were always underweight for their length, although one boy gained weight within the 50th percentile.

Nervous System

Each child had delayed mental and motor development and was considered mentally retarded.

Pathology

One boy died suddenly at 20 months of age. The autopsy showed hemorrhagic pneumonia and broad convolutions in the occipital-parietal area suggestive of pachygyria.

Laboratory Studies

Skull x-rays showed a prominent calvarium, shallow orbits, small facial bones, and a hypoplastic mandible in each boy (*Figures B and E*). The tubular bones were long and had thin cortices (*Figure F*). The most striking x-ray change was the acceleration of skeletal maturation. Each boy at the chronologic age of 3 to 6 months had a bone age by hand and wrist standards of 3 to 6 years (*Figures C and F*). Also, the middle phalanges of the fingers were widened and the distal phalanges were quite narrow. Each boy had a mild thoracolumbar scoliosis. Studies of thyroid function, urinary steroids and mucopolysaccharides, serum calcium, phosphorus and alkaline phosphatase, urinary and blood amino acids, and a rectal biopsy showed no abnormalities.

Treatment and Prognosis

Both boys had noisy respirations and recurrent respiratory infections. Each had feeding problems and relative failure to thrive.

Genetics

Neither boy had any similarly affected relatives.

Differential Diagnosis

Acceleration of skeletal maturation and a short, upturned nose are features of patients with the syndrome of peripheral dysostosis, nose hypoplasia, and mental retardation, but they have short stature at birth and a more generalized abnormality of the epiphyses, phalanges, metacarpals, and metatarsals (see page 268).

Reference

1. Marshall, R. E., Graham, C. B., Scott, C. R., and Smith, D. W. Syndrome of accelerated skeletal maturation and relative failure to thrive: a newly recognized clinical growth disorder. *J. Pediatr.*, **78**:95–101, 1971.

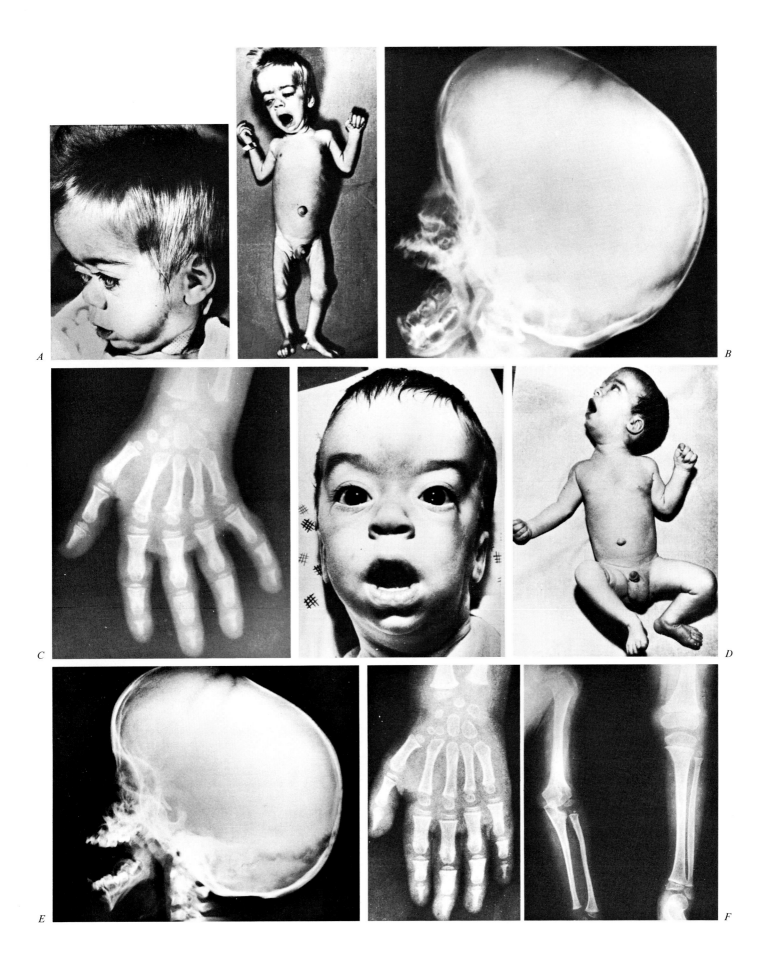

Plate VI-56. *A–C:* One boy at age 6 months showing bulging eyes, bushy eyebrows, and a low nasal bridge. His skull x-ray at 9 months shows a prominent frontal region. His left hand and wrist at age 16 months have a bone age of 6 years. *D–F:* The other boy at 7 months of age with a similar facial appearance. His skull x-ray at 11 months also shows a prominent frontal calvarium and shallow orbits. At 10 months his bone age was 6–7 years. At 11 months his tubular bones were long and had thin cortices. (*A–F:* From R. E. Marshall *et al.*, *J. Pediatr.*, **78:**95–101, 1971.)

Syndrome of Microcephaly, Peculiar Appearance, Spasticity, and Choreoathetosis

In 1968 Hooft, de Hauwere, and van Acker [1] described three siblings with microcephaly, a peculiar facial appearance, spasticity, choreoathetosis, and mental retardation.

Physical Features

HEAD: At the age of 4 months the head size of one infant was at the third percentile of normal. All three children had little increase in head size as they grew older. As a result, the microcephaly became more striking with increasing age.

FACE: The nose was prominent and the chin was retrognathic. Each of the children had epicanthal folds and strabismus. The eyes appeared to be widely spaced (*Figures A and B*).

EARS: The ears were large (*Figures A and B*).

LIMBS: The fingers were spindle-shaped.

Nervous System

All three children had severe mental retardation. Hypotonia, especially of the neck and back muscles, was the predominant feature in the first months of life. Hyperreflexia and spasticity were noted as early as 4 months of age. Choreoathetosis of the limbs and involuntary trunk movements occurred later, at about 2 to 3 years of age.

Pathology

Brain biopsies from each child showed similar mild histologic abnormalities in the white matter. There was slight pallor of the subcortical and laminar intracortical myelin system and acid-Schiff positive material in the molecular layer.

Laboratory Studies

Electroencephalograms showed a seizure pattern in one child. Skull x-rays revealed closure of the sutures and fontanels in two of the children when they were 4 and 7 months of age. The cranium was shortened in all directions. Amino acid, chromosome, and mucopolysaccharide screening tests revealed no abnormalities.

Genetics

The fact that three siblings were affected and the parents were normal is suggestive of autosomal recessive inheritance.

Differential Diagnosis

"True" or "pure" microcephaly is often associated with spasticity and is inherited as an autosomal recessive trait, but there is no associated choreoathetosis (see page 196).

Reference

1. Hooft, C., de Hauwere, R., and van Acker, K. J. Familial non-congenital microcephaly, peculiar appearance, mental and motor retardation, progressive evolution to spasticity and choreo-athetosis. *Helv. Paediatr. Acta,* **23**:1–12, 1968.

Syndrome of Cryptorchidism, Chest Deformities, Contractures, and Arachnodactyly

In 1970 van Benthem, Driessen, Haneveld, and Rietema [1] described three brothers with an apparently new syndrome of multiple deformities and severe mental retardation.

Physical Features

HEAD: All three boys had a long anteroposterior skull diameter (*Figure C*).

EARS: Each boy had ears of unequal size.

MOUTH: Two boys had a highly arched palate.

CHEST: A chest and sternal deformity became evident in the first year of life (*Figure C*).

GENITALIA: The testes of two of the boys were not palpable (*Figure D*). One also had hypospadias.

BACK: Each boy had kyphoscoliosis (*Figure E*).

LIMBS: All three had arachnodactyly. Two were noted to have contractures of the knees (*Figure C*).

SKIN: The subcutaneous tissue was absent or hypoplastic.

HEIGHT AND WEIGHT: One boy (Case 2) at age 10 years 9 months had a height of 124 cm and weight of 15.4 kg, both well below the third percentile.

Nervous System

Their neurologic abnormalities included muscular hypotonia, generalized muscular hypoplasia, convergent squint, a high-pitched squeaky voice, and slow psychomotor development. The 10-year-9-month-old was able to roll from side to side and sit with support; his IQ was 46.

Pathology

One boy (Case 3) had almost no subcutaneous fat tissue, pale and atrophic musculature, thin bronchi with deficient cartilaginous rings, and no testes. The longest surviving patient (Case 2), and the only one on whom neuropathologic information was available, had megalencephaly [2].

Laboratory Studies

One boy (Case 2) had a hypoplastic left main bronchus (*Figure F*). Chromosomal karyotype, urinary amino acid chromatography, urinary 17-ketosteroid levels, and protein-bound iodine in this boy showed no abnormalities.

Treatment and Prognosis

Each had recurrent atelectasis and pneumonia. They died at 8 months, 4½ years, and over 11 years of age [2].

Genetics

Not known. Either autosomal or X-linked recessive inheritance is possible.

Differential Diagnosis

1. Arachnodactyly, contractures, kyphoscoliosis, and a deformed chest were features of the child with the syndrome of blepharophimosis and congenital contractures, but she had blepharophimosis and an immobile face (see page 320).
2. Diseases characterized by congenital contractures are listed on page 320.

References

1. van Benthem, L. H. B. M., Driessen, O., Haneveld, G. T., and Rietema, H. P. Cryptorchidism, chest deformities, and other congenital anomalies in three brothers. *Arch. Dis. Child.,* **45**:590–92, 1970.
2. van Benthem, L. H. B. M. Personal communication, 1970.

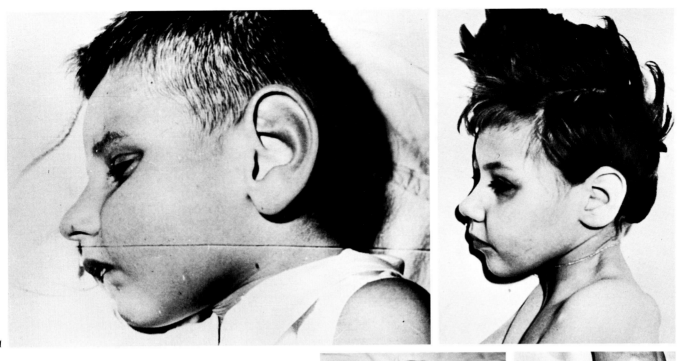

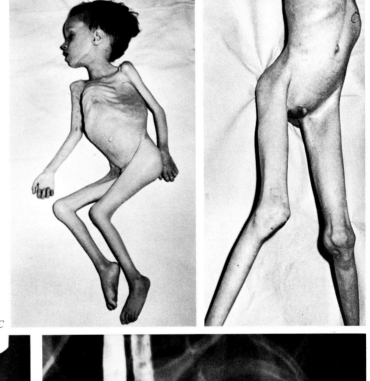

Plate VI-57. *A:* Shows microcephaly in the oldest of three affected siblings at 21 months. *B:* The second child at 5 years of age. Both she and her older brother had a prominent chin and backward sloping forehead. *C* and *D:* A $10\frac{3}{4}$-year-old boy (Case 2) with the second syndrome, showing his dolichocephaly, flattened and deformed chest, contracted knees, and cryptorchidism. *E:* His x-ray at 8 years showing scoliosis. *F:* A bronchogram at this age showing a long, hypoplastic left main bronchus. (*A* and *B:* From C. Hooft *et al., Helv. Paediatr. Acta,* **23:**1–12, 1968. *C:* From L. H. B. M. van Benthem *et al., Arch. Dis. Child.,* **45:**590–92, 1970. *D–F:* Courtesy of Dr. L. H. B. M. van Benthem, Heemskerk, The Netherlands.)

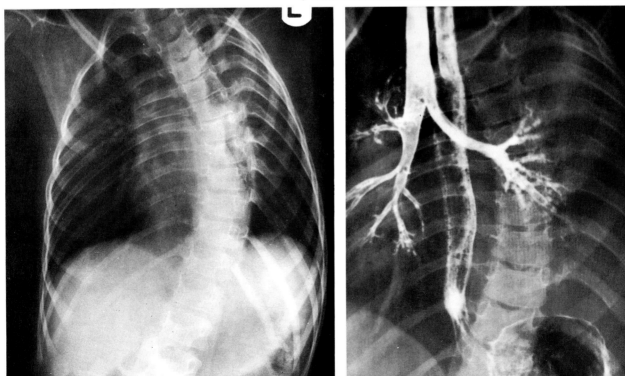

Syndrome of Microcephaly, Snub Nose, Livedo Reticularis, and Low-Birth-Weight Dwarfism

In 1971 Christian, Johnson, Biegel, Gresham, and Rosenberg [1] reported two sisters with low-birth-weight dwarfism and physical abnormalities including microcephaly, a snub nose, and livedo reticularis. This was thought to be a new genetic disorder.

Physical Features

HEAD: Both girls were microcephalic.

FACE: The striking facial feature was a short, broad, up-turned nose (*Figures A and B*).

EYES: At 4 years 8 months the older girl had coarse salt-and-pepper pigmentation of the retina.

LIMBS: Both girls had short tapering fingers, clinodactyly of the fifth finger, and calcaneovalgus foot deformities (*Figures A and B*).

DERMATOGLYPHICS: Both had distal axial triradii on the palms, a low digital ridge count and single fifth finger flexible crease. One girl had bilateral transverse palmar creases.

SKIN: Both girls had livedo reticularis in infancy (*Figure A*).

HEIGHT: Their heights were always well below the third percentile of normal.

WEIGHT: Both had birth weights of 1800 g.

Nervous System

The older girl's IQ at 4 years 8 months was 58; the IQ of the younger girl at 14 months was estimated to be 32 [2].

Pathology

The younger girl died suddenly at 21 months. Her thymus and lymph nodes were normal. The brain was small, but was normal except for one localized heterotopia.

Laboratory Studies

Both children had repeated infections in association with deficient humoral antibody production and delayed type hypersensitivity. Each girl consistently had elevated IgA levels for her age; the younger girl initially had low IgG levels. Both girls had a retarded bone age. Chromosome, amino acid, and urine mucopolysaccharide screening tests showed no abnormalities.

Genetics

Autosomal recessive inheritance was postulated.

Differential Diagnosis

1. Snub-nosed dwarfism, as discussed by Black [3], may be inherited as either a dominant or a recessive trait. In each type there is also a low birth weight, but only in the recessive type is the intelligence below normal.
2. Microcephaly, a short nose with anteverted nostrils, and short stature are features of patients with the Smith-Lemli-Opitz syndrome, but they often have a broad alveolar ridge, a wide medial canthus and ptosis, and do not have livedo reticularis (see page 312).

References

1. Christian, J. C., Johnson, V. P., Biegel, A. A., Gresham, E. L., and Rosenberg, G. J. Sisters with low birth weight, dwarfism, congenital anomalies, and dysgammaglobulinemia. *Am. J. Dis. Child.*, **122**:529–34, 1971.
2. Black, J. Low-birth-weight dwarfism. *Arch. Dis. Child.*, **36**:633–44, 1961.

Syndrome of Micromelia and Coarse Facial Features

In 1971 Rudiger, Schmidt, Loose, and Passarge described a brother and sister with coarse facial features, short extremities and digits, cleft soft palate, and a hoarse voice. They considered this a new genetic disorder.

Physical Features

FACE: Both children had a flat nasal bridge, stubby nose, epicanthal folds, and large mouth (*Figures C, D, and E*).

MOUTH: The boy had a cleft soft palate and uvula and the girl a cleft uvula.

NECK: Both children had a deep and hoarse cry.

EARS: There was no palpable cartilage in the external ears.

ABDOMEN: The boy had huge inguinal hernias (*Figure C*).

GENITALIA: His penis was short.

LIMBS: The limbs, hands, feet, fingers, and toes were shortened. The nails were very small. There were slight flexion contractures in the palms.

DERMATOGLYPHICS: Both children had transverse palmar creases and deep palmar skin folds.

HEIGHT: The boy's length at birth was 52 cm and at 4 months was 64 cm. The girl was 48 cm long at birth and 58 cm at 5 months.

WEIGHT: Their birth weights were normal.

Nervous System

Neither child showed any psychomotor development. The girl had myoclonic seizures.

Pathology

Both children had hydronephrosis and hydroureters. The ureterovesical junctions were stenotic due to muscular hypertrophy. The girl had a bicornuate uterus and ovaries with multiple cysts. The brains and bones showed no abnormalities.

Laboratory Studies

X-rays showed hypoplastic middle and distal phalanges in the fingers and no ossification of middle and distal phalanges of the toes (*Figure F*). Tests of thyroid function and chromosomal studies showed no abnormalities.

Treatment and Prognosis

Both children died at 5 months of age from pneumonia and respiratory insufficiency.

Genetics

Autosomal recessive inheritance was postulated.

Differential Diagnosis

1. Coarse facial features, short fingers and toes, small nails, and short stature are also features of the three children with the syndrome of absent fifth fingernails and toenails, short distal phalanges, and lax joints (see page 314).
2. Coarse facial features, a hoarse cry, and short limbs are features of infants with congenital hypothyroidism (see page 10).

Reference

1. Rudiger, R. A., Schmidt, W., Loose, D. A., and Passarge, E. Severe developmental failure with coarse facial features, distal limb hypoplasia, thickened palmar creases, bifid uvula, and ureteral stenosis: a previously unidentified familial disorder with lethal outcome *J. Pediatr.*, **79**:977–81, 1971.

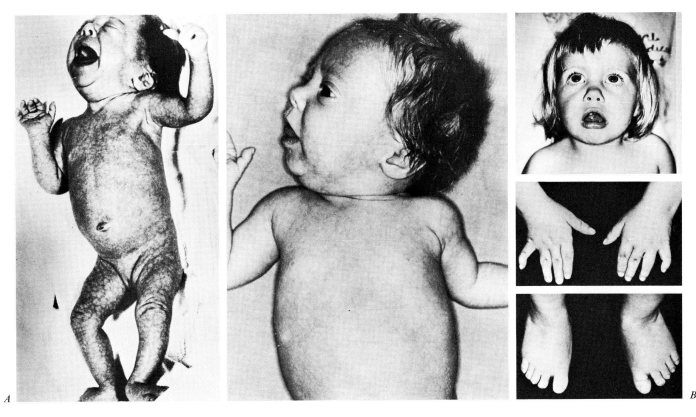

Plate VI-58. *A:* Shows in the younger girl the snub nose, calcaneo-valgus deformity, and livedo reticularis. *B:* The older girl with a snub nose, tapering fingers, and clinodactyly. *C* and *D:* Shows the coarse facial features and the large inguinal hernias in the boy with the second syndrome. *E:* His sister. *F:* Her x-rays showing shortened long bones and distal phalanges of the fingers and no ossification of the middle and distal phalanges of the toes. (*A* [*left*] and *B* [*bottom*]: From J. C. Christian *et al., Am. J. Dis. Child.,* **122:**529–34, 1971. *A* [*right*] and *B* [*top* and *middle*]: Courtesy of Dr. J. C. Christian, Indianapolis, Ind. *C, E* and *F* [*left*]: Courtesy of Dr. E. Passarge, Hamburg, Germany. *D, F* [*bottom* and *right*]: From R. A. Rudiger, *et al., J. Pediatr.,* **79:**977–81, 1971.)

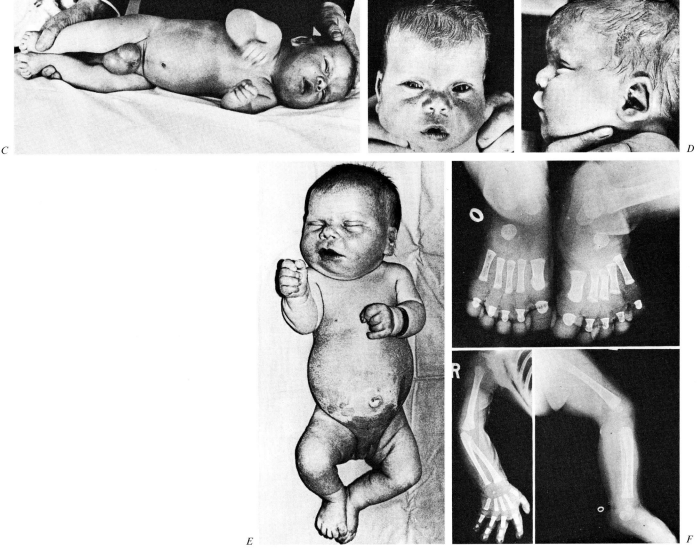

Syndrome of Micrognathia, Malformed Ears, Clubfoot, and Flexion Deformities (Pseudotrisomy 18)

At least six children have been described [1–5] who have the multiple anomalies that are considered typical of patients with chromosome 18 trisomy. At first the fact that these children had no demonstrable chromosomal abnormality was attributed to failure to detect the cell line with either trisomy 18 or duplication of part of a number 18 chromosome. However, extensive examinations have failed to reveal any chromosomal abnormality. Instead, a single mutant gene with autosomal recessive inheritance has been suggested as the cause, as three of the reported patients had a similarly affected sibling [2,4,*5].

Physical Features

HEAD: Three patients had either a prominent occiput or an elongated skull [1,2,4].

FACE: Five of the reported patients [1–5] had a small chin and either low-set or malformed ears (*Figures B, D, and E*).

NECK: Webbing of the neck was present in three patients [4,5] (*Figure F*).

CHEST: Three had either a short sternum or a shieldlike chest [4,5].

LIMBS: Four patients had flexion deformities of the fingers [1–4] (*Figure A*); two had flexion deformities of the knees [5]. Four patients had a clubfoot deformity [1,3,5].

DERMATOGLYPHICS: Two out of three patients examined had an increased number of digital arches [2–4].

Nervous System

All of the patients were retarded. Three had depressed Moro and suck reflexes and muscular hypotonia [4,5]. One patient had generalized muscular hypertonicity [2].

*Patient SC 120766/3465.

Pathology

Four patients had cardiac anomalies [1,2,5]. Three had genitourinary malformations [4,5].

Treatment and Prognosis

Two of the patients died within the first week of life [5]; one died at 3 months of age [4]; another patient died at 5 months of age [2].

Laboratory Studies

Chromosomal analysis was done on venous blood from all of the patients, on skin fibroblasts from two patients [3,5], and on both fibroblasts and bone marrow from one patient [2]. In none of these patients was there evidence of either 18 trisomy or translocation of extra chromosomal material.

Genetics

Autosomal recessive.

Differential Diagnosis

The same anomalies observed in these patients are also features of patients with chromosome 18 trisomy (see page 156).

References

1. Burks, J. L., and Sinkford, S. Clinical trisomy E syndrome (16–18): a cytogenetic enigma. *Clin. Pediatr. (Phila.)*, **3:**233–35, 1964.
2. Hook, E. B., and Yunis, J. J. Trisomy 18 syndrome in a patient with normal karyotype. *J.A.M.A.*, **193:**840–43, 1965.
3. deGrouchy, J. Chromosome 18: a topologic approach. *J. Pediatr.*, **66:**414–31, 1965.
4. Taylor, A. I. Autosomal trisomy syndromes. A detailed study of 27 cases of Edwards' syndrome and 27 cases of Patau's syndrome. *J. Med. Genet.*, **5:**227–52, 1968.
5. Simpson, J. L., and German, J. Developmental anomaly resembling the trisomy 18 syndrome. *Ann. Genet. (Paris)*, **12:**107–10, 1969.

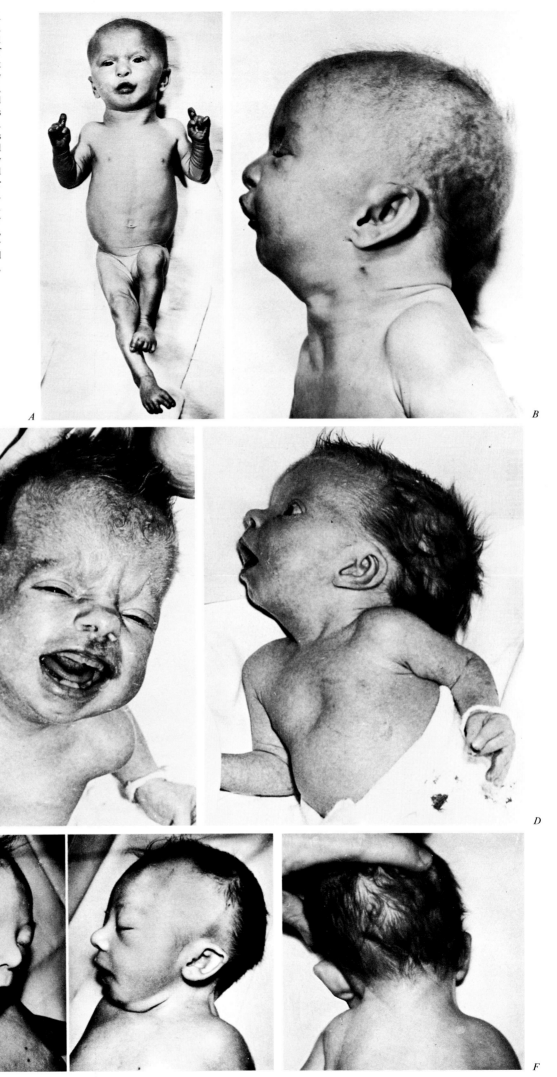

Plate VI-59. *A* and *B:* A 3-month-old female with a small chin, posteriorly rotated ears, and flexion deformities of her fingers. *C* and *D:* An infant with hypertelorism, a capillary hemangioma on the upper lip, small chin, posteriorly rotated ears, elongated skull, pectus excavatum, and webbed neck. *E* and *F:* Postmortem pictures of a 2-day-old male with a small chin, webbed neck, posteriorly rotated ears with overfolded helix, and a transverse palmar crease. (*A* and *B:* From E. B. Hook and J. J. Yunis, *J.A.M.A.,* **93:**840–43, 1965. *C* and *D:* Courtesy of Dr. A. I. Taylor, London, England. *E* and *F:* From J. L. Simpson and J. German, *Ann. Genet.,* **12:**107–10, 1969.)

A

B

C

D

E

F

Syndrome of Oral, Cranial, and Digital Anomalies

In 1969 Juberg and Hayward [1] described a sibship of six children in which five had anomalies of the oral cavity, cranium, and extremities. Two boys were severely affected, while three girls had similar, but fewer and less severe, anomalies. This was thought to represent a new genetic disorder.

Physical Features

HEAD: The head circumference of three of the children was below the third percentile of normal.

FACE: The two boys had a cleft lip (one unilateral, one bilateral) in association with a broad nasal bridge, a hypoplastic columella nasi, and deformed external nares (*Figures A and C*). One girl had an occult cleft lip and asymmetry of the external nares. She also had widely spaced eyes (*Figure E*).

MOUTH: Each boy had a cleft palate.

LIMBS: The boys had hypoplastic, inflexible, and distally placed thumbs (*Figure B*), and their forearms could not be completely extended. One of the girls was unable to flex her thumbs (*Figure F*). Four of the six children had minimal syndactyly of the second and third toes and medial curvature of the fourth toes (*Figure D*).

HEIGHT: Both boys were below the third percentile.

WEIGHT: Both boys and one of the girls weighed less than 2.4 kg at birth. When older, their weights were below the third percentile.

Nervous System

Two of the children had formal intelligence testing. One boy scored IQ's of 86 and 92 on two different tests and one girl, who had considerable difficulty with school work, had an IQ of 75 at age 11½ years [2].

Laboratory Studies

X-rays of the boys showed that the first metacarpals were small and the radius dislocated. One boy had a horseshoe kidney. Chromosomal studies of the parents and the boys showed no abnormalities.

Genetics

This syndrome was considered to be most likely due to an autosomal recessive mutant gene.

Differential Diagnosis

1. Cleft lip and palate, broad nasal bridge, syndactyly of toes 2–3, and renal anomalies were features of the two girls with the syndrome of hypertelorism, microtia, and facial clefting reported by Bixler and coworkers [3].
2. Cleft lip and palate and digital anomalies are features of patients with the popliteal pterygium syndrome, but they also have pterygia of the joints, hypoplasia of the external genitalia, and nail dysplasia [4].
3. A cleft lip and palate and various digit anomalies are features of patients with the oral-facial-digital (OFD I) syndrome, but they have a median cleft lip and numerous oral anomalies, and are usually females (see page 300).

References

1. Juberg, R. C., and Hayward, J. R. A new familial syndrome of oral, cranial, and digital anomalies. *J. Pediatr.,* **74**:755–62, 1969.
2. Hayward, J. R. Personal communication, 1969.
3. Bixler, D., Christian, J. C., and Gorlin, R. J. Hypertelorism, microtia and facial clefting. A newly described inherited syndrome. *Am. J. Dis. Child.,* **118**:495–500, 1969.
4. Hecht, F., and Jarvinen, J. M. Heritable dysmorphic syndrome with normal intelligence. *J. Pediatr.,* **70**:927–35, 1967.

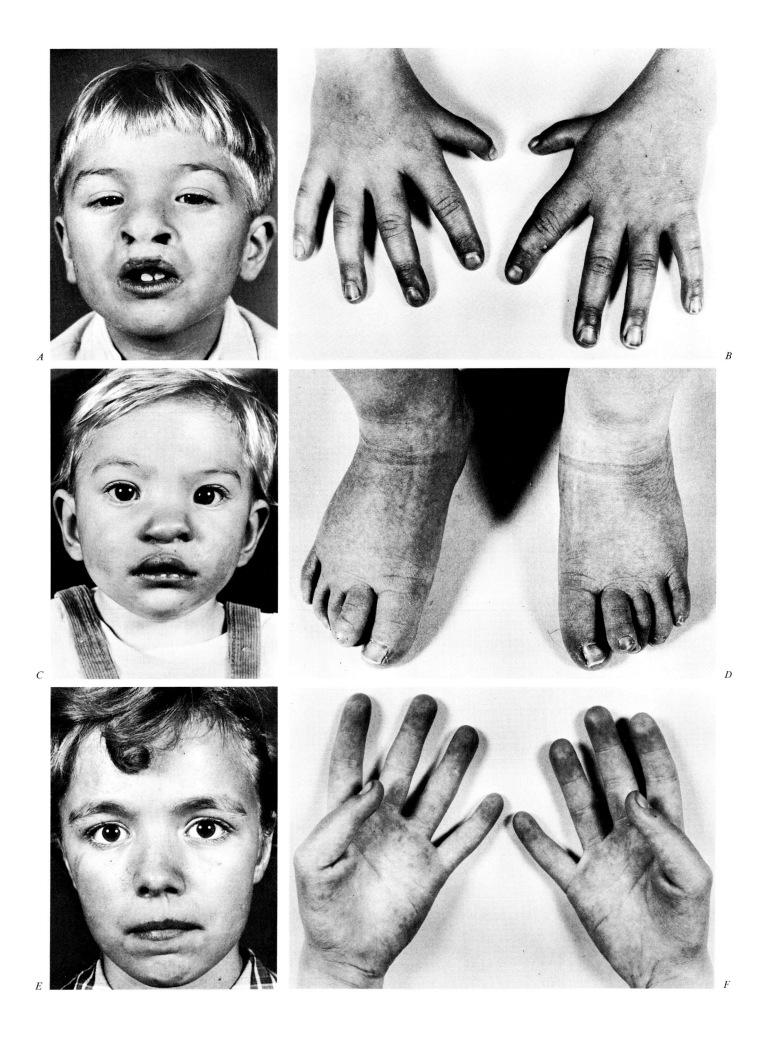

Plate VI-60. *A* and *B:* A 5-year-old boy with a repaired bilateral cleft lip, deformed tip of the nose, and broad nasal bridge. Both thumbs were small and distally placed. *C* and *D:* A 1⅓-year-old boy who had a unilateral cleft lip and palate, broad bridge of the nose, and medial deviation of toes 3 and 4. *E:* A girl with a left occult cleft lip and hypertelorism. *F:* The hands of another girl. Her thumbs had no interphalangeal flexibility. (*A–F:* From R. C. Juberg and J. R. Hayward, *J. Pediatr.,* **74:**755–62, 1969.)

339

Syndrome of Phocomelia, Flexion Deformities, and Facial Anomalies

In 1969 Herrmann, Feingold, Tuffli, and Opitz [1] described four children in two unrelated families with limb deformities, facial and eye anomalies, and silvery-blond hair. They noted two additional patients [2,3] described in 1906 and 1921. They considered this a new genetic disorder.

Physical Features

HEAD: All of the patients were microcephalic.

FACE: A downward palpebral slant, flat supraorbital ridges, and small chin were noted in the recently described patients [1]. Some also had hypoplastic cartilage in the tip of the nose (*Figures A and E*).

EYES: Three patients had cloudy corneas [1,2]; one also had microphthalmia [1].

EARS: The ear cartilage was considered hypoplastic in a brother and sister [1].

MOUTH: A highly arched palate was present in several patients. Two had a cleft lip and palate [1,3].

GENITALIA: Two brothers had congenital absence of the foreskin [3].

LIMBS: All patients had symmetric reductive malformations of the limbs. The upper arm limb deformities included phocomelia with the carpals articulating with the scapula [3], absence of the forearm bones and only a small portion of the humerus (*Figures B and C*), and shortening of the arm with radiohumeral synostosis (*Figure D*). Whenever the radius was small or absent, the thumb was also absent (*Figures C and F*). Patients with no ulna had either no fifth finger or a short, curved fifth finger (*Figure C*). The lower limb deformities included calcaneovalgus clubfoot with absent fibula and curved tibia (*Figure B*), absent tibia and fibula, articulation of the tarsals with the femurs, and weight bearing on the distal femoral condyles [3]. Flexion contractures were often present in the elbows, hips, and knees [1–3].

SKIN: Four of the infants had capillary hemangiomas on the face, ears, and neck.

HAIR: Three patients had fine, silvery-blond hair (*Figures A and E*).

HEIGHT: The height of all patients was well below the third percentile.

WEIGHT: The birth weights of three term infants were 1350, 1520, and 2100 g. The gestations of the first and third of these were estimated to be 42 and 43 weeks.

GROWTH AND DEVELOPMENT: The only adult had normal sexual maturation [3].

Nervous System

Three patients [1,3] were considered mentally retarded.

Pathology

In two brief autopsy summaries no cerebral or visceral malformations were noted [1,2].

Laboratory Studies

X-rays showed numerous skeletal malformations, primarily in the limbs; the clavicles and scapulae were small and malformed. Chromosomal studies on three patients showed no abnormalities.

Treatment and Prognosis

Two infants were stillborn [1,3], and one apparently died shortly after birth [2]. The oldest patient was 29 years old [3].

Genetics

Autosomal recessive inheritance seems likely, since siblings were affected in three families [1,3] and the parents were first cousins in one family [3].

Differential Diagnosis

1. Infants with the syndrome of tetraphocomelia, cleft lip and palate, and genital hypertrophy have more severe limb deformities and abnormal external genitalia (see page 344).
2. Reductive limb malformations and capillary hemangiomas are features of infants with thalidomide embryopathy, but they usually have asymmetric limb anomalies and do not have cleft lip, flexion contractures, cloudy corneas, or silvery-blond hair (see page 132).

References

1. Herrmann, J., Feingold, M., Tuffli, G. A., and Opitz, J. M. A familial dysmorphogenetic syndrome of limb deformities, characteristic facial appearance and associated anomalies: the "pseudothalidomide" or "SC-syndrome." *Birth Defects: Original Article Series*, Vol. V, No. 3, March, 1969, pp. 81–89. Williams & Wilkins Co., Baltimore.
2. Krueger, R. *Die Phocomelie.* August Hirschwald Verlag, Berlin, 1906.
3. O'Brien, H. R., and Mustard, H. S. An adult living case of total phocomelia. *J.A.M.A.*, **77**:1964–67, 1921.

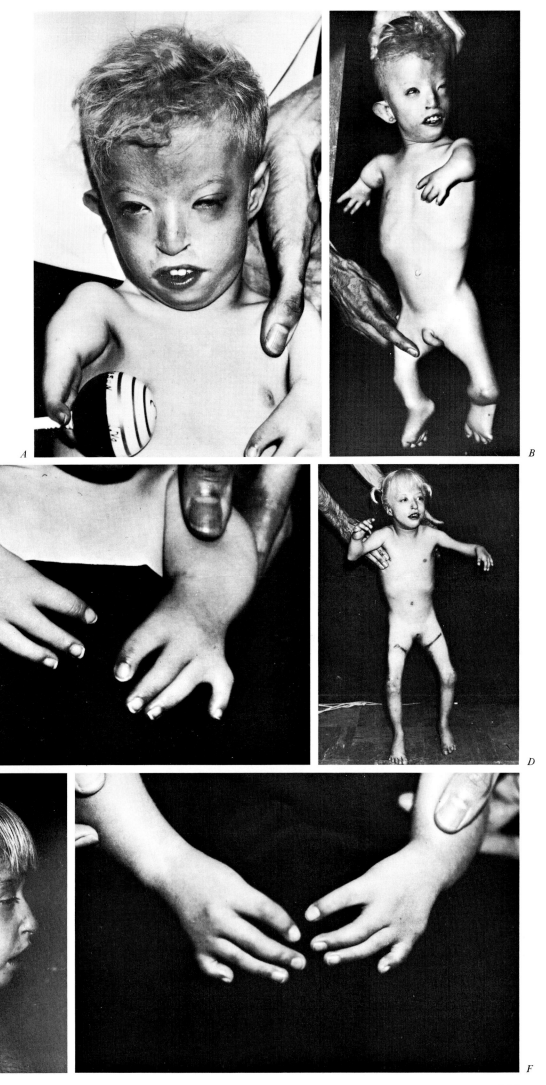

Plate VI-61. *A–C:* A boy with silvery-blond hair, a capillary hemangioma on the forehead, malformed ears and tip of the nose, and downward palpebral slant. He had no forearm bones or fibulae. He had no thumbs and his fifth fingers were short and curved. *D–F:* The sister of this boy. She also had a small chin, malformed nose and ears, and thin, silvery-blond hair. She had flexion contractures of the elbows and knees and no radii or thumbs. (*A–F:* Courtesy of Dr. J. M. Opitz, Madison, Wisc.)

Syndrome of Retinal Blindness, Polycystic Kidneys, and Brain Malformations

In 1969 Dekaban [1] reported a brother and sister with blindness, polycystic kidneys, and cerebellar and cerebral malformations. No similarly affected individuals have been reported.

Physical Features

HEAD: A small reducible midoccipital meningocele was present in the girl.

EYES: Both children had oscillatory eye movements in the first weeks of life and thereafter. At 3 years of age their optic discs were pale and the retinal vessels were narrow (*Figure B*).

SKIN: The girl had a small red nevus over her lumbar spine (*Figure A*).

Nervous System

Both children were considered to be congenitally blind and mentally retarded. The boy was moderately hypotonic and had brisk deep tendon reflexes. His pupils were moderately dilated and showed only slight constriction to strong illumination.

Pathology

The postmortem findings in the boy included absence of rods and a single layer of cones in the retina (*Figure D*), poorly myelinated optic nerves, hypoplasia of the vermis of the cerebellum, generalized immaturity of the cerebral neurons, polycystic kidneys, patent foramen ovale, heterotopic gastric mucosa in the esophagus, and fatty metamorphosis of the liver. The kidneys weighed 65 and 60 g. Numerous thin-walled cysts were visible through the capsule. The cortex of the kidney was markedly convoluted and had large fissures (*Figure C*). The renal cortex was very thin. The width from the tip of the papillae to the cortical surface was 1.1 cm [2]. The calyceal collecting system was dilated and extended far to the periphery. A piece of brain removed at the time of the repair of the girl's meningocele showed immaturity of the nerve cells.

Laboratory Studies

Electroretinograms showed little or no response in either patient. Pneumoencephalography showed slightly dilated lateral ventricles in both children. Communication between the ventricles and meningocele was demonstrated in the girl. She also had an enlarged cisterna magna and fourth ventricle. Intravenous pyelograms showed cystic spaces and calyceal clubbing in both children. Chromosomal analysis, done only on the second child, showed no abnormalities.

Treatment and Prognosis

These children died at 3 and 4 years of age.

Differential Diagnosis

1. Polycystic kidneys, encephaloceles, and cerebral malformations are features of infants with the Meckel syndrome, but they also have microphthalmia, cleft lip, and polydactyly (see page 292).
2. Three siblings with congenital blindness and polycystic kidney disease were described by Fairley and coworkers [3].
3. Two siblings with congenital blindness and renal dysplasia were described by Loken and associates [4].
4. Polycystic kidneys, cerebral malformations, and presumed blindness are features of infants with 18 trisomy, but they often have many other major and minor anomalies (see page 156).

References

1. Dekaban, A. S. Hereditary syndrome of congenital retinal blindness (Leber), polycystic kidneys and maldevelopment of the brain. *Am. J. Ophthalmol.,* **68:**1029–37, 1969.
2. Dekaban, A. S. Personal communication, 1970.
3. Fairley, K. F., Leighton, P. W., and Kincaid-Smith, P. Familial visual defects associated with polycystic kidney and medullary sponge kidney. *Br. Med. J.,* **1:**1060–63, 1963.
4. Loken, A. C., Hanssen, O., Halvorsen, S., and Jolster, N. J. Hereditary renal dysplasia and blindness. *Acta Paediatr.,* **50:**177–84, 1961.

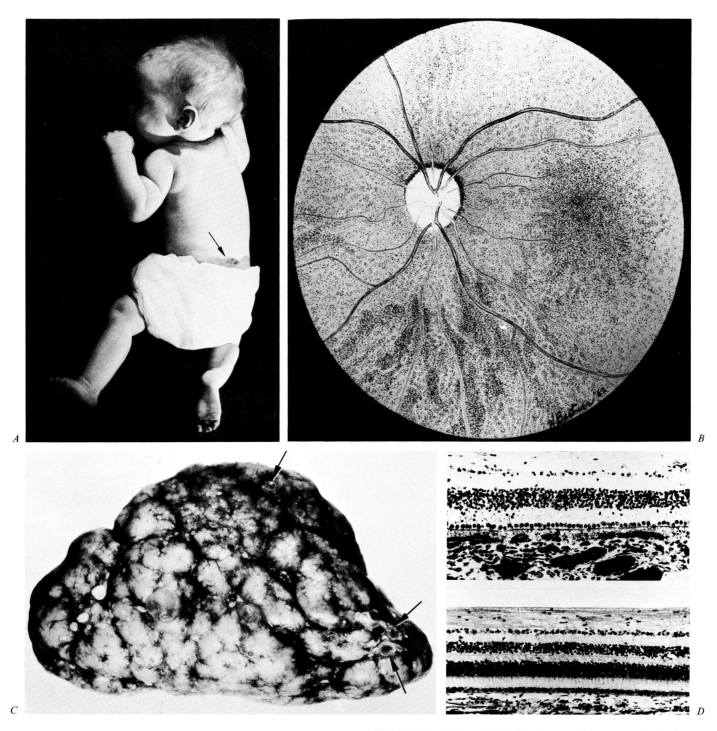

Plate VI-62. *A:* The affected girl whose small nevus over the lumbar spine is barely visible (*arrow*). *B:* A drawing of her retinal fundus showing the pale optic disc and narrow vessels. *C:* A kidney of the boy with marked convolutions and fissures. The thin-walled cysts (*arrows*) are scattered over the cortex. *D* (*top*): A photomicrograph of his retina near the macula showing no rods and only a single layer of cones (hematoxylin-eosin, × 210). *D* (*bottom*): Normal retina. (*A–C:* Courtesy of Dr. A. S. Dekaban, Bethesda, Md. *D:* From A. S. Dekaban, *Am. J. Ophthalmol.,* **68:**1029–37, 1969.)

Syndrome of Tetraphocomelia, Cleft Lip and Palate, and Genital Hypertrophy (Roberts Syndrome)

In 1919 Roberts [1] described a brother and sister with marked shortening of all limbs and cleft lip and palate. In 1966 Appelt, Gerken, and Lenz [2] reported another affected infant. A third infant was briefly described in 1970 [3]. Two families with five additional affected infants have been evaluated and compared with 12 previously reported patients [4].

Physical Features

HEAD: These infants are microcephalic.

FACE: The eyes protrude, are widely spaced, and there is a downward palpebral slant and a small mandible (*Figures A, B, E, and F*).

EYES: Three infants had a coloboma of the eyelid [2,4]. Three of 17 had either corneal opacities or cataracts [4].

EAR: Absent or hypoplastic ears were noted in 3 of 17 infants [4].

MOUTH: Cleft lip and palate with protrusion of the premaxilla has usually been present.

GENITALIA: The infant females often have a large clitoris (*Figures C and F*). The clitoris of one was 1.5 cm long; the labia minora were large and split [2]. Several infant males have had a large penis [1,4] (*Figures A and E*). They often have cryptorchidism.

LIMBS: The shortening of the limbs is symmetric and usually more severe in the arms. The humerus, radius, and ulna are either absent entirely or quite small. Two infants had only four fingers on each hand [2,4]. The tibia and fibula are usually absent and the femurs shortened. One infant had syndactyly of toes 4 and 5 [4] (*Figures A, E, and F*).

HEIGHT: One 9-year-old was 24 inches (62 cm) long [4].

WEIGHT: The birth weight is usually less than 2.2 kg in term pregnancies.

Nervous System

These infants are considered mentally deficient, but few data are available. One infant lay in an opisthotonic position [2]. The one long-term survivor is considered severely retarded [4]. Two of 17 had hydrocephalus [4].

Pathology

One infant [2] had a deformed base of the cranium and cribriform plate. Another infant female (*Figure F*) had a patent ductus arteriosus and foramen ovale and multiple cysts of one kidney. Her stillborn male sibling had a large anterior encephalocele protruding between the eyes and bilateral polycystic kidneys. In another family both affected infants had horseshoe kidneys [4]. Three of 17 had cardiac anomalies [4].

Laboratory Studies

X-rays showed the marked shortening or absence of the long bones in the limbs (*Figure D*). Absent or deformed metacarpals were usually associated with absent digits. Chromosomal studies in one patient showed no abnormalities [4]. A female infant [2] had a single sex chromatin body.

Treatment and Prognosis

All but one of these infants were either stillborn or died in the first days or weeks of life. The surviving child is now 9 years old [4].

Genetics

Autosomal recessive.

Differential Diagnosis

1. Patients with the syndrome of phocomelia, flexion contractures, and facial anomalies are distinguished by having less severe limb deformities, silvery-blond hair, and no genital anomalies (see page 340).
2. Infants with the thalidomide embryopathy usually have less severe limb deformities, often have microtia, and do not have facial or genital anomalies (see page 132).

References

1. Roberts, J. B. A child with double cleft of lip and palate, protrusion of the intermaxillary portion of the upper jaw and imperfect development of the bones of the four extremities. *Ann. Surg.*, **70**:252, 1919.
2. Appelt, H., Gerken, H., and Lenz, W. Tetraphokomelie mit Lippen-Kiefer-Gaumenspalte und Clitorishhypertrophie—ein Syndrom. *Pädiatrie und Pädologie*, **2**:119-24, 1966.
3. Temtamy, S. A., and Loutfi, A. H. Some genetic and surgical aspects of cleft lip/cleft palate problem in Egypt. *Cleft Palate J.*, **7**:578-94, 1970.
4. Freeman, M. V. R., German, J., Williams, D. W., Schimke, R. N., Temtamy, S. A., and Vachier, E. The Roberts syndrome. (In press.)

Plate VI-63. *A:* The first reported infant with short limbs, bilateral cleft lip, and large penis. *B–D:* Show in another infant the widely spaced eyes, downward eye slant, and large clitoris. The x-ray shows the small humerus, shortened femur, and absence of the radius, ulna, tibia, and fibula. *E:* The infant who has survived for many years. He has a large penis. *F:* His sister, who has a large clitoris. (*A:* From J. B. Roberts, *Ann. Surg.,* **70:**252, 1919. *B–D:* From Appelt *et al., Pädiatrie und Pädologie,* **2:**119–24, 1966. *E* and *F:* Courtesy of Dr. D. W. Williams, Denver, Col.)

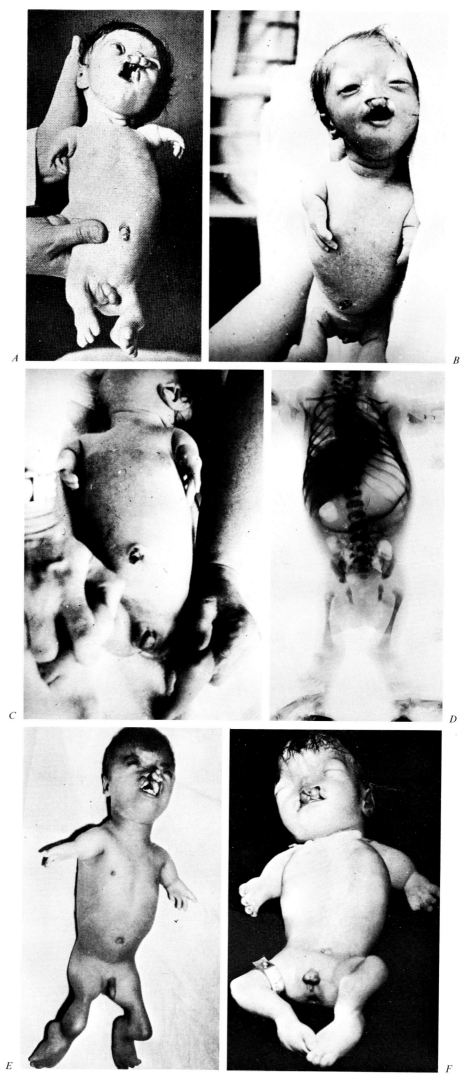

A

B

C

D

E

F

Telecanthus-Hypospadias Syndrome

In 1969 Opitz, Summitt, and Smith [1] described eight males in three families with a newly recognized syndrome of telecanthus, hypospadias, and other anomalies. The term *telecanthus* is used to describe any condition in which the distance between the medial canthi is increased [2].

Physical Features

HEAD: Two patients were brachycephalic and one had a prominent metopic suture.

FACE: Several patients had a prominent bridge of the nose. All had pronounced telecanthus (*Figures A, C, D, E, and F*); only one was shown to have true orbital hypertelorism by measurement of the interorbital distance on x-ray. One patient had a slight downward palpebral slant, and another had a slight upward slant (*Figure A*).

MOUTH: One boy had a cleft lip and palate.

EARS: The ears were posteriorly rotated in some of the patients (*Figure B*).

GENITALIA: The hypospadias varied from the mildest form, with the urethral opening on the ventral edge of the glans penis (*Figure D*), to third-degree hypospadias, with a chordee deformity and the urethral opening at the base of the penis. Three patients were cryptorchid with testes palpable in the inguinal region.

Nervous System

Five of the patients were mentally retarded, two having IQ's of 47 and 56.

Laboratory Studies

One patient had coarctation of the aorta and hypoplasia of the aortic arch. Excretory urograms in four patients and an intravenous pyelogram in one were normal.

Genetics

The telecanthus-hypospadias syndrome is transmitted as a dominant trait. Since male-to-male transmission has not been observed, it may be either X-linked or autosomal.

Differential Diagnosis

1. Telecanthus associated with many different anomalies, such as widow's peak, cranial asymmetry, imperforate anus, and hypospadias, was reported by Christian and coworkers [3] in eight individuals in five generations. Although their patients were not mentally retarded, this difference may be a reflection of phenotypic variability of the same mutant gene that is responsible for the telecanthus-hypospadias syndrome.

2. A family was reported by Juberg and Hirsch [4] in which eight members over five generations had telecanthus, with some also having cleft lip and palate, nasolacrimal duct abnormalities, and dental agenesis. Some were also mentally retarded.

3. Hypertelorism, a broad nose, and hypospadias are also features of some males with the 46,XY,4p— (see page 174) and 46,XY,5p— (see page 170) syndromes.

References

1. Opitz, J. M., Summitt, R. L., and Smith, D. W. The BBB syndrome. Familial telecanthus with associated congenital anomalies. *Birth Defects: Original Article Series,* Vol. V, No. 2, February, 1969, pp. 86–94. Williams & Wilkins Co., Baltimore.
2. Mustarde, J. C. Epicanthus and telecanthus. *Brit. J. Plast. Surg.,* **16**:346–56, 1963.
3. Christian, J. C., Bixler, D., Blythe, S. C., and Merritt, A. D. Familial telecanthus with associated congenital anomalies. *Birth Defects: Original Article Series,* Vol. V, No. 2, February, 1969, pp. 82–85. Williams & Wilkins Co., Baltimore.
4. Juberg, R. C. and Hirsch, R. Expressivity of heritable telecanthus in five generations of a kindred. *Am. J. Hum. Genet.,* **23**:547–54, 1971.

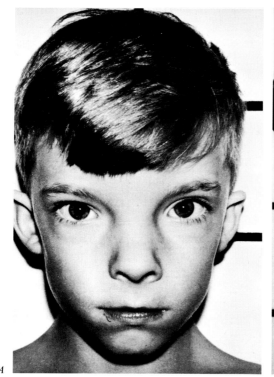

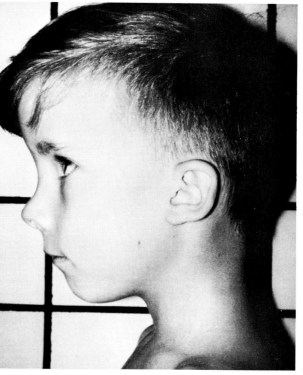

Plate VI-64. *A–C:* Two brothers with widely spaced eyes, wide and high bridge of the nose, and small chin. One boy had a prominent forehead. *D:* One of two brothers, both of whom had widely spaced eyes, epicanthal folds, and glandular hypospadias. *E:* Two boys with hypertelorism and hypospadias (one second-degree and the other third-degree) shown with their mother, who also had widely spaced eyes. The older boy had a prominent metopic suture. The mother and her younger son had normal intelligence. *F:* A brother of the woman shown in *E*. He had telecanthus and glandular hypospadias. (*A–F:* From J. M. Opitz *et al., Birth Defects: Original Article Series,* Vol. V, No. 2, February, 1969, pp. 86–94. Williams & Wilkins Co., Baltimore.)

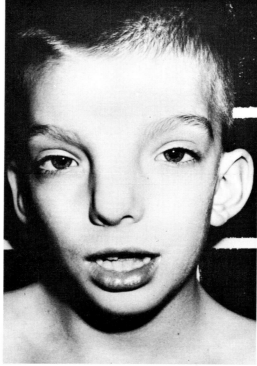

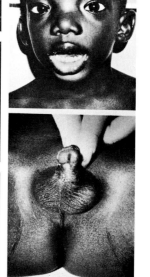

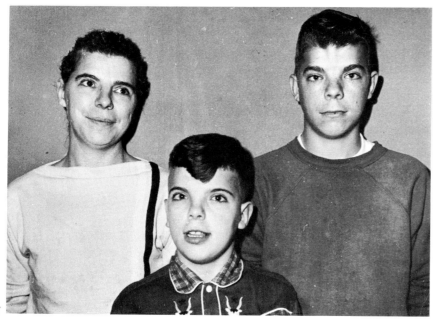

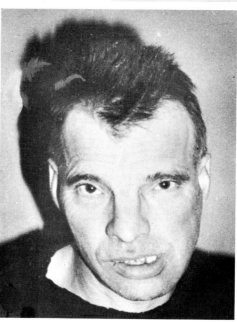

Treacher Collins Syndrome (Mandibulofacial Dysostosis, Franceschetti-Zwahlen-Klein Syndrome)

In 1889 Berry described a woman who had notched eyelids, a downward palpebral slant, and a cleft lip; her daughter also had a notched eyelid and a downward palpebral slant [1,2]. E. Treacher Collins [3] described in 1900 two patients with a similar appearance and emphasized the underdevelopment of the malar bones. Franceschetti and Zwahlen [4] in 1944 and Franceschetti and Klein [5] in 1949 described patients with this syndrome who had more severe facial anomalies and ear deformities. They introduced the term *mandibulofacial dysostosis*. While all of these authors seem to have been describing the same disorder, many different eponyms and terms continue to be used in different parts of the world. Two hundred cases were reviewed in 1964 [2].

Physical Features

FACE: A downward palpebral slant, eyelid colobomas, hypoplasia of the malar and zygoma areas, and a small, retracted chin are the most prominent facial features (*Figures A, B, C, D, E, and F*). The eyelid colobomas, which are present in most patients, are always in the outer third of the lower lid. The nose appears large because of the malar underdevelopment. Some patients also have narrow and thin alar cartilage. The mouth usually is large and the corners are turned downward. These facial anomalies may be asymmetric or even unilateral in some patients, but this is unusual.

EYES: Some patients have eye anomalies, such as microphthalmia, iris colobomas, and absence of the meibomian glands or the lower lacrimal puncta, but these are uncommon.

EARS: About half of the patients have abnormalities of the external ear and atresia of the external auditory meatus [6]. The external ear may be only mildly deformed, or it may be represented only by an undifferentiated soft mass (*Figures A, B, C, D, E, and F*). Middle and inner ear anomalies are frequent, especially in patients with external ear anomalies.

MOUTH: In association with the malar hypoplasia the palate is narrow and high and the teeth are crowded and poorly aligned. A cleft palate without a cleft lip is common.

Nervous System

Although some reported patients have been mentally retarded, most have normal intelligence. Many patients with middle and inner ear anomalies have a significant conductive hearing loss.

Laboratory Studies

Skull x-rays show poor development of the maxilla, malar bones, zygoma, mandible, middle ear ossicles, and paranasal sinuses. Chromosomal studies have shown no abnormalities.

Treatment and Prognosis

Hearing should be tested early, and hearing loss treated in infancy. Cosmetic surgery makes a striking improvement in the facial appearance of some patients.

Genetics

Autosomal dominant. Studies of several families have shown that this syndrome can be present in subtle forms so that a very mildly affected parent may have a severely affected child [6] (*Figures A and B*).

Differential Diagnosis

1. Patients with the syndrome of malformed low-set ears and conductive hearing loss can have a similar ear deformity, but do not have either malar hypoplasia or eyelid colobomas. This is due to an autosomal recessive mutant gene (see page 328).
2. Malformed external ears and a conductive hearing loss due to a dominant mutant gene are features of the family reported by Wildervanck [7]. However, these patients also had marginal ear pits and preauricular tags.
3. Macrostomia, mandibular hypoplasia, and external ear anomalies are features of patients with Goldenhar's syndrome, but they can usually be distinguished by the presence of epibulbar dermoids and vertebral anomalies (see page 284).
4. A hypoplastic mandible and cleft palate are features of patients with the Pierre Robin syndrome, but they do not have eyelid colobomas, malar hypoplasia, or ear anomalies (see page 304).

References

1. Berry, G. A. Note on a congenital defect (? coloboma) of the lower lid. *Roy. Lond. Ophthalmic Hosp. Rep.*, 12:255–57, 1889.
2. Rogers, B. O. Berry-Treacher Collins syndrome: a review of 200 cases. *Br. J. Plast. Surg.*, 17:109–37, 1964.
3. Collins, E. T. Case with symmetrical congenital notches in the outer part of each lower lid and defective development of the malar bones. *Trans. Ophthalmol. Soc. UK*, 20:190–92, 1900.
4. Franceschetti, A., and Zwahlen, P. Un syndrome nouveau: la dysostose mandibulo-faciale. *Bull. Schweiz. Akad. Med. Wiss.*, 1:60–66, 1944.
5. Franceschetti, A., and Klein, D. The mandibulo-facial dysostosis. A new hereditary syndrome. *Acta Ophthalmol. (Kobh.)*, 27:143–224, 1949.
6. Fazen, L. E., Elmore, J., and Nadler, H. L. Mandibulo-facial dysostosis (Treacher Collins syndrome). *Am. J. Dis. Child.*, 113:405–10, 1967.
7. Wildervanck, L. S. Marginal pits, pre-auricular appendages, malformations of the auricle and conductive deafness. *Acta Otolaryngol. (Stockh.)*, 54:553–60, 1962.
8. Ellwood, L. C., Winter, S. T., and Dar, H. Familial microtia with meatal atresia in two sibships. *J. Med. Genet.*, 5:289–91, 1968.

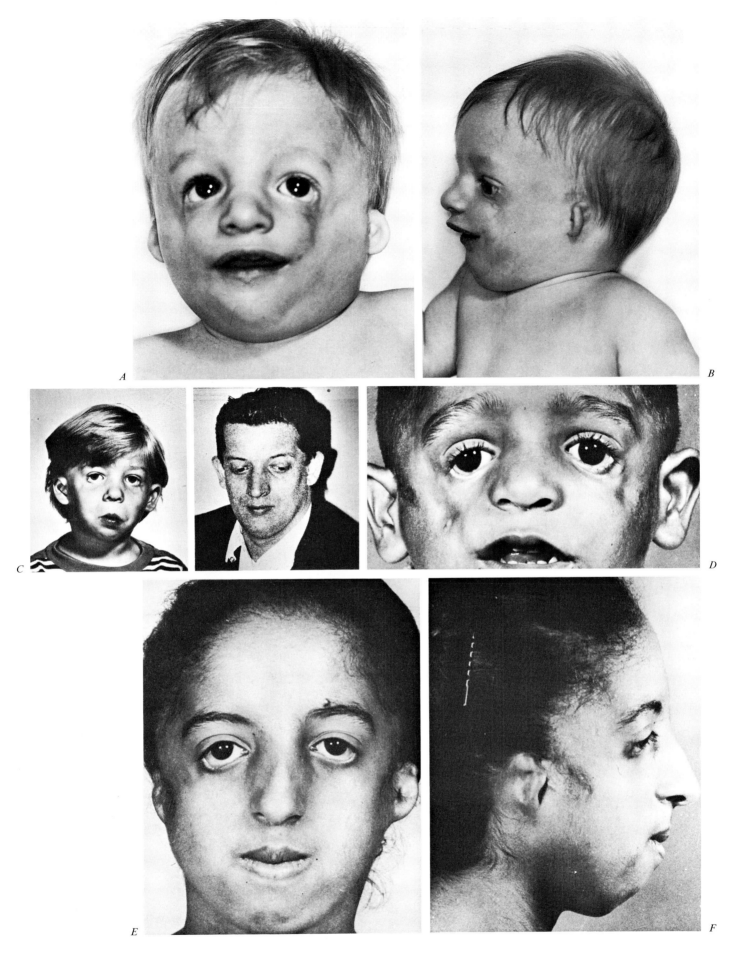

Plate VI-65. *A* and *B:* An infant with marked underdevelopment of the zygomas, maxillae, and mandible, a downward palpebral slant, notched lower eyelids, and rudimentary ears. *C:* This boy's less severely affected sister, who has normal ears, and his father, who has minimal hypoplasia of the facial bones, notching of the lower eyelids, and hearing loss. All affected members of this family have normal intelligence. *D:* A 4-year-old boy with downward palpebral slant more severe on the right. The right lower eyelid is notched and has no lashes. The left lower eyelid has no lashes on the medial two thirds.

E and *F:* A girl with less marked maxillary hypoplasia, but severe ear deformities and micrognathia, notching of the right lower eyelid, and absence of the lashes from the medial two thirds of both lower eyelids. (*A–C* [*right*]: From L. E. Fasen *et al., Am. J. Dis. Child.,* **113:**405–10, 1967. *C* [*left*]: Courtesy of Dr. H. L. Nadler, Chicago, Ill. *D:* From B. O. Rogers, *Br. J. Plast. Surg.,* **17:**109–37, 1964. *E* and *F:* From B. O. Rogers, *Plast. Reconstr. Surg.,* **41:**208–31, 1968; © 1968, Williams & Wilkins Co., Baltimore, Md.)

Trichorrhexis Nodosa with Mental Retardation

In 1968 Pollitt, Jenner, and Davies [1] described a brother and sister with short, stubbly hair, thin nails and tooth enamel, short stature, and mental retardation. The predominant hair abnormality was trichorrhexis nodosa. These patients were thought to represent a new clinical syndrome.

Physical Features

HEAD: Both children were microcephalic.

MOUTH: The tooth enamel was thin.

LIMBS: The nails were misshapen and spoonlike.

HAIR: The scalp and eyebrow hair was brittle, sparse, and stubbly (about 1 to 2 cm long) (*Figures A and C*). Alopecia occurred where there was excessive rubbing. The shafts of hair showed two changes: areas where it had split longitudinally into numerous small fibers (trichorrhexis nodosa) (*Figures B and D*) and areas where it was twisted in the long axis (pili torti). The hair surface was irregular and the normal pattern of scales was absent (*Figures E and F*).

HEIGHT AND WEIGHT: Both children had marked retardation of growth.

Nervous System

At the age of 5 years the girl could not speak and had a developmental age of 18 to 24 months. The boy, who could not walk without support at age 3 years, was considered less severely retarded than his sister.

Laboratory Studies

Urine, plasma, and fecal amino acids showed the normal patterns. Analysis of hair showed a low cystine content and no trace of argininosuccinic acid or its cyclic anhydrides. X-rays showed a small cranial vault and a retarded bone age. The chromosomal analysis was normal.

Differential Diagnosis

1. Trichorrhexis nodosa is a feature of argininosuccinic aciduria (see page 6) and kinky hair disease (see page 100), but each of these diseases is differentiated by the other physical features and the laboratory studies.
2. A mentally retarded brother and sister with fuzzy hair and a mild renal tubular aminoaciduria were recently reported [2].
3. Twisted hairs (pili torti) are short, broken, and of irregular shape. This condition is not associated with mental deficiency [3].
4. Trichorrhexis nodosa, pili torti, short stature, and mental deficiency were also features of the siblings reported by Tay [4], but they also had nonbullous congenital ichthyosiform erythroderma and a progeria-like appearance.

References

1. Pollitt, R. J., Jenner, F. A., and Davies, M. Sibs with mental and physical retardation and trichorrhexis nodosa with abnormal amino acid composition of the hair. *Arch. Dis. Child.,* **43:**211–16, 1968.
2. Mann, T. P. Mental retardation, abnormal hair and mild aminoaciduria, all of unknown aetiology, in siblings. *Proc. R. Soc. Med.,* **62:**328, 1969.
3. Nichamin, S. J. Twisted hairs (pili torti). *Am. J. Dis. Child.,* **95:**612–15, 1958.
4. Tay, C. H. Ichthyosiform erythroderma, hair shaft abnormalities, and mental and growth retardation. A new recessive disorder. *Arch. Dermatol.,* **104:**4–13, 1971.

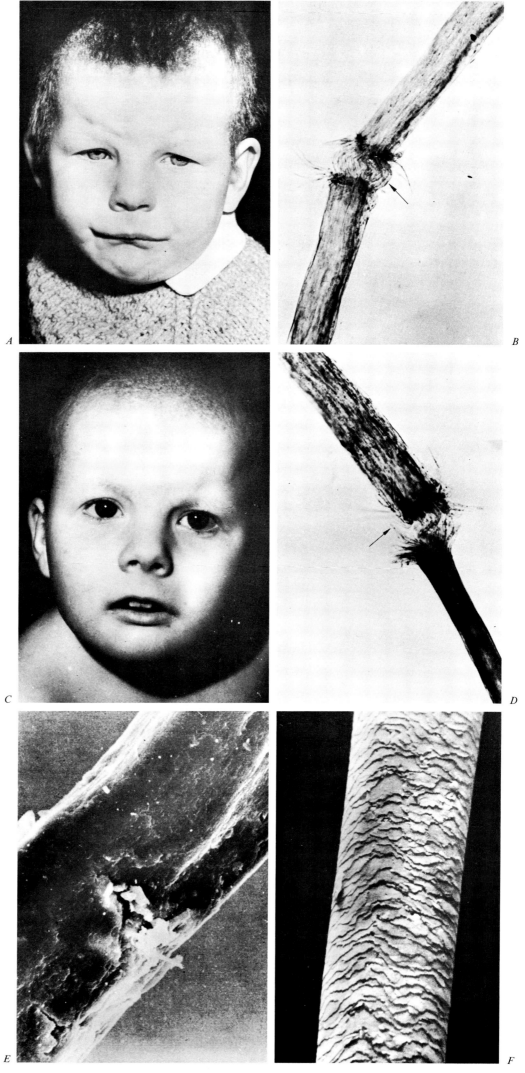

Plate VI-66. *A* and *C:* The affected brother and sister. Note their short scalp hair and sparse eyebrows and eyelashes. *B* and *D:* Light-microscope photographs of a hair of each child, showing where the shafts have broken and have brushlike ends (*arrows*). *E* and *F:* Electron micrograph of hair from the sister (*E*) showing the absence of the normal pattern of scales which is illustrated in electron-micrograph of a normal shaft of hair (*F*). (*A* and *C:* Courtesy of Dr. M. Davies, Bromsgrove, Worcestershire, England. *B, D–F:* Reprinted from R. J. Pollitt *et al., Arch. Dis. Child.,* **43:**211, 1968, by permission of the authors and editor.)

A

B

C

D

E

F

351

Chapter VII

Neurocutaneous Syndromes with Mental Retardation

Introduction

Diseases that affect both the skin and the nervous system are often classified as neurocutaneous disorders. The skin and the nervous system share a common embryologic origin from the ectodermal layer. As many of the neurocutaneous diseases are due to single mutant genes, it seems likely that the primary genetic abnormality affects both the skin and the nervous system. At this time the biochemical basis for any neurocutaneous disease is not known. One possible exception is xeroderma pigmentosum, in which an endonuclease deficiency has been identified [1].

Many, but not all, of the neurocutaneous syndromes are associated with mental retardation. Concerning those included in this chapter, several general observations can be made. First, some of these are among the most common genetic diseases. Neurofibromatosis is one of the most common disorders due to an autosomal dominant mutant gene, with the incidence estimated as 1:2500–3300 births. Second, either tumors or leukemia develop in the course of several of these diseases (ataxia telangiectasia, basal cell nevus syndrome, neurofibromatosis, tuberous sclerosis, and xeroderma pigmentosum). The cause of the tumor growth and malignancies is not known. Third, dramatic and serious defects occur in other organ systems of the affected individuals in many of these diseases. Eye anomalies are the most common. Skeletal anomalies, such as maxillary hypoplasia, cleft lip and palate, syndactyly, and ectrodactyly, are also frequent.

This group of neurocutaneous diseases is clearly heterogeneous. Any more specific classification awaits the delineation of the underlying biochemical abnormalities.

Reference

1. Cleaver, J. E. Xeroderma pigmentosum: a human disease in which an initial stage of DNA repair is defective. *Proc. Natl. Acad. Sci. USA,* **63:**428–35, 1969.

Ataxia-Telangiectasia
(Louis-Bar Syndrome)

In 1941 Madame Louis-Bar [1] described a patient with telangiectasia of the conjunctiva and skin and cerebellar ataxia. Subsequent reports of more than 150 patients have shown that sinopulmonary infections, immunologic deficiencies, mental deficiency, progressive neurologic deterioration, and a predisposition to malignancies are also features of this syndrome [2–5].

Physical Features

Skin: The telangiectases are usually evident between 3 and 4 years of age, often first seen in the exposed portion of the bulbar conjunctiva. Initially, these vessels are thin, bright red, symmetric streaks which resemble conjunctivitis; later, they enlarge and become tortuous (*Figure A*). The telangiectases spread eventually to involve the eyelids, the butterfly area of the face (*Figure F*), the external ears (*Figure B*), the neck, the antecubital (*Figure C*) and popliteal spaces, and, less frequently, the palate and the dorsum of the hands and feet. In general, the areas with the greatest exposure to the sun are the most affected. Within a few years the ears become inelastic, the skin of the face becomes tense and hidebound (*Figure F*), and the subcutaneous fat diminishes. The involved skin shows a mottled pattern of hyper- and hypopigmentation with cutaneous atrophy and telangiectasia. Basal cell carcinomas and senile keratoses occur. Almost all patients have seborrheic dermatitis. Follicular keratosis, nummular eczema, hirsutism, and recurrent impetigo and warts are other frequent skin lesions [2,3].

Nervous System

Ataxia becomes apparent in infancy, typically when the child begins to walk. It is the cerebellar type of ataxia that in the beginning affects mainly stance and gait. Choreoathetosis may be prominent in childhood and mask the ataxia. Later, dyssynergia and an intention tremor of the arms are prominent. Because of the steady progression of the ataxia and increased fatigability on walking, most patients are confined to a wheelchair before adolescence. Romberg's sign remains negative. Speech may begin normally, but becomes slow and slurred. With progression of the disease breath control becomes poor, the voice weak, and the speech indistinct. Oculomotor abnormalities, such as poorly sustained conjugate gaze, apraxia of eye movements, nystagmus, and strabismus, develop in many patients. The facial expression is usually relaxed, masklike, and inattentive (*Figures D, E, and F*) in contrast to the cheerful, alert appearance when smiling (*Figures D and F*). The smile is typically sweet and slow-spreading. Older children often drool excessively. The deep tendon reflexes become diminished and the plantar response flexor. The posture becomes more stooped, with drooped shoulders and the head bent forward. In the early stages of the disease, mental retardation is not evident. As the disease progresses the intelligence may drop below average, which suggests a failure of development of mental ability rather than true regression. Below-normal intelligence was present in one third of the 101 patients reviewed in one report [2]. The disposition usually remains pleasant.

Pathology

Neuropathologic findings include atrophy of the cerebellar cortex, chronic neuronal degeneration in the dentate and inferior olivary nuclei, demyelination of the posterior columns in the spinal cord, neuronal dystrophy in the medulla, and neuromelanosis and ballooning degeneration of neurons in the spinal ganglia [4]. Other common findings are absence or hypoplasia of the thymus, hypoplasia of lymphoid tissue, ovarian and anterior pituitary abnormalities, and a high incidence of malignancies, such as leukemia, lymphosarcoma, and basal cell carcinomas [2,5]. The cutaneous telangiectatic vessels branch from the subpapillar venous plexuses.

Laboratory Studies

These patients have deficient delayed-type hypersensitivity and a decrease in peripheral small lymphocytes. Various serum immunoglobulin abnormalities have been described, the most common being diminished levels of IgA and IgE [5]. An unusual form of diabetes mellitus, characterized by marked elevations of glucose and insulin, insulin resistance, and absence of glycosuria, has been reported [6]. Eight of 18 patients in one study [7] had antibodies to either thyroid, smooth muscle, parietal, or striated muscle cells.

Treatment and Prognosis

These patients have recurrent upper and lower respiratory, middle ear, and sinus infections; these are thought to be related to the immunoglobulin deficiencies. Bronchiectasis is a frequent complication. Most patients do not survive beyond 25 years of age. Pulmonary disease, malignancies, and debilitation are the most common causes of death.

Genetics

Autosomal recessive.

Differential Diagnosis

1. Cerebellar ataxia and erythematous skin lesions over the sun-exposed areas are features of patients with Hartnup's disease, but these patients do not have conjunctival or ear telangiectasia, and have a characteristic aminoaciduria (see page 24).
2. Wasting of the face, a progressive neurologic degeneration, and a butterfly rash with sun sensitivity are features of patients with Cockayne's syndrome, but they do not have cutaneous telangiectases (see page 82).
3. The cerebellar ataxia and progressive spinocerebellar degeneration make Friedreich's ataxia a frequent early diagnosis in patients with ataxia telangiectasia until the telangiectases are noticed (see page 92).

References

1. Louis-Bar, Mme. Sur un syndrôme progressif comprenant des télangiectasies capillaires cutanées et conjonctivales symétriques à disposition naevoïde et des troubles cérébelleux. *Confin. Neurol.*, **4**:32–42, 1941.
2. Boder, E., and Sedgwick, R. P. Ataxia-telangiectasia. A review of 101 cases. *Little Club Clinics in Developmental Medicine*, No. 8, Cerebellum, Posture and Cerebral Palsy, edited by Walsh, G. The National Spastics Society and Heinemann Medical Books, Ltd. London, 1963, pp. 110–18.
3. Reed, W. B., Epstein, W. L., Boder, E., and Sedgwick, R. Cutaneous manifestations of ataxia telangiectasia. *J.A.M.A.*, **195**:746–53, 1966.
4. Aguilar, M. J., Kamoshita, S., Landing, B. H., Boder, E. and Sedgwick, R. P. Pathological observations in ataxia telangiectasia. A report on five cases. *J. Neuropath. Exp. Neurol.*, **27**:659–76, 1968.
5. Ammann, A. J., Cain, W. A., Ishizaka, K., Hong, R., and Good, R. A. Immunoglobulin E deficiency in ataxia-telangiectasia. *N. Engl. J. Med.*, **281**:469–72, 1969.
6. Schalch, D. S., McFarlin, D. E., and Barlow, M. H. An unusual form of diabetes mellitus in ataxia telangiectasia. *N. Engl. J. Med.*, **282**:1396–1402, 1970.
7. Ammann, A. J., and Hong, R. Autoimmune phenomena in ataxia telangiectasia. *J. Pediatr.*, **78**:821–26, 1971.

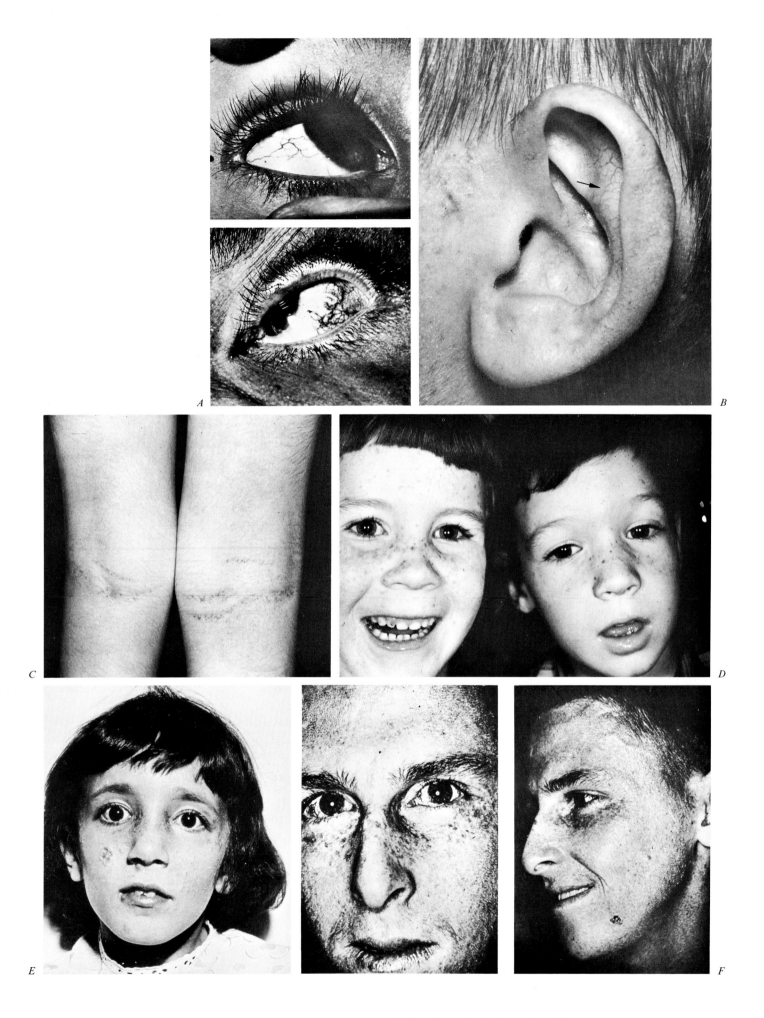

Plate VII-1. *A* (*top*): Shows early conjunctival telangiectases. *A* (*bottom*): Shows the more tortuous vessels in older telangiectases. *B* and *C:* Show telangiectases on the antihelix of the ear (*arrow*) and in the antecubital fossa of each arm. *D:* An affected sister and brother, aged 6 and 4 years. The girl (*left*) had a wide, cheerful-looking, but slow-spreading smile; her brother had a sad and dull facial appearance. Both had normal intelligence. *E:* Another child with an expressionless face. She had normal intelligence. *F:* An adult with tense facial skin, pigmented lesions below the eyes, prominent bulbar telangiectases, and a waxen smile. (*A* [*top*] and *D:* Courtesy of Drs. E. Boder and R. P. Sedgwick, Los Angeles, Calif. *B* and *C:* From E. Boder and R. P. Sedgwick, *Am. J. Dis. Child.,* **117:**317, 1969. *E:* From E. Boder and R. P. Sedgwick, *Pediatrics,* **21:**526–54, 1958. *F:* From W. B. Reed *et al., J.A.M.A.,* **195:**746–53, 1966.)

Basal Cell Nevus Syndrome

In 1951 Binkley and Johnson [1] reported the association of basal cell nevi and dental cysts in a mother and daughter. Further experience with more than 150 patients has shown that the nevi and dental cysts are only two features of a syndrome that also includes facial and skeletal anomalies, decreased responsiveness to parathormone, and dyskeratotic pitting of the hands and feet [2–5].

Physical Features

SKIN: Several types of skin tumors have been observed: solid, adenoid, cystic, morphealike, and superficial [2]. Most patients have either solid tumors or papules, which are usually located in the midportion of the face and on the neck and head (*Figures A, B, and C*). These papules may be present in infancy, but they are often not noticed until the teen-age or young adult years. They are either flesh-colored or pigmented, variable in size, and numerous. Crops of new lesions erupt periodically. They grow slowly and are often quiescent for months or years [3]. In addition to skin tumors, these patients often have small, superficial pits of the palms, soles (*Figure D*), fingers, and toes. These lesions are only a few millimeters in diameter, may be confluent, and may have either an erythematous or telangiectatic base. They usually appear in the second and third decade and are permanent.

FACE: Hypertelorism and a broad nasal root are common. Frontal and parietal bossing are often present. Swelling, tenderness, and other signs of mandibular cysts may develop during childhood. Most patients have jaw cysts, usually in the rami.

BACK: Several reported patients have had kyphoscoliosis [3].

LIMBS: A few reported patients have had short metacarpals and metatarsals; others have had polydactyly, syndactyly, and arachnodactyly [2].

GENITALIA: Some males have small external genitalia, cryptorchidism, and scanty pubic hair growth.

Nervous System

Several mentally retarded patients have been reported, but the incidence of subnormal intelligence is not known. A few patients have had hydrocephalus [2–4].

Pathology

The skin tumors cannot be differentiated by histologic studies from ordinary basal cell cancers. The mandibular cysts, which may be single or multiple, are lined with stratified squamous epithelium and surrounded by a thick fibrous capsule (*Figure E*). Several patients have had ovarian fibromas. A few have had a medulloblastoma [2,3].

Laboratory Studies

About 75 percent of the patients have skeletal anomalies, the most common being bifurcation of ribs. Lamellar calcification of the falx cerebri, falx cerebelli, or dura has been found in 35 percent of the patients over 14 years of age [2] (*Figure F*). A subnormal response to intravenous parathyroid hormone has been documented in some, but not all, of the patients who have been studied [2–4].

Treatment and Prognosis

Surgical removal of the facial lesions is recommended for patients in the teen-age years or older. For the numerous lesions on other parts of the body, electrodesiccation and curettage are recommended. Topical 5-fluorouracil may also be used. X-ray therapy is contraindicated. Prolonged exposure to sunlight seems to play no role in causing these tumors. The rate of growth and the number of tumors do not diminish with increasing age [3].

Genetics

Autosomal dominant.

Differential Diagnosis

1. Multiple benign cystic epitheliomas have a similar appearance, but they do not have either calcification or an abundance of sulfated acid mucopolysaccharides. Also, patients with benign cystic epitheliomas do not have jaw cysts or rib anomalies [5].
2. Cerebral calcifications, short metacarpals and metatarsals, and hyporesponsiveness to parathyroid hormone are features of patients with pseudohypoparathyroidism, but they also have basal ganglia calcification and hypocalcemia and do not have skin tumors or jaw cysts (see page 50).
3. Cerebral calcifications and skin tumors are features of patients with tuberous sclerosis, but they usually have other skin lesions, such as adenoma sebaceum, white macules, and shagreen patches, which clearly differentiate them (see page 380).

References

1. Binkley, G. W., and Johnson, H. H., Jr. Epithelioma adenoides cysticum: basal cell nevi, agenesis of the corpus callosum and dental cysts. *Arch. Dermatol.,* **63**:73–84, 1951.
2. Gorlin, R. J., Vickers, R. A., Kelln, E., and Williamson, J. J. The multiple basal-cell nevi syndrome. An analysis of a syndrome consisting of multiple nevoid basal-cell carcinoma, jaw cysts, skeletal anomalies, medulloblastoma, and hyporesponsiveness to parathormone. *Cancer,* **18**:89–104, 1965.
3. Howell, J. B., Anderson, D. E., and McClendon, J. L. Multiple cutaneous cancers in children: the nevoid basal cell carcinoma syndrome. *J. Pediatr.,* **69**:97–103, 1966.
4. Berlin, N. I., Van Scott, E. J., Clendenning, W. E., Archard, H. O., Block, J. B., Witkop, C. J., and Haynes, H. A. Basal cell nevus syndromes. *Ann. Intern. Med.,* **64**:403–21, 1966.
5. Graham, J. H., Mason, J. K., Gray, H. R., and Helwig, E. B. Differentiation of nevoid basal cell carcinoma from epithelioma adenoides cysticum. *J. Invest. Dermatol.,* **44**:197–200, 1965.

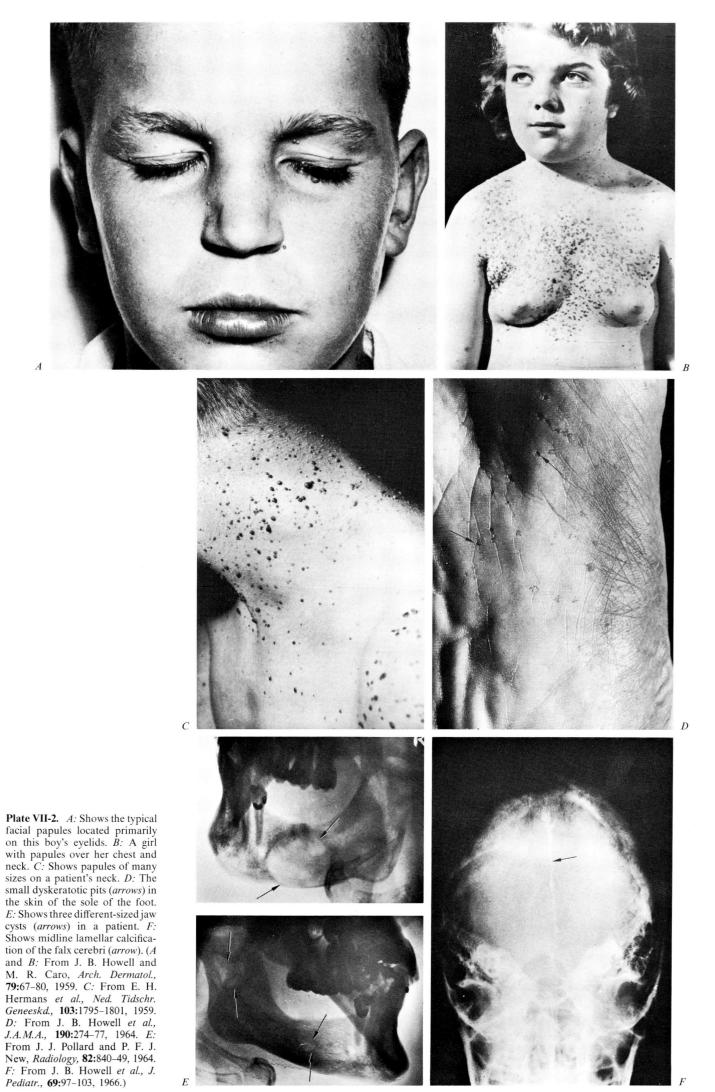

Plate VII-2. *A:* Shows the typical facial papules located primarily on this boy's eyelids. *B:* A girl with papules over her chest and neck. *C:* Shows papules of many sizes on a patient's neck. *D:* The small dyskeratotic pits (*arrows*) in the skin of the sole of the foot. *E:* Shows three different-sized jaw cysts (*arrows*) in a patient. *F:* Shows midline lamellar calcification of the falx cerebri (*arrow*). (*A* and *B:* From J. B. Howell and M. R. Caro, *Arch. Dermatol.,* **79:**67–80, 1959. *C:* From E. H. Hermans *et al., Ned. Tidschr. Geneeskd.,* **103:**1795–1801, 1959. *D:* From J. B. Howell *et al., J.A.M.A.,* **190:**274–77, 1964. *E:* From J. J. Pollard and P. F. J. New, *Radiology,* **82:**840–49, 1964. *F:* From J. B. Howell *et al., J. Pediatr.,* **69:**97–103, 1966.)

Ectodermal Dysplasia, Hypohidrotic Type with Maxillary Hypoplasia

Hypohidrotic ectodermal dysplasia is characterized by decreased functioning of the sweat and sebaceous glands, hypotrichosis, and dental and facial anomalies. In view of the different modes of inheritance reported [1–4], there must be several mutant genes which cause hypohidrotic ectodermal dysplasia with maxillary hypoplasia.

Physical Features

SKIN: The skin is soft, dry, and thin. There are wrinkles around the mouth and eyes. The periorbital area is often darker in color than the rest of the body (*Figures A and C*). Eczema is common. Sweating is either decreased or entirely absent [3–6].

HAIR: The newborn has almost no lanugo hair. At all ages the scalp hair is fine, short, and stiff. The eyebrows and eyelashes may be scanty or absent. In adults the pubic and axillary hair is scanty; the beard is usually normal.

TEETH: The teeth are conical and malformed; often several teeth are missing.

NAILS: The nails are usually normal.

FACE: Frontal bossing, a short nose, a flat nasal bridge, and underdevelopment of the maxilla are the characteristic features (*Figures A, B, C, E, and F*). The lips and chin are prominent [3–6].

EYES: The conjunctiva is moist, but lacrimal secretions are diminished. Many patients have photophobia.

MOUTH: The oral, nasal, pharyngeal, and laryngeal mucosa is atrophic and dry, resulting in crusting and a purulent, foul-smelling discharge and hoarseness.

Nervous System

Many reported patients have subnormal intelligence, but the severity is quite variable [1–3,6]. The retardation may be caused by brain damage from the episodes of extremely high body temperature which these patients experience throughout their lives.

Pathology

Skin biopsies show a diminished number of sweat and sebaceous glands [6].

Laboratory Studies

Decreased sweat production can be demonstrated by iontophoresis or the use of silver nitrate plates. Absence of epidermal ridge sweat pores can be demonstrated with the use of a stereomicroscope [7].

Treatment and Prognosis

Because of their intolerance to heat due to decreased sweat production, these patients must avoid hot environments and strenuous exercise. Respiratory infections are common. Eye drops are necessary to prevent corneal scarring. Frequent nasopharyngeal irrigations with normal saline decrease the foul-smelling discharge, irritation, and injury to the mucosa [3,5].

Genetics

Autosomal dominant and recessive and X-linked recessive inheritance have each been demonstrated in different families [1–4]. In families with the X-linked recessive mutant gene, the carrier females may have a decreased number of epidermal ridge sweat pores [7].

Differential Diagnosis

1. Hypotrichosis and dental anomalies are features of patients with hidrotic ectodermal dysplasia, but they have normal sweat production, dystrophic nails, palmar hyperkeratosis, and normal intelligence [8].
2. Maxillary hypoplasia and diminished sweating occurred in the family reported by Marshall [9], but these patients also had myopia, cataracts, and decreased hearing, and did not have dental or hair abnormalities.
3. Maxillary hypoplasia and a flat nasal bridge are features of many disorders, including Apert's syndrome (see page 222), Crouzon's disease (see page 230), XXXXY syndrome (see page 190), and 18q— syndrome (see page 160), but they are distinguished by other physical features and the fact that they have normal sweating and no skin or hair abnormalities.

References

1. Halperin, S. L., and Curtis, G. M. Anhidrotic ectodermal dysplasia associated with mental deficiency. *Am. J. Ment. Defic.*, **46:**459–63, 1942.
2. Perabo, F., Velasco, J. A., and Prader, A. Ektodermale Dysplasie vom anhidrotischen Typus. 5 neue Beobachtungen. *Helv. Paediatr. Acta,* **11:**604–39, 1956.
3. Rossman, R. E. The ectodermal dysplasias. *Cutis,* **4:**1246–48, 1968.
4. Parant, M., Cayron, R., and Ragot et Boublil, C. M. Un cas d'anodontie appartenant à une dysplasie ectodermique avec anhydrose et hypotrichose. *Rev. Stomatatol. Chir. Maxillofac.,* **70:**461–70, 1969.
5. Hartwell, S. W., Pickrell, K., and Quinn, G. Congenital anhidrotic ectodermal dysplasia. *Clin. Pediatr. (Phila.),* **4:**383–86, 1965.
6. Reed, W. B., Lopez, D. A., and Landing, B. Clinical spectrum of anhidrotic ectodermal dysplasia. *Arch. Dermatol.,* **102:**134–43, 1970.
7. Frias, J. L., and Smith, D. W. Diminished sweat pores in hypohidrotic ectodermal dysplasia: a new method for assessment. *J. Pediatr.,* **72:**606–10, 1968.
8. Williams, M., and Fraser, F. C. Hidrotic ectodermal dysplasia—Clouston's family revisited. *Can. Med. Assoc. J.,* **96:**36–38, 1967.
9. Marshall, D. Ectodermal dysplasia. Report of kindred with ocular abnormalities and hearing defect. *Am. J. Ophthalmol.,* **45:**143–56, 1958.

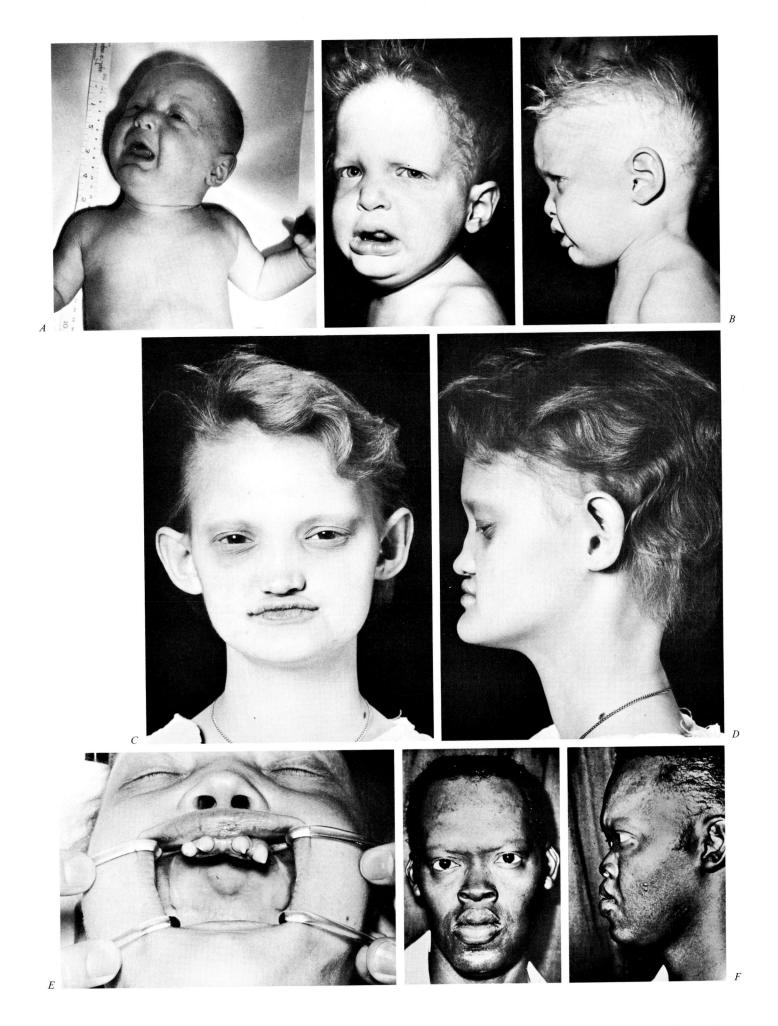

Plate VII-3. *A* and *B:* A boy with X-linked recessive anhidrotic ectodermal dysplasia at ages 3 months and 2 years showing sparse and fine hair, frontal bossing, slight maxillary hypoplasia, and abnormal teeth. He had normal intelligence. *C–E:* One of two identically affected sisters with anhidrosis, short, fine hair, maxillary hypoplasia, pouting lips, dark wrinkles around the eyes, and only four conical teeth. *F:* A man with the X-linked recessive form, showing pouting lips, mild maxillary hypoplasia, flattening of the nasal bridge, and scant eyebrows and lashes. (*A* and *B:* Courtesy of Dr. Y. E. Hsia, New Haven, Conn. *C–E:* From S. W. Hartwell *et al., Clin. Pediatr.* [*Phila.*], **4:**383–86, 1965. *F:* From R. E. Rossman, *Cutis,* **4:**1246–48, 1968.)

Focal Dermal Hypoplasia (Goltz' Syndrome)

In 1962 Goltz, Peterson, Gorlin, and Ravits [1] described three girls with congenital skin defects, nodules of herniated subcutaneous fat, abnormal pigmentation, and digit and eye anomalies. While this syndrome had been described before 1962, it is often designated Goltz' syndrome. More than 40 cases have been described [2–6].

Physical Features

SKIN: The skin lesions, which may involve the face, trunk, and limbs, are present at birth. The most characteristic findings are streaks of thin skin and herniation of nodules of fat (*Figure E*). Another common finding is depressed or atrophic areas with either hypo- or hyperpigmentation (*Figures A and B*) and telangiectasia. Angiofibromas are often present on the lips (*Figure D*), vulva, and anus.

HAIR: The hair is usually thin, sparse, and short.

TEETH: Most patients have small teeth with deficient enamel. Absent and extra teeth and malalignment have also been described [2,4].

NAILS: Thin, dystrophic nails are common (*Figure F*).

HEAD: Out of 33 patients, 6 had microcephaly and 1 hydrocephalus [6].

EYES: Seven of 15 patients in one review [2] had eye anomalies, which included microphthalmia (*Figure D*), colobomas, and strabismus.

GENITALIA: A few females have had hypoplastic external genitals [6].

BACK: Scoliosis was present in 4 of 33 patients [6].

LIMBS: Many patients have skeletal anomalies, the most common of which involve the digits, such as syndactyly, polydactyly, clinodactyly, absent digits, and ectrodactyly (*Figures C and F*).

HEIGHT AND WEIGHT: Most of the reported patients have been short and thin.

DERMATOGLYPHICS: Dermal ridge hypoplasia has been observed on the digits and hypothenar areas [4].

Nervous System

The incidence of mental retardation has not been established, but it has occurred in a few instances. Two patients, a child [1] and an adult [6], were severely retarded. Another child, who seemed as an infant [5] to have normal develop-ment, had an IQ of less than 60 at 5 years of age [7]. One patient had severe combined sensory and conductive hearing loss [2].

Pathology

The essential change is the presence in the dermis of apparently normal adipose cells. The extent of the dermal collagen hypoplasia varies from site to site in the same patient. The epithelial structures and epidermis are normal.

Genetics

Almost all of the reported patients have been females [6], which suggests that this disorder either is usually lethal in males or is not as easily recognized in males.

Differential Diagnosis

1. Atrophic skin with hyperpigmentation and telangiectasia, short hair, and poor nail development are features of the Rothmund-Thomson syndrome, but these patients do not usually have any skin lesions at birth, have no dermal hypoplasia, and have atrophic changes in the epidermis (see page 368).
2. Linear streaks of hyperpigmentation and eye anomalies occur in incontinentia pigmenti, but the initial lesions are vesicles and bullae and these are not usually present at birth (see page 362).
3. Other skin lesions which resemble angiofibromas and may occur on the lips and gluteal area are warts and condyloma accuminata, but these lesions are lobulated and usually have a gray or white color [2].

References

1. Goltz, R. W., Peterson, W. C., Gorlin, R. J., and Ravits, H. G. Focal dermal hypoplasia. *Arch. Dermatol.,* **86:**708–17, 1962.
2. Holden, J. D., and Akers, W. A. Goltz's syndrome: focal dermal hypoplasia. *Am. J. Dis. Child.,* **114:**292–300, 1967.
3. Daly, J. F. Focal dermal hypoplasia. *Cutis,* **4:**1354–59, 1968.
4. Goltz, R. W., Henderson, R. R., Hitch, J. M., and Ott, J. E. Focal dermal hypoplasia syndrome. A review of the literature and report of two cases. *Arch. Dermatol.,* **101:**1–11, 1970.
5. Lever, W. F. Hypoplasia cutis congenita. *Arch. Dermatol.,* **90:**340, 1964.
6. Warburg, M. Focal dermal hypoplasia. Ocular and general manifestations with a survey of the literature. *Acta Ophthalmol.,* **48:**525–36, 1970.
7. Cloherty, J. P. Personal communication, 1970.

Plate VII-4. *A C:* A newborn female with no left eye, areas of hypopigmentation on the face and legs, and a split-foot deformity. *D–F:* A 13-year-old girl with a small right eye, an angiofibroma of the lip, areas of marked protrusion of subcutaneous fat on her legs, deformed fingers and toes, and hypoplastic nails. Patchy depigmentation was present on her face, legs, hands, and feet. (*A–C:* Courtesy of Dr. G. W. Hazard, Hyannis, Mass. *D* and *F* [*top*]: Courtesy of Dr. W. A. Akers, San Francisco, Calif. *E* and *F* [*bottom*]: From J. D. Holden and W. A. Akers, *Am. J. Dis. Child.,* **114:**292–300, 1967.)

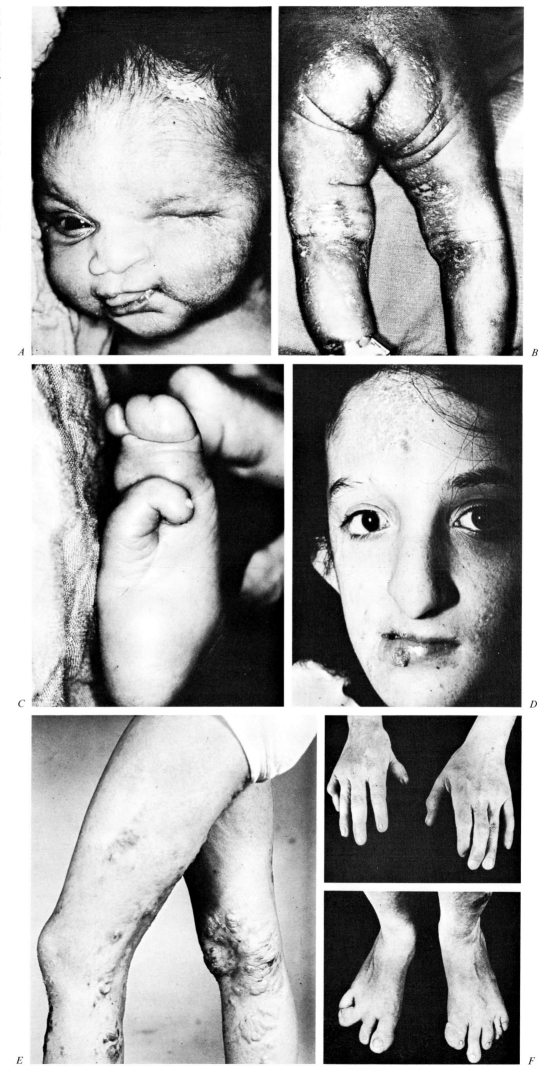

Incontinentia Pigmenti
(Bloch-Sulzberger Syndrome)

The term *incontinentia pigmenti* is used to designate a dermatologic lesion that progresses from vesicles and bullae to hyperkeratosis and finally to streaks of pigmentation. Because incontinentia pigmenti refers only to the end stage of this disease, it is considered by some [1] an inappropriate term. Bloch [2] in 1926 and Sulzberger [3] in 1927 described a patient with these end-stage pigmentary changes, as well as spasticity and mental retardation. This syndrome, which includes dermal, skeletal, and nervous system abnormalities, has now been described in more than 300 patients [4,5].

Physical Features

SKIN: The initial lesions, which usually develop in the first months of life, are bullae and vesicles with an erythematous base (*Figures A, B, and C*). They are usually arranged in lines or groups and located on the trunk and extremities. These lesions are often pruritic and may develop into pustules. The lesions may persist or come and go for several months. They are gradually replaced by verrucous and hyperkeratotic lesions (*Figure D*) which appear at the site of the original blebs; these lesions constitute the second stage of the skin changes. The third type of lesion is the gray or brown pigmentation and dermal fibrosis which develops after the keratotic crusts are lost (*Figures E and F*). The time required for the transition of the skin lesions may be a few weeks or several years. In general, the pigmented lesions persist for several years and fade very slowly, leaving either normal-looking or slightly atrophic and depigmented areas [1,5].

HAIR: Patchy, scarring alopecia is common [4,5].

TEETH: The teeth are often either missing, late in erupting, or malformed, especially conical. In a study of 20 patients, 19 had dental anomalies [5].

NAILS: The nails may be thin, poorly developed, or even replaced by hyperkeratotic plugs.

HEAD: Microcephaly is frequently observed.

EYES: Many different eye anomalies, including microphthalmia, corneal opacities, cataracts, retinal detachment, optic atrophy, and strabismus, have been described. In one review [4], about one third of the patients had eye abnormalities; the most common finding was a mass in the posterior chamber of the eye.

Nervous System

In a review of 145 patients, 43 had neurologic abnormalities, including hemiparesis, spastic tetraplegia, seizures, and mental deficiency [4]. In a study of 24 patients, 4 had paresis and 3 were mentally deficient (2 had retarded parents) [5].

Pathology

The bullae of the early skin lesions are located within the epidermis, and the fluid in the blebs contains large numbers of eosinophils. The number of tissue mast cells and the skin histamine content are increased. The second stage is characterized by hyperkeratosis and acanthosis with lymphocytic infiltrations of the dermis. In the pigmentary stage the melanophages in the upper dermis are loaded with melanin. The epidermis may be either thickened or atrophic [1]. Few neuropathologic studies have been reported. In a report on two patients [6] it was noted that one had no brain abnormalities and the other had micropolygyria of the cortex, unilateral pyramidal hypoplasia, and several small areas of sclerotic atrophy and neuronal loss in the central white matter.

Laboratory Studies

Eosinophilia, accounting for as much as 50 percent of the peripheral white blood cells, is present during the stage of bullae and blisters [1]. A variety of skeletal anomalies, such as hemivertebrae and wide, fused, or bifid ribs, have been described.

Treatment and Prognosis

Only supportive skin care is helpful. The lesions eventually disappear.

Genetics

Almost all of the reported cases have been females; there is doubt as to the diagnosis in some reported males [1]. It has been suggested [7] that the disease is due to an X-linked mutant gene, which is dominant in females and lethal in males. It has also been postulated [4] that the mutant gene has an X-linked dominant mode of inheritance.

Differential Diagnosis

1. Patients with epidermolysis bullosa dystrophica (recessive form) have vesicles in infancy and scarring alopecia, but normal teeth and nails. The vesicles develop at sites of trauma; and keloid scar formation, hyperpigmentation, and depigmentation occur during healing. This disorder affects both males and females.

2. Linear areas of dermal hypoplasia with hyperpigmentation and anomalies of the hair, teeth, nails, and eyes are features of patients with focal dermal hypoplasia. However, the dermal hypoplasia is associated with nodules of herniated fat, and there are no bullae or vesicular lesions (see page 360).

3. Reticular hyperpigmentation and hyperkeratosis are also features of Naegeli's syndrome; however, there are no bullae or vesicles, no associated ectodermal or ocular anomalies, and both males and females are affected [8].

References

1. Asboe-Hansen, G. Incontinentia pigmenti—bullous keratogenous and pigmentary dermatitis with blood eosinophilia in newborn girls. *Cutis,* **4:**1341–44, 1968.
2. Bloch, B. Eigentümliche bisher nicht beschriebene Pigmentaffektion (Incontinentia pigmenti). *Schweiz. Med. Wochenschr.,* **7:**404–405, 1926.
3. Sulzberger, M. B. Über eine bisher nicht beschriebene congenitale Pigmentanomalie (Incontinentia Pigmenti). *Arch. Dermatol. Syph.* (*Berl.*), **154:**19–32, 1927.
4. Pfeiffer, R. A. Das Syndrom der Incontinentia Pigmenti (Bloch-Siemens). *Munch. Med. Wochenschr.,* **101:**2312–16, 1959.
5. Carney, R. G., and Carney, R. G., Jr. Incontinentia pigmenti. *Arch. Dermatol.,* **102:**157–62, 1970.
5a. Morgan, J. D. Incontinentia pigmenti (Bloch-Sulzberger syndrome). *Am. J. Dis. Child.,* **122:**294–300, 1971.
6. O'Doherty, N. J., and Norman, R. M. Incontinentia pigmenti (Bloch-Sulzberger syndrome) with cerebral malformation. *Dev. Med. Child Neurol.,* **10:**168–74, 1968.
7. Lenz, W. Zur Genetik der Incontinentia Pigmenti. *Ann. Paediatr.* (*Basel*), **196:**149–65, 1961.
8. Naegeli, O. Familiärer Chromatophorennävus. *Schweiz. Med. Wochenschr.,* **8:**48–49, 1927.

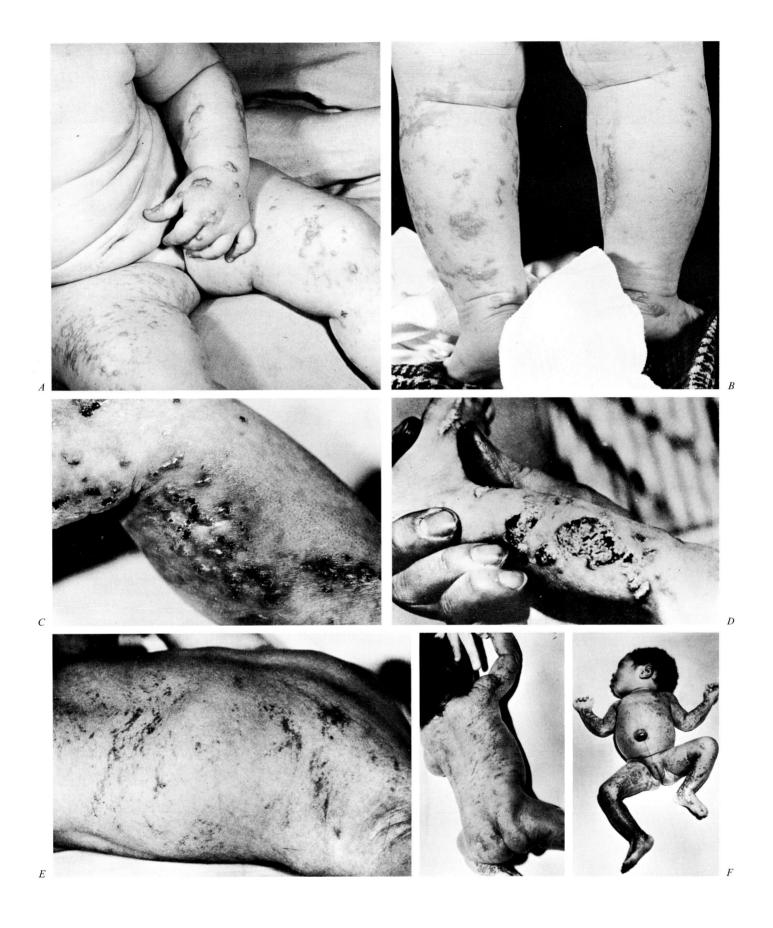

Plate VII-5. *A* and *B:* An infant with numerous vesicles, some in linear streaks. *C:* Shows vesicles, bullae, and pustules on the leg of another child. *D:* Shows the second stage of the disease, consisting of verrucous and hyperkeratotic lesions at the site of the original vesicles. *E:* The third stage, linear hyperpigmentation, shown here on the chest and abdomen. *F:* An infant with widespread linear hyperpigmentation. (*A* and *B:* Courtesy of Dr. T. B. Fitzpatrick, Boston, Mass. *C–E:* From G. Asboe-Hansen, *Cutis,* **4:**1341–44, 1968. *F:* From W. A. Lieb and D. Guerry, III, *Am. J. Ophthalmol.,* **45:**265–71, 1958.)

Linear Sebaceous Nevus with Convulsions and Mental Retardation

In 1962 Feuerstein and Mims [1] described two unrelated boys with linear nevi of the face associated with convulsions and mental retardation. Since then at least nine more patients have been described [2–9].

Physical Features

SKIN: The skin lesions are similar to the organoid nevus, also called the nevus sebaceus of Jadassohn. These lesions are present at birth. There are often yellow-orange papules which form a patch or linear streak in the middle of the forehead, extending down the nose (*Figures A, C, and E*). Some patients have large pigmented nevi on the neck (*Figures B, C, and F*), trunk, back, and extremities (*Figure D*).

HAIR: Some patients have had areas of alopecia [3–5,9].

EYES: Four patients have had lipodermoids of the conjunctivae [2,4,5] (*Figure C*); vascularization of the cornea and iris and choroid colobomas have also been noted [2,4].

Nervous System

Some, but not all, of the reported patients have been retarded. Seizures usually begin in the first months of life. One child [2] had hydrocephalus and dilatation of a lateral ventricle; another [7] had hydrocephalus *ex vacuo* and a third [4] had unilateral cortical atrophy.

Pathology

In general, skin biopsies show thickening and hyperplasia of the epidermis and hyperplasia of sebaceous glands.

Laboratory Studies

Electroencephalograms showed focal spikes in three patients [1,6] and more generalized and severe abnormalities in four others [2,4,7,9]. One patient [9] had an increased level of spinal fluid protein. One [7] had a generalized aminoaciduria and vitamin D–resistant rickets. One child [2] had coarctation of the aorta.

Genetics

No similarly affected family members have been reported.

Differential Diagnosis

1. The sebaceous or organoid nevus, not associated with mental retardation and seizures, is a common lesion involving most of the skin constituents and usually located on the scalp. These lesions show underdevelopment in infancy, hyperplasia at puberty, and benign and malignant tumor growth in adulthood [10].

2. Facial papules, seizures, and mental retardation are features of tuberous sclerosis, but the facial papules (adenoma sebaceum) are not present at birth and, when present, have a butterfly distribution (see page 380).

References

1. Feuerstein, R. C., and Mims, L. C. Linear nevus sebaceus with convulsions and mental retardation. *Am. J. Dis. Child.,* **104:**675–79, 1962.
2. Marden, P. M., and Venters, H. D. A new neurocutaneous syndrome. *Am. J. Dis. Child.,* **112:**79–81, 1966.
3. Monahan, R. H., Hill, C. W., and Venters, H. D. Multiple choristomas, convulsions and mental retardation as a new neurocutaneous syndrome. *Am. J. Ophthalmol.,* **64:**528–32, 1967.
4. Moynahan, E. J., and Wolff, O. H. A new neuro-cutaneous syndrome (skin, eye and brain) consisting of linear naevus, bilateral lipo-dermoid of the conjunctivae, cranial thickening, cerebral cortical atrophy and mental retardation. *Br. J. Dermatol.,* **79:**651–52, 1967.
5. Lantis, S., Leyden, J., Thew, M., and Heaton, C. Nevus sebaceus of Jadassohn. *Arch. Dermatol.,* **98:**117–223, 1968.
6. Solomon, L. M., Fretzin, D. F., and Dewald, R. L. The epidermal nevus syndrome. *Arch. Dermatol.,* **97:**273–85, 1968.
7. Sugarman, G. I., and Reed, W. B. Two unusual neurocutaneous disorders with facial cutaneous signs. *Arch. Neurol.,* **21:**242–47, 1969.
8. Bianchine, J. W. The nevus sebaceus of Jadassohn. A neurocutaneous syndrome and a potentially premalignant lesion. *Am. J. Dis. Child.,* **120:**223–28, 1970.
9. Lovejoy, F. H., Jr. Personal communication, 1970.
10. Mehregan, A. H., and Pinkus, H. Life history of organoid nevi. *Arch. Dermatol.,* **91:**574–88, 1965.

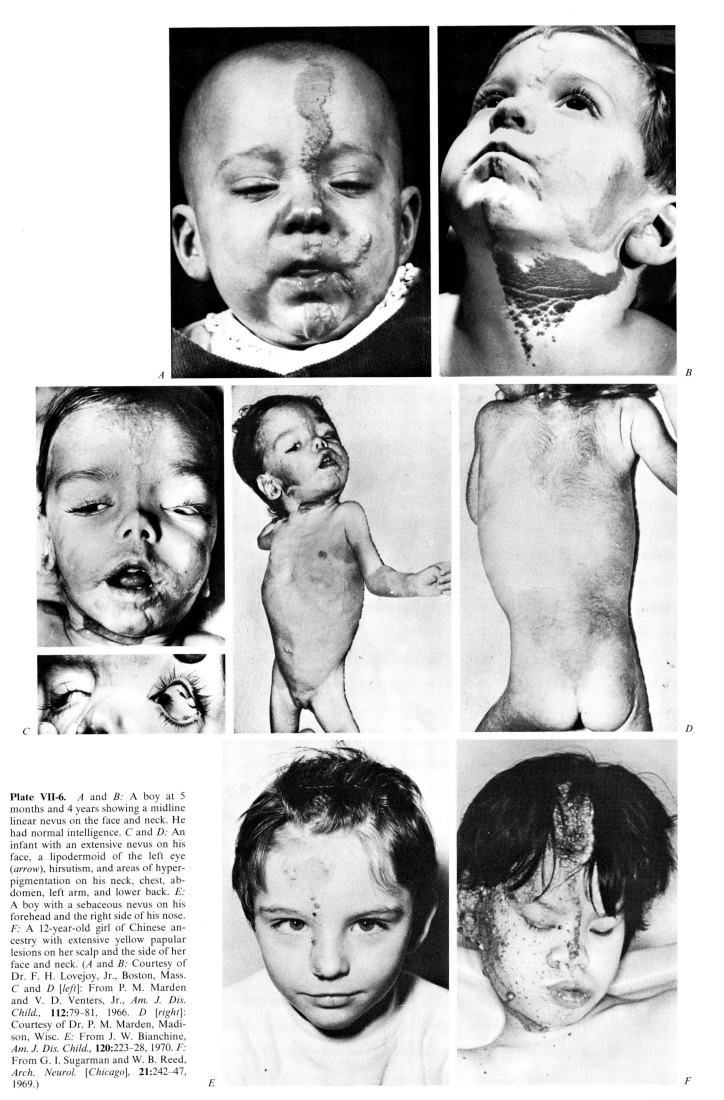

Plate VII-6. *A* and *B:* A boy at 5 months and 4 years showing a midline linear nevus on the face and neck. He had normal intelligence. *C* and *D:* An infant with an extensive nevus on his face, a lipodermoid of the left eye (*arrow*), hirsutism, and areas of hyperpigmentation on his neck, chest, abdomen, left arm, and lower back. *E:* A boy with a sebaceous nevus on his forehead and the right side of his nose. *F:* A 12-year-old girl of Chinese ancestry with extensive yellow papular lesions on her scalp and the side of her face and neck. (*A* and *B:* Courtesy of Dr. F. H. Lovejoy, Jr., Boston, Mass. *C* and *D* [*left*]: From P. M. Marden and V. D. Venters, Jr., *Am. J. Dis. Child.,* **112:**79–81, 1966. *D* [*right*]: Courtesy of Dr. P. M. Marden, Madison, Wisc. *E:* From J. W. Bianchine, *Am. J. Dis. Child.,* **120:**223–28, 1970. *F:* From G. I. Sugarman and W. B. Reed, *Arch. Neurol.* [*Chicago*], **21:**242–47, 1969.)

Neurofibromatosis
(von Recklinghausen's Disease)

In 1882 von Recklinghausen [1] first reported the clinical and pathologic features of neurofibromatosis. Subsequent studies have shown this to be a common clinical syndrome of skin pigmentation and central and peripheral nervous system tumors. It is considered the most common neurocutaneous syndrome; the incidence is estimated to be 1:2500–3300 births [2].

Physical Features

SKIN: Patches of increased pigmentation, usually pale yellow or light brown (cafe-au-lait spots), are one of the two common skin lesions. These spots are usually irregular in outline and oval in shape, although many different shapes occur [3] (*Figures A and B*). They are often present at birth and are usually the first physical sign of neurofibromatosis [4]. They increase in size and number during the first and second decades. Since multiple cafe-au-lait spots are unusual in normal children, it has been suggested that a child with five or more spots having a diameter of at least 0.5 cm should be considered as having neurofibromatosis until proven otherwise [5]. In a study of 149 persons with neurofibromatosis it was found that 78 percent had six or more cafe-au-lait spots; 5 percent had none [2]. Based on the results of this study it was suggested that any person with more than six cafe-au-lait spots exceeding 1.5 cm in broadest diameter must be presumed to have neurofibromatosis even in the absence of a positive family history. Another helpful clinical sign is the presence of freckles in the axilla (*Figure B*), a finding that is almost always diagnostic of neurofibromatosis. (One child with progeria is the only known exception to this rule [6].)

Skin tumors are the other common manifestation. These tumors usually appear in late childhood or early adolescence and are either cutaneous or subcutaneous. The cutaneous tumors are discrete nodules that may be either gelatinous or firm in consistency (*Figure C*). The size varies from a few millimeters to 1 or 2 cm. The shape is quite variable—flattened, sessile, pedunculated, conical, or lobular. Initially, these tumors may be purplish in color, but later they are flesh-colored. With compression the soft tumors may invaginate, which is called "buttonholing." The total number of cutaneous tumors may be only a few or several thousand. The subcutaneous tumors are firm, discrete nodules which are most often found on the face, cranium, neck, or chest. They are often attached to a peripheral nerve (*Figure D*). They may be associated with a great overgrowth of subcutaneous tissue which feels like a bag of strings or worms. This overgrowth may cause hideous disfigurement.

EYES: Pulsatile exophthalmos may occur in association with a defect in the orbit and a retroocular growth of neural tissue (*Figure E*).

BACK: Scoliosis is frequent. Nine of 46 children in one study [4] had scoliosis.

LIMBS: Some patients have localized overgrowth of an entire limb, a digit, or a portion of a bone.

GROWTH AND DEVELOPMENT: Isosexual precocious puberty has been observed in several patients [7].

Nervous System

Mental deficiency is considered a common finding in neurofibromatosis, but the incidence is not known. In a study of 46 children, 11 were retarded or had slow development [4]. Many patients have abnormalities of cranial nerve function due to gliomas of the acoustic, trigeminal, and optic nerves. Spinal root tumors and meningiomas are occasionally present.

Pathology

The cafe-au-lait spots have a normal number of melanocytes; the increased pigmentation is due to an excess of melanosomes in the malpighian cells. Giant pigment granules may be seen in the malpighian cells and the melanocytes. These granules are present in both the areas of normal skin color and the areas of hyperpigmentation [3]. The cutaneous tumors consist of elongated connective tissue cells which lack the support of normal dermal collagen. Studies using two different glucose-6-phosphate dehydrogenase genes as markers showed that the tumors in two women had a multiple cell origin [8a]. The nerve root tumors usually contain a mixture of fibroblasts and Schwann cells. More differentiated tumors, such as pheochromocytomas, sarcomas, glioblastomas and meningiomas, also occur. Neuropathologic studies of 10 patients with neurofibromatosis showed abnormalities of cerebral development, including disorders of cortical architecture and neuronal heterotopias [8]. The 5 patients with mental subnormality had more severe abnormalities than the 5 with normal intelligence. Several patients have had renal artery dysplasia in association with hypertension [8b].

Treatment and Prognosis

Surgical removal of tumors is recommended when they cause mechanical damage due to local growth, when they are disfiguring, and, of course, when they are malignant.

Genetics

Autosomal dominant.

Differential Diagnosis

1. Large cafe-au-lait spots similar to those seen in neurofibromatosis may occur in patients with Albright's syndrome of polyostotic fibrous dysplasia. However, these patients often have associated bone cysts; they do not have skin tumors, and giant pigment granules are rarely seen in their malpighian cells and melanocytes [3].
2. Acoustic neuromas occur in individuals with few or no cafe-au-lait spots and subcutaneous tumors. They have been considered as having "central neurofibromatosis" [9].
3. Several patients with the syndrome of cafe-au-lait spots, pulmonary stenosis, and mental deficiency have been described [10].

References

1. von Recklinghausen, F. *Über die Multiplen Fibrome der Haut and ihre Beziehung zuden Multiplen Neuromen.* A. Hirschwald, Berlin, 1882, p. 138.
2. Crowe, F. W., Schull, W. J., and Neel, J. V. *A Clinical, Pathological and Genetic Study of Multiple Neurofibromatosis.* Charles C Thomas, Publisher, Springfield, Ill., 1956.
3. Benedict, P. H., Szabó, G., Fitzpatrick, T. B., and Sinesi, S. J. Melanotic macules in Albright's syndrome and in neurofibromatosis. *J.A.M.A.*, 205:618–26, 1968.
4. Fienman, N. L., and Yakovac, W. C. Neurofibromatosis in childhood. *J. Pediatr.*, 76:339–46, 1970.
5. Whitehouse, D. Diagnostic value of the café-au-lait spot in children. *Arch. Dis. Child.*, 41:316–19, 1966.
6. Fitzpatrick, T. B. Personal communication, 1969.
7. Saxena, K. M. Endocrine manifestations of neurofibromatosis in children. *Am. J. Dis. Child.*, 120:265–71, 1970.
8. Rosman, N. P., and Pearce, J. The brain in multiple neurofibromatosis (von Recklinghausen's disease): a suggested neuropathological basis for the associated mental defect. *Brain*, 90:829–38, 1967.
8a. Fialkow, P. J., Sagebiel, R. W., Gartler, S. M., and Rimoin, D. L. Multiple cell origin of neurofibromatosis. *N. Engl. J. Med.*, 284:298–300, 1971.
8b. Bourke, E., and Gatenby, P. B. B. Renal artery dysplasia with hypertension in neurofibromatosis. *Br. Med. J.*, 3:681–82, 1971.
9. Young, D. F., Eldridge, R., and Gardner, W. J. Bilateral acoustic neuroma in a large kindred. *J.A.M.A.*, 214:347–53, 1970.
10. Watson, G. H. Pulmonary stenosis, café-au-lait spots and dull intelligence. *Arch. Dis. Child.*, 42:303–307, 1967.
11. Brasfield, R. D., and Das Gupta, T. K. Von Recklinghausen's disease: a clinicopathological study. *Ann. Surg.*, 175:86–104, 1972.

Plate VII-7. *A:* Melanotic macules that stop at the midline, cover large areas, or have irregular borders are considered features of Albright's syndrome of polyostotic fibrous dysplasia, and yet all three patients pictured had neurofibromatosis. *B:* A girl with multiple pigmented nevi, freckles on the neck and in the axilla, and a tumor of a sympathetic nerve ganglion in her neck. *C:* A man with numerous skin tumors of various shapes and sizes. *D:* Two isolated tumors located on peripheral nerves. *E, F:* A body with pulsatile exophthalmos and ptosis of the right eye shown at 6 and 13 years of age. His pneumoencephalogram shows marked asymmetry and enlargement of the calvarium, lateral cerebral ventricles, the temporal horn (*arrows*), and the orbit on the right side. He also has elevation and stretching of the right lesser sphenoid wing. (*A* [*left*]: From F. Albright, *J. Clin. Endocrinol. Metab.,* **7:**307–24, 1947. *A* [*center and right*]: From P. H. Benedict *et al., J.A.M.A.,* **205:**618–22, 1968. *B* [*right*]: From K. M. Saxena, *Am. J. Dis. Child.,* **120:**265–71, 1970. *C, D,* and *E* [*top*]: Courtesy of Dr. G. R. Hogan, Boston, Mass.)

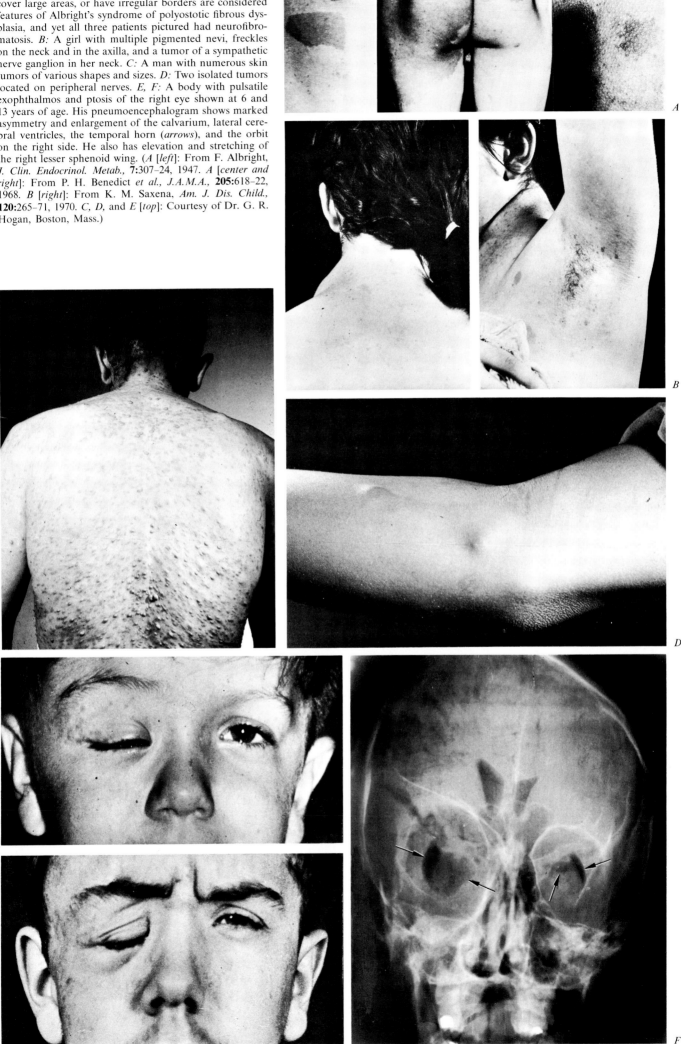

Rothmund-Thomson Syndrome (Poikiloderma Congenitale)

In 1868 Rothmund [1] described several children from an interrelated isolated community in the Alps with cataracts and a peculiar marmorization of the skin. In 1923 Thomson [2] described two sisters with poikiloderma congenitale, which appeared as a red, tense swelling of the skin in infancy and later as punctate atrophy. Although these patients did not have cataracts, the skin biopsy showed a type of hyperkeratosis similar to that described by Rothmund. By 1966 more than 50 patients had been described [3].

Physical Features

SKIN: The first skin lesion is a diffuse, bright pink or red color of the cheeks, which is soon replaced by macular and reticular patterns with lines spreading out and producing a marmoreal appearance. These lesions may be present at birth, but are usually first noticed between the third and sixth months of life. They begin on the face and spread to the ears, buttocks, and extremities, and then to the rest of the body. Later, striae and telangiectases appear. Several types of lesions may be seen in the same area—linear telangiectases, punctate atrophy, depigmentation, and brown pigmentation (*Figures C, D, E, and F*). The child may develop bullae on exposure to sunlight, but ulceration and crusting do not ordinarily occur [3,4].

HAIR: About half of the patients have sparse or short hair, eyebrows, and eyelashes. Some have total alopecia [4] (*Figures A, D, and E*).

TEETH: Abnormalities of teeth, such as microdontia, malformations, and failure of eruption, are frequent.

NAILS: The nails are abnormal in a fourth of the patients [4]. They may be either rough, ridged, and heaped up or small and atrophic (*Figures C and F*).

HEAD: Several patients have had microcephaly. Frontal bossing has also been described.

FACE: A flat bridge of the nose is often noted (*Figure E*).

EYES: Cataracts, usually bilateral, have been reported in about half of the patients (*Figure B*). They develop rapidly over a period of a few weeks or months, and usually are noted between the ages of 3 and 6 years. However, cataracts may appear as early as 4 months of age and occasionally have not developed until the third or fourth decade. Degenerative lesions of the cornea have also been described [4,5].

GENITALIA: Males often have small external genitalia and cryptorchidism (*Figures A and D*).

BACK: Scoliosis has been present in a few patients.

LIMBS: Many patients have skeletal anomalies. Those reported include short distal phalanges, shortening or asymmetry of the extremities, syndactyly, ectrodactyly, absence of metacarpals, rudimentary ulna and radius, and pelvic deformities. No specific pattern of anomalies is consistently present.

HEIGHT: Short stature is common.

GROWTH AND DEVELOPMENT: Both males and females may have poor development of secondary sex characteristics. Females often have amenorrhea and are sterile [4].

Nervous System

Several reported patients were mentally retarded [3,4], but the overall incidence is not known.

Pathology

The histopathology of the skin lesions is not diagnostic. The most consistent findings are hyperkeratosis, atrophy of the epidermis, and areas of increased or decreased pigmentation.

Treatment and Prognosis

The skin lesions are progressive during the first few months and years of life, but after that remain stationary. In adults carcinomatous changes of the skin may occur. The cataracts have been successfully removed [5].

Genetics

Autosomal recessive.

Differential Diagnosis

1. The initial lesion on the cheeks resembles atopic eczema, but the progressive changes and lack of response to treatment clearly differentiate it.
2. Reticulate hyperpigmentation of the skin and dystrophy of the nails are features of patients with dyskeratosis congenita, but they also have leukoplakia of the mucous membranes and pancytopenia, and do not develop cataracts [6].
3. Hyperpigmentation, atrophy of the skin, and telangiectases occur in patients with xeroderma pigmentosa, but they also develop warty and malignant growths, and do not have cataracts or dystrophy of the hair, nails, and teeth (see page 382).
4. Cataracts and a butterfly rash after sun exposure are features of patients with Cockayne's syndrome, but they also have a degenerative neurologic disease and do not have nail or tooth dystrophy (see page 82).
5. Patients with congenital erythropoietic porphyria have photosensitivity of the skin often associated with a vesicular or bullous eruption which leaves depressed pigmented scars. However, they are readily distinguished by their intermittent red urine, red-brown teeth, hypertrichosis, and splenomegaly [7].

References

1. Rothmund, A. Über Kataract in Verbindung mit einer eigentümliche Haut degeneration. *Arch. Ophthalmol.*, **14**:159–66, 1868.
2. Thomson, M. S. An hitherto undescribed familial disease. *Br. J. Dermatol.*, **35**:455–62, 1923.
3. Silver, H. K. Rothmund-Thomson syndrome: an oculocutaneous disorder. *Am. J. Dis. Child.*, **111**:182–90, 1966.
4. Taylor, W. B. Rothmund's syndrome—Thomson's syndrome. *Arch. Dermatol.*, **75**:236–44, 1957.
5. Wahl, J. W., and Ellis, P. P. Rothmund-Thomson syndrome. *Am. J. Ophthalmol.*, **60**:722–26, 1965.
6. Bryan, H. G., and Nixon, R. K. Dyskeratosis congenita and familial pancytopenia. *J.A.M.A.*, **192**:203–208, 1965.
7. Schmid, R. The porphyrias. In *The Metabolic Basis of Inherited Disease*, 2nd ed. Stanbury *et al.* (eds.). McGraw-Hill Book Co., New York, 1966, pp. 813–70.

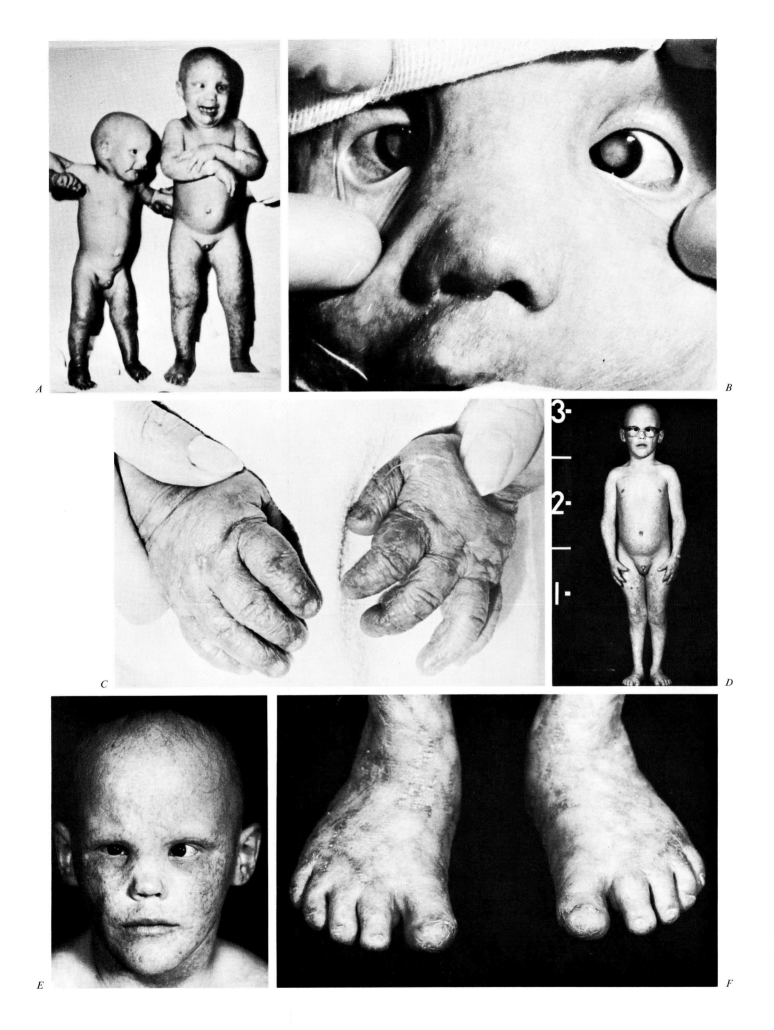

Plate VII-8. *A–C:* Two brothers, aged 17 and 30 months, who showed alopecia, marmorization, pigmentation and atrophy of the skin, small nails, and small external genitalia. The close-up view of the eyes of the older boy shows the mature cataracts and absence of cilia. Only the older boy was considered mentally retarded. *D–F:* A 7⅔-year-old boy with short stature (height 38 in., or 98 cm), reticulated hyperpigmentation, strabismus, flat nasal bridge, and rudimentary or absent toenails. He had normal intelligence. (*A:* From H. K. Silver, *Am. J. Dis. Child.,* **111:**182–90, 1966. *B* and *C:* From J. W. Wahl and P. P. Ellis, *Am. J. Ophthalmol.,* **60:**722–26, 1965. *D–F:* Courtesy of Dr. W. A. Lafrance, Montreal, Canada.)

Sjögren-Larsson Syndrome

In 1957 Sjögren and Larsson [1] reported 28 patients with a new hereditary disorder consisting of congenital ichthyosis, spasticity, and mental retardation. Although the first group of patients was found in an inbred Swedish population, this disease has now been described in many ethnic groups and many parts of the world [2–5].

Physical Features

SKIN: The skin lesions in the reported patients have not been identical. In the original Swedish patients [2] the lesions were like nonbullous congenital ichthyosiform erythröderma. There was generalized scaling ichthyosis of the neck, trunk, and extremities, which was more noticeable in the axillae and flexural areas of the extremities (*Figures A and B*). Moderate hyperkeratosis and desquamation were present on the palms and soles (*Figure C*). The erythema was more often noted in the very young patients. By contrast, the American patient reported by Gilbert and coworkers [3] had lesions like lamellar ichthyosis. At birth the child only had thick skin. When 2½ years old he had generalized ichthyosis that was more marked on his arms and legs. The scales were large and gray-brown. The palms and soles were involved (*Figures D and E*). In all patients [2,3] sweating was either sparse or absent over the entire body.

HAIR: The scalp hair may be normal or thin. Usually there is no loss of eyebrows or eyelashes.

TEETH: A few reported patients have had deficient enamel [2].

NAILS: The nails are normal.

EYES: Fundal changes have been described in about a quarter of the patients, but the nature of the lesion has varied considerably. In general, there is degeneration of the pigmentary epithelium that is most evident in the region of the macula (*Figure F*). This has been observed in 2-year-olds, but more often in adults [3].

Nervous System

These patients are usually severely retarded. In addition, they have spasticity, primarily in the legs, although the deep tendon reflexes in the arms are slightly hyperactive. Some patients have seizures.

Pathology

The skin biopsies in some patients [2] have shown a basket-weave pattern in the stratum corneum, few sweat glands, and diminished or absent stratum granulosum; these are the typical changes of ichthyosis erythroderma. Others [3] have shown a slightly papillomatous epidermis with hyperkeratosis and hypergranulosis compatible with lamellar ichthyosis.

Laboratory Studies

No abnormalities of amino acids or chromosomes have been consistently observed [2,4], although the incomplete studies on one large kindred [5] suggested an associated aminoaciduria.

Genetics

Autosomal recessive.

Differential Diagnosis

1. Congenital ichthyosiform erythroderma and lamellar ichthyosis both occur as isolated autosomal recessive traits unassociated with spasticity or mental retardation [6].
2. Patients with Refsum's syndrome may have ichthyosis and retinal changes, but they also have normal intelligence, polyneuritis, and an elevated serum phytanic acid level [7].
3. Ichthyosis and mental retardation are also features of patients with the X-linked syndrome of ichthyosis and hypogonadism (see page 378).

References

1. Sjögren, T., and Larsson, T. Oligophrenia in combination with congenital ichthyosis and spastic disorders: a clinical and genetic study. *Acta Psychiatr. Scand.*, **32** (Suppl. 113):1–112, 1957.
2. Heijer, A., and Reed, W. B. Sjögren-Larsson syndrome. *Arch. Dermatol.*, **92**:545–52, 1965.
3. Gilbert, W. R., Jr., Smith, J. L., and Nyhan, W. L. The Sjögren-Larsson syndrome. *Arch. Ophthalmol.* (*Chicago*), **80**:308–16, 1968.
4. Selmanowitz, V. J., and Porter, M. J. The Sjögren-Larsson syndrome. *Am. J. Med.*, **42**:412–22, 1967.
5. Witkop, C. J., Jr., and Henry, F. V. Sjögren-Larsson syndrome and histidinemia: hereditary biochemical diseases with defects of speech and oral functions. *J. Speech Hear. Disord.*, **28**:109–23, 1963.
6. Esterly, N. The ichthyosiform dermatoses. *Pediatrics*, **42**:990–1004, 1969.
7. Steinberg, D., Vroom, F. Q., Engel, W. K., Cammermeyer, J., Mize, C. E., and Avigan, J. Refsum's disease—a recently characterized lipidosis involving the nervous system. *Ann. Intern. Med.*, **66**:365–95, 1967.

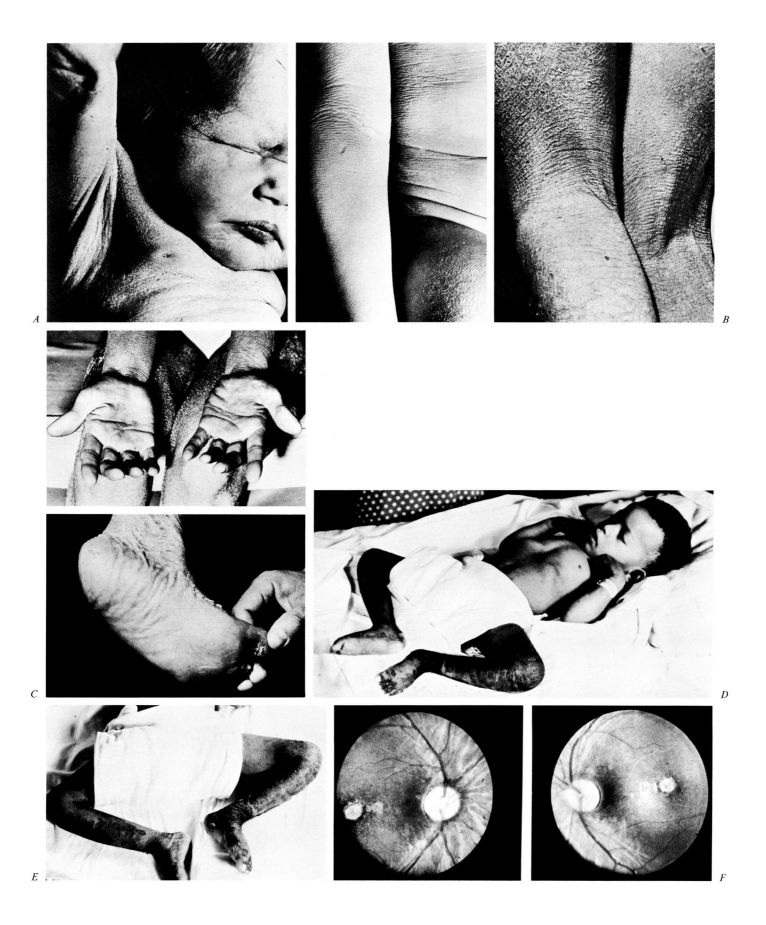

Plate VII-9. *A:* A 4-day-old infant with generalized ichthyosis and erythema. She later developed spasticity of the legs. *B:* Shows thickening and scaling of the skin in the antecubital fossa and the popliteal spaces. *C:* Shows thickening and a few areas of desquamation on the palms and soles. *D–F:* A 2⁷⁄₁₂-year-old Negro boy with spastic diplegia, contractures, generalized ichthyosis, and retinal lesions in each macular area. The scaling of the skin was most severe on his hands and legs. (*A:* From A. Heijer and W. B. Reed, *Arch. Dermatol.* [*Chicago*], **92:**545–52, 1965. *B* [*left*]: From W. B. Reed and A. Heijer, *Am. J. Dis. Child.,* **116:**653–54, 1968. *B* [*right*] and *C:* Courtesy of Dr. W. B. Reed, Burbank, Calif. *D–F:* From W. R. Gilbert *et al., Arch. Ophthalmol.* [*Chicago*], **80:**308–16, 1968.)

Sturge-Weber Syndrome (Encephalofacial Angiomatosis)

In 1879 Sturge [1] described a child who had a port-wine stain on the right side of her face and scalp, glaucoma of the right eye, and seizures affecting only the left side of her body. In 1922 Weber [2] reported the intracranial calcifications in a woman with spastic hemiplegia, a large port-wine stain over the face, chest, arms, and back, and unilateral glaucoma. Over 250 reported patients were reviewed in 1960 [3].

Physical Features

SKIN: The facial port-wine stain (nevus flammeus) is present at birth. It is often confined to half of the face in a pattern similar to that of the branches of the trigeminal nerve (*Figure C*). However, it may be bilateral and present on other parts of the body (*Figures A and B*). The stain is sharply demarcated and flat; the intensity of the color decreases with age. In many patients the area of the stain becomes thickened and verrucous with age.

EYES: The most common eye lesion is a choroidal angioma (*Figure E*). This is often associated with glaucoma and an enlarged globe (*Figures A, C, and F*).

MOUTH: In the area of the port-wine stain there are often angiomas of the mouth, nose, and throat. These areas may appear to be overgrown. The soft tissue and bone are enlarged and there is early eruption of teeth (*Figures A and C*).

Nervous System

Most patients have focal motor seizures. They may also have spastic hemiplegia, hemiatrophy, and homonymous hemianopia contralateral to the facial lesions. Mental retardation is very common; in one series of 35 patients, 19 were retarded [4]. The severity of the retardation is quite variable.

Pathology

The essential pathology is angiomatosis of the skin and the leptomeninges. The areas of meningeal thickening with venous angiomatosis are usually found over the occipital lobe and on the same side as the facial nevus, although other areas of the brain may be involved. The cortical and subcortical regions may have increased vascularity and be atrophic and sclerotic. In the affected areas of the cortex there are loss of neurons and fibers, extensive gliosis, pericapillary fibrosis, and deposition of calcium and iron in both the capillary walls and the cortical parenchyma. The cortical calcification follows cerebral convolutions. Both the atrophic changes and the calcium deposits increase in size as the child grows older [5]. Malformations of the cerebral and cerebellar cortex, including micropolygyria and agyria, were noted in one patient [6].

Laboratory Studies

Most of the patients have intracranial calcifications. These are usually on the same side as the facial nevus and have the appearance of double curvilinear ("railroad track" or "tram line") densities (*Figure D*). These lesions are usually not visible on x-ray in the first 2 years of life. The electroencephalogram often shows a depression of cortical activity on the affected side; spike waves are sometimes, but not always, present. Cerebral atrophy with unilateral dilatation of the ventricle and widening of the subarachnoid sulci may be demonstrated on the affected side by pneumoencephalography.

Treatment and Prognosis

The extent of the intracranial angiomas cannot be correlated with the size of the facial nevus. Some patients whose seizures were difficult to control with anticonvulsants have benefited from surgical excision of the affected parts of the cerebral cortex [4].

Genetics

No increased incidence of this syndrome among the relatives of the affected patients has been reported.

Differential Diagnosis

1. Capillary hemangiomas are a common facial nevus in the newborn, but the lesions are usually located on the forehead and eyelids and not in the pattern of trigeminal nerve distribution.
2. Retinal angiomas and intracranial calcifications are seen in patients with the von Hippel–Lindau syndrome, but there is no facial nevus or cortical railroad track calcifications or mental deficiency [7].
3. Intracranial calcifications are seen in patients with congenital toxoplasmosis (see page 124), cytomegalovirus (see page 122) and perinatal herpes (see page 130) infection, tuberous sclerosis (see page 380), and pseudohypoparathyroidism (see page 50), but the location and pattern in each are different from the Sturge-Weber syndrome.

References

1. Sturge, W. A. A case of partial epilepsy, apparently due to a lesion of one of the vasomotor centres of the brain. *Trans. Clin. Soc. London,* **12**:162–67, 1879.
2. Weber, F. P. Right-sided hemi-hypotrophy resulting from right-sided congenital spastic hemiplegia, with a morbid condition of the left side of the brain, revealed by radiograms. *J. Neurol. Psychopath.,* **3**:134–39, 1922.
3. Alexander, G. L., and Norman, R. M. *The Sturge-Weber Syndrome.* John Wright & Sons, Ltd., Bristol, 1960.
4. Peterman, A. F., Hayles, A. B., Dockerty, M. B., and Love, J. G. Encephalotrigeminal angiomatosis (Sturge-Weber disease). Clinical study of thirty-five cases. *J.A.M.A.,* **167**:2169–76, 1958.
5. Chao, D. H.-C. Congenital neurocutaneous syndrome of childhood. III. Sturge-Weber disease. *J. Pediatr.,* **55**:635–49, 1959.
6. Nellhaus, G., Haberland, C., and Hill, B. J. Sturge-Weber disease with bilateral intracranial calcifications at birth and unusual pathologic findings. *Acta Neurol. Scand.,* **43**:314–47, 1967.
7. Melmon, K. L., and Rosen, S. W. Lindau's disease. Review of the literature and study of a large kindred. *Am. J. Med.,* **36**:595–617, 1964.

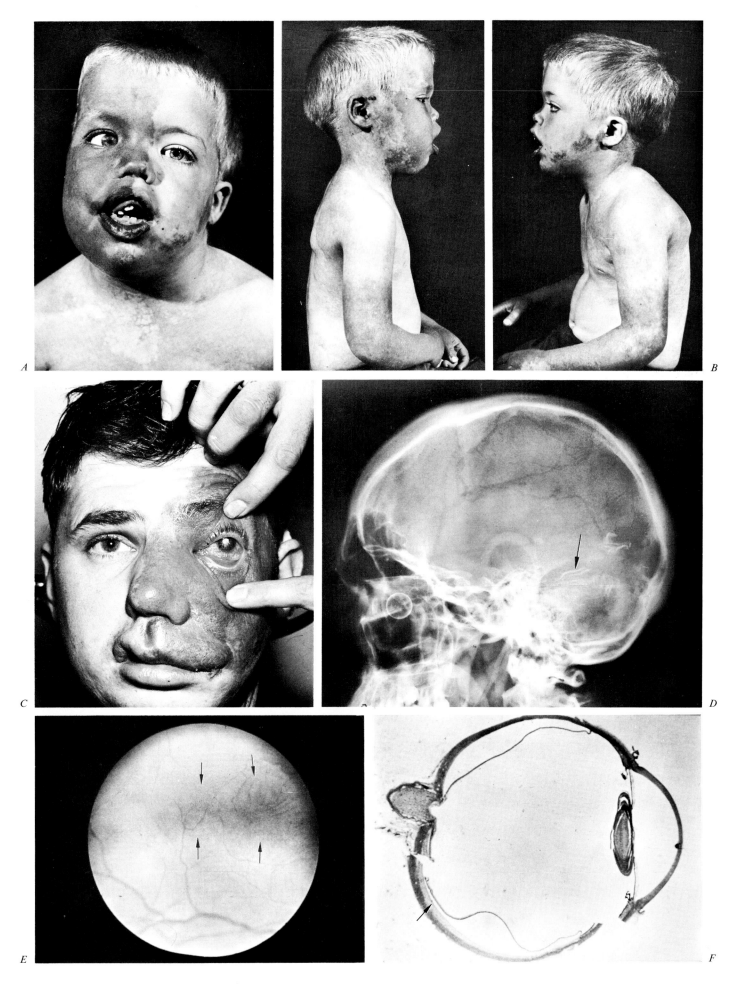

Plate VII-10. *A* and *B:* A boy with a large port-wine stain over the right side of his face, chest, and back and a small area on the left side of his face. He also had glaucoma of his right eye (the miotic pupil is the result of medication) and hyperplasia of the right half of the maxillary ridge. *C* and *D:* A 25-year-old man with lifelong blindness in his left eye, a port-wine stain, and thickened skin on the nose and lip. In his left eye he had a calcified cornea and cataract, band keratitis, and small angiomas of the iris. The skull x-ray after the removal of his left eye showed the eye prosthesis and the double lines of calcification in the occipital region (*arrow*). He had normal intelligence. *E:* A retinal fundus photograph showing the slight elevation and darker pigmentation due to a choroid hemangioma (*arrows*). *F:* A cross section of a glaucomatous eye showing the cupped optic nerve head, detached retina, and area of the choroid hemangioma (*arrow*). (*C:* Courtesy of Dr. D. G. Cogan, Boston, Mass. *E* and *F:* Courtesy of Retina Associates, Boston, Mass.)

373

Syndrome of Ectrodactyly, Cleft Lip and Palate, and Ectodermal Dysplasia

In 1970 Rudiger, Haase, and Passarge [1] reported a child with ectrodactyly, cleft lip and palate, and anhidrotic ectodermal dysplasia. They referred to other patients with similar anomalies and suggested that these had a previously undescribed disorder. At least seven more patients have been studied [2,3], including one published case report [4].

Physical Features

SKIN: Light pigmentation and dry skin have been noted in several patients.

HAIR: The hair was fine, soft, and blonde. Two patients [1,2] had sparse scalp hair (*Figures A and C*). The eyebrows and eyelashes were also sparse.

TEETH: Small, malformed, and absent teeth were noted, especially in the upper teeth (*Figure E*).

NAILS: The nails of some patients [2,4] were thin and brittle, and others [1] were normal.

EYES: Blepharitis and corneal erosions were noted in some of the patients [1,2].

MOUTH: Four patients had a bilateral cleft lip and palate [1,2]. One did not [4].

LIMBS: Ectrodactyly was the most common anomaly in the hands and feet (*Figures A, D, and F*). Some patients had associated syndactyly and absent or curved or shortened digits.

Nervous System

Some, but not all, of these patients have subnormal intelligence [1,2].

Laboratory Studies

X-rays of the hands and feet show many abnormalities of the carpals, tarsals, metacarpals, and metatarsals (*Figure B*). No sweat production could be elicited in one patient [1]. Absence of one kidney was shown by pyelography in one patient [4]. Chromosomal studies have shown no abnormalities.

Treatment and Prognosis

Some of these patients have required treatment for recurrent purulent rhinitis and blepharitis and corneal erosions [1,2].

Genetics

None of the patients has had any similarly affected relatives.

Differential Diagnosis

1. Limb deformities and ectodermal dysplasia are features of the siblings described by Freire-Maia [5], but they had severe tetramelia and ear deformities.
2. Ectrodactyly is also a feature of the patients with the syndrome of ectromelia and ichthyosis (see page 376).
3. Ectrodactyly and teeth anomalies are features of the patients with the syndrome of ectrodactyly, anodontia, and lacrimal duct abnormality [6].
4. Individuals with ectrodactyly and cleft lip and palate, but no ectodermal dysplasia, have been reported [7].

References

1. Rudiger, R. A., Haase, W., and Passarge, E. Association of ectrodactyly, ectodermal dysplasia, and cleft lip-palate. The EEC syndrome. *Am. J. Dis. Child.*, **120**:160–63, 1970.
2. Bixler, D. Personal communication, 1970.
3. Pruzansky, S. Personal communication, 1970.
4. Rosselli, D., and Gulienetti, R. Ectodermal dysplasia. *Br. J. Plast. Surg.*, **14**:190–204, 1961.
5. Freire-Maia, N. A newly recognized genetic syndrome of tetramelic deficiencies, ectodermal dysplasia, deformed ears, and other abnormalities. *Am. J. Hum. Genet.*, **22**:370–77, 1970.
6. Levy, W. J. Mesodermal dysplasia: a new combination of anomalies. *Am. J. Ophthalmol.*, **63**:978–82, 1967.
7. Walker, J. C., and Clodius, L. The syndrome of cleft lip, cleft palate and lobster claw deformities of hands and feet. *Plast. Reconstr. Surg.*, **32**:627–36, 1963.

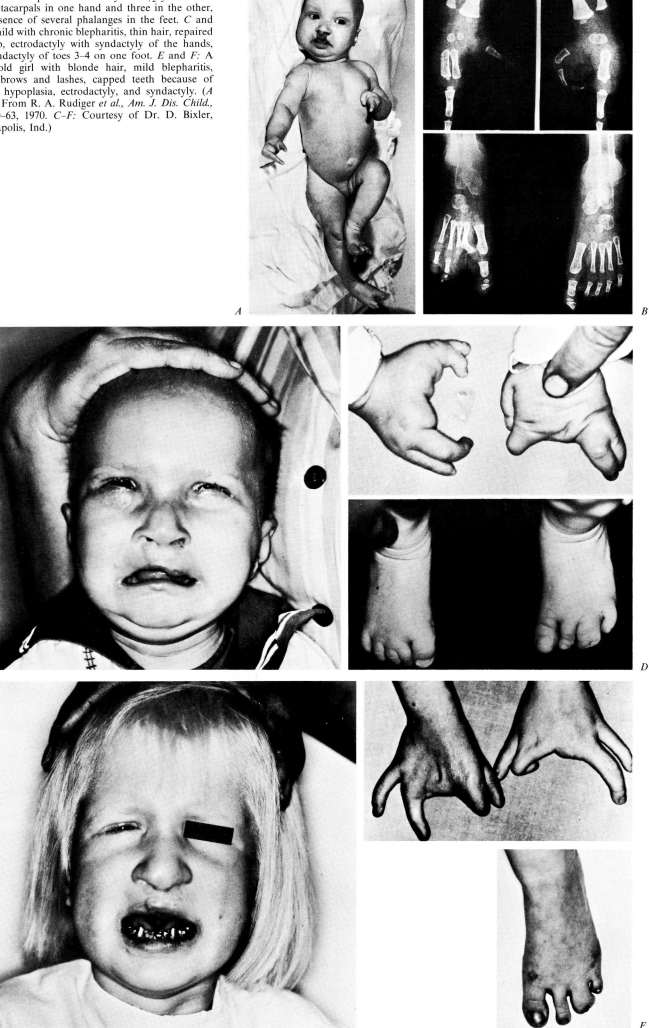

Plate VII-11. *A* and *B:* A 6-month-old girl with ectrodactyly of the hands and feet, bilateral cleft lip, and sparse scalp hair. The x-rays at 2½ years show two metacarpals in one hand and three in the other, and absence of several phalanges in the feet. *C* and *D:* A child with chronic blepharitis, thin hair, repaired cleft lip, ectrodactyly with syndactyly of the hands, and syndactyly of toes 3–4 on one foot. *E* and *F:* A 5-year-old girl with blonde hair, mild blepharitis, sparse brows and lashes, capped teeth because of enamel hypoplasia, ectrodactyly, and syndactyly. (*A* and *B:* From R. A. Rudiger *et al., Am. J. Dis. Child.,* **120:**160–63, 1970. *C–F:* Courtesy of Dr. D. Bixler, Indianapolis, Ind.)

A

B

C

D

E

F

Syndrome of Ectromelia and Ichthyosis

In 1963 Rossman, Shapiro, and Freeman [1] described a child with unilateral ichthyosiform erythroderma and limb anomalies on the same side. Since then four more similarly affected patients have been reported [2–4].

Physical Features

SKIN: The skin lesion in each patient has been dry, scaly, and often erythematous. The usual diagnosis is ichthyosiform erythroderma. The area involved has been the entire arm and leg on the same side as the limb anomalies. The skin lesion covers the body to the midline anteriorly and sometimes posteriorly. It extends up either to the axilla or to the scalp and ear on the same side as the limb anomalies (*Figures A, B, D, E, and F*).

NAILS: On the side with the skin lesions the nails are usually thickened (*Figure B*).

HEAD: One child [2,5] had asymmetry of the cranium and face, being smaller on the side with the deformities (*Figure A*).

MOUTH: One child [1] had a cleft lip.

LIMBS: Only the arm and leg on one side of the body have been abnormal. The most common findings have been either a smallness or absence of one or both limbs. On the limbs that are small and shortened the digits have been shortened and malformed (*Figure B*) or only one digit has remained (*Figure D*).

Nervous System

One child's intelligence quotient was estimated to be 66 at age 14 months [2] and 84 at 28 months of age [5]. Another child [1] had normal intelligence at age 12 years [6].

Pathology

Biopsies of the skin lesion in three patients [1,3,4] showed hyperkeratosis, parakeratosis, and acanthosis. Two affected siblings [3] died at 2 and 3 days of age, and both were found to have cardiac malformations, including single ventricle as well as other anomalies. All of the abdominal organs were normal; their brains were not examined.

Laboratory Studies

One child [2,5] had enlargement of the lateral cerebral ventricle and cortical atrophy on the same side as the skin and limb abnormalities (*Figure E*). Another child [1] had hydroureter and hydronephrosis on the same side as the skin lesion. A third child [4] had a polycystic kidney only on the normal side of the body. X-rays have shown absence or hypoplasia of the long bones as is clinically apparent. They also have shown rib anomalies and, on the side with limb anomalies, hypoplasia of the pelvis and scapula. Chromosomal studies on lymphocytes and skin fibroblasts have shown no abnormalities.

Treatment and Prognosis

There is no effective treatment of the skin condition. The limb anomalies necessitate the use of prostheses.

Genetics

In view of the occurrence of this disorder in siblings [3], it may be due to an autosomal recessive mutant gene.

Differential Diagnosis

Nonbullous congenital ichthyosiform erythroderma unassociated with limb anomalies is inherited as an autosomal recessive disorder. However, these patients have a generalized skin involvement, including the face [7].

References

1. Rossman, K. E., Shapiro, E. M., and Freeman, R. G. Unilateral ichthyosiform erythroderma. *Arch. Dermatol.,* **88:**567–71, 1963.
2. Carter, C. H., Howard, F. H., and Connolly, J. Unilateral ichthyosiform erythroderma. Report of a case. *Clin. Pediatr. (Phila.),* **7:**605–606, 1968.
3. Falek, A., Heath, C. W., Jr., Ebbin, A. J., and McLean, W. R. Unilateral limb and skin deformities with congenital heart disease in two siblings: a lethal syndrome. *J. Pediatr.,* **73:**910–13, 1968.
4. Cullen, S. I., Harris, D. E., Carter, C. H., and Reed, W. B. Congenital unilateral ichthyosiform erythroderma. *Arch. Dermatol.,* **99:**724–29, 1969.
5. Shear, C. S. Personal communication, 1970.
6. Shapiro, E. M. Personal communication, 1970.
7. Esterly, N. B. The ichthyosiform dermatoses. *Pediatrics,* **42:**990–1004, 1968.

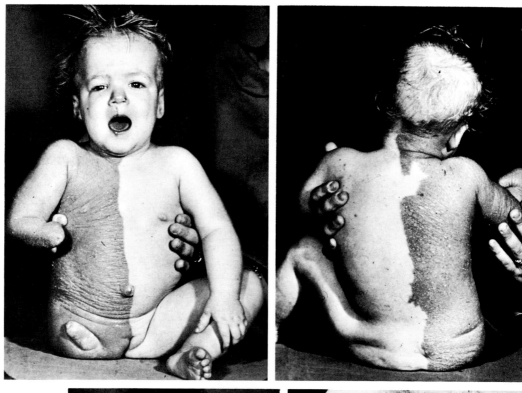

Plate VII-12. *A* and *B*: A 4-year-old girl with a repaired cleft lip, absence of the right leg, amelia of the right arm, and a rough, scaly erythematous skin lesion over the right half of her body. She has normal intelligence. *C–E*: A 3⅔-year-old girl with a similar scaly skin over much of the right side of her body. She has five fingers, the fifth being pedunculated, and two toes separated by a deep cleft. Her pneumoencephalogram shows an enlarged right lateral ventricle. *F*: One of two siblings with scaly skin over the left side, shortened left arm and leg each ending in a single digitlike structure. (*A* and *B*: Courtesy of Dr. E. M. Shapiro, Pasadena, Tex. *C–E*: Courtesy of Dr. C. S. Shear, Miami, Fla. *F*: From A. Falek *et al.*, *J. Pediatr.*, **73**:910–13, 1968.)

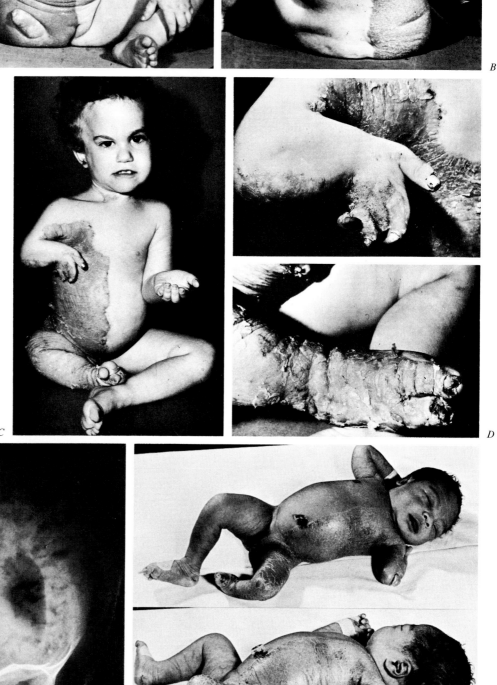

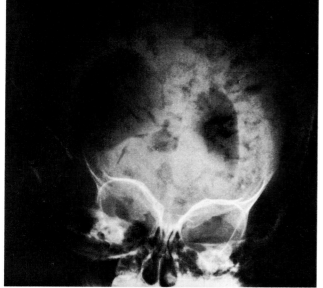

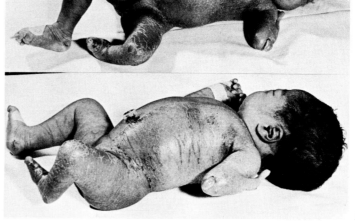

Syndrome of Ichthyosis and Hypogonadism

In 1960 Lynch, Ozer, McNutt, Johnson, and Jampolsky [1] described a family in which five males in three generations had congenital ichthyosis and secondary hypogonadism. In 1969 Maurer and Sotos [2] briefly described another family with ten affected males. This was considered a new hereditary disorder.

Physical Features

SKIN: The ichthyosis was present on many areas of the body, but in the first family most often over the extensor surfaces of the limbs (*Figures A, B, and C*).

GENITALIA: The testes and penis were small. There was no evidence of any pubertal changes in the adults (*Figures A, B, and D*).

Nervous System

All but one of the patients in the second family had mild mental retardation. Most also had anosmia [2]. Neither intelligence estimates nor anosmia was mentioned in the first report [1].

Pathology

Skin biopsies showed congenital ichthyosis; no additional information was given [1]. Testis biopsies showed generalized atrophy, absent or decreased Leydig cells, and immature tubules (*Figure E*).

Laboratory Studies

Urinary gonadotropins in adults were below normal. A decreased ACTH reserve was proven in one family [2]. Chromosomal karyotypes were normal.

Treatment and Prognosis

Treatment of one patient [1] with human chorionic gonadotropin produced androgenic effects and testicular enlargement; Leydig cells were present in the testes biopsy after treatment. This response was evidence that the hypogonadism was secondary to a primary gonadotropin deficiency.

Genetics

X-linked recessive.

Differential Diagnosis

1. Ichthyosis may also be an X-linked recessive abnormality not associated with either hypogonadism or mental retardation [3].
2. Hypogonadotropic hypogonadism and mental retardation were also features of the two brothers with the syndrome of testicular deficiency and mental retardation, but they had gynecomastia and did not have ichthyosis (see page 60).
3. Anosmia and hypogonadism are also features of males with Kallmann's syndrome, an X-linked recessive form of hypogonadotropic hypogonadism [4]. These patients do not have ichthyosis.

References

1. Lynch, H. T., Ozer, F., McNutt, C. W., Johnson, J. E., and Jampolsky, N. A. Secondary male hypogonadism and congenital ichthyosis: association of two rare genetic diseases. *Am. J. Hum. Genet.*, **12**:440–47, 1960.
2. Maurer, W. F., and Sotos, J. F. Sex-linked familial hypogonadism and ichthyosis. (Abstract.) Society for Pediatric Research, Atlantic City, 1969, p. 181.
3. Esterly, N. B. The ichthyosiform dermatoses. *Pediatrics*, **42**:990–1004, 1968.
4. Nowakowski, H., and Lenz, W. Genetic aspects in male hypogonadism. *Recent Progr. Horm. Res.*, **17**:53–95, 1961.

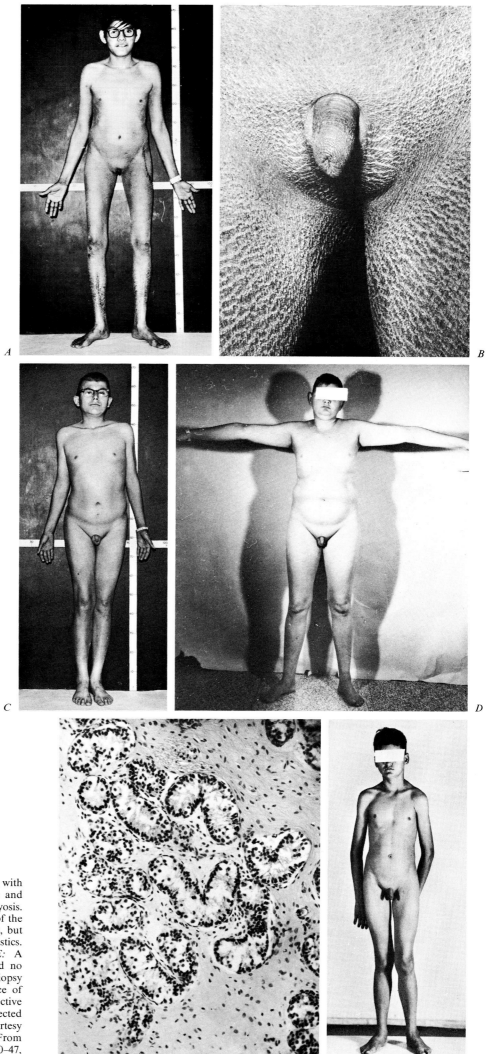

Plate VII-13. *A* and *B:* A 31-year-old man with striking hypogonadism, absence of pubic and axillary hair, hyperpigmentation, and ichthyosis. *C:* A 16-year-old boy, a maternal nephew of the first patient, with less striking skin changes, but a similar lack of secondary sexual characteristics. He had normal intelligence. *D* and *E:* A 19-year-old obese boy with ichthyosis and no secondary sexual characteristics. His testis biopsy showed a lack of spermatogenesis, absence of Leydig cells, and hyalinization of the connective tissue in some areas. *F:* The similarly affected maternal cousin of the boy in *D.* (*A–C:* Courtesy of Dr. J. F. Sotos, Columbus, Ohio. *D–F:* From H. T. Lynch *et al., Am. J. Hum. Genet.,* **12:**440–47, 1960.)

Tuberous Sclerosis

The clinical syndrome of tuberous sclerosis is often said to consist of a classic triad of seizures, mental retardation, and adenoma sebaceum. Reports concerning scores of patients studied over the past 100 years have added many other features, such as white macules, brain tumors, and retinal phakomas, to this syndrome and have shown that affected patients need not have the classic triad. The incidence of tuberous sclerosis is not known, but it was estimated as 1:20,000 to 1:40,000 in North Carolina [1].

Physical Features

SKIN: The first visible skin lesions are usually white macules, which are present at birth. These lesions are dull white, measure more than 1 cm in diameter, number from a few to several dozen, and may be on any part of the body. The shape may be oval or linear; the most characteristic is the lance-ovate shape, which is similar to the configuration of the mountain ash leaf (*Figures A, B, E*). Most patients have these ash leaf macules, although in fair-skinned individuals it may be necessary to use ultraviolet light (a Wood's lamp) to find them [2]. There was adenoma sebaceum in 83 percent of the patients in a study of 71 patients [3]. These are discrete flesh-colored or pink nodules about 1 to 7 mm in diameter, which are often present by 5 years of age but rarely at birth. The typical locations are the nasolabial folds, cheeks, and chin (*Figures B and D*). Less common skin lesions are the shagreen patch (*Figures D and E*), periungual and subungual fibromas (*Figure F*), and areas of hyperpigmentation. The shagreen patch is a tan, irregular, slightly raised area of fibrous induration that is usually located over the lumbosacral area.

EYES: In one series [3], over half of the patients had retinal nodules, which are phakomas of the fundus composed of glial fibers and large cells. These lesions may be present in infancy. The most common lesions are small, round, flat, or slightly raised, and may be located in any part of the retina. Less common, but more suggestive of tuberous sclerosis, are large nodules over, under, or close to the optic nerve head. Other less frequent ocular abnormalities are conjunctival nodules, cataracts, pigmentary retinopathy, and phthisis bulbi [1,4,5].

Nervous System

The incidence of mental retardation varies according to the age of the patients and the method of ascertainment, which in many studies has been through institutions for the retarded. Of 71 patients seen at the Mayo Clinic, 38 percent had average intelligence [3]. All types of seizures occur. Some patients have infantile spasms and akinetic seizures in infancy before other features of this syndrome have appeared.

Pathology

Hamartomas are often present in the brain, kidneys, and heart. In the brain these smooth, firm, and pearly white or gray nodules usually involve the cerebrum, but they may also be present in the cerebellum, midbrain, and spinal cord. Nodules in the ependymal lining of the ventricles can cause obstructive hydrocephalus. The cerebral nodules are composed of masses of glial tissue in which large, multinucleated glial and nerve cells are scattered; more than half are calcified. A few reported patients had brain tumors with the histology

similar in each and consisting of mixtures of spongioblasts and gemistocytic astrocytes [6]. The kidney hamartomas are usually bilateral, multiple, and quite variable in size. Co-existing polycystic disease of the kidneys has also been observed [7]. Rhabdomyomas of the heart were present in 8 of 31 autopsies in one series [4]. These tumors are one of the most common causes of death in childhood in patients with tuberous sclerosis. Two types of bone changes have been noted: cysts, especially of the phalanges; and irregular cortical thickening, most often in the metatarsal and metacarpal bones. The adenoma sebaceum and subungual lesions are angiofibromas. The shagreen patch is composed of a dense sclerotic bundle of collagen. The white macules show reduced melanin deposition on melanosomes [2].

Laboratory Studies

Skull x-rays show calcifications (*Figure C*) most often in the area of the basal ganglia. In general, the incidence increases with age. Sclerotic plaques in the bony cranial vault may also be seen. Electroencephalograms are frequently abnormal and vary according to the age of the patient; the hypsarrhythmia pattern is common in infants with infantile spasms.

Treatment and Prognosis

Two features of this syndrome merit emphasis: first, a patient may have skin lesions, intracranial calcifications, and seizures and still have average intelligence; and second, some patients have a steady decrease in the IQ with increasing age. Many patients have died before adulthood because of status epilepticus or cardiac or renal tumors. In general, the seizures become more easily controlled with increasing age. The removal of large adenoma sebaceum and shagreen patches greatly helps the appearance of some patients (*Figure D*).

Genetics

Autosomal dominant.

Differential Diagnosis

1. Intracranial calcifications and fundal abnormalities are features of patients with rubella (see page 118), cytomegalovirus (see page 122) and herpesvirus infections (see page 130), and congenital toxoplasmosis (see page 124).
2. Intracranial calcifications, seizures, and retinal angiomas are features of patients with the Sturge-Weber syndrome, but they also have capillary hemangiomas on the face (see page 372).

References

1. Paulson, G. W., and Lyle, C. B. Tuberous sclerosis. *Dev. Med. Child Neurol.,* **8**:571–86, 1966.
2. Fitzpatrick, T. B., Szabó, G., Hori, Y., Simone, A. A., Reed, W. B., and Greenberg, M. H. White leaf-shaped macules. *Arch. Dermatol.,* **98**:1–6, 1968.
3. Lagos, J. C., and Gomez, M. R. Tuberous sclerosis: reappraisal of a clinical entity. *Mayo Clin. Proc.,* **42**:26–49, 1967.
4. Reed, W. B., Nickel, W. R., and Campion, G. Internal manifestations of tuberous sclerosis. *Arch. Dermatol.,* **87**:715–28, 1963.
5. Grover, W. D., and Harley, R. D. Early recognition of tuberous sclerosis by funduscopic examination. *J. Pediatr.,* **75**:991–95, 1969.
6. Kapp, J. P., Paulson, G. W., and Odom, G. L. Brain tumors with tuberous sclerosis. *J. Neurosurg.,* **26**:191–202, 1967.
7. Wenzl, J. E., Lagos, J. C., and Albers, D. D. Tuberous sclerosis presenting as polycystic kidneys and seizures in an infant. *J. Pediatr.,* **77**:673–76, 1970.

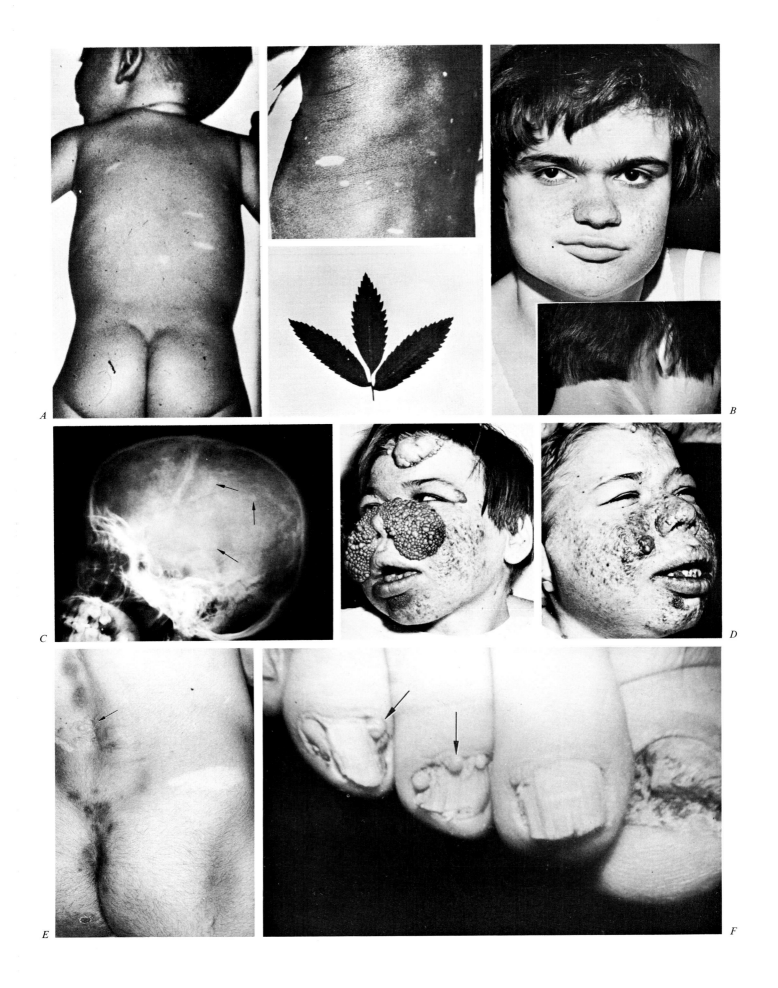

Plate VII-14. *A:* Two infants with many white macules scattered over their backs. Several of the macules have the shape of a mountain ash leaf. A silhouette of part of an ash leaf is shown in the insert. *B* and *C:* An 18-year-old girl with adenoma sebaceum in a butterfly pattern over her nose and on her chin. The white macule on her neck was noted at birth, but no causation for her seizures was suggested until years later, when the adenoma sebaceum and calcifications (*arrows*) on the lateral skull x-ray appeared. *D:* A grossly disfigured 22-year-old woman with extensive confluent papules over the nose and a large shagreen patch on the forehead, and a smaller fibrous tumor on her left upper eyelid. She is shown a year later after treatment of the lesions. *E:* Shows on the lower back of a 20-year-old man both the shagreen patch (*arrow*) and a large white macule. *F:* Shows periungual fibromas on the toes (*arrows*). (*A* [*left*]: Courtesy of Dr. T. B. Fitzpatrick, Boston, Mass. *A* [*right*]: From T. B. Fitzpatrick, *Arch. Dermatol.* [*Chicago*], **98:**1–6, 1968. *D:* From S. A. M. Johnson, *Arch. Dermatol.* [*Chicago*], **90:**229–31, 1964. *F:* Courtesy of Dr. G. R. Hogan, Boston, Mass.)

Xeroderma Pigmentosum

In 1874 Hebra and Kaposi [1] described the syndrome of sunlight hypersensitivity, freckles, and skin cancers. The association of these features with microcephaly, hypogonadism, and subnormal intelligence was reported by de Sanctis and Cacchione [2] in 1932. While patients with xeroderma pigmentosum and mental retardation are sometimes said to have the xerodermic idiocy of de Sanctis and Cacchione, these patients do not have a separate disorder, but rather have the more severe manifestations of the syndrome of xeroderma pigmentosum [3,4]. By 1954 over 360 patients with xeroderma pigmentosum had been reported [5].

Physical Features

SKIN: The first skin lesions usually appear in infancy or childhood, although they may not appear until adulthood. The initial changes are erythema after exposure to sunlight. The first definite signs of the disease are small pigmented lesions, resembling freckles, on the exposed parts of the body, which become more pronounced on exposure to sunlight (*Figures A, B, C, D, and E*). They fuse and form areas several centimeters in diameter. Interspersed among the pigmented lesions are white, parchmentlike, atrophic areas (*Figures D, E, and F*). These are sometimes covered with fine scales. The white areas may coalesce and form cicatriform patches. Telangiectases are usually present in these areas, and sometimes small angiomas as well. Pedunculated growths develop from the pigmented spots and may be present before there are any atrophic changes (*Figure F*). These growths vary in size and may be flat or convex. Later, the lesions undergo malignant changes.

EYES: Photophobia with excessive tearing occurs early in the course of the disease. Later, atrophy of the eyelid results in epilation of the cilia and either ectropion or entropion. Symblepharon and ankyloblepharon often develop. The bulbar conjunctiva may become dry and injected. Corneal ulceration and iritis occur in patients with exposed and unprotected eyes.

GENITALIA: Small external genitalia are frequently noted.
HEIGHT: These patients may be below normal in height.
GROWTH AND DEVELOPMENT: Delayed or deficient sexual maturation is often described in the more severely affected patients, but the incidence is not known [3].

Nervous System

In a study of 33 patients [4], about half had subnormal intelligence. The most common neurologic findings are microcephaly, spasticity, cerebellar ataxia, and sensorineural deafness [3,6].

Pathology

A biopsy of the affected area shows an absence of the granular cell layer and a dense overlying keratin layer. Melanin pigmentation is patchy and irregular. These patients can develop many different types of carcinomas, such as angiosarcomas, fibrosarcomas, lymphomas, and melanomas. Few neuropathologic studies have been reported. In one patient [6] there was cerebral and olivopontocerebellar atrophy.

Laboratory Studies

Patients with xeroderma pigmentosum are sensitive to light of wavelength 280 to 310 nanometers. Studies in skin fibroblasts on the repair of ultraviolet radiation damage to deoxyribonucleic acid have shown that the repair replication of DNA is either absent or greatly reduced in comparison to normal fibroblasts. This may be due to an enzyme deficiency (endonuclease) involved in early DNA repair [8]. A convenient diagnostic test is the demonstration of a lack of unscheduled DNA synthesis in a skin biopsy following the intradermal injection of tritiated thymidine and exposure to ultraviolet light [9]. Studies of chromosomes and serum and urinary amino acids have shown no consistent abnormalities.

Treatment and Prognosis

Exposure to sunlight must be avoided. Obviously, skin tumors are removed when there is evidence of malignancy.

Genetics

Autosomal recessive. A rapid method suited for prenatal diagnosis has been developed [9a].

Differential Diagnosis

1. Multiple nevi and basal cell carcinomas on the sun-exposed areas are features of patients with the basal cell nevus syndrome, but they do not have either freckles or atrophic areas of skin, and frequently have jaw cysts. It is an autosomal dominant disorder (see page 356).
2. Hypersensitivity to the sun, short stature, and a predisposition to malignancies are features of patients with Bloom's syndrome, but they do not develop extensive skin hyperpigmentation and atrophy or warty growths, and their chromosomes show increased chromosomal breakage [10].

References

1. Hebra, F., and Kaposi, M. *On Diseases of the Skin.* New Sydenham Society, London, 3:252, 1874.
2. de Sanctis, C., and Cacchione, A. L'idiozia xerodermica. *Riv. Sper. Freniatr.,* 56:269–92, 1932.
3. Reed, W. B., May, S. B., and Nickel, W. R. Xeroderma pigmentosum with neurological complications. *Arch. Dermatol.,* 91:224–26, 1965.
4. El-Hefnawi, H., Gawad, M. S. A., and Rasheed, A. Neuropsychiatric manifestations in xeroderma pigmentosum. *Gaz. Egypt. Soc. Dermatol. Venereol.,* 2:6–22, 1967.
5. Moore, C., and Iverson, P. C. Xeroderma pigmentosum showing common skin cancer plus melanocarcinoma controlled by surgery. *Cancer,* 7:377–82, 1954.
6. Reed, W. B., Landing, B., Sugarman, G., Cleaver, J. E., and Melnyk, J. Xeroderma pigmentosum. Clinical and laboratory investigation of its basic defect. *J.A.M.A.,* 207:2073–79, 1969.
7. Lynch, H. T., Anderson, D. E., Smith, J. L., Jr., Howell, J. B., and Krush, A. J. Xeroderma pigmentosum, malignant melanoma and congenital ichthyosis. *Arch. Dermatol.,* 96:625–35, 1967.
8. Cleaver, J. E. Xeroderma pigmentosum: a human disease in which an initial stage of DNA repair is defective. *Proc. Natl. Acad. Sci. USA,* 63:428–35, 1969.
9. Epstein, W. L., Fukuyama, K., and Epstein, J. H. Early effects of ultraviolet light on DNA synthesis in human skin *in vitro. Arch. Dermatol.,* 100:84–89, 1969.
9a. Regan, J. D., Setlow, R. B., Kaback, M. M., Howell, R. R., Klein, E., and Burgess, G. Xeroderma pigmentosum: a rapid sensitive method for prenatal diagnosis. *Science,* 174:147–50, 1971.
10. German, J. Bloom's syndrome. I. Genetical and clinical observations in the first twenty-seven patients. *Am. J. Hum. Genet.,* 21:196–227, 1969.

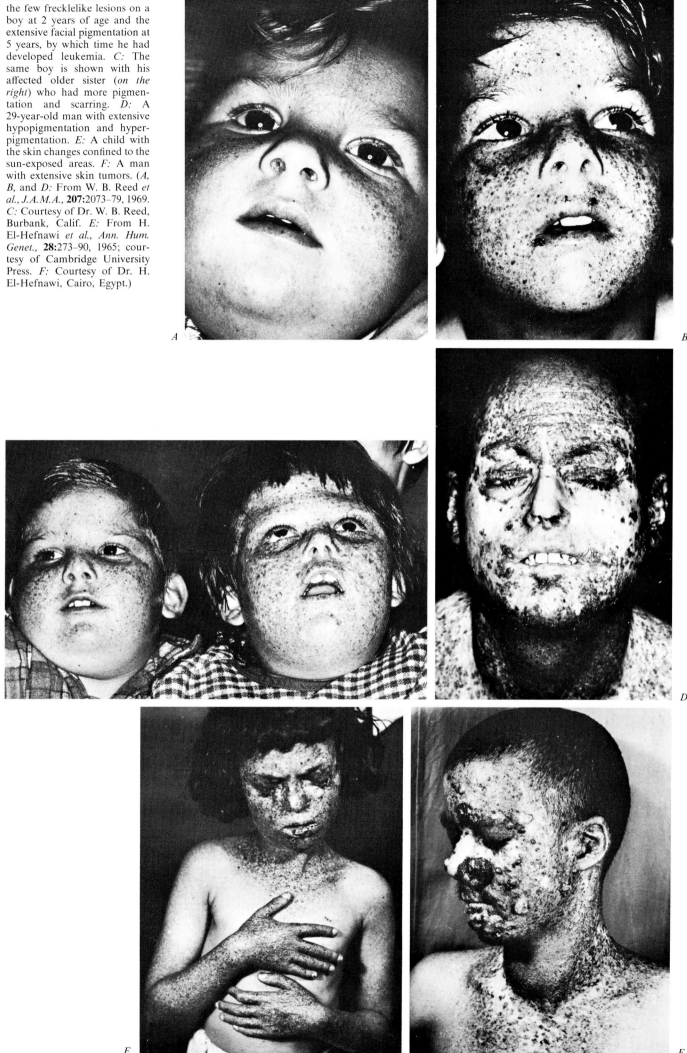

Plate VII-15. *A* and *B:* Shows the few frecklelike lesions on a boy at 2 years of age and the extensive facial pigmentation at 5 years, by which time he had developed leukemia. *C:* The same boy is shown with his affected older sister (*on the right*) who had more pigmentation and scarring. *D:* A 29-year-old man with extensive hypopigmentation and hyperpigmentation. *E:* A child with the skin changes confined to the sun-exposed areas. *F:* A man with extensive skin tumors. (*A, B,* and *D:* From W. B. Reed *et al., J.A.M.A.,* **207:**2073–79, 1969. *C:* Courtesy of Dr. W. B. Reed, Burbank, Calif. *E:* From H. El-Hefnawi *et al., Ann. Hum. Genet.,* **28:**273–90, 1965; courtesy of Cambridge University Press. *F:* Courtesy of Dr. H. El-Hefnawi, Cairo, Egypt.)

Index

Alzheimer type II cells, argininosuccinic aciduria, 6
Amenorrhea. *See also* Puberty
  familial hormonal disorder associated with mental deficiency, deaf-mutism, and ataxia, 86
  myotonic dystrophy, 106
  Prader-Labhart-Willi syndrome, 48
  Rothmund-Thomson syndrome, 368
  XO syndrome, 178
Amethopterin. *See* Aminopterin and amethopterin embryopathy
Amino acids, cerebrospinal fluid. *See* Cerebrospinal fluid, amino acids
Aminoaciduria
  argininosuccinic aciduria, 6
  galactosemia, 14
  Hartnup disease, 24
  homocystinuria, 26
  linear sebaceous nevus with convulsions and mental retardation, 364
  oculocerebrorenal syndrome of Lowe, 248
  phenylketonuria, 46
  Wilson's disease, 64
Aminopterin and amethopterin embryopathy, 134
  differentiated from
    acrocephalosyndactyly, absent digits, and cranial defects, syndrome, 134, 238
    cloverleaf skull deformity, 134
Ammonemia, argininosuccinic aciduria, 6
Amniocentesis. *See* Prenatal diagnosis
Anemia
  aplastic, Fanconi's anemia, 282
  battered child syndrome, 142
  galactosemia, 14
  hemolytic, Wilson's disease, 64
  hypoplastic, congenital rubella syndrome, 118
  normochromic normocytic, de Lange syndrome, 276
  osteopetrosis, infantile form, 264
  Wolman's disease, 66
Anencephaly
  aminopterin and amethopterin embryopathy, 134
  genetic counseling, meningomyelocele, 212
  thalidomide embryopathy, 132
Angiofibromas
  focal dermal hypoplasia, 360
  tuberous sclerosis, 380
Angiomas
  Sturge-Weber syndrome, 372
  xeroderma pigmentosum, 382
Angiosarcomas, xeroderma pigmentosum, 382
Anhidrosis. *See* Sweating, absent or reduced
Aniridia. *See also* Iris
  aniridia, cerebellar ataxia, and oligophrenia, syndrome, 102
  oculocerebral syndrome with hypopigmentation, 246
Anophthalmia. *See also* Eyes
  chromosome 13 trisomy, 164
  focal dermal hypoplasia, 360
  Goldenhar's syndrome, 284
  Meckel syndrome, 292
  thalidomide embryopathy, 132
  X-linked, 242
    differentiated from
      chromosome 13 trisomy, 166, 242
      cryptophthalmos, 242
Anosmia. *See also* Hyposmia
  Engelmann's disease, 262
  ichthyosis and hypogonadism, syndrome, 378
  Kallmann's syndrome, 378
Anus
  imperforate
    chromosome 13, deletion of long arm and ring D, 168
    extra small acrocentric chromosome, syndrome, 176
    thalidomide embryopathy, 132
Aorta. *See also* Congenital heart disease
  arch right-sided, facial dysmorphism, right-sided aortic arch, and mental deficiency, syndrome, 326
  coarctation
    linear sebaceous nevus with convulsions and mental retardation, 364

telecanthus-hypospadias syndrome, 346
  XO syndrome, 178
hypoplasia
  hypercalcemia, elfin facies, supravalvular aortic stenosis, and mental retardation, syndrome, 54
  telecanthus-hypospadias syndrome, 346
stenosis, hypercalcemia, elfin facies, supravalvular aortic stenosis, and mental retardation, syndrome, 54
Apert's syndrome, 222, 224
  differentiated from
    Carpenter's syndrome, 224, 232
    Chotzen's syndrome, 224, 226
    chromosome 18, deletion of long arm, 160
    cloverleaf skull, 234
    Crouzon's disease, 224, 230
    ectodermal dysplasia, hypohidrotic type with maxillary hypoplasia, 358
    Mohr type acrocephaly, 224
    Pfeiffer's syndrome, 224, 228
    Rubinstein-Taybi syndrome, 306
    Waardenburg type acrocephaly, 224
Aqueduct of Sylvius
  forked, meningomyelocele, 212
  stenosis
    Apert's syndrome, 222
    familial aqueductal stenosis and basilar impression, 200
    meningomyelocele, 212
    X-linked aqueductal stenosis, 200
Arachnodactyly
  basal cell nevus syndrome, 356
  blepharophimosis and congenital contractures, syndrome, 320
  cryptorchidism, chest deformities, contractures, and arachnodactyly, syndrome, 332
  homocystinuria, 26
  Marfan's syndrome, 26
Arachnoid cysts in the posterior fossa, differentiated from Dandy-Walker syndrome, 202
Arch tibial pattern, chromosome 21 trisomy, 150
Arginine transport defective, oculocerebrorenal syndrome of Lowe, 248
Argininosuccinase deficiency, argininosuccinic aciduria, 6
Argininosuccinic aciduria, 6
  differentiated from
    kinky hair disease, 6, 100
    trichorrhexis nodosa with mental retardation, 6, 350
Arhinencephaly
  chromosome 13, deletion of long arm and ring D, 168
  chromosome 13 trisomy, 164
  chromosome 18, deletion of short arm, 162
  chromosome 18 trisomy, 156
  cyclopia, ethmocephaly, and cebocephaly, 206
  holotelencephaly with cleft lip and hypotelorism, 208
  Meckel syndrome, 292
Arms. *See* Limbs; Short-limbed dwarfism
Arnold-Chiari malformation
  cranium bifidum with encephalocele, 210
  meningomyelocele, 212
Arthritis, gouty, Lesch-Nyhan syndrome, 30
Arthrogryposis. *See* Joint, contractures
Arthrogryposis multiplex congenita, 76, 78
  differentiated from several other conditions with joint contractures, 78
  encephalopathic type, 78
  myopathic type, 76
  neuropathic type, 76
  nodular fibrosis of the anterior spinal nerve roots, 78
Arylsulfatase A, metachromatic leukodystrophy, 36
Aspermia. *See* Seminiferous tubules, atrophied
Asphyxiating thoracic dystrophy, differentiated from Ellis–van Creveld syndrome, 280
Asymmetry
  body, Silver-Russell syndrome, 310
  face
    Apert's syndrome, 222
    chromosome 5, deletion of short arm, 170

Carcinoma (predisposition to). *See also* specific name
  ataxia-telangiectasia, 354
  Fanconi's anemia, 282
  macroglossia, omphalocele, visceromegaly, and neonatal hypogly-
    cemia, syndrome, 56
  xeroderma pigmentosum, 382
Cardiac anomalies. *See* Congenital heart disease
Cardiovascular malformations. *See* Congenital heart disease
Caries. *See* Dental caries
Carotenemia, congenital hypothyroidism, 10
Carotid artery anomalies, dyschondroplasia, facial anomalies, and
    polysyndactyly, syndrome, 322
Carpal bones
  anomalies, ectrodactyly, cleft lip and palate, and ectodermal dys-
    plasia syndrome, 374
  fused, acrocephaly, cleft lip and palate, radial aplasia, and absent
    digits, syndrome, 240. *See also* Capitate-hamate bone fusion
  reduced in number, Fanconi's anemia, 282
Carpenter's syndrome, 232
  differentiated from
    acrocephalosyndactyly, absent digits, and cranial defects, syn-
      drome, 238
    Apert's syndrome, 222, 232
    Chotzen's syndrome, 226
    chromosome 5, deletion of short arm, 170
    dyschondroplasia, facial anomalies, and polysyndactyly, syn-
      drome, 322
    Laurence-Moon syndrome, 288
    Mohr syndrome, 232
    Noack's syndrome, 232
Cataracts
  cerebrohepatorenal syndrome, 270
  cerebrotendinous xanthomatosis, 80
  chromosome 13, deletion of long arm and ring D, 168
  chromosome 13 trisomy, 164
  chromosome 18 trisomy, 156
  Cockayne's syndrome, 82
  congenital rubella syndrome, 118
  congenital toxoplasmosis, 124
  Conradi's disease, 272
  extra small acrocentric chromosome, syndrome, 176
  Flynn-Aird syndrome, 90
  galactosemia, 14
  G monosomy, 154
  Hallermann-Streiff syndrome, 286
  homocystinuria, 26
  incontinentia pigmenti, 262
  Laurence-Moon syndrome, 288
  mannosidosis, 34
  Marinesco-Sjögren syndrome, 102
  myotonic dystrophy, 106
  Norrie's disease, 244
  perinatal herpesvirus infection, 130
  pseudohypoparathyroidism, 50
  Rothmund-Thomson syndrome, 368
  Rubinstein-Taybi syndrome, 306
  Smith-Lemli-Opitz syndrome, 312
  tetraphocomelia, cleft lip and palate, and genital hypertrophy,
    syndrome, 344
  tuberous sclerosis, 380
Catlike cry
  chromosome 4, deletion of short arm, 174
  chromosome 5, deletion of short arm, 170
  chromosome 18 trisomy, 170
Cat's eye syndrome. *See* Extra small acrocentric chromosome syn-
    drome
Caudate nucleus. *See also* Basal ganglia; Globus pallidus; Putamen
    atrophy; Substantia nigra
  atrophy, Huntington's chorea, 96
  shrunken and discolored, Wilson's disease, 64
Cebocephaly
  chromosome 13 trisomy, 164
  chromosome 18, deletion of short arm, 162
  holotelencephaly, 206
Cephaloskeletal dysplasia, 318

Ceramide excess in tissues, Farber's lipogranulomatosis, 88
Cerebellar ataxia. *See* Ataxia, cerebellar
Cerebellum. *See also* Dandy-Walker malformation
  anomalies
    cerebrohepatorenal syndrome, 270
    chromosome 13 trisomy, 164
    chromosome 18 trisomy, 156
    cloverleaf skull, 234
    Dandy-Walker syndrome, 202
    dysmorphogenesis of joints, brain, and palate, 278
    Meckel syndrome, 292
    Möbius syndrome, 296
    retinal blindness, polycystic kidneys, and brain malformations,
      syndrome, 342
  atrophy. *See also* Neuronal lipidoses
    ataxia-telangiectasia, 354
    cerebrotendinous xanthomatosis, 80
    Cockayne's syndrome, 82
    kinky hair disease, 100
    Hallervorden-Spatz disease, 94
    mannosidosis, 34
    Marinesco-Sjögren syndrome, 102
    mucopolysaccharidosis III, 42
    oculocerebrorenal syndrome of Lowe, 248
  hamartomas, tuberous sclerosis, 380
Cerebral gigantism, 8
  differentiated from
    acromegaloid features, hypertelorism, and pectus excavatum,
      syndrome, 8
    acromegaly, 8
Cerebral palsy, differentiated from metachromatic leukodystrophy, 36
Cerebral ventricle(s)
  dilated or enlarged. *See also* Hydrocephalus
    Alpers' disease, 74
    arthrogryposis multiplex congenita, neuropathic type, 76
    brain dysgenesis, microcephaly, and skeletal dysplasia, syndrome,
      318
    cerebrohepatorenal syndrome, 270
    Chotzen's syndrome, 226
    chromosome 4, deletion of short arm, 174
    chromosome 5, deletion of short arm, 172
    congenital sensory neuropathy with anhidrosis, 254
    elastic tissue deficiency, corneal dystrophy, grimacing, and mental
      retardation, 320
    familial amyotrophic dystonic paraplegia, 84
    happy puppet syndrome, 258
    kinky hair disease, 100
    linear sebaceous nevus with convulsions and mental retardation,
      364
    lissencephaly syndrome, 198
    mannosidosis, 34
    retinal blindness, polycystic kidneys, and brain malformations,
      syndrome, 342
    Smith-Lemli-Opitz syndrome, 312
    spongy degeneration of the central nervous system in infancy,
      112
    Sturge-Weber syndrome, 372
    Tay-Sachs disease, 62
  single. *See also* Arhinencephaly
    chromosome 13 trisomy, 166
    chromosome 18, deletion of short arm, 162
    cyclopia, ethmocephaly, and cebocephaly, 206
    holotelencephaly, 206
    holotelencephaly with cleft lip and hypotelorism, 208
    Meckel syndrome, 292
Cerebrohepatorenal syndrome, 270
  differentiated from
    chromosome 21 trisomy, 150, 270
    congenital hypothyroidism, 10
    Conradi's disease, 270, 272
    glycogenosis, type II, 20
    lissencephaly, 198
    microphthalmos, corneal opacity, mental retardation, and spas-
      ticity, syndrome, 250
    oculocerebrorenal syndrome of Lowe, 248, 270

393

403

elbow contractures, corneal opacities, pointed nose, and mental retardation, syndrome, 324

extra small acrocentric chromosome, syndrome, 176

Lesch-Nyhan syndrome, 30

meningomyelocele, 212

mucopolysaccharidosis I, 38

otopalatodigital syndrome, 302

Seckel's bird-headed dwarfism, 308

Smith-Lemli-Opitz syndrome, 312

thalidomide embryopathy, 132

XXXX syndrome, 180

Hirschsprung's disease, chromosome 21 trisomy, 150

Hirsutism

absent fifth fingernails and toenails, short distal phalanges, and lax joints, syndrome, 312

ataxia-telangiectasia, 354

de Lange syndrome, 276

G_{M1} gangliosidosis, 22

leprechaunism, 290

lipodystrophy, 32

mucopolysaccharidosis I, 38

mucopolysaccharidosis II, 40

Rubinstein-Taybi syndrome, 306

Histamine content of skin increased, incontinentia pigmenti, 362

Histidinemia, frequency in Massachusetts newborns, 4

Histiocytosis, visceral, G_{M1} gangliosidosis, 22

Hoarseness. *See* Cry, hoarse

Holotelencephaly with cleft lip and hypotelorism, 208

differentiated from

chromosome 13 trisomy, 166, 206, 208

chromosome 18, deletion of short arm, 162, 206, 208

Meckel syndrome, 206, 208, 292

median cleft face syndrome, 206, 208, 294

Holt-Oram syndrome

differentiated from

chromosome 13, deletion of long arm and ring D, 168

thalidomide embryopathy, 132

Homocystine excess in homocystinuria, 26

Homocystinuria, 26

differentiated from Marfan's syndrome, 26

mentally retarded in Northern Ireland, 4

prenatal diagnosis, 26

Horseshoe kidney. *See also* Kidney

Fanconi's anemia, 282

oral, cranial, and digital anomalies, syndrome, 338

XO syndrome, 178

Humerus, shortened. *See* Short-limbed dwarfism

Hunter's syndrome. *See* Mucopolysaccharidosis II

Huntington's chorea, 96

differentiated from

Hallervorden-Spatz disease, 94, 96

late-onset metachromatic leukodystrophy, 36, 96

neuronal lipidoses without sphingolipid accumulation, 96, 110

Wilson's disease, 64, 96

Hurler's syndrome. *See* Mucopolysaccharidosis I

Hutchinson's teeth, congenital syphilis, 126

Hydranencephaly, 204

differentiated from

Dandy-Walker syndrome, 202, 204

dysmorphogenesis of joints, brain, and palate, 204, 278

oral-facial-digital syndrome, 204, 300

porencephaly, 204

X-linked aqueductal stenosis, 200, 204

Hydrencephaly. *See* Hydranencephaly

Hydrocephalus. *See also* Cerebral ventricles, dilated; Head, enlarged; Intracranial pressure increased; Megalencephaly

achondroplasia, 260

Alexander's disease, 72

aminopterin and amethopterin embryopathy, 134

Apert's syndrome, 222

basal cell nevus syndrome, 356

battered child syndrome, 140

cerebral gigantism, 8

chromosome 18 trisomy, 158

cloverleaf skull, 234

congenital cytomegalovirus, 122

congenital toxoplasmosis, 124

Conradi's disease, 272

cranium bifidum with encephalocele, 210

Dandy-Walker syndrome, 202

differentiated from Alexander's disease, 72

dysmorphogenesis of joints, brain, and palate, 278

ectromelia and ichthyosis, syndrome, 376

familial aqueductal stenosis and basilar impression, 200

Farber's lipogranulomatosis, 88

focal dermal hypoplasia, 360

linear sebaceous nevus with convulsions and mental retardation, 364

meningomyelocele, 212

microcephaly, hypogonadism, and mental deficiency, syndrome, 58

mucopolysaccharidosis, I, 38

II, 40

III, 42

oculocerebrorenal syndrome of Lowe, 248

oral-facial-digital syndrome, 300

perinatal herpesvirus infection, 130

Pierre Robin syndrome, 304

stenosis of the aqueduct of Sylvius, 200

tuberous sclerosis, 380

X-linked aqueductal stenosis, 200

Hydronephrosis. *See also* Kidney

chromosome 13 trisomy, 164

cryptophthalmos syndrome, 274

ectromelia and ichthyosis, syndrome, 376

Fanconi's anemia, 282

Lesch-Nyhan syndrome, 30

micromelia and coarse facial features, syndrome, 334

Hydroxysteroid excretion low. *See* Urinary 17-ketosteroids low

Hyperaminoaciduria. *See* Aminoaciduria

Hyperammonemia

argininosuccinic aciduria, 6

differentiated from Alpers' disease, 74

Hypercalcemia, elfin facies, supravalvular aortic stenosis, and mental retardation, syndrome, 54

Hypercholesterolemia

differentiated from cerebrotendinous xanthomatosis, 80

XXY syndrome, 184

Hyperglycemia. *See* Diabetes mellitus

Hyperinsulinism. *See* Insulin level increased

Hyperkeratosis

ectromelia and ichthyosis, syndrome, 376

Flynn-Aird syndrome, 90

Hartnup disease, 24

incontinentia pigmenti, 362

Rothmund-Thomson syndrome, 368

Sjögren-Larsson syndrome, 370

Hyperkeratotic lesions, incontinentia pigmenti, 362

Hyperlipemia

differentiated from cerebrotendinous xanthomatosis, 80

lipodystrophy, 32

macroglossia, omphalocele, visceromegaly, and neonatal hypoglycemia, syndrome, 56

XXY syndrome, 184

Hyperlipogenesis, Prader-Labhart-Willi syndrome, 48

Hyperlipoproteinemia, type II, Cockayne's syndrome, 82

Hyperphenylalaninemia, transient, prematurity, 46

Hyperpigmentation

areas

ataxia-telangiectasia, 354

focal dermal hypoplasia, 360

neurofibromatosis, 366

tuberous sclerosis, 380

generalized

adrenocortical atrophy and diffuse cerebral sclerosis, 114

Fanconi's anemia, 282

Hartnup disease, 24

incontinentia pigmenti, 362

lipodystrophy, 32

Hypertelorism. *See also* Medial canthus

acrocephalosyndactyly, absent digits, and cranial defects, syndrome, 238

congenital herpesvirus, 130
congenital rubella, 118, 380
congenital toxoplasmosis, 124, 380
linear sebaceous nevus with convulsions and mental retardation, 364, 380
Sturge-Weber syndrome, 372, 380
Turner's syndrome, 178
Tyrosinemia, neonatal, 46
differentiated from phenylketonuria, 46

Ulna
rudimentary, Rothmund-Thomson syndrome, 368
short, in acrocephaly, cleft lip and palate, radial aplasia, and absent digits, syndrome, 240
Ulnar deviation of hands
cerebrohepatorenal syndrome, 270
chromosome 18 trisomy, 156
dyschondroplasia, facial anomalies, and polysyndactyly, syndrome, 322
Umbilical artery (single)
chromosome 18 trisomy, 156
dysmorphogenesis of joints, brain, and palate, 278
Umbilical hernia
absent fifth fingernails and toenails, short distal phalanges, and lax joints, syndrome, 314
chromosome 13 trisomy, 164
chromosome 18 trisomy, 156
chromosome 21 trisomy, 150
congenital hypothyroidism, 10
cryptophthalmos syndrome, 274
fucosidosis, 12
I-cell disease, 28
lipodystrophy, 32
macroglossia, omphalocele, visceromegaly, and neonatal hypoglycemia, syndrome, 56
marked acceleration of skeletal maturation and facial anomalies, syndrome, 330
mucopolysaccharidosis, I, 38
II, 40
Ungual tufts missing, pycnodysostosis, 266
Urate deposits in kidney, Lesch-Nyhan syndrome, 30
Uric acid excess, Lesch-Nyhan syndrome, 30
Uric acid tophi in ears, Lesch-Nyhan syndrome, 30
Urinary amino acid. See Aminoaciduria
Urinary argininosuccinic acid excess, argininosuccinic aciduria, 6
Urinary arylsulfatase A activity deficient, metachromatic leukodystrophy, 36
Urinary chorionic gonadotropins. See also Eunuchoid appearance; Hypogonadism; Urinary 17-ketosteroids low
compatible to height-age, cerebral gigantism, 8
elevated
Prader-Labhart-Willi syndrome, 48
Silver-Russell syndrome, 310
testicular deficiency and mental retardation, 60
XXXXY syndrome, 190
XXXY syndrome, 188
XXY syndrome, 184
XXYY syndrome, 186
reduced
familial hormonal disorder associated with mental deficiency, deaf-mutism, and ataxia, 86
ichthyosis and hypogonadism, syndrome, 378
Laurence-Moon syndrome, 288
microcephaly, hypogonadism, and mental deficiency, syndrome, 58
Prader-Labhart-Willi syndrome, 48
Urinary copper, Wilson's disease, 64
Urinary dermatan sulfate elevated, mucopolysaccharidosis I and II, 38, 40
Urinary dopamine excretion low, Huntington's chorea, 96
Urinary estrogens reduced, in familial hormonal disorder associated with mental deficiency, deaf-mutism, and ataxia, 86
Urinary galactose elevated, galactosemia, 14

Urinary heparan sulfate elevated, mucopolysaccharidosis I, II, and III, 38, 40, 42
Urinary homocystine elevated, homocystinuria, 26
Urinary homovanillic acid, familial dysautonomia, 256
Urinary hydroxysteroids low. See Urinary 17-ketosteroids low
Urinary indican elevated, Hartnup disease, 24
Urinary indole acetic acid elevated, Hartnup disease, 24
Urinary 17-ketosteroids low. See also Eunuchoid appearance; Hypogonadism; Urinary chorionic gonadotropins
adrenocortical atrophy and diffuse cerebral sclerosis syndrome, 114
familial hormonal disorder associated with mental deficiency, deaf-mutism, and ataxia, 86
microcephaly, hypogonadism, and mental deficiency, syndrome, 58
Prader-Labhart-Willi syndrome, 48
testicular deficiency and mental retardation, syndrome, 60
XXYY syndrome, 186
Urinary mucopolysaccharides elevated
brain dysgenesis, microcephaly, and skeletal dysplasia, syndrome, 318
metachromatic leukodystrophy, 36
mucopolysaccharidosis I, II, and III, 38, 40, 42
Urinary phenylpyruvic acid, phenylketonuria, 46
Urinary pregnandiol reduced, in familial hormonal disorder associated with mental deficiency, deaf-mutism, and ataxia, 86
Urinary sulfatides, metachromatic leukodystrophy, 36
Uterus
bicornuate
cryptophthalmos syndrome, 274
micromelia and coarse facial features, 334
leprechaunism, 290
biseptate, chromosome 13 trisomy, 164
small, XXXXX syndrome, 182
Uvula cleft. See also Cleft lip; Cleft palate
Apert's syndrome, 222
and cleft palate
blepharophimosis and congenital contractures, syndrome, 320
Goldenhar's syndrome, 284
micromelia and coarse facial features, 334
XXXXY syndrome, 190
Noonan's syndrome, 298
Pfeiffer's syndrome, 228
Pierre Robin syndrome, 304

Valgus position of hands, in acrocephaly, cleft lip and palate, radial aplasia, and absent digits, syndrome, 240
Varicose veins, XXYY syndrome, 186
Varus deformity of foot, in acrocephaly, cleft lip and palate, radial aplasia, and absent digits, syndrome, 240
Vasopressin-insensitive diabetes insipidus, in hypercalcemia, elfin facies, supravalvular aortic stenosis, and mental retardation, syndrome, 54
Veins prominent, lipodystrophy, 32
Vena cava, inferior and superior with common entrance, in blepharophimosis and congenital contractures, syndrome, 320
Ventral hernia, cryptophthalmos syndrome, 274
Ventricle of heart single. See also Congenital heart disease; Heart
Carpenter's syndrome, 232
ectromelia and ichthyosis, syndrome, 376
Ventricular system, dilated cerebral ventricles. See Hydrocephalus
Vermis aplastic or hypoplastic. See Cerebellum, anomalies
Verrucous lesions, incontinentia pigmenti, 362
Vertebrae. See also Lumbar vertebrae; Sacrum
anomalies
absent fifth fingernails and toenails, short distal phalanges, and lax joints, syndrome, 314
cloverleaf skull, 234
congenital hypothyroidism, 10
Conradi's disease, 272
extra small acrocentric chromosome, syndrome, 176
fucosidosis, 12
Goldenhar's syndrome, 284
meningomyelocele, 212
Noonan's syndrome, 298
otopalatodigital syndrome, 302